MAN & ENVIRONMENT

THIRD EDITION   A HEALTH PERSPECTIVE

ANNE NADAKAVUKAREN

Illinois State University

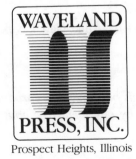

WAVELAND

PRESS, INC.

Prospect Heights, Illinois

For information about this book, write or call:

Waveland Press, Inc.
P.O. Box 400
Prospect Heights, Illinois 60070
(708) 634-0081

TABLE OF CONTENTS

PREFACE

Man and Environment: A Health Perspective is intended as a text for introductory level courses in environmental health or human ecology, presenting a broad survey of the major environmental issues facing society during this last decade of the 20th century. The book combines an overall ecological concern with specific elements related to personal and community health, emphasizing the inter-relatedness of the two and conveying to students an awareness of how current environmental issues directly affect their own lives.

Commencing with a rudimentary discussion of general ecological principles, the text focuses primarily on our present population-resources-pollution crisis and explains why human health and welfare depend on a successful resolution of these challenges. Intended for a one-semester course, the text consists of 16 chapters and is divided into three main sections, each with its own introduction. Discussion within each chapter covers general aspects of the subject in question, while specific illustrative examples are treated in box inserts. In order to give students a perspective on the kinds of actions being taken to deal with identified problems, a brief description of federal statutes dealing with particular environmental issues is included wherever appropriate. Appendices at the end of the book summarize federal environmental legislation since 1970, describe the various federal agencies dealing with environmental and health issues, and list names and addresses of major non-governmental environmental organizations for the benefit of those students who wish to obtain further information or to become actively affiliated with such groups. The ability of citizens to influence public policy is stressed throughout the book, a basic purpose of the text being to provide students with sufficient information and insight into environmental problems to enable them to understand and participate in the public decision-making processes which will profoundly influence health and environmental quality in the decades ahead.

I would like to express my sincere gratitude to those who helped me make this book possible: to Heinz Russelmann, Director of the Environmental Health Program at Illinois State University, whose encouragement, suggestions, and painstaking review of the manuscript were of invaluable assistance; to my colleagues Phil Kneller and Tom Bierma whose critical review of the sections on foodborne disease and radon was extremely helpful; to Becky Anderson whose classroom experience using the text enabled her to give valuable suggestions on content and scope; to Cheryl Newton, Environmental Protection Specialist at USEPA, Region V (Chicago), for constructive comments on the topic of auto emission controls; to Linn Haramis at Illinois Dept. of Public Health for his review of the passage on Lyme disease; to Art Carlson at Illinois Dept. of Nuclear Safety for reviewing coverage of medical X-rays; to Dr. Harry Huizinga, Dept. of Biological Sciences, Illinois State University, for his comments on schistosomiasis; to Dr. Richard Hogan, Chairman of the Department of Biological Sciences at East Texas State University, for reviewing the chapter on Radiation; to Neil Rowe, publisher of Waveland Press, for his cooperation and help; and especially to my husband and daughters for their loving support and understanding during the course of this project.

Anne Nadakavukaren

PART I

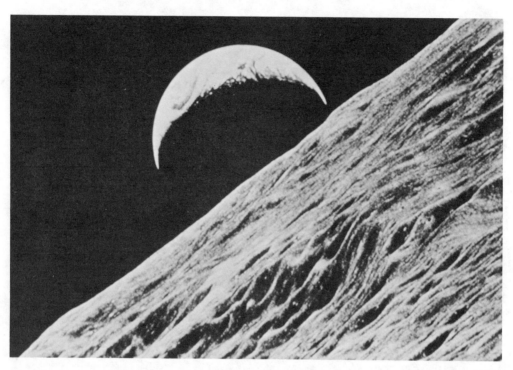

Earth's uniqueness as an "Oasis in Space" is dramatized in this photo taken from the moon. In an otherwise lifeless universe, our planet appears hauntingly beautiful and fragile. The space program has reinforced human awareness of the need to protect and preserve the life support systems which sustain us. [*NASA*]

MAN AND NATURE
Is conflict inevitable?

"Only within the moment of time represented by the
present century has one species—man—acquired
significant power to alter the nature of his world."
—Rachel Carson

Human beings, as a species, are unquestionably the dominant form of life on
earth today. Inhabiting every continent, roaming the seas, exploring space,
creating glittering cities and festering slums, taming rivers, bringing water to the
desert, harnessing the atom, tinkering with the gene—man often deceives
himself into believing he is all-powerful, a creature apart from the rest of nature.
Yet a half-million years of cultural evolution cannot alter the fact that man, like
all other living organisms, is inextricably bound up in the web of interdepen-
dency and interrelationships which characterize life on this planet. Human
health, well-being, and indeed survival are ultimately dependent on the health
and integrity of the whole environment in which man lives. Today the natural
world which we share with all other forms of life on this planet is under
unprecedented attack, not by some outside forces of evil, as in a science fiction
movie, but rather by a wide range of human activities and the sheer pressure of
human numbers. Sometimes unwittingly, sometimes with full awareness of the
consequences of our actions, we are rapidly altering the basic foundations of the
environment which sustains us.

Will the abuses currently being heaped upon the environment by man
ultimately lead to collapse of the entire system? This question has been a hot
topic of debate for at least the past two decades as levels of pollution, depletion
of resources, destruction of land, and the population spiral continue to mount.
In 1977, then-President Carter directed the Council on Environmental Quality
and the Department of State, working with other appropriate agencies, to make
a study of probable changes in the world's population, natural resources, and
environment through the end of the century. The results of this study, intended
to serve as the basis for long-range planning, were published in 1980 as "The
Global 2000 Report to the President of the U.S.: Entering the 21st Century".

Among the trends cited as posing very difficult problems within the near
future are the following:

3

1. *Population*—World population growth rates will have scarcely changed by 2000 A.D. The present world population of 4.8 billion will grow to 6.3 billion by the end of the century. While the rate of growth will slow very slightly, growth in total numbers each year will be faster than it is now—about 100 million being added each year in 2000. A full 90% of this growth will occur in the poorest countries which are finding it difficult to provide the amenities to their present populations.

2. *Food Production*—Worldwide, food production is projected to increase by 90% between 1970 and 2000. In per capita terms this would amount to about a 15% increase over the same period if food supplies were evenly apportioned. However, the largest portion of this increase will occur in the richer countries whose populations for the most part are already well fed. In the food-short countries of South Asia, the Middle East, and tropical Africa, per capita food consumption will remain at present inadequate levels or even decline. During the same time period, real prices for food are expected to double. Hopes for increasing production by expanding acreage offer little promise, since arable land will increase by only 4%; most of the additional output of food will have to come from higher yields.

3. *Natural Resources*—Nonfuel mineral resources appear sufficient to meet demand through 2000, but further discoveries and investments will be needed to maintain reserves. Some mineral resources may become uneconomic because of rising prices. Three-fourths of the world's mineral production will continue to be consumed by the industrial countries. Fossil fuel resources and uranium theoretically will last several centuries, but they are not evenly distributed and pose serious environmental and economic problems. The demand for firewood, the source of fuel for about one-quarter of the earth's people, will exceed supplies before the end of the century.

4. *Water*—Shortages will become more severe; population growth alone will result in a doubling of water demand by 2000 and still greater increases will be necessary to improve standards of living. Over-pumping of ground-water, poor land use practices which increase runoff, and pollution of existing water supplies all reduce the availability of water at a time of rising need.

5. *Forests*—Loss of forests will continue over the next 20 years as demand for timber, pulp, and firewood increases. Most of the loss will occur in the biologically rich tropical forests of Asia, Africa, and South America. By 2000 nearly half of the remaining forest cover in those areas will have been destroyed.

6. *Wildlife*—Rates of extinction will increase sharply, resulting in the loss of hundreds of thousands of species (perhaps 20% of all species on earth), especially in the tropical forest regions.

7. *Pollution*—Increased emissions of carbon dioxide and chlorofluoro-carbons in the atmosphere are threatening to alter the world's climate and upper atmosphere significantly by 2050. Acid rain from the burning of fossil fuels is affecting ever-wider areas with damage to lakes, soils, and crops. Toxic and radioactive wastes continue to be spewn into the air, dumped into waterways, or carelessly buried, presenting health and safety problems in a growing number of countries.

The authors of this much-publicized report concluded that:

"If present trends continue, the world in 2000 will be more crowded, more polluted, less stable ecologically, and more vulnerable to disruption than the world we live in now. Serious stresses involving population, resources, and environment are clearly visible ahead. Despite greater material output, the world's people will be poorer in many ways than they are today.
   For hundreds of millions of the desperately poor, the outlook for food and other necessities of life will be no better. For many it will be worse. Barring revolutionary advances in technology, life for most people on earth will be more precarious in 2000 than it is now—unless the nations of the world act decisively to alter current trends."

This gloomy outlook is not a prediction of inevitable future events, but rather a projection of what can reasonably be expected if very real problems are ignored. It describes conditions which are likely to develop if there are no changes in public policies, institutions, or rates of technological advance. Fortunately, we do not have to sit back as passive spectators to the despoliation of our environment and the impoverishment of our society. Much can be done to limit the impact of advanced technology on the natural world and to incorporate environmental considerations into national policy-making. To a great extent the technical know-how to prevent further deterioration exists—what is needed most is a societal commitment to get the job done. The most important decisions being made in the environmental health arena today are political decisions, balancing ecological concerns with economic and social considerations. Individuals wishing to become involved in protecting and enhancing environmental quality will find their efforts most effective when directed toward influencing environmental policy-making by legislative bodies at the federal, state, and local levels. To be a successful eco-advocate, however, requires a thorough understanding of the nature of our environmental crisis, how the present situation developed, what the human impact of these threats may be, and what action has already been taken in an attempt to restore and maintain a quality environment. These are the issues this book will attempt to address in the belief that a well-informed, politically active citizenry is an essential ingredient in achieving the policies and programs which will prevent the Global 2000 projections from becoming reality.

1

Introduction to Ecological Principles

"The most important fact about Spaceship Earth: an instruction book didn't come with it."
—Buckminster Fuller

When astronauts Neil Armstrong and "Buzz" Aldrin became the first humans to land on the moon and gazed back at their home planet more than 200,000 miles away, they were filled with a sense of wonder at the beauty and uniqueness of Earth. Of all the heavenly bodies of which we are aware, our planet is neither the largest nor the smallest, the hottest nor the coldest, yet it *is* extraordinary in one vital respect—in all the universe Earth is the only planet known to support life. Within that narrow film of air and water which envelops the surface of the globe, extending vertically from the deepest ocean trenches more than 36,000 feet below sea level to about 30,000 or more feet above sea level, exists what ecologists call the Biosphere—that portion of the earth where life occurs.

For all practical purposes, the physical extent of the biosphere is even more limited than just described. Even though the deep ocean trenches do possess a number of bizarre aquatic species and certain fungal spores and pollen grains may be found floating in the upper reaches of the atmosphere, by far the greatest number of living things are found in the region extending from the permanent snow line of tropical and subtropical mountain ranges (about 20,000 feet above sea level) to the limit of light penetration in the clearest oceans (about 600 feet deep). Here a vast assemblage of plant, animal, and microbial life can be found—perhaps as many as 10 million different species living today. These species interact both with each other and with their physical environment; over very long periods of time they become modified in response to environmental pressures and, in turn, they themselves modify their physical surroundings.

Inter-relatedness of Life: A Product of Evolutionary Adaptation

The first living organisms on earth (probably forms similar to bacteria) are now thought to have arisen more than 3.5 billion years ago on a planet whose environment was considerably different from that of the present-day world. The life activities of those early organisms, feeding upon and reacting with the chemical compounds in the waters where they first arose, were responsible for the creation of the modern atmosphere, which made possible the emergence of higher forms of life. The first primitive organisms evolved in a world devoid of atmospheric oxygen but rich in carbon dioxide. This carbon dioxide in turn provided a carbon source for the evolutionarily more advanced photosynthetic organisms which could produce their own food by utilizing the sun's energy to convert carbon dioxide and water into carbohydrates, releasing oxygen as a waste product. It was through the action of such photosynthetic organisms that the earth's atmosphere gradually became an oxygen-rich one, permitting the development of the types of life with which we're familiar today. In this way, the life activities of one group of organisms profoundly altered the environment and created conditions which facilitated the emergence of other forms of life. The ability of living things to modify their surroundings and the tendency of other organisms to respond positively or negatively to such changes has been a constant feature of evolutionary progression throughout the ages and remains so today.

Ecosystems

Recognizing the fundamental unity which encompasses living organisms and the non-living (or "abiotic") components of the environment, scientists established the concept of the *Ecosystem* as the basic functional unit in ecology. Essentially, the term ecosystem refers to any natural area where living things are interacting with the chemical and physical factors in the environment. The concept of ecosystems is a broad one, its main usefulness being to emphasize interdependence of the biotic and abiotic components of an area. The size of an ecosystem can vary widely: a fallen tree covered with moss and fungi, providing shelter and food for burrowing insects and microbes, can be regarded as an ecosystem; so can a family-room aquarium, a suburban backyard, a mountain lake, a cow pasture, a rocky ocean shore, or, indeed, the entire planet Earth. Any of these widely diverse situations can be considered an ecosystem so long as living and non-living elements are present and interacting to achieve some sort of functional stability.

Box 1-1

"Operation Cat Drop"

The results of drastic changes in a community (e.g. disappearance of deer, bear, etc., when a forest is clearcut by loggers) are easily observable and predictable. Less obvious, though often equally significant in the long run, are the sorts of changes which can be unwittingly wrought within an ecosystem simply by removing or modifying one of its constituent parts. Let's look at an example of how this can happen:

A major focus of public health programs in tropical areas of the world has been the controlling of infectious diseases such as malaria. Malaria is a highly debilitating, sometimes fatal ailment caused by a protozoan transmitted to humans by the bite of anopheline mosquitoes. Malaria was the scourge of the tropics, directly responsible for millions of deaths annually, until the advent of the insecticide DDT at the end of the Second World War. Since that time, widespread use of DDT and related products has been responsible for greatly reducing the numbers of malaria-carrying mosquitoes in areas where the disease is endemic. In this manner, malaria rates were rapidly lowered, with a corresponding increase in the health and well-being of populations in those regions. However, the spraying programs sometimes were accompanied by unexpected and undesired side effects. Early in the 1950s health workers decided to spray huts in a Malaysian village with DDT in order to kill the mosquitoes responsible for infecting up to 90% of the villagers with malaria. Soon after the huts were sprayed, their thatched roofs began rotting and collapsing. Investigations revealed that this was the result of a boom in the populations of thatch-eating moth larvae whose natural predators, a type of wasp, had been killed by the same DDT that felled the mosquitoes. To compound the problem, cockroaches living in the huts were not killed by the spraying, but they did absorb DDT and when they were eaten by the omnipresent geckos (a type of small lizard found on the walls inside most houses in the tropics), the DDT further accumulated in their bodies. By the time the housecats ate geckos which had eaten the cockroaches, the DDT had reached such high concentrations that most of the cats died. With the demise of the village cats, the rat population exploded, and with their increase came the threat of plague and typhus, epidemic diseases associated with rat-borne fleas and lice. The final chapter in this odd tale was a venture launched by the World Health Organization called "Operation Cat Drop," whereby cats were parachuted into villages to kill the rats!

This particular episode may sound somewhat bizarre, but in just such ways human disruption of delicately balanced ecological relationships, often done with the best of intentions, has resulted in suprisingly far-reaching effects. In our attempts to "control nature" we must never forget that the intricate interdependencies which have evolved over the millennia among the biotic communities of the earth cannot be altered without provoking a corresponding change somewhere else in the ecosystem.[1]

Biotic Community

The most familiar classification system used for grouping plants and animals is one based upon presumed evolutionary relationships—lions, tigers, and leopards being grouped in the cat family; wheat, corn, and rice in the grass family, and so forth. However, ecologists tend to arrange species on the basis of their functional association with each other. A natural grouping of different kinds of plants and animals within any given habitat is termed by ecologists a

Biotic Community.

"Biotic community," like "ecosystem", is a broad term which can be used to describe natural groupings of widely differing sizes, from the various microscopic diatoms and zooplankton swimming in a drop of pond water to the hundreds of species of trees, wild flowers, ferns, insects, birds, mammals, etc., found in an Appalachian forest. Biotic communities have characteristic trophic structures and energy flow patterns and also have a certain taxonomic unity, in the sense that certain species tend to exist together.

Individuals of the same species living together within a given area are collectively referred to as a *Population.* Such populations constitute groups more or less isolated from other populations of the same species. A population within the biotic community of a region is not a static entity but is continually changing in size and reshuffling its hereditary characteristics in response to environmental changes and to fluctuations in the populations of other members of the community.

The community concept is one of the most important ecological principles because (1) it emphasizes the fact that different organisms are not arbitrarily scattered around the earth with no particular reason as to why they live where they do, but rather that they dwell together in an orderly manner; and (2) by illuminating the importance of the community as a whole to any of its individual parts, the community concept can be used by man to control a particular organism, in the sense of increasing or decreasing its numbers. As an illustration of what is meant by the latter, consider the plight of the black-footed ferret, officially classified as an endangered species. The sharp decline in the population of this weasel-like animal, an inhabitant of grassland communities of the high plains of the western U.S., has resulted from large-scale extermination by ranchers of the prairie dogs which constitute the ferrets' major food item. Although no ill-will was harbored against the ferret, disruption of the biotic community of which the animal is a part has been just as devastating to its survival as direct shooting would have been. The realization that the success of any particular species is dependent on the integrity of its biotic community as a whole has profound implications for human welfare at a time of unprecedented interference with natural systems.

Ecological Dominants

Although all members of a biotic community have a role to play in the life of that community, it is obvious that certain plants or animals exert more of an effect on the ecosystem as a whole than do others. As George Orwell might have put it, "All animals are equal, but some animals are more equal than others." Those organisms which exert a major controlling influence on the community are known as *Ecological Dominants.* Such dominants comprise those species which largely control the flow of energy through the community; if they were to be removed from the community, much greater changes in the ecosystem would result than if a non-dominant species were to be removed. For example, when farmers chop down the dominant hardwood trees in an eastern forest to clear the land for cultivation, the changes produced by this removal (i.e. loss of animal species which depended on the trees for food and shelter, loss of shade-loving plants which proliferated under the canopy, change in soil microbiota, raising of soil temperature, increase in soil erosion, etc.) are much more pronounced than would be the changes brought about when the farmers' children wander into the forest and pick all of the trilliums and lady slippers they find growing there. In either case, the stability of the ecosystem is upset, but the loss of several species of spring wildflowers, while unfortunate, has much less effect on the forest community as a whole than does the loss of the dominant oaks, maples, and beeches.

In most terrestrial biotic communities certain plants comprise the dominant species because not only do they provide food and shelter for other organisms but also because they directly affect and modify their physical environment. That is, they contribute to a build-up of topsoil, moderate fluctuations of temperature, improve moisture retention, affect the pH of the soil, etc. As a general rule, the number of dominant species within a community becomes progressively fewer as one moves toward the poles and greater the closer the community is to the tropics. While a northern coniferous forest may consist of only spruces or firs, a jungle in Sumatra may have a dozen or more tree species that could be considered dominants. In addition to the effects of latitude on number of dominants in a community, one can also generalize that dominant species are fewer in regions where climatic conditions are extreme, i.e. tundra and deserts.[2]

Biomes

The species composition of any particular biotic community is profoundly affected by the physical characteristics of the environment, particularly temperature and rainfall. The kinds of plants and animals one would see while touring Yellowstone National Park would differ significantly from those found on a trek through the Amazon. Ecologists have divided the terrestrial communities of the world into general groupings called *Biomes,* areas which can be recognized by the distinctive life forms of their dominant species. In most cases, the key characteristic of a biome is its dominant type of vegetation. We might define a biome as *a complex of communities characteristic of a regional climatic zone.* Each biome has its own pattern of rainfall, its own seasons, its own maximum and minimum temperatures, and its own changes of daylength, all of which combine to support a certain kind of vegetation. Since climatic zones change in a relatively uniform pattern as one moves from the poles toward the equator, the earth's biomes form more or less continuous latitudinal bands around the globe. Starting at the polar regions, let's take a brief look at the major biomes of the earth (Note: ecologists list numerous sub-divisions of the biomes described here, but for our purposes these general groupings will suffice):

Tundra

the northernmost of the world's land masses, tundra is characterized by permanently frozen subsoil called "permafrost". In this biome rainfall is quite low, about 8″ annually, but because the permafrost doesn't allow moisture to penetrate beyond the upper few inches of soil, the tundra in summer is dotted with numerous lakes and bogs—and probably the world's most voracious mosquitoes! The tundra is windy, with only a few stunted trees. The dominant vegetation here consists of moss, lichens, grass, and some small perennials. Animal life is limited in the number of species but very abundant in the number of individuals. These include caribou or reindeer, birds, insects, polar bears, lemmings, foxes, rabbits, and fish. Reptiles and amphibians are absent. The tundra is basically a very fragile environment. Because of the slow rates at which tundra plants grow and decompose (due to the low temperatures and the characteristics of permafrost), the thick, spongy matting of lichens, grasses, and sedges that typify tundra is especially slow to recover from disturbance. Tracks of vehicles or animals can remain visible for decades. Great care must be taken in building on tundra because heat from structures will melt the permafrost and cause uneven settling, which often badly distorts the buildings. Until recently the tundra was relatively unexploited, but with the construction of the Alaska oil pipeline and similar kinds of mineral development in Canada and Siberia, that situation has changed.

Taiga

a Russian word for "swamp forest", the taiga is sometimes called the **Northern Coniferous Forest.** This biome covers much of Canada, Scandinavia, and the USSR. As the name implies, the dominant vegetation here consists of conifer trees which have needlelike leaves which stay on the trees for 3 to 5 years. These include spruces, firs, hemlocks, and pines. Some deciduous trees such as aspens, alders, and larches are also prominent. In general, the trees are much less diverse in number of species than those in the deciduous forests farther south and the soils have a different kind of humus and are more acid. Precipitation in the taiga is only moderate, but because drainage is poor lakes, ponds, and bogs are common here. Animals of the taiga include bears, moose, lynxes, weasels, wolverines, and a variety of birds. Because of the huge stands of just one or two species of conifers, the taiga provides an opportunity for periodic outbreaks of pests like the spruce budworm which can defoliate huge areas of forest. Perhaps because of the lack of diversity of species, taiga populations tend to undergo "boom or bust" cycles fairly regularly.

Temperate Deciduous Forest

this biome occurs in a belt south of the taiga where climate is milder and where rainfall is abundant relative to the amount of evaporation. This is the biome familiar to most of us because it is the one in which Western, as well as Chinese and Japanese, civilization developed. Soil types and elevations vary widely within this biome. Maples, beech, oaks, and hickories are common trees; many species of ferns and flowering herbaceous plants are found also. The deciduous forest has a great variety of mammals, birds, and insects, as well as a modest number of reptiles and amphibians. Because of the annual leaf drop, deciduous forests generate soils rich in nutrients, which in turn support a multitude of soil microbes. When such forests are cleared, the richness of the soils can be maintained if great care is taken to see that their supplies of nutrients and decaying organic matter are preserved (in a sense, raising crops or grazing animals is akin to mining the soil, since the nutrients leave along with the crops, meat, wool, or whatever is removed). All too often, however, short-term careless exploiters have allowed soils to deteriorate or have ignored opportunities to improve them. Unfortunately, economic considerations often lead individuals who are exploiting an ecosystem to use short-term strategies that are disastrous for humanity in the long run.

Grasslands

in regions where annual rainfall is not sufficient to sustain the growth of trees and evaporation rates are high we find the grasslands of the world. These may be called by different names in various countries: prairie, veldt, savannah, steppe, pampas, llanos. All are characterized by the dominance of grasses and herds of grazing animals. Carnivores also abound, such as coyotes, lions, etc., as do rodents and many species of reptiles. The grassland biome has a higher concentration of organic matter in its soil than does any other biome, the amount of humus in grassland soil being about 12 times greater than that in forest soils. The extraordinary richness of grassland soil has led to the establishment of extremely successful agricultural ecosystems in the grassland areas. However, these systems can break down rapidly if careful soil husbandry is not practiced. The interlaced roots and creeping underground stems of grasses form a turf that prevents erosion of the soil. When the turf is broken with a plow or over-grazed, the soil is exposed to the erosive influences of wind or water, resulting in such calamities as the "Dust Bowl" of the Great Plains in the 1930s.

Desert

areas receiving less than 10″ annual precipitation are classified as deserts. These areas are concentrated in the vicinity of 30° north and 30° south latitude. Lack of moisture is the essential factor shaping the desert biome. Most deserts are quite hot in the daytime and, because of the sparse vegetation and resultant rapid re-radiation of heat, quite cold at night. Desert plants and animals are characterized by species which can withstand prolonged drought. Among plants such adaptations include waxy cuticle on stems or leaves, reduction in leaf size, and spiny growths to repel moisture-seeking animals. Plants may appear to be widely spaced, but if their roots were visible, the ground between them would be seen to be laced with a shallow root system to take maximum advantage of any rain which does fall. Proportionately more annual plants are found in the desert biome than in any other; because their seeds often require abrasion or a rain heavy enough to leach out inhibiting chemicals, the desert appears to bloom almost overnight after a heavy rain. For the most part, desert animals are active at night, remaining under cover during the heat of the day. Desert soils contain little organic matter and must ordinarily be supplied with both water and

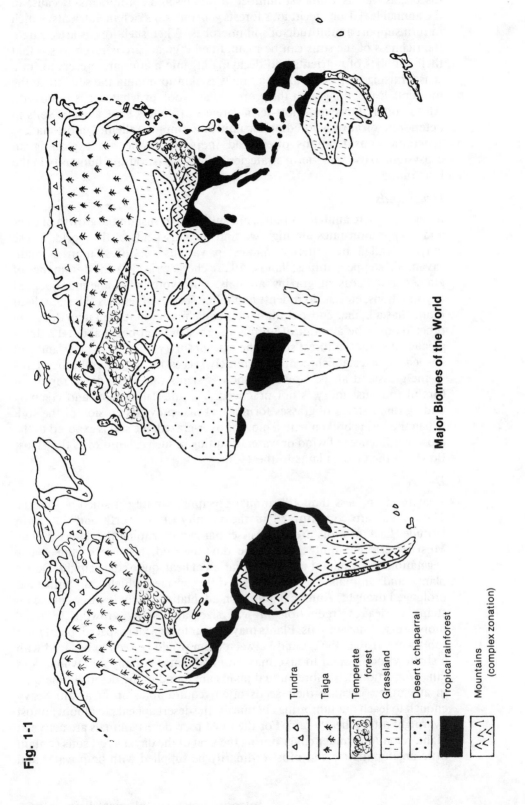

Fig. 1-1

Major Biomes of the World

Tundra

Taiga

Temperate
forest

Grassland

Desert & chaparral

Tropical rainforest

Mountains
(complex zonation)

nitrogen fertilizer if they are to be cultivated. Human activities have already produced a great increase in the amount of desert and wasteland, removing many once-productive acres from cultivation. Occasional years of good rainfall cause people to forget that the desert is inherently a very fragile environment.

Tropical Rain Forest

this biome is found in Central and South America, central Africa, South and Southeast Asia. It is characterized by high temperatures and high annually rainfall; 100 inches or more of annual precipitation is common in this biome. Year-round temperature variation is slight. Tropical rain forests are characterized by a great diversity of plant and animal species and by four distinct layers of plant growth—the top canopy of trees reaching 200 feet or more; a lower canopy of densely intertwined treetops at about 100 feet; a sparse understory, and only a very few plants growing at ground level. A wide variety of epiphytic plants can be found. Both plant and animal species exist in greater diversity in the tropical rain forest than anywhere else in the world, though numbers of individuals of a particular species are usually limited. To most people, the luxuriant growth of a tropical jungle implies a rich soil and one hears many glowing promises of the agricultural riches to be reaped by turning the Amazon or Congo River basins into farmland. The truth of the situation is far different, however. Tropical forest soils in general are exceedingly thin and nutrient-poor. They cannot maintain large reserves of minerals needed for plant growth, primarily because heavy rainfall and a high rate of water flow through the ground to the water table leach them from the soil. The leaching process leaves behind large residues of insoluble iron and aluminum oxides in the upper levels of tropical forest soils, a process termed "laterization". With the exception of certain fertile river valleys, primitive slash-and-burn agriculture is the only type suitable to most areas of the tropical rain forest. Unfortunately, this fragile ecosystem is being destroyed more rapidly than any other biome under the pressure of expanding human populations and in some cases, such as in Brazil, as a direct consequence of governmental actions.

Note: In areas where there are substantial variations in altitude, the biomes differ at different elevations. This is primarily because the temperature of the air decreases about 6°C for every 1000 meter increase in altitude and because, especially in desert areas, rainfall increases with altitude.[3]

This brief survey of biome characteristics should make it obvious that various regions differ in their ability to return to an ecologically stable condition once they have been disrupted by human activities. Thus it should not be surprising that certain practices are far more devastating to the local ecology in some areas than they are in others. For example, strip mining in the flat or gently-rolling lands of Illinois, Indiana, and Ohio is certainly disruptive to the environment, yet with proper soil reclamation practices the land can be restored to productive uses once mining has ceased. In the arid regions of the High Plains and Southwest, however, exploitation of fossil fuel reserves by strip mining presents a real threat that the acres thus despoiled could never recover and would remain permanent wastelands.

Ecological Niches

Within any biotic community each species occupies its own particular place in space and time, different from that of any other member of the community. Through the processes of evolution and natural selection, plants and animals have become increasingly better adapted to the specific environments in which they live. In order to reduce competition between species for food and living space, groups of organisms have become increasingly specialized for life in a particular ecological niche, the term "niche" signifying not only the physical space that the species occupies, but also its way of life, including structural adaptations, physiological responses, and patterns of behavior. The "Principle of Competitive Exclusion", basic to ecological theory, holds that when two species are competing for the same limited resources, only one will survive. Only when the environmental resources in a given locality are partitioned among the co-inhabiting species by means of niche diversification is direct competition minimized, thus permitting coexistence of species.

The effects of species competition are well illustrated by the present-day distribution of the two most common species of domestic rats. The roof rat *(Rattus rattus)* was the most prevalent house rat in Europe and the North American colonies until about the mid-1700s; it was an extremely widespread species, notorious in history as the carrier of plague ("Black Death") which decimated the population of Europe during the Middle Ages. When the Norway rat *(Rattus norvegicus),* a migrant from central Asia, appeared in Europe in the 1700s and began competing with the roof rat for the same territory, its more aggressive habits resulted in the displacement and disappearance of the roof rat throughout most of its former range. Only under very special conditions are the two now found in the same area, an example of this being in one eastern U.S. seaport where roof rats live in the top of a grain elevator while Norway rats live in the bottom, probably because roof rats are better climbers than Norway rats. Thus only when these species are able to modify their behavior and feeding habits through niche diversification can they continue to exist within the same geographic area.[4]

In other situations species may utilize the same physical space but minimize competition by restricting their feeding activities to different times of day. Within any given area one can find some species which are diurnal (active during the day), such as most birds, grazing animals, many insects, etc.; other species which are nocturnal (active at night)—most snakes, many predators such as foxes, lions, wolves, owls, raccoons, skunks, etc.; and still others which prefer the in-between hours of dawn and dusk. Structural modifications among species allow animals inhabiting the same general area to utilize different foods. The finches of the Galapagos Islands, immortalized by Charles Darwin, were very similar in appearance and obviously evolved from the same parental stock, but modifications in their beak structure permitted each species to utilize a different type of food—insects, small seeds, medium-sized seeds, or large seeds, depending on the size and shape of the beak—and thus to coexist within the same geographical area. The principles of niche diversification can be seen on the human body itself, where competition for the same resources has been minimized by three common types of lice, each of which lays claim to a specific region of the human anatomy and exhibits distinctive behavioral patterns (see Box 1-2).

Examples of niche diversification illustrate the fact that throughout evolutionary history ecosystems have become exceedingly complex through increasingly effective adaptation of organisms to their environment and through a fine-tuning of relationships among organisms within any natural community. Such a complex ecosystem is generally quite stable unless something happens to change that environment to which the organisms have become so well adapted. The processes of natural selection and adaptation are too slow to permit the vast majority of organisms to adjust quickly to such radical changes in their surroundings. As a result, the animal and plant populations in such disrupted situations generally die out or move elsewhere and the previously stable ecosystem collapses or, at a minimum, becomes less varied and less stable.

Limiting Factors

Why do corn plants thrive in central Illinois but not in Norway? Why don't ferns grow in the Mohave Desert? Why is the poison produced by the botulism bacterium *(Clostridium botulinum)* sometimes present in canned green beans but never in fresh ones? The reason why living things occur and thrive where they do depends upon a variety of conditions. Sometimes those conditions are quite obvious: summer temperatures in Norway are not hot enough nor is the growing season long enough to produce a bountiful corn harvest; lack of water and shade make survival of ferns impossible in a desert environment. In some cases the factors which control where a plant or animal lives are not quite so apparent: *Clostridium botulinum* can multiply and produce its deadly toxin only in an environment where oxygen is absent, hence it may present a threat in improperly canned foods, but seldom in fresh ones.

Environmental conditions which limit or control where an organism can live are called **Limiting Factors.** Obviously not every factor in an organism's environment is equally important in determining where that plant or animal can live. Components which are relatively constant in amount and moderately abundant are seldom limiting factors, particularly if the individual in question has a wide limit of tolerance. On the other hand, if an individual has a narrow limit of tolerance for a factor which exists in low or variable amounts, then that factor might indeed be the crucial determinant in where the organism can live. For example, most higher forms of life require a plentiful supply of oxygen to carry out their metabolic activities. Nevertheless, even though oxygen is essential, because it is so abundantly present and readily available to most land plants and animals (with the exception of some parasites and organisms living underground) it is almost never a limiting factor in terrestrial communities. On

Box 1–2

A Tale of Three Lice

The human body provides food and shelter (albeit unwillingly!) to three varieties of lice which can co-exist on the same host by restricting their activities to specific parts of the human anatomy.

The better-known of the two species involved, *Pediculus humanus* occurs in two forms often classified as distinct subspecies: *P. humanus humanus,* commonly known as the body louse and notorious in history as the carrier of typhus fever, feeds on parts of the body below the neck; *P. humanus capitis,* or head louse, confines its activities to the head and neck. The fact that the two are almost identical in appearance (the body louse is slightly larger and sometimes lighter in color) and occasionally interbreed indicates their close relationship, but niche diversification is quite apparent in their different behavioral patterns. Head lice cement their eggs to the hairs of the scalp, while body lice usually glue theirs to fibers of clothing; in fact, body lice spend most of their time on clothing, coming into contact with the body only when taking a blood meal. For this reason, body lice are much more common in cool countries where people wear several layers of clothing than in the tropics where little or no clothing is worn (in the latter, however, lice may infest beads and necklaces). In addition, the body louse lays more eggs, lives longer, and is more resistant to starvation than the head louse. Because ordinary laundering of clothing with hot water destroys both eggs and adults of *P. humanus humanus,* higher standards of personal hygiene have greatly reduced the incidence of body lice in the U.S. in recent decades.

The crab louse, *Phthirus pubis,* is a species which is specialized for life among the widely-spaced, coarse hairs of the pubic areas primarily, but may be found also on hairy chests and in the armpits; in addition, crab lice are frequently observed to inhabit the eyebrows and eyelashes (head lice are common behind the ears and on the scalp, but are not found around the eyes). A bluish coloration directly above the eyebrows is an indication of the presence of crab lice, since they feed in a very localized area and cause hemorrhages under the skin. Unlike body and head lice which constantly move about, crab lice tend to settle at one spot, grasping hairs with their legs, inserting their mouthparts, and then feeding off and on for many hours at a time. Spread chiefly by sexual contact, the incidence of *P. pubis* has risen significantly in recent years in response to increasing levels of sexual permissiveness.[5]

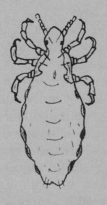

Pediculus humanus

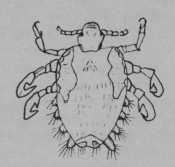

Phthirus pubis

the other hand, lack of oxygen can definitely be a limiting factor for a number of aquatic organisms. The larvae of certain insects such as mayflies and caddisflies, as well as important game fish such as brook trout, simply die or move elsewhere when levels of dissolved oxygen in a waterway drop below a critical point.

Although the Massachusetts Indians who taught the Pilgrims to bury a dead fish in each hill of corn must have intuitively understood the concept, the idea of limiting factors was first formulated in 1840 by the German biochemist Justus Liebig while studying problems of fertility in agricultural soils. Liebig was experimenting with the use of inorganic chemical fertilizers in place of manures then currently in use and found that crop yields were affected not so much by the nutrients needed in large quantities, such as carbon dioxide and water, since these were generally present in plentiful supply, but by some mineral, such as copper, needed in minute amounts but lacking from particular soils. From this observation he proclaimed his famous "Law of the Minimum", stating that "the growth of a plant is dependent on the amount of foodstuff which is presented to it in a minimum quantity." Succeeding generations of ecologists have expanded Liebig's concept to include not only mineral nutrients but also such things as light, temperature, pH, water, oxygen supply, and soil type as possible limiting factors to the distribution of organisms.

Further investigations revealed a complicating fact: when some factor other than the minimum one is available in very high concentrations, this may moderate the rate at which the critical one is used. For example, plants growing in the shade require less zinc than those growing in the sun. Thus shade-grown plants are less affected by a zinc-deficient soil than are plants of the same species growing in full sunlight. Also, some organisms can substitute a chemically-similar nutrient for one which is deficient, as can be seen in certain molluscs which partially substitute strontium for calcium in their shells when amounts of calcium are low.

To make matters more complex, by the early 20th century it became clear that the old adage, "If a little bit is good, then more must be better," was quite untrue so far as the needs of living things were concerned. The concept of the Law of the Minimum was broadened by the American ecologist Victor Shelford who demonstrated that too much of a limiting factor can be just as harmful as not enough. Organisms have both an ecological maximum and minimum, the range in between these two extremes representing that organism's Limits of Tolerance.

Limits of Tolerance

Subsequent investigations in regards to tolerance ranges have revealed a great deal about why certain species live where they do. Not surprisingly, those plants and animals which have a wide range of tolerance for all factors are the ones which have the widest distribution. However, some organisms can have a wide tolerance range for some factors but a narrow range for others and thus their distribution will be accordingly more limited. Not all stages of an animal's or plant's life cycle are equally sensitive to the effect of limiting factors. Among many spore-forming bacteria, for example, high temperatures which would be almost instantly fatal for actively growing cells have no effect on the spore stage unless the duration of exposure is fairly long. In general, the most critical period when environmental factors are most likely to be limiting (i.e. when the range of tolerance is narrowest) is during the reproductive period. Susceptibility of the young to conditions which adult organisms could tolerate with little difficulty is well established in regards to one of our major environmental problems at present, that of acid rainfall. The low pH levels which are blamed for the near-total disappearance of many species of fish in lakes throughout eastern Canada, northeastern U.S., and parts of Scandinavia have been shown to be **lethal to fish eggs and fingerlings, but not to adult fish. Thus the effects of acid rain on aquatic life are much less dramatic than the effects of, for example, a** chemical spill into a river. Rather than a massive, immediately visible (and smelly!) fish kill, the fish in an acidifying lake simply fail to reproduce and become less and less abundant, older and older, until they die out completely. Other examples of the vulnerability of the reproductive stage include the observations that while adult cypress trees can grow either on dry ground or with their bases continually submerged in water, cypress seedlings can only develop in moist, unflooded soil. Similarly, some adult marine animals such as blue crabs can tolerate fresh water which is slightly salty and so are frequently found in rivers some distance upstream from the sea. Their young, however, can thrive only in salt water, so reproduction and permanent establishment of these organisms in rivers cannot occur. Just as the very young of lower forms of life display less tolerance to environmental extremes than do adults, the same situation applies with humans. Many widespread environmental toxins have been shown, some in tragic ways, to have a much more devastating effect on developing fetuses and young children than on adults. The drug thalidomide and organic mercury are just two substances which have been ingested by pregnant women with no harmful effects on themselves but with disastrous results on their unborn children. Levels of air pollution which are largely ignored by the adult population can cause severe respiratory distress in infants and children. It's important for us to keep in mind the qualifications to the range of tolerance concept when we hear official assurances that exposure to this or that substance is "safe". What is safe for one segment of the population may be far from safe for others.

Energy Flow Through the Biosphere

Living things are dependent for their existence not only on proper soil and climate conditions but also on some form of energy; a basic understanding of the flow of energy through the ecosystem is fundamental to the study of how that system functions.

The ultimate source of all life activities, from the unfolding of a flower bud to the 100-meter dash of an Olympic athlete is, of course, the sun. Some 93 million miles (150 million km) from the earth, the sun emits vast amounts of electromagnetic radiation which, traveling through space at a rate of 186,000 miles (300,000 km) per second, takes about 9 minutes to reach the earth's surface. There is no energy loss as the sun's radiation travels through space, but since its intensity decreases inversely as the square of the distance from the sun, the amount of solar radiation intercepted by the earth is but one two-billionth of the sun's total energy output. On this seemingly tiny portion all life on earth depends. More than half the incoming radiation is unusable by living things, however. Electromagnetic radiation consists of several different wavelengths. Of the total amount of energy received from the sun, 9% is in the form of short-wave, high-energy ultraviolet rays, 50% in the form of long-wave infra-red waves (heat waves), and 41% as visible light. Only those wavelengths within the visible spectrum, particularly those in the red and blue range, can be absorbed and utilized by green plants. These, through the process of photosynthesis, convert solar energy into the energy of chemical bonds. The complex and still not entirely understood mechanism whereby plants harness certain wavelengths of sunlight and use this energy to join molecules of carbon dioxide and water to form the simple sugar glucose, releasing oxygen in the process, makes the existence of all higher forms of life possible. The transfer of this captured energy from organism to organism is basic to the functioning of ecosystems. Before examining the paths of energy flow, however, let us take a brief look at some physical laws which control and limit the amount of energy available to living things.

Laws of Thermodynamics

An understanding of many problems in both environmental science and energy technology depends on a basic conception of the principles which govern how energy is changed from one form into another. Known as the first and second laws of thermodynamics, these principles can be summarized as follows:

1. *The First Law of Thermodynamics,* sometimes called the Law of Conservation of Energy, states that energy can neither be created nor destroyed, even though it may be changed from one form into another. Solar energy which is absorbed by rocks or soil or water on the earth's surface is converted into the heat energy which, because of temperature differentials and the earth's rotation, gives rise to winds and water currents which are a form of *Kinetic Energy.* When such kinetic energy accomplishes work such as the raising of water by wind, then it has been changed into *Potential Energy,* so-called because the latent energy of a water droplet in a cloud or at the top of a dam can be converted into some other kind of energy when it falls. In the same way, light energy absorbed by the chlorophyll molecules in a leaf is converted into the potential energy of chemical bonds within carbohydrates, proteins, and fats. As light energy passes from one form to another, it may appear that most of it is eventually

lost or consumed (how often have we heard references to that misnomer, "energy consumption"?). This is a misconception, however, for if one maintained a global balance sheet it would show that all the energy which enters the biosphere as light is re-radiated and leaves the earth's surface in the form of invisible heat waves. The form of energy leaving the system is different from the incoming radiation, but no energy has been either created or destroyed during its passage through the biosphere.

2. *The Second Law of Thermodynamics* states that with every energy transformation there is a loss of *usable* energy (that is, energy that can be used to do work). Put another way, all physical processes proceed in such a way that the *availability* of the energy involved decreases (note that the availability, not the total amount, of energy is what decreases—the latter would be a violation of the First Law). The Second Law introduces the concept of *Entropy*, the idea that all energy is moving toward an ever less available and more dispersed state. This process will continue until all energy has been transformed to heat distributed at a uniform temperature throughout the solar system—at which point the stable state will have been achieved.

The Second Law has some interesting implications concerning ecological relationships. Perhaps the most important of these is the fact that no type of energy transformation is ever 100% efficient—there will always be a significant energy loss involved whenever energy is transferred from one organism to another. This explains why we need a continued input of energy to maintain ourselves and why we must consume substantially more than a pound of food in order to gain a pound of weight. In addition, because a given quantity of energy can be used only once, the ability to convert energy into useful work cannot be "recycled". Thus energy, unlike the essential minerals and gases, moves in a unidirectional way through ecosystems, becoming ever more dispersed and eventually being degraded to heat. Bearing these fundamental physical laws in mind, let's now take a more detailed look at the flow of energy through the biotic community.

Food Chains

One way of describing the movement of energy through the ecosystem is to use the concept of a *Food Chain.* Basically, a food chain involves the transfer of food energy from a given source through a series of organisms, each of which eats the next lower individual in the chain. In terms of energy flow, the living components of the ecosystem can be subdivided into three broad categories:

Producers—the green plants which convert the sun's energy into food energy. On land the major producers are the flowering plants and the conifers; in water they are mainly the diatoms, microflagellates, and green algae.
Consumers—animals; primary consumers are the herbivores and secondary consumers are the carnivores.

Decomposers—primarily bacteria and fungi, some insects. Decomposers are essential for recycling detritus back into the soil where it is once again available for use by producer organisms. No community could exist very long without decomposers.

There are basically three types of food chains. The most familiar of these, called a *Grazing Food Chain* (or "predator chain"), may be typified by a grass-rabbit-fox association which starts with a plant base and proceeds from smaller to larger animals. Less conspicuous but equally important is the *Detritus Food Chain*, where dead organic matter (detritus) is broken down by microorganisms, primarily bacteria. Small animals eat particles of this detritus, securing energy largely from assimilation of the energy-rich bacteria. The small animals, in turn, become a source of energy for larger consumers. A prime example of a detritus food chain accounting for a substantial portion of an ecosystem's energy flow can be found in the salt marsh habitat of many coastal areas. Here plants such as marsh grass die and are washed into estuaries where they are decomposed by microbes into finely divided particles which are then consumed by such primary consumers as fiddler crabs, molluscs, etc. These, in turn, may be eaten by secondary consumers such as raccoons, water birds, or other crabs.

A variation on grazing food chains can be seen in certain *Parasitic Chains*, in which energy flows from larger to smaller animals (e.g. dogs which provide an energy source for fleas which in turn are fed upon by parasitic protozoans). In energy terms, however, there is no fundamental difference between a parasitic food chain and a grazing food chain, since a parasite is basically a "consumer".

Pyramid of Numbers

Through the interactions of the community, a unidirectional flow of energy occurs from producers to primary consumers, secondary consumers, etc. Each of these stages of consumption is called a *Trophic Level*, defining the *relative position occupied by an organism in a food chain*. If we examine a food chain in terms of the animals and plants which constitute it, it becomes apparent that these forms can be arranged into what is called a "pyramid of numbers". At the bottom of the pyramid are multitudes of energy-producing plants, then a smaller number of herbivores that feed upon them, then a still smaller number of primary carnivores, followed by an even smaller number of secondary carnivores. The animals at the top of the heap, the final consumers, are usually the largest in the community, while those organisms at the bottom of the pyramid, the producers, are usually the smallest, but much more abundant. In addition, the organisms at the lower trophic levels usually reproduce more rapidly and more prolifically than those higher up, so there is seldom danger of a predator eating itself out of its food supply. It should be noted, however, that in those cases where the size of the producer organisms is very large and the size of the primary consumers is small (e.g. a cherry tree being munched upon by hundreds of caterpillars), the shape of the pyramid of numbers may be inverted.

Introduction to Ecological Principles   23

Pyramid of Biomass

Just as the numbers of individual organisms in a community is generally greatest at the lower trophic levels, so the living weight, or **Biomass** (measured as dry weight per unit area), is generally greatest at the producer trophic level. In the same way, biomass of the primary consumers will be greater than that of the secondary consumers, etc., so the ecological biomass pyramids used to portray weight relationships among trophic levels will often look identical to those of numbers pyramids. Biomass, which in effect is an indicator of the amount of energy stored within an ecosystem, varies widely from one type of biotic community to another. For example, the amount of biomass in a tropical rainforest far exceeds that in a comparable area of abandoned field, while open ocean water is relatively poor in terms of biomass.

Although biomass pyramids, like numbers pyramids, usually have a broad base and tapered apex, in those situations where the organisms at the producer level are much smaller than the consumers, the shape of the biomass pyramid may be upside-down. This occurs because the "standing crop biomass" (the total dry weight of organisms present at any one moment in time) which can be maintained by a steady flow of energy in a food chain depends to a large extent on the size of the individual organisms. The smaller the organisms are, the greater is their metabolic rate per gram of biomass. Thus the smaller the organism, the smaller the biomass which can be supported at a given trophic level; in the same way, the larger the organism, the larger the amount of biomass at any one point in time. This is why in, say, an aquatic ecosystem the biomass of the blue whale would be far greater than the biomass of the microscopic diatoms and zooplankton on which it feeds. The biomass pyramid which illustrates the energy relationships in such a situation would be an inverted one. This doesn't mean that the producer organisms are defying the laws of nature; it simply reflects the fact that the tiny phytoplankton have very high metabolic rates and that they reproduce much more rapidly than do whales, having complete turnovers in their populations within very short time periods.

Pyramid of Energy

Whereas pyramids of numbers tend to exaggerate the importance of small organisms and pyramids of biomass often understate their role, pyramids of energy give the best picture of energy flow through a food chain, showing what actually is happening within the biotic community. As was mentioned earlier, light energy from the sun is captured by green plants and stored in the form of chemical bonds in the molecules of starch, glucose, fats, etc. However, as the Second Law of Thermodynamics states, only a portion of the energy stored by one trophic level is available to the next higher one, since a considerable amount is lost at every stage of transformation. Thus when cows graze in a pasture, some of the chemical bond energy in the grass is converted into the muscle tissue which represents stored food in the cow. The largest portion of energy derived from the grass, however, is lost in the form of waste heat during respiration. A lesser amount is lost as unassimilated food materials in feces or urine and as organic material which is not eaten by the next higher trophic level (i.e. just as people do not eat every part of a cow or pig, so many animals leave certain parts of their prey unconsumed; such "rejects" constitute an energy loss to the food chain).

At each transfer of energy within a food chain, approximately 90% (sometimes a big more, sometimes less) of the chemical energy stored in organisms of the lower level is lost and therefore unavailable to the higher level. Since the total amount of energy entering the food chain is fixed by the photosynthetic activities of plants (and plants are less than 1% efficient, on the average, in converting solar energy into chemical energy), obviously more usable energy is available to organisms occupying lower positions in the food chain than to those at higher trophic levels. Expressing this concept in simpler terms, one might say, for example:

10,000 lbs. corn → 1,000 lbs. beef → 100 lbs. human

By moving man one step lower in the food chain, ten times more energy becomes directly available:

10,000 lbs. corn → 1,000 lbs. human

In very simplified terms, this explains why countries like China and India are largely vegetarian. In order to produce enough food to sustain many millions of people, such nations cannot afford the luxury of wasting the amount of energy involved in the raising of animals for meat. Some people feel that at a time when massive food shortages are a fact of life in many parts of the world, Americans have a moral responsibility to abstain from our predilection for corn-fed beef and use our fertile Mid-West acres for the production of crops which humans can eat directly. From another viewpoint, the above equation indicates why populations which, because of their habitat, are almost exclusively dependent on meat as a food source cannot permit their numbers to grow very large. One important factor contributing to the small population size of Eskimo groups is that these people exist as top carnivores of a relatively long food chain:

diatoms → zooplankton → fish → seals → Eskimos

Such energy flow patterns indicate that if Americans want to retain meat as a major component of their diet, they cannot permit population levels to increase substantially.

The preceding observations should make it readily apparent that food chains are limited by energy considerations to usually four, sometimes five, trophic levels. A food chain of unlimited length is a physical impossibility, because the higher the feeding level, the less energy there is available within a given area. An animal which is a high level consumer must range over wide areas in order to find enough food to support itself. Eventually the point is reached where the energy required to secure the food is greater than the energy obtained by eating it. At such a point no more organisms can be supported and the upper limits of the food chain have been reached.

Fig. 1-2

Food Pyramid

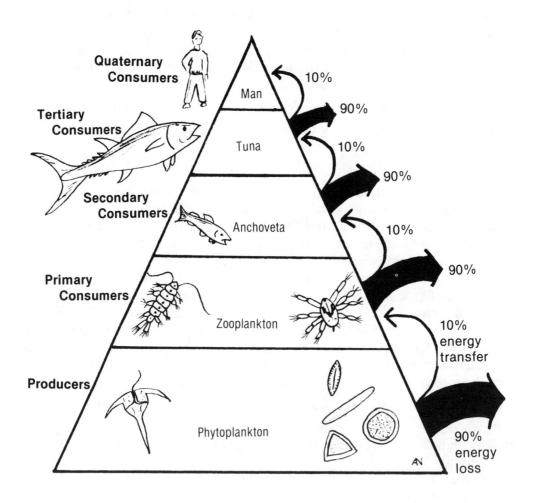

Of course in most real communities the actual structure of trophic levels is much more complex than the food chain concept portrays. A "food web" would be a more accurate depiction, since many organisms feed on many different species and in some cases on more than one trophic level. Humans, for example, can be quaternary or tertiary consumers by eating fish, secondary consumers when dining on roast turkey, or primary consumers when munching on peanut-butter sandwiches. The many interlocking food chains tend to promote stability for organisms at the higher levels, providing them with alternative food sources should one or more of the prey species become less abundant. In general, the more complex the food web, the more stable the ecosystem is likely to be.

Biogeochemical Cycling

Every home gardener who maintains a compost pile in his backyard intuitively understands the basic principles of biogeochemical cycling. All living organisms are dependent not only on a source of energy, but also on a number of inorganic materials which are continuously being circulated throughout the ecosystem. These materials provide both the physical framework which supports life activities and the inorganic chemical building-blocks from which living molecules are formed. When such molecules are synthesized or broken down, changed from one form into another as they move through the ecosystem, the elements of which they are composed are not lost or degraded in the same way in which energy moving through a food chain is lost. Indeed, the manner in which inorganic materials move through ecosystems differs fundamentally from the movement of energy through those same systems in that matter, unlike energy, is conserved within the ecosystem, its atoms and molecules being used and reused indefinitely.

The cycling of earth materials through living systems and back to the earth is called *Biogeochemical Cycling*. Of the 92 naturally-occurring chemical elements, about 40 are essential to the existence of living organisms and hence are known as *Nutrients*. Some of these nutrients are fairly abundant and are needed in relatively large quantities by plants and animals. Such substances are termed *Macronutrients* and include carbon, hydrogen, oxygen, nitrogen, phosphorus, potassium, calcium, magnesium, and sulfur. Others which are equally necessary but are required in much smaller amounts are called *Trace Elements*. These include such substances as iron, copper, manganese, zinc, chlorine, and iodine. The perpetuation of life on this planet is ultimately dependent on the repeated recycling of these inorganic materials in more or less circular paths from the abiotic environment to living things and back to the environment again. Such cycling involves a change in the elements from an inorganic form to an organic molecule and back again. Biogeochemical cycles are important because they help retain vital nutrients in forms usable by plants and animals and because they help to maintain the stability of ecosystems.

Organisms have developed various adaptations to enable them to capture and retain nutrients. As we've seen in our discussion of biomes, plants in both the tropical rainforest and in desert regions have widespread, shallow root systems which permit them quickly to absorb water and the mineral nutrients which it carries in dissolved form before these can be lost through rapid run-off, competition from other organisms, or evaporation. In the tropical rainforest, for example, virtually all the mineral nutrients are retained in plant tissues and the topsoil of this biome is extremely nutrient-poor. If nutrient cycling did not occur, amounts of necessary elements would constantly decrease and would make the development of stable plant and animal populations impossible, since there is no constant addition to the source of nutrients from outside (as there is of energy in the form of sunlight).

There are basically two types of biogeochemical cycles—gaseous and sedimentary—depending on whether the primary source for the nutrient involved happens to be air and water (gaseous cycle) or soil and rocks (sedimentary cycle).

Gaseous Cycles

The elements moved about by gaseous cycles, primarily through the atmosphere but to a lesser degree in water, recycle much more quickly and efficiently than do those in the sedimentary cycle. Gaseous cycles pertain to only four elements: carbon, hydrogen, oxygen, and nitrogen. These four constitute about 97.2% of the bulk of protoplasm and so are of vital importance to life. An examination of two of these, the cycles of carbon and nitrogen, give an idea of the complexity of gaseous cycles.

Carbon Cycle: Carbon atoms are the basic units of all organic compounds and hence, along with water, could be considered the most important component of biological systems. The principal inorganic source of carbon is the carbon dioxide found in the atmosphere and dissolved in bodies of water (the concentration of carbon dioxide dissolved in water is about 100 times greater than the amount present in the atmosphere; for this reason, carbon dioxide is much more accessible to aquatic organisms than to species living on land). Another large source of inorganic carbon lies in storage within deposits of fossil fuels—coal, oil, gas—but the largest amount of all occurs in the form of carbonate sediments such as limestone, formed under the seas and gradually uplifted during slow geologic processes.

Carbon dioxide is made available to living organisms through the process of photosynthesis, whereby green plants utilize solar energy to combine carbon dioxide and water, ultimately producing carbohydrates into proteins, fats, and complex sugars. Animals obtain the carbon they need by eating plants and re-synthesizing these into new carbon-containing compounds. Completion of the cycle, the break-down of organic molecules to release inorganic carbon dioxide, is accomplished by several different pathways: 1) through the processes of respiration, whereby plants and animals take in oxygen and release carbon dioxide as a waste product; 2) through the decay of dead organisms or of animal wastes, whereby bacteria and fungi decompose the carbon-containing organic molecules, releasing large amounts of carbon dioxide through their respiratory activities; 3) natural weathering of limestone; and 4) by the combustion of organic fuels (coal, oil, gas, wood). The last of these sources of inorganic carbon is causing growing concern among scientists who note that while the amount of atmospheric carbon remained relatively stable for millions of years, it has been increasing steadily since the onset of the Industrial Revolution and has particularly accelerated during the past century.

Nitrogen Cycle: The major reservoirs of nitrogen in the ecosystem are the 78% of free nitrogen gas which makes up our atmosphere and the nitrogen stored in rock-forming minerals. Atmospheric nitrogen, however, is biologically inert and cannot be utilized as such by most green plants. Nitrogen in the air can be returned to the soil and converted to a form accessible to plants in one of two ways:

1. lightning passing through the atmosphere can convert nitrogen to nitrogen oxide; when nitrogen oxide is dissolved in water it can be acted upon by certain bacteria in the soil which convert it into nitrate ions which can be absorbed by plant roots.
2. fixation of atmospheric nitrogen by *Rhizobium* sp. bacteria which live in symbiotic association with leguminous plants inside root nodules, converting nitrogen to nitrates; certain species of free-living soil bacteria and some blue-green algae also have the ability to fix free nitrogen into nitrates.

Of these two methods, nitrogen-fixation of atmospheric nitrogen by bacteria is by far the most significant way of making nitrogen available to other organisms. To complete the nitrogen cycle, nitrogenous wastes in the form of dead organisms, feces, urine, etc., are decomposed to ammonia by other types of soil bacteria; ammonia in turn is acted upon by nitrifying bacteria which form more nitrates. Such nitrates may be taken up again by plants or further broken down by another group of microorganisms called de-nitrifying bacteria, which act upon nitrates to produce free nitrogen which is once again returned to the atmosphere.

Sedimentary Cycles

Many of the elements which are essential for plant and animal life occur most commonly in the form of sedimentary rocks from which recycling takes place very slowly. Indeed, such sedimentary cycles may extend across long periods of geologic time and for all practical purposes constitute what are essentially one-way flows. In comparison with gaseous cycles, sedimentary cycles seem relatively simple in nature. Iron, calcium, and phosphorus are examples of nutrients whose cycling occurs via the basic sedimentary pattern. A brief look at the phosphorus cycle will give an idea of the transformations involved.

Phosphorus Cycle: Phosphorus, a key element in the nucleic acids DNA and RNA, as well as a component of the organic molecules which govern energy transfer within living organisms, occurs principally in the form of phosphate rock deposits. Smaller, though locally significant, amounts occur where quantities of excrement from fish-eating birds accumulate (e.g. the guano deposits on islands off the coast of Peru) or in deposits of fossil bones. When such phosphate reservoirs are exposed to rainfall, phosphorus ions dissolve and can be absorbed by plant roots and incorporated into vegetative tissue. At the same time, much phosphorus is effectively lost from the ecosystem through run-off to the sea. Animals obtain the phosphorus they need by eating plants. When animals excrete waste products or when they die and decay, phosphates are returned to the soil where they once again become available for uptake by plants or are lost by downhill transport into the sea. Within the shallow coastal areas some of this phosphorus is taken up by the marine phytoplankton which constitute the ultimate source of phosphorus for fish and sea birds. However, much of the phosphorus entering the sea is carried by currents to the deeper marine sediments where it is inaccessible to living organisms and may remain locked up for millions of years until future geologic upheavals. The large amounts of phosphate being produced commercially today for use as fertilizers come from the mining of phosphate rock. Unfortunately, much as in the case of oil or coal, such phosphate deposits constitute an essentially non-renewable resource, since the processes responsible for their creation occurred millions of years in the past. In recent years the use of phosphate fertilizers has been increasing at an annual rate of 5%. If this trend continues, the known supply and reserves of phosphates will be exhausted within 90 years.

The fact that the general pattern in sedimentary cycling is a downhill one, where materials tend to move through ecosystems into relatively inaccessible geologic pools, poses some interesting implications for the stability of ecosystems. The loss of soluble mineral nutrients from upland areas to the lowlands and oceans is curbed only by local biological recycling mechanisms which prevent downhill loss from outpacing the release of new materials from underlying rocks. Such local recycling depends upon the return of dead organic material to the soil where break-down and reuse of materials can occur. Human disruption of this process, through wide-scale removal of potential nutrients (e.g. by logging, which removes trees which would otherwise have died and decayed in place; grazing of livestock which consume local resources but whose flesh, wool, bones, etc., will be disposed of elsewhere), accelerates the impoverishment of certain ecosystems where essential mineral nutrients are already in short supply. In such situations the lowlands are not benefitted either, for the increased flow of materials they receive generally pass into the sea and out of biological circulation before they can be assimilated. Concern about the long-range stability of ecosystems demands that we begin to pay more careful attention to the biological recycling of inorganic materials which move in sedimentary cycles.

Change in Ecosystems

The fact that ecosystems undergo dramatic change over vast periods of time is now well-accepted. Geologists have shown us how mountains are worn down and washed to the seas, forming thick layers of underwater sediments which eons later may be uplifted by immense tectonic pressures to form new mountains; deserts expand and retreat as rainfall patterns shift, and periodically great glacial ice sheets move southward, changing the face of the earth. As land forms and climate change, it is not surprising that the biotic communities within the affected ecosystems change also. It is now recognized that the biotic communities in past geologic eras differed greatly from those existing today. What is less well understood is that present ecosystems have a dynamic quality of their own, their component communities changing in an orderly sequence within a given area, a process known as *Ecological Succession*.

Succession

In our discussion of biomes it was shown that each climatic zone is associated with a certain dominant plant type which ecologists term the *Climax Community*. By "climax" we mean *a relatively stable community achieved by a population of organisms in a given climatic area*. In theory it's all well and good to think of such communities as large homogeneous areas in which the composition of organisms is relatively uniform, but such ideal situations are difficult to find in the modern world. Most areas of virgin hardwood forest are now gone, replaced by farms, open pastureland, cut-over woodlots, etc. The former vast expanses of prairie are now mainly corn and wheat fields; many tropical rain forests have been converted to tea and rubber estates or paddy fields, and so forth. Even in regions where animals and plants tend to be in a more natural condition over large areas, there are still deviations from the climax community in areas of extensive rock outcrops, on overgrazed land, in areas swept by forest fires, etc. Regions such as these may have very few organisms of any kind or may possess a community unlike that of the climax for the region. Although at a casual glance such a community appears quite stable, if one could observe it over a period of many years one could see it changing, slowly but surely, in the direction of the climax community. Depending on the particular location involved, the change might take a very long time or it might be completed within a few decades, but in either case the process of change would follow a definite pattern. The phenomenon of gradual, orderly, and predictable change in the composition of communities toward the climax type is known as *Succession*. The concept of succession involves four components:

1. There is a dynamic shifting in the species composition of the community.
2. Species change is orderly and predictable.
3. Sequence of change is directional, each succeeding community type becoming more like the climax type in physical characteristics.
4. The ultimate community type is the climax community.

The concept can be more easily understood if we look at some specific examples of succession in action. Imagine that a volcanic eruption has completely destroyed all life in an area, leaving nothing but bare lava. Will the surface of the rock remain barren forever? Of course not; over a period of time, perhaps hundreds or even thousands of years if the climate is cold or dry, faster if it is warm and wet, changes in the biotic communities occupying the surface of the rock will change it beyond recognition. Such a sequence of change, proceeding from a stage where no community has existed previously (e.g. glacial till left by retreating ice sheets, sandy lake shore, gash on mountainside left by rock slide, etc.) is termed *Primary Succession*

At first the only factors that can change the nature of the rock's surface are physical ones. Rain falls, combining with carbon dioxide in the air to form a dilute solution of carbonic acid. Bit by bit, this gradually begins to wear down the rocky surface. If the climate is a northern or temperate one, freezing and thawing may occur, helping to split the rock further. Wind erosion may also play a part. Soon spores of algae and fungi come through the air from surrounding areas and colonies of lichens are established on the rock surface. The life processes of these organisms hasten the deterioration of the rock and when the lichens die, their dead organic matter contributes toward building up a thin layer of soil. The primitive plants (lichens) of the first stage of succession are called *Pioneer Plants*. Such organisms must be tolerant of severe climatic conditions and be largely self-sustaining. Interestingly, plants which are so tolerant of adverse physical conditions are often intolerant of other organisms. Once the lichens have helped to corrode the rock, create a small amount of soil, and maintain better moisture conditions, mosses take over and crowd out the lichens. These may form a dense cover, attracting insects and other small invertebrates. The mosses continue to build up deposits of organic matter and soil as more rock is broken away and as the old mosses and lichens die. The most significant change that these organisms can produce in an environment is that created by their own dead bodies. As decayed organic material accumulates, erosion of the rock slows down, but herbaceous plants move in and take over. Insects will be the main form of animal life at this stage, but some small mammals and reptiles may be present also. Eventually saplings of trees and shrubs will take hold, and since the taller plants furnish shade and act as a windbreak, the moisture conditions of the soil and near-soil atmosphere improve. Gradually the shrubs become the dominant plants, shading out most of the herbs. Corresponding animal types may change also, insects perhaps becoming fewer but birds increasing in number. As the shrub stage matures, sapling trees begin to predominate. Shade-loving plants proliferate under the canopy. With maturation of the forest, the climax community has been re-established and a relatively stable condition achieved. It is important to note that during the successional process, it is not only the composition of the biotic community that is changing—the physical environment has been substantially altered as well. Thus succession represents a dynamic process in which abiotic factors influence the plants and animals of the community and these in turn modify the physical habitat.

A less extreme, and more common, situation than primary succession is that exemplified by *Secondary Succession*. In this case, succession proceeds from a

Nature provided ecologists with a unique opportunity to observe at first hand the progress of primary succession when, on August 27, 1883, after several weeks of minor eruptions, the small volcanic island of Krakatoa blew itself out of the water. An island of the Indonesian archipelago lying between Java and Sumatra, Krakatoa exploded with several tremendous blasts which scientists speculate may have been the loudest noises ever heard on earth, audible as far away as Australia and Sri Lanka. The eruption blew six cubic miles of rock into the air and completely destroyed all life on the island, leaving only a peak completely covered with volcanic ash and rock. The explosion generated tidal waves which killed an estimated 36,000 people living in coastal areas of nearby islands and threw clouds of dust as high as 17 miles into the atmosphere. The volcanic dust was responsible for the famous red sunsets visible worldwide during the following two years.

As a spectacular example of nature's powers, the destruction of Krakatoa has no parallel in history; its importance to the scientific community, however, was the opportunity it provided biologists to observe how vegetation and animal life develop and change during the course of succession in a tropical rain forest ecosystem.

In spite of the fact that the remains of Krakatoa were separated from the large land masses of Java and Sumatra by about 30 miles of ocean, new life reached the island by both sea and air and the re-establishment of a new biotic community quickly began. During the year following the explosion, erosion of the ash by the heavy monsoon rains etched deep gullies into the surface of the land. Only three years later, however, visitors to the island found most of the rock and ash covered with a thin layer of blue-green algae, the pioneer plants, while large sections of the lower part of the island already were occupied by a number of herbaceous plant species, mostly ferns. Fourteen years later when the next group of botanical explorers arrived, they found well-developed vegetation throughout the island. Tropical beach plants such as the coconut palm had rooted along the shore; inland, tall grasses and scattered shrubs had replaced the ferns. Another expedition 23 years after the explosion documented the development of a woodland of casuarina trees behind the shrub community along the shore, while grasses, small trees and shrubs still dominated the interior. Higher up toward the peak, scattered trees with an understory of ferns were noted. After 36 years the fringe of beach plants and casuarinas were gone, replaced by mixed woodland; above this woodland, tropical grasses still predominated, though scattered rain forest-type trees could be found. Finally, after 50 years, the entire island was covered with a woodland similar to the one which had first developed along the beach; in addition, by this time over 1200 animal species had become established. How many more years it will take before the climax forest is attained remains to be seen. Life on Krakatoa is now abundant but has not yet achieved ecological stability. If experience in other disturbed climax communities is any guide, it will probably be many more centuries before Krakatoa hosts a flora and fauna similar to those which existed there prior to 1883.

state in which other organisms are still present; new life doesn't have to start from scratch, so to speak. Examples of secondary succession are legion— abandoned farms or pastureland growing up into forest, revegetation of an area burned over by a forest fire, vacant city lot going to weeds, etc. In such cases succession begins at a more advanced stage but proceeds, like primary succession, in a unidirectional, predictable way toward the climax community.

Fig. 1-3

Primary Succession

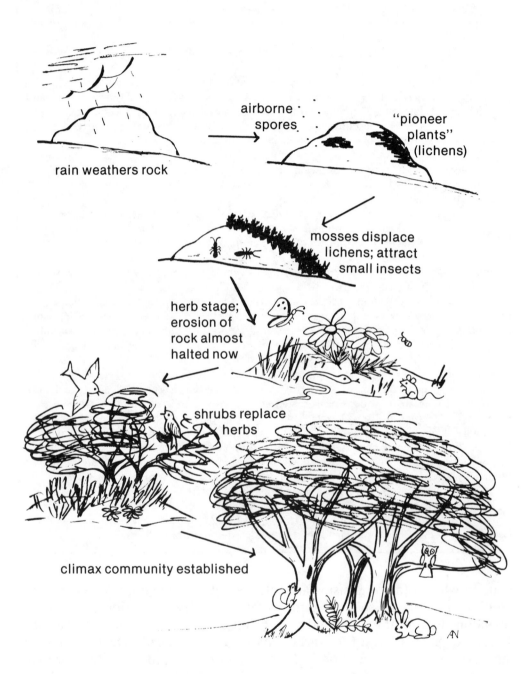

airborne spores

rain weathers rock

"pioneer plants" (lichens)

mosses displace lichens; attract small insects

herb stage; erosion of rock almost halted now

shrubs replace herbs

climax community established

Fig. 1-4

Aquatic Succession

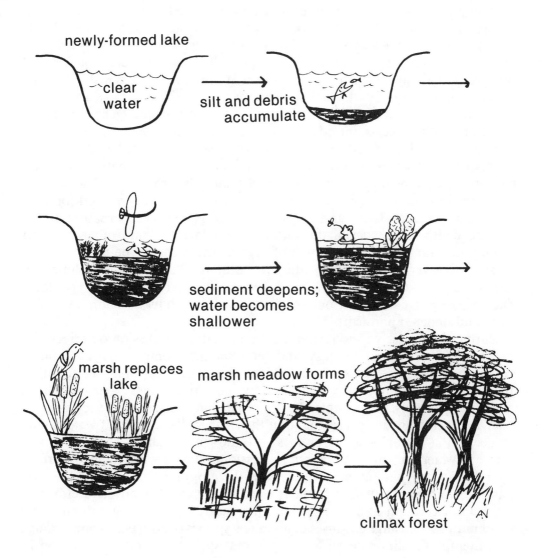

newly-formed lake

clear water

silt and debris accumulate

sediment deepens; water becomes shallower

marsh replaces lake

marsh meadow forms

climax forest

Thus far we've only referred to terrestrial succession, but the same concept applies to most enclosed bodies of water as well. A newly-formed lake (e.g. one left behind by a retreating glacier) will generally have clear water with little or no vegetation or debris. Gradually silt and dead materials are deposited on the lake botton. The sides of the lake may also be eroded by wave action and thus help fill in the deeper parts of the basin. Around the edges of the lake rooted aquatic plants such as water lilies and pickerel weed, rushes, cat-tails, etc., become established. With the accumulation of dead organic material, the supply of nutrients necessary for the growth of algae and microorganisms is increased and they flourish accordingly, providing a food source for fish and other large animals. This process of nutrient enrichment is called *Eutrophication*. The speed with which this phenomenon occurs is greatly accelerated when human-produced substances such as phosphate detergents, chemical fertilizers, or sewage is introduced. Eventually, as the lake becomes more completely filled with sediment, the whole area is converted into a marsh. Terrestrial grasses and moisture-tolerant plants subsequently move in, converting the marsh into a meadow, and finally the grasses are displaced by trees, resulting in a climax community. The length of time required for such succession to take place varies widely, depending on such variables as the original depth of the basin, the rate of sedimentation, and other physical conditions which affect the growth of organisms. It should be mentioned in passing, however, that not all aquatic succession results in the establishment of a terrestrial climax community. In cases where the body of water is very large and deep or where there is strong wave action, a stable aquatic community may form and undergo no further change.

During the course of succession, as the preceding discussion describes, the number of species, the biomass, and the structural complexity of the biotic community increases. Interestingly, humans have generally preferred to utilize the kinds of communities characterized by the earlier stages of succession. In aquatic ecosystems, for example, the desirable food and game fish such as trout, bass, and perch are all species found in the clear, well-oxygenated water found in deep, non-eutrophic lakes or in swiftly-flowing streams. The carp which thrive in waters at a more advanced successional stage are less highly regarded. In relation to land communities, the development of agriculture and pastoralism have resulted in humans exerting increasingly effective efforts to maintain succession at an early, simplified stage. By replacing natural biotic communities with large expanses of just a few species of crop plants and through the attempt to eliminate such competitors as insects, rodents, and birds, agricultural man has further simplified biotic communities, often undermining the stability of ecosystems in the process.

The stresses which humans are today imposing upon natural ecosystems extend far beyond the biological simplification of agricultural communities, however. The toxic pollutants being discharged into the air and water in unprecedented amounts are subjecting biotic communities to pressures with which they are evolutionarily unequipped to cope. Perhaps even more serious, the sheer increase in numbers of humans and their domestic animals is creating physical pressures which in many parts of the world are changing ecosystems in ways which are severely detrimental not only to the biological communities which inhabit them but to human long-term interests as well.

References:

[1]Harrison, Gordon, "Operation Cat Drop", *Natural History,* December 1968.

[2]Odum, Eugene P., *Fundamentals of Ecology,* W. B. Saunders Co., 1959.

[3]Ehrlich, Paul R., Anne H. Ehrlich, and John P. Holdren, *Ecoscience: Population, Resources, Environment,* W. H. Freeman and Company, 1977.

[4]Pratt, Harry D. and Robert Z. Brown, *Biological Factors in Domestic Rodent Control,* U.S. Department of Health, Education and Welfare, Public Health Service, Center for Disease Control, 1976.

[5]Pratt, Harry D. and Kent S. Littig, *Lice of Public Health Importance and Their Control,* U.S. Department of Health, Education, and Welfare, Public Health Service, Center for Disease Control, 1973.

[6]Strahler, Arthur N., and Alan H. Strahler, *Environmental Geoscience,* Hamilton Publishing Company, 1973.

2

Population Dynamics

..."Be fruitful and multiply and fill the earth and subdue it"...
—Genesis 1:28

"Growth for the sake of growth is the ideology of the cancer cell."
—Edward Abbey

"Standing room only" is a phrase used only half in jest to describe the possible human predicament on this finite planet if present growth rates continue unchecked indefinitely into the future. Population projections for the year 3000 A.D., if growth rates hold steady at their present 1.8%, reveal that total world population at that time would be one billion billion people, a number which would squeeze 1700 humans onto every square yard of the earth's surface, including oceans, deserts, and polar ice caps. Obviously such figures represent an exercise in the absurd. Common sense observation of the world around us reveals that when populations of any organism explode, be they swarms of migratory locusts, an outbreak of tent caterpillars, lemmings marching toward the sea, or whatever, something, sooner or later, brings that population back into a state of relative equilibrium with its environment. There is no reason to suppose that man, any more than locusts, caterpillars, or lemmings, can defy the laws of Nature by multiplying indefinitely. Certain ecological principles govern the ways in which populations change in size; the study of such changes—population dynamics—is of great practical importance to humans who wish to be able to predict or control the size of populations of other organisms or, even more important today, to forecast trends in human population growth and, if possible, guide such growth into ecologically sustainable patterns.

Population Attributes

As we saw in Ch. 1, a biotic community is made up of populations of a number of different species which are bound together by an intricate web of relationships, interacting with each other and with the physical environment. Any population, be it that of leopard frogs in a farm pond, lions on the Serengeti Plain, or humans overcrowding Spaceship Earth, exhibits certain measurable group attributes which are unique to that population. Such group attributes include birth and death rate, age structure, population density, spatial distribution, and so forth. Knowing what these characteristics are for any given population is helpful in predicting how that population will change in response to changes in the environment.

Basically, assessing dynamic changes within a population largely revolves around keeping track of additions to that population from births and immigration and of losses from the same group due to deaths and emigration. Age structure of the population also must be taken into account in those species, such as Man, where generations tend to overlap.

Limits to Growth

More than 100 years ago Charles Darwin observed in his *Origin of Species* that all organisms have a tendency to produce many more offspring than will survive to maturity. Indeed, in nature a given population of organisms tends to maintain relatively stable numbers over a long period of time. Although a single oyster may produce up to 100 million eggs at one spawning, an orchid release a million seeds, or one mushroom be responsible for hundreds of thousands of fungal spores drifting through the air, nevertheless the world has not yet been overwhelmed with oysters, orchids, or mushrooms. Even much less prolific species theoretically could give rise to staggering numbers of offspring. Darwin himself cited the example of the slow-breeding elephant (gestation period of 600-630 days), showing that the progeny from a single pair would number 19 million after 750 years, assuming that all survived to reproductive age.

Obviously the increase of populations as described above could only occur in a situation where no forces act to slow the growth rate—a scenario which is virtually non-existent in the real world, at least for any extended period of time.

The maximum growth rate which a population could achieve in an unlimited environment is referred to as that population's *Biotic Potential*. In reality of course no organism ever reaches its biotic potential because of one or more factors which limit growth long before population size attains its theoretical maximum. Such limiting factors include: food shortages, overcrowding, disease, predation, and accumulation of toxic wastes. Taken together, the environmental pressures which limit a population's inherent capacity for growth are termed **Environmental Resistance**. Environmental resistance is generally measured as the difference between the biotic potential of a population and the actual rate of increase as observed under laboratory or field conditions.[1]

Population Growth Forms

Earlier in this century a number of population biologists were curious to discover what would happen to a population if most of the usual factors of environmental resistance were removed. They devised carefully controlled laboratory experiments to chart growth curves for populations where limitation of resources, predation, parasites and the like which normally contribute to high death rates would not come into play. Their findings revealed that populations exhibit characteristic patterns of increase which biologists call population growth forms. Experimentation with a wide variety of organisms has revealed two basic patterns, described as the S-curve and the J-curve.

S-Curve

A classic study in population dynamics was carried out by the Russian, G. F. Gause, in 1932 using a population of the protozoan, *Paramecium caudatum.* Gause placed one paramecium into an aquarium with a broth of bacterial cells suspended in water to provide a food supply and then carefully observed the subsequent growth of that population. He found that numbers of paramecia increased rather slowly for the first few days, then increased very rapidly for a period; finally the rate of increase began to slow down and gradually levelled off as the upper limits of growth were reached and a steady-state equilibrium was achieved. The growth pattern thus revealed is that of an S-curve (sigmoid curve), the upper limit, called the **Upper Asymptote**, indicating that point at which increased mortality has brought birth and death rates into balance once again (in the case of Gause's paramecia, increased mortality was due to the fact that as the organisms became increasingly crowded in the culture, the constant food supply became too limited to support them all). The population density at the upper asymptote thus represents an equilibrium level between the biotic potential of that population and the environmental resistance. Thus the upper asymptote of the S-curve is often referred to as the **Carrying Capacity** of that environment—the limit at which that environment can support a population.

J-Curve

The sigmoid growth pattern, typical of populations as diverse as microorganisms, plants, and many types of birds and mammals as well, results from the gradually increasing pressures of environmental resistance as the density of population increases. Another type of population growth form, more dramatic because it frequently results in the population "crashes" which attract journalistic attention, can be represented by what is known as a J-curve. In this

Fig. 2-1

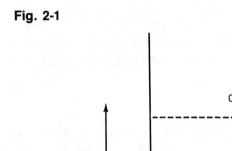

S-Curve

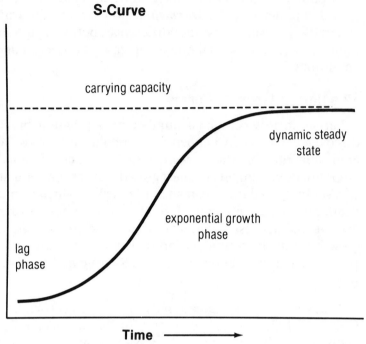

carrying capacity

dynamic steady
state

**Number of
Organisms**

exponential growth
phase

lag
phase

Time ⟶

J-Curve

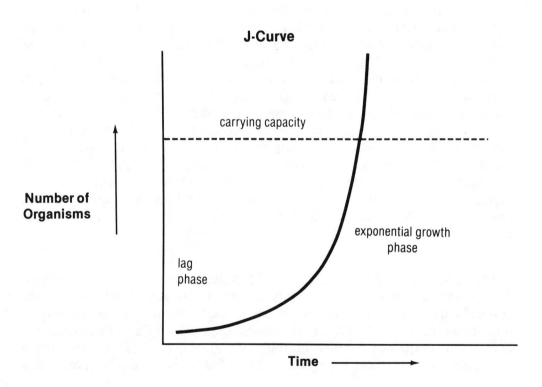

carrying capacity

**Number of
Organisms**

exponential growth
phase

lag
phase

Time ⟶

type of situation population growth increases at rapid exponential rates up to or even beyond the carrying capacity of the environment. In this situation the environmental resistance becomes effective only at the last moment, so to speak, and as a result populations which have overshot the carrying capacity suffer die-backs or "population crashes." This type of pattern is frequently seen in many natural populations such as lemmings, algal blooms, certain insects, etc. It should be apparent that the early phases of growth represented by S- and J- curves are identical: a preliminary "lag" phase, during which time the rate of increase is relatively slow, followed by a logarithmic, or exponential, growth phase during which not only do the actual numbers grow rapidly, but the *rate* of increase is also increasing (in the manner of compound interest). Thus basically a J-curve can be considered an incomplete S-curve since the sudden imposition of limiting effects halts growth before the self-limiting effects within a population become apparent.

Homeostatic Controls

Food shortage, excess predation, and disease are not the only factors which can cause populations to decline. Extensive research has shown that a number of self-regulating factors, or *Homeostatic controls*, in the form of behavioral, physiological, and social responses within a population are also very important in controlling the size of a given population. Each population appears to have an optimal density, and if this optimum is exceeded a number of stress-related responses become evident. For example, it has been observed that among the snowshoe hares of northern Canada population crashes occur at regular 9-10 year intervals even in the absence of predators, disease, or human hunting pressures. Researchers have found that during the rapid die-off phase of these oscillations large numbers of hares suffer a stress-induced degeneration of their livers, resulting in inadequate glycogen reserves. The animals may then exhibit "shock disease", lapsing into convulsions, coma, and ultimately death.[2]

Classic studies on the effects of overcrowding in rats have shown that even when abundant food is present, self-regulating mechanisms induce population crashes when rat populations exceed a certain density. When crowded, rats begin to exhibit abnormally hostile behavior; social interactions become pathological and fighting intensifies, often with results fatal to one of the combatants. Some individual males become hyperactive and hypersexual, attempting to mate without the customary courtship rituals and often mounting males, non-receptive females, and juveniles indiscriminately. Pregnant females under such conditions frequently abort; if the young are born alive they are frequently killed by the mother or die as a consequence of neglect. It has been suggested that the cause of such deviant behavior can be traced to the effects of crowding-induced stress on the functioning of the endocrine system which regulates hormone levels in animals. Whether the response of rats to crowding is indicative of what we can expect among human populations as our species continues to increase is open to question, but there are many who point to rising levels of violence and aggression in many parts of the world as ominous portents.

Box 2-1

"Boom-and-Bust" Cycles of the North

In the relatively simple biotic communities of the far north, violent fluctuations in the size of populations occur with predictable regularity. Species exhibiting these regular oscillations in population size are referred to as "cyclic species" and, as would be expected, exhibit the J-shaped growth curve. Such cyclic species give regions such as the taiga their "boom-and-bust" character and have provided population ecologists with some tantalizing research problems. One of the best-studied examples of cyclic oscillations is that of lemmings, voles, and mice—small herbivores of the tundra—and their predators, the Arctic fox and snowy owl. The populations of these species fluctuate widely at 3-4 year intervals. Population explosions of the lemmings across broad areas of tundra both in North America and Eurasia are followed closely by corresponding "booms" in the populations of foxes and owls in response to the great increase in their food supply, which consists almost exclusively of these small mammals. The exponentially increasing lemming population depletes the vegetation on which the animals feed. This leads to massive starvation and a precipitous population "bust" when the carrying capacity of the environment is exceeded. Soon afterwards, the populations of foxes and owls plummet also; foxes starve in large numbers while the owls migrate southward, never to return. The greatly reduced lemming population takes about 3 or 4 years to attain a population peak once again, and thus the cycle of boom-and-bust is perpetuated.[3]

Human Population Growth

Undoubtedly the reason for much of the current upsurge of interest in population dynamics stems from the fact that the human species is experiencing an unprecedented population explosion, with growth rates resembling those depicted on a J-curve. There are many people who strongly feel that the foremost environmental problem we face today, and perhaps the one which is most difficult to tackle, is human overpopulation. The explosive growth of the human species is probably the most significant event of the past million years. No other occurrence, geological or biological, has posed a threat to earthly life comparable to that of human over population. We have little hope of significantly reducing other types of environmental degradation if present rates of population increase are not reversed.

Until very recently, people who warned of an impending crunch or advocated even the mildest measures to restrain birth rates were either ridiculed, castigated, or ignored. Laboratory experiments with rats and mice, plotting of exponential curves, and the like were of interest to population biologists but didn't strike any particular chord with the public at large. After the great strides forward in agricultural productivity evidenced during the last century, the predictions of Thomas Malthus were dismissed as invalid pronouncements of the "gloomy prophet" (see Box 2–2). Indeed, as late as the 1930s, the main population concern was that the dip in the American birth rate experienced during the Depression years indicated serious depopulation in this country.

However, after World War II and especially since the early and middle 1960s, concern about population growth began to be manifested. Such concern was

---

Box 2–2

The Gloomy Prophet: Thomas Robert Malthus (1766-1834)

Of all commentators on the subject of population growth, none has had a greater impact than the economist-clergyman, Thomas Malthus. Living in the waning years of the Age of Reason, an era of optimistic faith in the perfectibility of man, when philosophers looked forward to a future where peace would prevail between men and nations and all poverty and oppression would vanish, young Malthus viewed the human situation in a very different light. His contemporaries regarded population growth as highly desirable for both economic and political power. Malthus, however, in a brilliantly logical treatise published in 1798 under the title, "An Essay on the Principle of Population as It Affects the Future Improvement of Society," dashed all rosy hopes of a utopian future and substituted instead a dreary, chilling vision. Malthus argued that growth of populations is not an unmitigated blessing. With mathematical precision he demonstrated that whereas populations have an inherent tendency to grow geometrically (2, 4, 8, 16, 32, etc.), agricultural production increases only arithmetically (1, 2, 3, 4, 5, etc.). Thus population growth will always tend to outpace additions to the food supply, thereby condemning the bulk of mankind to a marginal standard of living and frequent bouts of famine, war, and disease. Stating that man cannot live without food and observing that "the passion between the sexes is necessary and will remain nearly in its present state," Malthus concluded that visions of an increasingly perfect society were doomed to failure.

Not surprisingly, such views were not well received, though they certainly attracted a great deal of attention and discussion and exerted some effect on social policies of the time, being used as a justification by the rich for abolishing the existing poor law system and severely restricting aid to the indigent.

Population growth continued to accelerate during the 19th century, but a number of developments which Malthus had not anticipated prevented the mass misery he had predicted from occurring and led to a discounting of his "dismal theorem." Improvements in agricultural technology and the opening of the American prairies to grain production allowed greatly increased food production in the Western nations to keep pace with or even exceed the number of new mouths being added. As a result, Malthus' warnings were largely forgotten.

In recent years, however, spiralling growth rates in the food-deficit nations of the Third World have led to renewed speculation on the intrinsic soundness of Malthus' theory. In addition, just within the last decade, we have begun to recognize that in our efforts to boost food supply for growing populations we may be irreparably damaging the long-term ability of the biosphere to sustain life. We are today confronted with the disquieting possibility that Western technology has not disproved Malthus, but that there simply has not yet been sufficient time to test his gloomy prophesies.

precipitated by the awareness that intensive efforts to improve living standards and national stability in the developing nations were being largely nullified by the rapid population growth in those countries. Since the mid-1960s, heightened awareness of the world-wide nature of this problem has led to initiation of population policies and programs by scores of national governments, as well as by the United Nations and many private organizations and institutions. In order to understand why the situation was recognized so belatedly and why there's such a sense of urgency now, we need to look at some demographic facts.

Historical Trends in Human Population Growth

Assuming that the first humans appeared on earth between 1.5 million and 600,000 years ago, we can estimate that somewhere between 60 and 100 billion people have inhabited the planet at some time. Today the earth supports about 5.2 billion human inhabitants—close to 5% of all who have ever lived. We don't have enough information to estimate accurately what populations were before 1650 A.D., but we can make some educated guesses based on circumstantial ev-

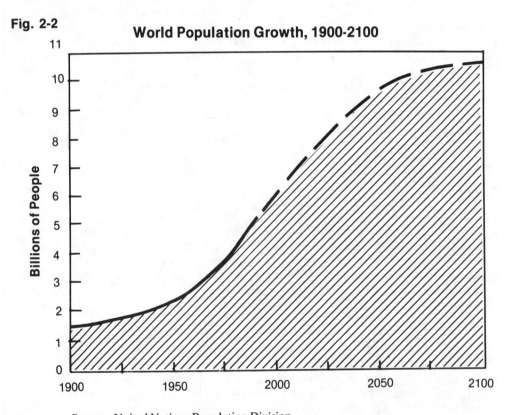

Fig. 2-2

World Population Growth, 1900-2100

Source: United Nations Population Division

idence (e.g. number of people who could be supported on X square miles by hunting and gathering, by primitive agriculture, etc.). On this basis, it's been calculated that the total human population of 8,000 B.C. was about 5 million people. By the beginning of the Christian Era, when agricultural settlements had become widespread, world population is estimated to have risen to about 200-300 million, and increased to about 500 million by 1650. It then doubled to one billion by 1850, to 2 billion by 1930, and to 4 billion by 1975; by the late 1980s, world population passed the 5 billion mark and continues to climb. Thus not only has world population been increasing steadily (with minor irregularities) for the past million years, but the rate of increase has also increased.

Doubling Time

Perhaps the best way to describe growth rate is in terms of "doubling time"—the time required for a population to double in size. During the period from 8000 B.C. to 1650 A.D., the population doubled about every 1500 years. The next doubling took 200 years, the next 80 years, and the next, 45 years.

Fig. 2-3

DOUBLING TIME OF WORLD POPULATION		
Date	Estimated Human Population	Doubling time (in years)
8000 B.C.	5 million	1500
1650 A.D.	500 million	200
1850 A.D.	1 billion	80
1930 A.D.	2 billion	45
1975	4 billion	36

Historical evidence indicates that the increase in human numbers did not occur at a steady, even pace but rather that three main surges in growth occurred; one around 600,000 years ago with the evolution of culture (developing and learning techniques of social organization and group and individual survival); the next about 8000 B.C. with the agricultural revolution; and the most recent beginning about 200 years ago with the onset of the industrial-medical-scientific revolution.[4] Bearing in mind the fact that changes in the size of populations occur when birth and death rates are out of balance, one can reasonably conclude that each of these spurts indicates that the story of human population growth is not primarily a story of changes in birth rates, but of changes in death rates. Let's now take a closer look at some of the demographic facts which help to explain our current population dilemma.

Birth and Death Rates

Birth rates are generally expressed as the number of babies born per 1000 people per year. The total number of births during the year is divided by the estimated population at the midpoint of the period. For example, there were 3,855,000 babies born in the U.S. during the 12-month period ending July 1, 1988. At the midpoint of that year, the population of the United States was 244,799,000. Therefore, the United States' birth rate for 1988 is calculated as 15.8.[5] Birth rate figures are sometimes confused with *Fertility Rates*, a figure which represents the number of births per 1000 women between the ages of 15 and 44. The fertility rate of a population gives a better indication of birth trends than does crude birth rate because it compensates for differences in sex ratio (in some countries there may be a disproportionately large female population because of wars or migration of male workers) and for differences in age composition. For example, two populations might have identical crude birth rates but greatly differing fertility rates if one had a small proportion of its population 15 to 44 years old, a majority of whom bore a child that year, while the other group had a large proportion of its population in that age group, but only a small percentage of them gave birth within the same time period.

In the U.S. both birth rates and fertility rates fell together during the 1960s, indicating that not only were fewer babies being born relative to the entire population than was true during the 1950s, but also fewer babies were born relative to the number of women in the childbearing years. In 1970 the fertility rate began to rise briefly due to the rising proportion of women in their twenties (the prime reproductive period); by 1974, however, a significant change in reproductive behavior became apparent and for the first time ever fertility in the U.S. dropped below replacement level. Despite the greater refinement of information given by fertility rates, birth rates are more readily available and more widely quoted and our subsequent discussion will be confined to these.

Death rates are calculated in the same way as birth rates, being expressed as the number of deaths per 1000 people per year.

Growth Rates

Since birth rates represent additions to a population and death rates represent subtractions, a change in population size is represented by the difference between the two, i.e. by the *Growth Rate* of that population. Growth rates can be calculated quite simply by subtracting the death rate from the birth rate. Take the case of Guatemala for example: with a 1988 birth rate of 41 and a death rate of 9, the growth rate of Guatemala's population will be 41 minus 9 or 32 per 1000 population. This is called the "rate of natural increase" (migration is not taken into consideration here). Because growth rate is normally expressed as a per cent, not per 1000 as in birth and death rates, Guatemala would have a growth rate of 3.2% annually.

Fig. 2-4 1989 POPULATION DATA FOR SELECTED COUNTRIES

Region or Country	Population (millions)	Birth Rate	Death Rate	Growth Rate	Doubling Time-yrs.
WORLD	5,234	28	10	1.8	39
AFRICA	646	45	15	2.9	24
Egypt	54.8	38	9	2.8	24
Ethiopia	49.8	44	23	2.1	33
Ghana	14.6	44	13	3.1	22
Kenya	24.1	54	13	4.1	17
Nigeria	115.3	46	17	2.9	24
South Africa	38.5	35	9	2.6	27
Zaire	34.9	45	15	3.1	23
ASIA	3,061	28	9	1.9	36
Bangladesh	114.7	43	15	2.8	25
China	1,103.9	21	7	1.4	49
India	835	33	11	2.2	32
Iran	53.9	44	10	3.4	20
Japan	123.2	11	6	0.5	141
Philippines	64.9	35	7	2.8	25
Thailand	55.6	24	7	1.7	41
Turkey	55.4	30	8	2.2	32
Vietnam	66.8	34	8	2.6	27
LATIN AMERICA	438	29	7	2.1	33
Argentina	31.9	22	9	1.4	51
Brazil	147.4	28	8	2.0	34
Colombia	31.2	28	7	2.1	34
Cuba	10.5	17	6	1.1	62
Mexico	86.7	30	6	2.4	29
Nicaragua	3.5	43	8	3.5	20
Peru	21.4	29	8	2.1	33
Venezuela	19.1	28	4	2.4	29
NORTH AMERICA	275	16	9	0.7	97
Canada	26.3	15	7	0.8	92
U.S.	248.8	16	9	0.7	98
EUROPE	499	13	10	0.3	269
France	56.1	14	10	0.4	161
Germany, W.	61.5	10	11	–0.1	–
Hungary	10.6	12	14	–0.2	–
Italy	57.6	10	9	0.0	2,310
Poland	38.2	16	10	0.6	114
Spain	39.2	11	8	0.3	210
Sweden	8.5	13	11	0.2	367
U.K.	57.3	14	11	0.2	289
USSR	289	20	10	1.0	70

Source: Population Reference Bureau, 1989 World Population Data Sheet

Growth rate is the critical factor to look at to get a quick impression of what is happening to a particular population. It is entirely possible that a country could have a traditionally high birth rate and still have a relatively low growth rate if the death rate is high also. In fact, just such a situation was characteristic of most human societies until only a few hundred years ago.

When the average person hears that Guatemala (or Algeria or Malawi, etc.) has a population growth rate of 3.2%, the number in question may fail to make an appropriate impact, since most of us find it difficult to conceptualize what a

Box 2–3

Riddle of the Magic Lily Pond

In his book, "The Twenty-Ninth Day", Lester Brown recounts a simple yet vivid illustration of the doubling time concept, one which very effectively dramatizes how quickly a given scenario can shift from a condition of abundance to one of scarcity when growth rates are increasing exponentially.

Recalling a French childhood riddle, Brown describes a mythical lily pond containing but one lily pad. Each day, however, the number of leaves doubles, so that on the second day there are two lily pads, on the third day four, on the fourth day eight, and so on. The question posed is: If the lily pond is completely full on the 30th day, when is it half-full? The answer, of course: the 29th day.

The relevance of this riddle to the present world situation is that in terms of Earth's carrying capacity, many authorities consider our global lily pond to be half full already. The implications for tomorrow should be clear.

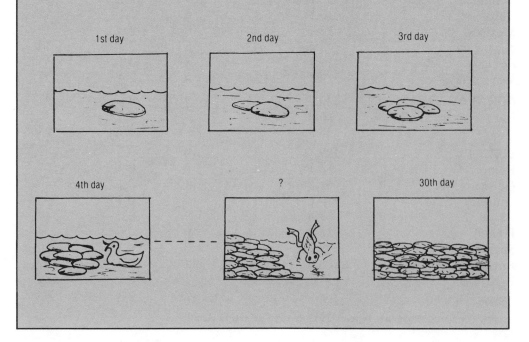

3.2% growth rate means in human terms. Besides, 3.2% really doesn't sound like very much! However, when expressed in terms of doubling time, the importance of growth rates takes on a new perspective. By calculating the annual growth rate of a population and then referring to a conversion table, we can learn what the doubling time of that population will be:

GROWTH RATE	DOUBLING TIME
0.5%	140 years
0.8%	87 years
1.0%	70 years
2.0%	35 years
3.0%	24 years
4.0%	17 years

Thus, with an annual growth rate of 3.2%, the population of Guatemala will double in a mere 21 years. In human terms this means that *just to maintain present standards of living* (which for the bulk of the population are none too high, though better than those of many other developing countries), *everything* in Guatemala needs to be doubled in 21 years—food production, provision of jobs, educational facilities, medical personnel, public services, and so forth. Whether such a herculean task can be accomplished remains to be seen; certainly the leaders of Guatemala (and of a great many other nations whose doubling times are similarly brief) face a formidable challenge in the decades ahead, especially at a time when the "revolution of rising expectations" has created a demand among the electorate for an improvement in their standard of living, not just maintenance of the status quo.

Population Explosion

With a basic understanding of what birth, death, and growth rates imply, let us now turn our attention to the crucial question of why growth rates have so accelerated during the past several generations. Obviously an increase in world growth rate can be caused by only one of two things: either the birth rate has increased or the death rate has decreased, resulting in a widening gap between the two. Surveying the history of human population growth (an admittedly risky enterprise, particularly for the prehistoric period), we can say with a fair degree of certainty that birth rates throughout the world remained fairly steady at about 40-50 per 1000 until relatively modern times. (Recently some anthropologists doing research among contemporary hunter-gatherer societies have forwarded the idea that, prior to the agricultural revolution, birth rates among primitive peoples were lower than among subsequent agricultural societies. This they attribute to environmental restraints causing such groups to attempt to space the births of their children). That women in many societies continue to bear children at traditionally high levels can be readily perceived by glancing at the current birthrates of most of the nations of Africa and many in Asia and Latin America as well.

With birth rates having apparently held steady during most of human history, we must look then to changes in death rates to explain why growth rates have shot upwards. Each of the three major changes in human lifestyle mentioned earlier effected a decline in the death rate. Cultural advances among prehistoric man probably reduced the death rate to some slight degree, but the consequences of this cultural evolution were minor compared with the changes wrought by the agricultural revolution. The increase in food supply, the more settled mode of existence, and the general rise in living standards are thought to have reduced mortality rates and increased life expectancy to some degree over that of primitive peoples.

Even so, the gains were gradual until about 200-300 years ago when improvements in public sanitation, advances in agriculture, and the control of infectious disease resulted in a precipitous decline in death rates, particularly in regards to infant and child mortality.

The growth in human numbers which resulted from these improved conditions was not, of course, a steady, uninterrupted rise. Wars, famine, and disease provoked periods of sharp population declines among localized groups. Certainly the most spectacular reversal of the overall trend toward increasing population size was the impact of bubonic plague (the notorious "Black Death" of the Middle Ages) on the societies of Europe. Plague first reached the Continent in 1348 A.D. and within 2 years had killed approximately 25% of the total population. Successive outbreaks of the disease continued to sweep across Europe during the next several decades, during which time the population of England dropped by nearly one-half (two-thirds of the student body at Oxford University died during one episode of plague), and many regions in both Europe and Asia were similarly decimated. Nearly constant warfare and the disease and famine which frequently accompanied such conflict also had a negative influence on population growth. Particularly devastating in terms of civilian suffering was the Thirty Years' War (1618-1648), during which time it is estimated that as many as one-third of the inhabitants of Germany and Bohemia died as a direct result of the war. Outside of Europe, warfare, even prior to the World Wars of the 20th century, resulted in enormous loss of life. Conquest and subjugation of native American civilizations by European colonizers, tribal warfare in Africa, the Moghul invasion of Hindu India, centuries of internal strife in China—all resulted in high death rates and sometimes severe depopulation within the affected groups. Perhaps the most extreme example of a population being decimated by warfare involves the most bloody, savage war ever fought in South America. This 5-year conflict which ended in 1870 pitted the combined forces of Brazil, Uruguay, and Argentina against those of Paraguay. The result was virtual extinction for the Paraguayans, whose army was outnumbered 10 to 1 and included 12-year-old boys fighting alongside their grandfathers. Within a 5-year period, the population of Paraguay dropped from an estimated 525,000 to 221,000, of whom slightly less than 29,000 were men. A new generation of Paraguayans was sired courtesy of the Brazilian army of occupation![6]

Nevertheless, such examples, while tragic in terms of individual suffering, and occasionally disastrous to certain ethnic groups or nationalities (e.g. the total extermination of native Tasmanians by white settlers), represented only minor aberrations from the general upward trend of human numbers when viewed from a global perspective. In general, world population has increased more or less steadily, at first quite slowly but subsequently faster and faster, from ancient times right up to the present.

Demographic Transition

By the latter half of the 19th century, Western Europe began to witness a demographic phenomenon unlike any that had occurred previously anywhere in the world. Toward the end of the 1700s and early in the 1800s, as the Industrial Revolution began transforming an entire way of life, death rates, as we have seen, started to fall gradually in response to a more adequate food supply, improved medical knowledge, better public sanitation, etc. As a result, growth rates predictably accelerated, and during the early years of the 19th century Western Europe experienced a population boom. This led, among other things, to massive emigration to the Western Hemisphere, but by approximately 1850 another rather surprising trend became apparent—throughout the industrializing nations of that era, birth rates began to fall for the first time since the agricultural revolution. The Scandinavian countries (which were among the first to compile accurate demographic records) provide a good example of the changes which were occurring. In Denmark, Norway, and Sweden the combined birth rate was about 32 in 1850; by 1900 it had dropped to 28 and today stands at 12, one of the lowest in the world. Elsewhere in Western Europe similar declines were becoming apparent. This phenomenon—the falling of both birth and death rates which has characteristically followed industrialization— marked the onset of the *Demographic Transition*, a trend which has carried on and accelerated into the 20th century. By the 1930s, decreases in the birth rates in some countries had outpaced decreases in death rates, though actual birth rates remained somewhat higher than death rates.

Reasons for the demographic transition are still being debated, but the cause for declining birth rates probably centers on the realization by married couples that in an industrial society children are an economic liability; they are expensive to feed, clothe, and educate; they reduce family mobility and make capital accumulation more difficult. In rural areas of Europe, population pressures on a finite amount of land and the modernization and mechanization of farms which reduced the amount of manual labor needed, all combined to bring about a reduction in rural birth rates also. In addition, during the late 1800s and into the 20th century, a trend toward later age at the time of marriage undoubtedly had an effect in reducing birth rates.

The decline in both birth and death rates which marked the demographic transition in Western Europe became noticeable in both Eastern Europe and North America several decades later. Although birth rates in the latter have still not fallen as low as those in the nations where the demographic transition began, the trends are quite clearly in the same direction.

Incomplete Demographic Transition

In the nations of Asia, Africa, and Latin America where traditional societies were only marginally influenced by the dynamic economic and social changes occurring in Europe and North America, demographic patterns changed very little until early in the present century. In the areas under the control of imperial powers, improvements in public sanitation and an imposed peace between formerly warring factions within the subject nations permitted a gradual increase in population levels. This gradual decline in death rates in the underdeveloped countries took a quantum leap in the years immediately following World War II as a consequence of the rapid export of modern drugs and public health measures from the industrialized nations to the Third World countries. Virtually overnight, the widely applauded introduction of "death control" into traditional cultures produced the most rapid, widespread change known in the history of population dynamics. The situation in Sri Lanka (formerly Ceylon) is a good case in point:

Prior to World War II, a major killer in many tropical countries was the mosquito-borne parasitic disease, malaria. In Sri Lanka a malaria epidemic during 1934-35 may have been responsible for half the deaths occurring in the country that year (Sri Lanka had a death rate of 34 during that time period). Not only were many victims killed directly, but many others were so debilitated by their bouts with the recurring cycles of chills and fever that they became more susceptible to other illnesses as well. Thus malaria was a contributory cause of death in some cases, a primary cause in others. In 1945, at the end of the Second World War, the death rate in Sri Lanka stood at 22. During the following year, 1946, one of the great technological innovations to rise out of the global conflict was introduced into Sri Lanka—the synthetic chemical insecticide DDT. Widescale spraying with DDT brought rapid control over the mosquitoes, with a corresponding plunge in the incidence of malaria. As a result, the death rate on the island was cut by more than half within a decade and has continued to drop since then to its present low of 6. As a consequence, the number of Sri Lankans has soared upwards.

Victory over malaria, yellow fever, smallpox, cholera, and other infectious diseases has been responsible for similar decreases in death rates throughout most of the underdeveloped world. This trend has been most pronounced among children and young adults. In a sample of 18 underdeveloped areas, the average decline in death rates between 1945 and 1950 was 24%. This decline in death rates is different in kind from the long-term slow decline that occurred throughout most of the world following the agricultural revolution. It is also different in kind from the comparatively more rapid decline in death rates in the Western world over the past century. The difference is that it is a response to a spectacular environmental change in the underdeveloped countries largely

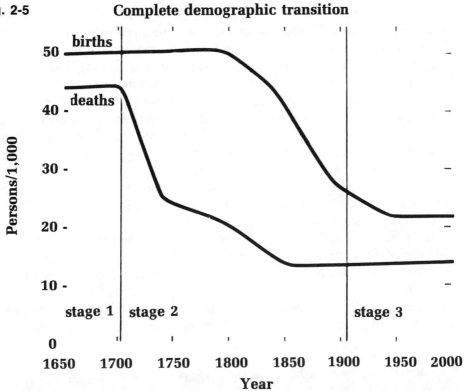

Fig. 2-5   **Complete demographic transition**

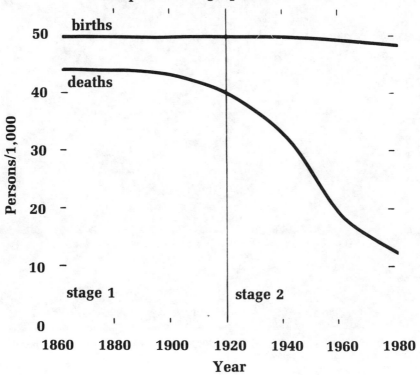

Incomplete demographic transition

through control of infectious diseases, not a fundamental change in their institutions or general way of life. Furthermore, the change did not originate within these countries, but was brought about from the outside. The factors that led to a demographic transition in the West were not and are not present in the underdeveloped nations. Instead, a large proportion of the world's people have moved rapidly from a situation of high birth and death rates to one of high birth and low death rates, a situation referred to as an *Incomplete Demographic Transition*. This, in essence, is the cause of what biologist Paul Ehrlich refers to as the "Population Bomb."

Thus have we arrived at the present situation where the bulk of world population growth is occurring in Third World countries which are already finding it difficult to support their existing populations.

Until recently, demographers assumed that societies currently experiencing rapid rates of population increase would, like Europe and North America, witness a significant decline in birth rates as rising incomes and better living conditions resulted in a general desire for smaller families. However, after nearly 40 years of explosive population growth, many Third World nations appear to be trapped in the mid-stage of their demographic transition, unable to attain

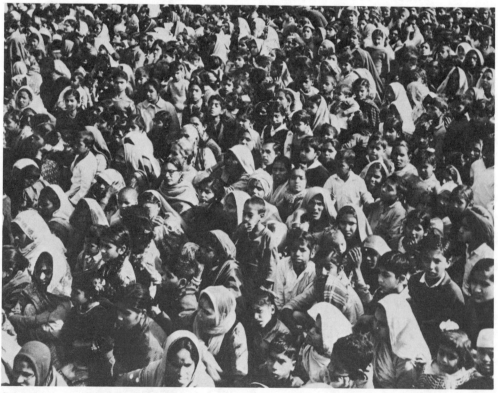

Calcutta is a city which exemplifies the poverty and congestion which results from India's population crisis. [*Agency For International Development*]

the social and economic progress essential to reducing birth rates. The world is today witnessing a sharp demographic polarization between nations where population growth is slow (1.0% or less) and living standards are improving, and countries where rapid population growth rates (2.2% or higher) continue to prevail and living conditions are deteriorating. The demographic middle ground has all but vanished, with slightly under half the world's people living in low-growth regions, the remainder in rapid-growth areas. The concern among population experts, who agree that an incomplete demographic transition cannot continue indefinitely, is that the pressure of human numbers is overwhelming the natural life-support systems in high-growth countries. As demands for food, water, fuel, and living space continue to escalate, the resource base itself is being consumed. The decline in incomes and living standards anticipated as a consequence of exceeding the local environment's carrying capacity may well trigger a rise in death rates and thrust such nations backward into the high birth/high death rate situation characteristic of the pre-Demographic Transition era.

Age Structure

It's relatively easy to comprehend the significance of birth and death rates so far as population growth is concerned, but there are other characteristics of a population which are important also.

Age structure refers to the number of people in different age categories within a given population. In countries where populations are growing rapidly because of high birth rates and declining death rates, a large percentage of the population is made up of young people; in many Third World countries nearly half the population is under the age of 15. In Western Europe, by contrast, there are proportionately many more people in the middle and older age groups. In countries where children comprise a large segment of the population, there hasn't been time yet for individuals born during the period of "death control" to reach the older age groups where death rates are higher than those of the younger age categories. In most of these countries the greatest decreases in death rates among infants and children occurred late in the 1940s and the large numbers of children born in that period reached their peak reproductive years in the 1970s. Their children, in turn, will further inflate the lower tiers of the population structure. Eventually either population control will lower birth rates in these countries or famine, disease, etc., will once again increase mortality rates. In the absence of such calamities, death rates in the extraordinarily young populations of the underdeveloped nations may temporarily fall below those of the industrialized countries.

One of the most significant features of age structure of a population is the proportion of people who are economically productive in relation to those who are dependent on them (arbitrarily considered to be those persons between 15 and 59). The proportion of dependents in the underdeveloped countries is much higher than in the developed nations, presenting an additional heavy burden to

Box 2–4
Are Europeans an Endangered Species?

"In demographic terms, Europe is vanishing. Twenty years or so from now, our countries will be empty, and no matter what our technological strength, we shall be incapable of putting it to use."

—Jacques Chirac, 1984

The above lament by the then-Prime Minister of France reflected a century of national concern about the population stagnation inherent in his country's low birthrate. Few demographers would echo Chirac's alarmist pronouncements, correctly pointing out the slowness and momentum of any significant change in population size, as well as the notorious inability of demographers to predict future childbearing patterns. Nevertheless, current fertility trends portend inevitable population decline in Europe, as birth rates continue to decline in nations all across the continent. After reaching a post-World War II peak exceeding 2.5 children per woman in 1965, fertility rates have fallen below replacement level in all European countries except Albania, Ireland, Malta, Poland, and the USSR. In Austria, Denmark, Hungary, and West Germany, deaths already exceed births, resulting in a slow but steady decline in the size of their populations—a trend which will soon be evident in East Germany, Italy, Sweden, Belgium, Bulgaria, and the United Kingdom as well (concerns about these trends should be allayed somewhat by the realization that even if unusually low fertility rates continue to prevail, it will be from 42 to 131 years, depending on the country in question, before population size falls to the level prevailing in those nations at the beginning of World War II). According to the most recent U.N. projections, the population of Europe as a whole will rise only marginally from its present 499 million, reaching 509 million by the year 2000, 512 million in 2025, then stabilizing and gradually beginning a slow decline. As birthrates fall, the age structure of European societies will shift upward. The U.N. estimates that by 2025 one out of every 5 Europeans will be 65 or older and that the working age population which must support these senior citizens will be steadily shrinking.

The consequences of an aging and dwindling population have been the subject of heated debate between European pronatalists and antinatalists for nearly 2 decades and raise issues which may be of relevance in North America as well, since similar demographic trends loom on our horizon. Spokesmen for the pronatalist viewpoint, such as Prime Minister Chirac, raise the cry, "No children, no future." They view the emerging female preference for personal development and a profession as destructive to family life and a form of collective suicide. They fear loss of world influence and European cultural identity as non-European populations continue rapid growth. They warn that with too few young men being produced for military service, young women may have to be recruited and they foresee the possible collapse of Europe's elaborate social welfare system as the demands of swelling numbers of the elderly overwhelm the ability of a proportionally smaller workforce to support them.

Discounting such worries as grossly exaggerated, opponents of the pronatalist position insist that Europe need never fear for lack of leadership and innovation as long as it ensures that a substantial fraction of its young people receive a good education—something that is easier to accomplish when the population is not growing rapidly. They charge that talk of maintaining national military strength is reminiscent of a fascist past and a hindrance to greater European solidarity. Welcoming the greater individual freedom which lower fertility rates provide, they oppose any measures aimed at encouraging increased childbearing. Reflective of such attitudes was a polemic in the German feminist journal EMMA which proclaimed, "*All attempts to influence the decision of women for motherhood must again and again be confronted with the demand for self-determination; in concrete terms: my belly is mine!"* Philosophically, antinatalists feel it would be wrong to encourage national population growth at a time when global overpopulation is perceived as a serious problem. Pointing out that economic strength is more important than population size or military might in determining a country's international standing, they stress that economic integration, rather than an attempt to boost fertility, is the way to safeguard Europe's position in the world. They point to technological advances in the workplace as reducing the need for an expanding human workforce, and insist that as long as productivity increases, funding social security systems will pose no problem.

For the most part, European politicians have been hesitant to choose sides in this debate, knowing that any position they might take would offend large blocs of voters. Several nations, most notably France and several East European countries, have implemented economically costly incentives to encourage childbearing, but for the most part such programs have had minimal long-term effects on fertility. Regardless of the rantings of political leaders, the emphasis of young Europeans on individual rights and self-fulfillment makes it highly unlikely that fertility rates will rebound anytime soon. Thus although Europeans are certainly not about to join the Siberian tiger or the black-footed ferret on the "endangered" list, a long-term population decline for most of the continent's nations appears irrevocable and is now well underway. [7]

those countries as they struggle for economic development. The high percentage of people under 15 is also indicative of the explosive growth potential of their populations. In most developing nations this percentage is 40-45%, in some as high as 50%. By contrast, the percentage under 15 in most industrialized countries is 20-30%. In the U.S., for example, there are two people of working age for every one who is too young or too old to work; in Mexico and Nigeria there is only one. Thus underdeveloped countries have a much greater proportion of people in their pre-reproductive years. As they grow up and marry, the size of the childbearing fraction of the population will increase tremendously and their children will further inflate the size of the youngest age groups. The existence of such large numbers of young people means that even if great progress were made immediately in reducing the number of births per female in those countries, it would still be some 30 years before such birth control could significantly slow down population growth.

Population Density

Mankind is quite obviously not evenly distributed over the face of the earth. Population density is usually expressed in terms of numbers of individuals per square mile or kilometer. Assessing how crowded or uncrowded a country is on the basis of density figures can be quite misleading, because such statistics take no account of areas which are uninhabited or uninhabitable. Thus a nation like Egypt has 99% of its people squeezed into 3.5% of its area. Overpopulation is usually thought of, not in relation to the absolute size of the population, but to its density and the extent of the resource base on which that population is dependent. Until fairly recent times, pressures caused by increasing population

Fig. 2-6
Age Structure Pyramids of Developing and Developed Regions

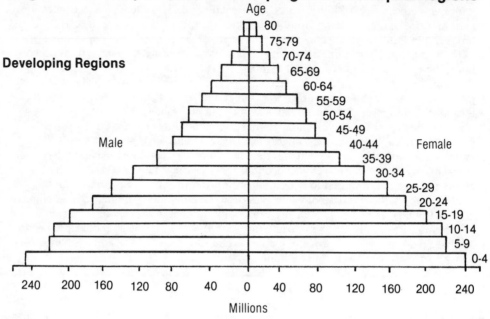

Developing Regions

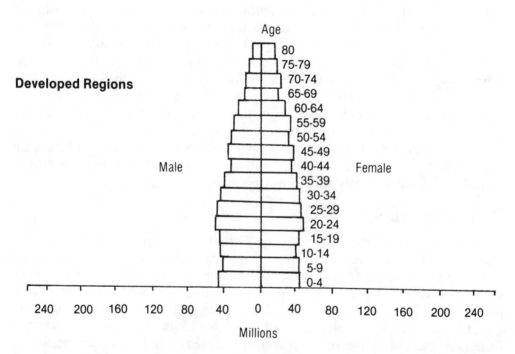

Developed Regions

Source: United Nations, *Demographic Indicators of Countries: Estimates and Projections as Assessed in 1980.*

Box 2–5

Africa's Baby Boom

Nowhere are the reverberations of the population explosion more deafening than on the continent of Africa, particularly in those nations south of the Sahara. From Senegal in the west to Somalia in the east, from Mauritania to Malawi, African population growth projections into the 21st century have assumed frightening proportions. While birth rates are gradually falling in most of the developing countries of Asia and Latin America, they remain at traditionally high levels throughout Africa (with the sole exception of Zimbabwe, where the birth rate has experienced a modest decline). Some sub-Saharan nations have even witnessed slight *increases* in fertility, thanks to improved maternal health care, a decline in the breast-feeding of infants, and an easing of traditional taboos against sexual intercourse soon after childbirth. At the same time, thanks to government efforts at improving standards of health and nutrition, previously high death rates have declined sharply, propelling growth rates upward.

If awards were given for the world's highest birth rate, fastest growth rate, and shortest doubling time, all the gold medals would go to sub-Saharan Africa. Benin, Kenya, Malawi, Niger, and Rwanda all have birthrates in excess of 50. The region as a whole is growing at a rate of 3% annually, but many individual nations exceed the regional average. The distinct front-runner in the population race is the East African nation of Kenya, growing at the unprecedented rate of 4.1% each year. Kenya also wins the prize for shortest doubling time—in just 17 years this nation of 24 million will be home to 48 million souls. Ironically, the only factor preventing African growth rates from soaring even higher is the continent's unhappy distinction in possessing the world's highest infant mortality rates as well. Although the situation is markedly better than it was a few decades ago, infant mortality in Africa today averages 110 per thousand, as compared to 10 in the U.S. and 5 in Japan.

The stresses that continued high rates of population growth are imposing on economic development and ecological stability in Africa are now attracting international attention. The World Bank, looking at U.N. projections which show Africa's population mushrooming from its present 646 million to 872 million by the turn of the century, has expressed its concern that the explosive rate of population growth in Africa is slowing development and sharply reducing the possibility of raising living standards on the continent. Consequently, the Bank has declared that stemming population growth will be its "highest priority" in sub-Saharan Africa. Efforts by international agencies to promote fertility control programs in Africa have recently been augmented by a growing commitment on the part of many national governments in the region. Until just a few years ago, many African leaders actively favored high rates of population growth, equating large numbers with political and economic strength. That attitude is now rapidly changing, as governments observe the impact uncontrolled growth is having on efforts at national development. Nigeria, the most populous nation on the continent, in 1985 became the first African country to adopt a national policy aimed at lowering fertility; since then, ten additional countries have followed Nigeria's example and plan to implement similar policies of their own. Elsewhere in most nations of the region, with or without officially adopted policy goals, family planning efforts are underway or at least being considered.[8]

No matter how successful these programs are, however—and most currently are reaching only a small percentage of fertile women—African populations will continue to grow rapidly for many years. With fully 45% of the African population age 15 or younger, the built-in momentum for future growth ensures that Africa's baby boom will continue for at least several more generations. Perhaps an even more formidable obstacle to the growth-dampening efforts of national leaders is the fact that the overwhelming majority of

African couples *want* large families. Surveys conducted among married women in Kenya regarding desired family size reveal that the average Kenyan mother wants (and usually has) 7-8 children; similar attitudes are expressed throughout the continent. "Our richness is in children", affirms a young mother of 3 in a village near Nairobi. "Children are a gift from God", agrees a civil servant in Ethiopia, adding the warning that "God will punish you if you do not accept His gift." Unless and until changing socioeconomic conditions alter prevailing views on desired family size, Africa will retain its position as the fastest-growing region in the world.

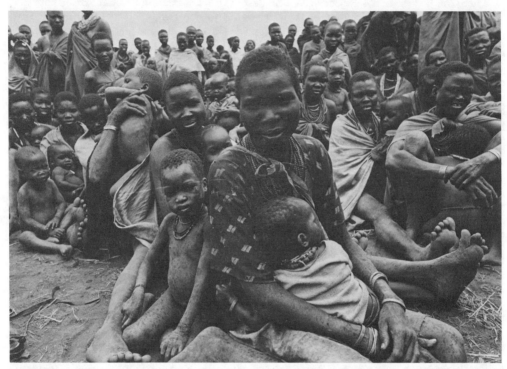

Mothers and children waiting for food at the UNICEF relief station in Kadepo. [*World Bank Photo/Yosef Hadar*]

densities were generally eased by migration from more crowded to less crowded regions (i.e. witness the massive movement of Europeans to the New World during the past several hundred years). In today's world of fiercely guarded political boundaries and increasingly strict immigration quotas, this traditional safety valve is scarcely a solution to present problems. Unfortunately there are few, if any, places left on earth today which have the capacity to sustain a large influx of immigrants and the tragic fact is that in the years ahead we may see an increasing number of homeless "boat people" doomed to drifting from port to port like modern-day "Flying Dutchmen", with no nation willing to provide a haven.

Urbanization

The "urban explosion", referring to the tremendous increase in the population of metropolitan areas, has been one of the most marked phenomena related to the over-all growth of human populations during the 20th century. Urbanization is, of course, one of the oldest of demographic trends, having its birth in the small settled communities made possible by adoption of an agricultural way of life. The first true cities are believed to have arisen in Mesopotamia about five or six thousand years ago, but growth of urban areas proceeded rather slowly during the millennia that followed. Increase in size of urban populations depended almost entirely on an influx of new residents from the surrounding countryside. Due to extremely poor sanitary conditions and crowded living conditions, mortality rates in these urban centers were higher than birth rates and not until recent times have urban centers become self-sustaining in terms of population growth.

The advent of the industrial revolution gave a tremendous impetus to the growth of cities and the rate of increase has continued to accelerate ever since. As an example of the great population shift which has occurred, consider the change in rural-urban ratios in the U.S.: in 1800 a mere 6% of all Americans lived in an urban area: the number of city dwellers increased to 15% by 1850 and 40% by 1900. In 1988, 74% of the U.S. population lived in cities.

In the world as a whole, population increased by a factor of 2.6 during the years between 1800 and 1950; during that same time period the number of people living in cities over 20,000 population grew from 22 million to over half a billion—a factor of 23. In the largest cities (100,000 or more) of the industrialized countries, the growth was even more rapid, increasing by a factor of 35. By 1950, 29% of the world's people lived in cities; by 1988 the percentage of urban dwellers in the world as a whole had risen to 45 and is expected to reach 50% by 2000 A.D.

In recent years this urban expansion in the developed world has slowed somewhat, but since 1900 has accelerated at a great rate in the nations of Asia, Africa, and Latin America. U.N. projections into the future indicate no slow down in the mass movement to the cities in the poorer countries, forecasting that almost 60% (or 1.2 billion people) of total population growth in such nations between now and the end of the century will occur in urban areas. Most of this increase will take place in already existing cities, with staggering impact on the ability of those municipalities to provide even the rudiments of a decent standard of living. Much of the population growth in Third World cities occurs in the euphemistically labelled "uncontrolled settlements"—slum areas and shantytowns spreading like ugly cancerous growths around the periphery of almost every large city in the developing world. More than a quarter of the inhabitants of Calcutta, Mexico City, Baghdad, Rio de Janeiro, Seoul, and Taipei already live in such uncontrolled settlements, a portion that rises to nearly one-half in Izmir and Ankara in Turkey, Maracaibo in Venezuela, and Bombay, India. These uncontrolled settlements are growing even faster than the urban areas as a whole, doubling in size every 5-7 years.[9] This means that in the future, ever larger segments of the urban population will be living in the squalor and hopelessness which characterize these shantytowns.

In most cases the trend to the cities seems to be caused by the hope for a better, more comfortable life, and though most migrants continue to live in abject poverty, nearly all seem to prefer to remain there rather than return to the deprivation of their rural home villages. Historically, urbanization seems to have the universal effect of breaking down the traditional cultures of those who migrate to the cities, where anonymity is the main feature. The overwhelming majority of urban dwellers in the Third World are migrants who have brought their peasant culture with them. They generally lack the specialized education and skills required to penetrate the city's complex social web. Migrants inevitably find that their limited skills make them incapable of contributing to the economy and consequently they are scarcely any better off than before. Many migrants form modified village societies within the city and thus tend to transfer aspects of village culture to the city. This may explain why the reproductive rates and attitudes of the inhabitants of these cities closely resemble those of their rural relatives.

The rapid increase in the populations of Third World cities presents a number of very serious problems which government officials are going to find extremely difficult to manage. Two of the most pressing needs, if disease outbreaks are to

---

Box 2–6

Mexico City: Urbanization Run Rampant

When Hernando Cortez gazed down upon Montezuma's capital of Tenochtitlan in the Valley of Mexico late in the fall of 1519, he was immensely impressed by the size and beauty of the city. It is doubtful, however, that even in his wildest dreams Cortez could have imagined that this Aztec center of 100,000 souls would, in a span of less than 500 years, explode into the world's most populous urban area. Today Mexico City is home to 18 million people and continues to grow at such a rate (between 3–5% annually) that the city is projected to have a population of about 30 million by the year 2000—more than any other metropolis in the world.

The rapid growth of cities during the late 20th century, sometimes referred to as the "urban explosion," has been particularly dramatic in nations of the developing world. U.N. projections indicate that within the next 20 years 45 urban areas in the less developed countries will have populations over 5 million; of these, fully 11 will boast figures over 20 million. As one of the fastest growing, Mexico City provides us with a living example of what we can expect in urban areas throughout the Third World as an ever-larger percentage of humanity become city dwellers.

When the conquistadores arrived in what is today Mexico City, they marveled at the natural beauty spread before them. Bernal Diaz del Castillo, a soldier who served under Cortez and who subsequently wrote the most illuminating account of the Conquest, undoubtedly expressed the sentiments of his colleagues as he described gardens full of

---

beautiful and aromatic plants, a crystal-clear lake (Texcoco), and remarked, ". . . when I beheld the scenes that were around me, I thought within myself that this was the garden of the world!" (Diaz del Castillo, *The True History of the Conquest of Mexico*). Diaz del Castillo would have difficulty in recognizing the city today. Hillsides are denuded of trees and the once-lovely Lake Texcoco is now dry and dusty. The demands of a mushrooming population for water have forced the government to drill more and more wells, and due to overpumping of groundwater, the earth is subsiding and the city gradually sinking (35 feet in the past 70 years). Mexico City ranks among the world's worst in terms of air quality, pollution having increased by 30% between 1976-1980. Most of this comes from the city's two million autos, virtually none of which have pollution control devices. Articles in the Mexican press regularly decry the environmental damage caused by too-rapid population growth and call for controls on pollution, reducing noise levels, reforesting the barren valley, and augmenting the city's water supply.

In response, the Mexican government recently announced a plan to control further pollution, to improve drinking water quality, and to plant 50 million trees a year. The basic problem, however, is the pressure of continuing population growth on a finite amount of land. Although Mexico's birth rate has dropped during the last 15 years, the total Mexican population will continue to increase well into the next century. The Latin American Demographic Center projects a Mexican population of 116 million by 2000, a figure which could soar to 174 million by 2025. Such numbers guarantee a continuation of current pressures.

be prevented, will be the provision of safe drinking water and sewage disposal. Even at current population levels a World Health Organization survey in 1975 revealed that 24% of Third World urban residents had no house water connections nor even access to a standpipe. Where expansion of service is occurring, it is taking place more rapidly in the relatively affluent middle-income neighborhoods than in the poverty-ridden uncontrolled settlements. Another report published in 1976 revealed that only 3.3% of city dwellers in such countries lived in homes which were connected with a sewage treatment system; another 23.7% had homes connected to a sewage system which simply funneled excrement to a waterway; 42.1% relied on outhouses, septic tanks, or buckets, while the remaining 30.9% had no facilities whatsoever and were forced to perform their bodily functions along the roadside or in open ditches.[10] As urban populations continue to expand, provision of such basic services will undoubtedly lag even further behind, increasing the threat of epidemic disease and worsening already serious problems of water pollution. Air quality, already at critical levels in many Third World capitals, will continue to deteriorate as the number of old, poorly-maintained automobiles and pollutant-emitting motorbikes, scooters, and motorcycles continue to rise. Pressures on municipal authorities to provide jobs, housing, transportation, and social facilities will mount inexorably within the coming years and will present those societies with economic and environmental challenges which may prove impossible to meet.

Fig. 2-7

WORLD'S 15 LARGEST CITIES: 1985		
Rank	Urban area	Population (in millions)
1.	Tokyo/Yokohama, Japan	18.82
2.	Mexico City, Mexico	17.30
3.	Sao Paulo, Brazil	15.88
4.	New York, U.S.A.	15.64
5.	Shanghai, China	11.96
6.	Calcutta, India	10.95
7.	Buenos Aires, Argentina	10.88
8.	Rio de Janeiro, Brazil	10.37
9.	London, United Kingdom	10.36
10.	Seoul, Korea	10.28
11.	Bombay, India	10.07
12.	Los Angeles, U.S.A.	10.05
13.	Osaka/Kobe, Japan	9.45
14.	Beijing, China	9.25
15.	Moscow, USSR	8.97

WORLD'S 15 LARGEST CITIES: 2000		
Rank	Urban area	Population (in millions)
1.	Mexico City, Mexico	25.82
2.	Sao Paulo, Brazil	23.97
3.	Tokyo/Yokohama, Japan	20.22
4.	Calcutta, India	16.53
5.	Bombay, India	16.00
6.	New York, U.S.A.	15.78
7.	Shanghai, China	14.30
8.	Seoul, Korea	13.77
9.	Teheran, Iran	13.58
10.	Rio de Janeiro, Brazil	13.26
11.	Jakarta, Indonesia	13.25
12.	Delhi, India	13.24
13.	Karachi, Pakistan	12.00
14.	Beijing, China	11.17
15.	Dacca, Bangladesh	11.16

Source: "*The Prospects of World Urbanization*", Population Studies No. 101, United Nations, New York, 1987

Population Projections

The obvious question to anyone looking at a graphic representation of human numbers soaring toward infinity on the upswing of a J-curve is, "How long can this continue?" and "Where will population stabilize?" The inherent assumption, and one which is validated by the results of numerous animal experiments in population dynamics, is that such growth rates cannot continue forever. Within the last few years, in fact, statistical evidence indicates that population growth rates peaked in the early 1970s at about 2.1% and are now declining slowly, standing at 1.7–1.8% since the mid-1980s. Nevertheless, although a growth rate decrease is heartening, in terms of absolute numbers population will be growing faster during the remainder of this century than it is right now, due to the enormous size of the present population base. By the year 2000, world population will be increasing by 100 million people each year (90 million of whom will be residents of Third World countries) compared with 87 million a year in the late 1980s.

The United Nations, an organization logically quite interested in future world growth patterns, regularly publishes projections of population size for the next several decades. Such projections are not just extrapolations of present trends into the future, but take into consideration trends in fertility, mortality, migration, etc. (they do not consider the possibility of major disasters such as a nuclear war, however). The U.N. presents three sets of projections—low, medium, and high—all of which assume that there will be some lowering of fertility rates (a substantial drop in fertility is assumed for the low projection, a less significant decline for the high projection) in regions where these are currently quite high. Recently revised U.N. projections estimate that global population should stabilize at 14.2 billion in the year 2100.

Because different areas of the world exhibit quite diverse fertility patterns, some regions will achieve population stability long before others do. As can be seen in the Population Data chart, Italy has already attained a growth rate of 0, while East and West Germany now have negative growth rates.

Looking at population projections on a regional basis, the countries of South Asia (India, Pakistan, Bangladesh) will experience the largest population increase, adding 2.7 billion people to their present 1.4 billion before numbers stabilize around 2100. At the other extreme, European populations should peak by 2030 with a total of half a billion people, only slightly more than the present figure. Africa, with the world's highest growth rate, will be second only to Asia in total numbers. Together, Africa and the nations of South Asia will account for fully 60% of the world's total population at the time of stabilization. Latin America is currently growing at a rate second only to Africa, a rate which will cause a doubling of its population in only 32 years. North America, like Europe, has a relatively low growth rate, and, barring an unanticipated change in fertility trends, should reach zero population growth early in the next century.

Obviously, making population projections is a risky business. In the past, particularly during the 1950s and 1960s, projections tended to err on the low side rather consistently. For example, in 1957 the U.N. medium projection for world population in 1970 was 3,480,000,000. By 1968, however, world population had already passed 3.5 billion. The accuracy of recent forecasts will depend not only on fertility trends but also on mortality rates. A number of

Fig. 2-8   Projected Population Size at Stablization,
Selected Countries

Country	Population in 1986	Annual Rate of Population Growth	Size of Population at Stabi-lization	Change from 1986
	(million)	(percent)	(million)	(percent)
Slow Growth Countries				
China	1,050	1.0	1,571	+ 50
Soviet Union	280	0.9	377	+ 35
United States	241	0.7	289	+ 20
Japan	121	0.7	128	+ 6
United Kingdom	56	0.2	59	+ 5
West Germany	61	−0.2	52	− 15
Rapid Growth Countries				
Kenya	20	4.2	111	+455
Nigeria	105	3.0	532	+406
Ethiopia	42	2.1	204	+386
Iran	47	2.9	166	+253
Pakistan	102	2.8	330	+223
Bangladesh	104	2.7	310	+198
Egypt	46	2.6	126	+174
Mexico	82	2.6	199	+143
Turkey	48	2.5	109	+127
Indonesia	168	2.1	368	+119
India	785	2.3	1,700	+116
Brazil	143	2.3	298	+108

Source: World Bank, *World Development Report 1985* (New York: Oxford University Press, 1985).

demographers fear that an increase in death rates may be as influential in curbing growth as a decrease in birth rates. Already there is evidence that in widely scattered areas of the underdeveloped world child mortality rates are rising due to increasing levels of malnutrition. There is a real danger that mounting human pressures on already over-taxed ecosystems may cause a collapse in the food-producing capabilities of many regions.

In its 1988 assessment of world population prospects, the United Nations revised upward its projections of future world population size at the turn of the century to 6.2 billion. This was necessary because an earlier projection of 6.1

Fig. 2-9

World Population Growth, 1950-2000

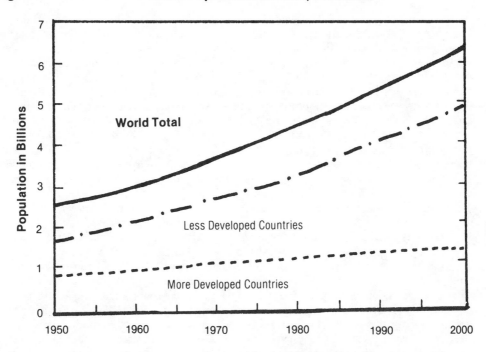

Source: United Nations, *World Population Prospects As Assessed in 1980,* Population Studies No. 78.

Box 2-7

U.S. Prospects For ZPG: The Impact of Immigration

Give me your tired, your poor
Your huddled masses, yearning to breathe free,
The wretched refuse of your teeming shore,
Send these, the homeless, tempest-tossed to me:
I lift my lamp beside the golden door.

The inspirational words of Emma Lazarus inscribed on the Statue of Liberty have greeted successive waves of immigrants to American shores and extend a national welcome to newcomers from a country which has long been proud of its "melting pot" tradition. In an age when many governments allow few, if any, permanent immigrants to settle within their borders, the U.S. has admitted approximately 600,000 legal immigrants and refugees annually for the past decade—and estimates that close to half a million illegal aliens have entered each year as well. This number exceeds the total of immigrants accepted annually by all other nations combined and comes close to equalling the number of new arrivals in 1907 and 1914, the peak years of immigration to the U.S., when over 1.2 million newcomers streamed through the "Golden Door".

Although we are truly a "nation of immigrants", Americans historically have exhibited an ambivalent attitude toward immigration policy. We have congratulated ourselves for providing a place of refuge and an opportunity for a "fresh start" for millions of hopeful newcomers and have rightly stressed the many contributions to American life made by the diverse peoples who have settled here. At the same time we question the nation's ability to continue absorbing additional millions, worrying whether the influx will exacerbate existing social and economic problems.

In the past, controversy over immigration policy focused primarily on ethnic quotas (until 1965, the system heavily favored immigrants of northwestern European origin and almost totally excluded Asians) and on concerns that hard-working new arrivals would drive down wages, take away jobs that might otherwise go to citizens, or, conversely, that unskilled immigrants would go on welfare and become a burden to taxpayers. More recently, however, a new element has been added to the policy debate pertaining to immigration law reform. Immigration's impact on American population growth is now being recognized as the single most important variable in our country's demographic future—the factor which will largely determine the ultimate population size of this country and the date at which population stabilization occurs.

Changes in population size occur only through fluctuations in the ratio between birth and death rates or as a result of changes in net migration (the difference between emigration and immigration). In the vast majority of countries today, immigration's impact on total population size is negligible. Such is not the case in the United States, however. While numbers of new arrivals rose significantly throughout the 1980s, American fertility rates have remained stable at below-replacement levels (1.8 births per woman) for the past 2 decades. Consequently, immigration is now having a disproportionate impact on U.S. population growth, accounting for approximately one-third of the total increase each year. Assuming a continuation of current child-bearing trends, by the 2030s natural increase in the U.S. will come to a halt and the level of net immigration will determine the total amount of population growth each year thereafter.

Policymakers wrestling with immigration reform proposals would do well to note demographers' projections of future U.S. population size, depending on legally-sanctioned levels of annual immigration. Current figures indicate that if net migration is held constant at 500,000 each year, U.S. population size will increase to 295 million by 2040, then begin a slow decline to 277 million by 2080 as the fertility of immigrants gradually falls to approximate that of native-born women. However, if a more liberal immigration policy prevails, allowing annual net migration of 1 million (a number close to the present figure, if illegal immigrants are included), then by 2080 American population size will reach 340 million and continue to climb.

Although the nation has yet to adopt a national population policy, as long ago as 1972 the President's Commission on Population Growth and the American Future concluded: "*Recognizing that our population cannot grow indefinitely and appreciating the advantages of moving now towards the stabilization of population, the Commission recommends that the nation welcome and plan for a stabilized population.*" Do Americans agree with the President's Commission that at some time, preferably sooner rather than later, zero population growth is desirable? If so, policymakers must seriously consider lowering the ceiling on annual immigration, taking U.S. fertility trends into account, in order to attain the agreed-upon goal.[11]

billion assumed a larger fertility decline in China and India during the 1980s than actually occurred. Thus even a modest slowdown in reducing birthrates in these two demographic giants can have a major impact on overall world population figures.

While most long-range projections show global population growth halting around the year 2100, the ability of natural ecosystems to support a substantial rise in human numbers for another century or so has been questioned. Since most of the expected increase will occur in the poorest countries which already are finding it difficult to support their current millions, many observers insist that population growth needs to be stabilized long before it reaches the theoretical levels projected by the U.N.

Reflecting the sentiments of a growing number of his colleagues throughout the developing world, a Kenyan official recently remarked:

"If more and more people keep pouring into a country that can only deliver so much, you can expect political unrest, serious shortage of food and everything else that people need to live, and in general, chaos."

REFERENCES

[1] Odum, Eugene P., *Fundamentals of Ecology,* W.B. Saunders Company, 1959.

[2] Farb, Peter, *Ecology,* Life Nature Library, Time Inc., 1963.

[3] Odum, op. cit.

[4] Ehrlich, Paul R., Anne H. Ehrlich, and John P. Holdren, *Ecoscience: Population, Resources, Environment,* W.H. Freeman and Company, 1977.

[5] "Population Update", *Population Today,* Population Reference Bureau, vol. 16, no. 12, December 1988.

[6] Herring, Hubert, *A History of Latin America,* Alfred A. Knopf, 1960.

[7] van de Kaa, Dirk J., "Europe's Second Demographic Transition", *Population Bulletin,* vol. 42 no. 1, March 1987.

[8] Haymaker, John, "Nigerian Government Seeks Public Support for Population Policy", *POPLINE,* World Population News Service, vol. 10, February 1988.

[9] Council on Environmental Quality and the Department of State, *The Global 2000 Report to the President of the U.S.: Entering the 21st Century,* Pergamon Press, Inc., 1980.

[10] Ibid.

[11] Bouvier, Leon F. and Robert W. Gardner, "Immigration to the U.S.: The Unfinished Story", *Population Bulletin,* vol. 41, no. 4, November 1986.

3
Population
Control

"We need to make a world in which fewer children are born, and in which we take better care of them."
—Dr. George Wald

Studies of population dynamics clearly indicate that no population can sustain limitless growth, raising the as-yet unanswered question of what will eventually bring a halt to still-climbing human numbers? Basically, one of two factors could effect a drop in growth rates: a *decrease* in birth rates or an *increase* in death rates. Either change would result in a narrowing of the gap between births and deaths which has been responsible for the unprecedented growth in human population witnessed during the past century. A decrease in the death rate caused the population explosion and a number of demographic experts gloomily predict that a reversal of this trend in the future will bring a halt to further growth. They point to an observable rise in infant mortality rates due to the increasing frequency of malnutrition; to the possibility of global pandemics as population densities increase; and to the growing likelihood of military confrontations as nations compete for dwindling resources.

However, no rational individual would advocate starvation, epidemics, or war as a means of ending the population explosion. The humane approach to a very real problem lies instead in attempts to reduce growth by lowering birth rates to the point at which they will be in approximate equilibrium with death rates, thereby achieving a stabilization of population size, popularly referred to as ZPG ("zero population growth").

73

Early Attempts at Family Limitation

Although most traditional cultures have consistently encouraged prolific child-bearing, records indicate that during stressful periods of famine, war, or civil upheaval many couples throughout history have attempted in various ways to prevent unwanted births. While some of the methods employed were based on nothing more than superstition, others were moderately effective and continue to be used today.

One of the oldest documented means of contraception, referred to in the Old Testament story of Onan (Genesis 38:9), is that of withdrawal (coitus interruptus), whereby the man withdraws his penis from the vagina prior to ejaculation. Since a keen sense of timing is essential to the success of this method, withdrawal has the highest failure rate of any major method of birth control, but it does have the advantage of requiring no drugs or devices nor access to medical personnel for its use—and it costs nothing. Where couples are highly motivated not to have children, it can be fairly successful and, in fact, is believed to be the method by which European couples substantially reduced birthrates in that part of the world during the early years of the demographic transition. Even now, in such countries as Yugoslavia, Bulgaria, Czechoslovakia, Turkey, Spain, and Italy, withdrawal remains the most popular method of contraception.[1]

Crude barriers to the cervix, similar in concept to the modern diaphragm or cervical cap, were used by women in ancient Egypt who fashioned such devices out of leaves, cloth, wads of cotton fibers, or even crocodile dung![2]

Herbal concoctions were used for contraceptive purposes in many societies and although it long was fashionable among researchers to dismiss such brews as totally useless, recently it has been found that some of the plants used are, in fact, remarkably effective in preventing pregnancy. A group of researchers at the College of Pharmacy of the University of Illinois has done a literature search of botanical and anthropological references and has confirmed claims of fertility control for more than 4000 plant species, 370 of which have been identified by computer analysis as being particularly promising for development of contraceptive substances. Attracting the greatest interest is a Mexican shrub called zoapatle, a member of the sunflower family, whose reputation in folklore as an effective birth control agent has been scientifically confirmed in laboratory tests on both animals and humans. Ortho Pharmaceuticals has already taken out patents on prostaglandin-like molecules isolated from zoapatle, hoping to develop a successful "morning-after pill" from the plant extract. Another candidate, the motherwort plant, a native of China, has been used as a contraceptive for over 2000 years and is now undergoing scrutiny by the World Health Organization.[3]

The use of condoms dates back at least to the 16th century when the use of fine linen sheaths to be worn on the penis during intercourse were recommended as a means of preventing the spread of venereal disease. By the 17th century condoms made of lamb intestines were introduced for the express purpose of preventing conception and by the 18th century were reportedly available for use by patrons at all the finer houses of prostitution in Europe. With the advent of vulcanized rubber by the mid-1800s, a truly effective male contraceptive became available for the masses, though rubber condoms were not widely used until World War I when they were distributed among the troops as protection against venereal disease.[4]

Other birth-control practices with a similarly long history include douching (flushing out the vagina with a water solution immediately after intercourse), almost totally ineffective in spite of its popularity, and breast-feeding of infants—quite an effective means of suppressing the onset of ovulation following childbirth and thereby helpful in spacing pregnancies.

When attempts such as the above failed, as they frequently did, women commonly resorted to abortion, a very ancient practice believed to have been the most prevalent method of family limitation throughout history.

As a last resort, unwanted children in past centuries frequently fell victim to infanticide—the deliberate killing of babies, particularly girl babies, immediately after birth. This practice was quite common in ancient Greece and in several Asian countries up until fairly recent times, especially during periods of famine.

Modern Family Planning Movement

The origins of the modern family planning movement in the U.S. can be traced to the publication in 1832 of a contraceptive textbook, "Fruits of Philosophy", written by Dr. Charles Knowlton who won renown as the first person in this country to be jailed for advocating birth control. The development of the diaphragm in the 1840s further stimulated public interest in contraceptive techniques and although proponents of birth control were viciously persecuted by so-called "societies for the suppression of vice", the resultant notoriety only enhanced sales of birth control literature. Open discussion of sex or reproductive matters was still taboo during those years of Victorian morality, however, and an "establishment" back-lash against the growing birth control movement was reflected in the passage in 1873 of the Comstock Law, a federal mandate which prohibited sending birth control information or devices through the mail, such items being defined as "obscene".

Toward the end of the 19th century, the burgeoning feminist movement lent support to the concept of family planning, stressing the health burdens imposed on women by too many children born too close together. An outstanding pioneer of family planning in America was Margaret Sanger, a nurse in New York City who was appalled by the extent of poverty and death due to over-large families and abortions among the people with whom she worked. Recognizing that the Comstock Law prevented such people from obtaining the contraceptive information they so badly needed, she launched a personal crusade to overturn that legislation. In 1914 she founded the National Birth

Box 3–1

Abortion

Regarded as the most widely practiced method of family limitation throughout history, abortion remains today a method of last resort when contraceptives are unavailable, unused, or fail. On a worldwide basis, rough estimates suggest there are between 40-60 million abortions annually. In the U.S., the number of legal abortions each year has remained relatively stable at 1.6 million since the mid-1980s; added to these, Planned Parenthood reports an additional 20,000 illegal abortions per year. The subject of intense current controversy, abortion was not always legally prohibited. Among ancient Greeks and Romans no social or criminal stigma was attached to abortion; during the early Christian era abortion was viewed as murder only after the soul became "animated"—a time established as 40 days after conception for males and 80 days for females. Under English common law, which prevailed in the U.S. as well as in England, life was regarded as beginning with "quickening," or the first perception of fetal movement by the mother, generally occurring around the beginning of the 5th month. Prior to that time, no penalties accrued to abortion; even after quickening, abortion was not regarded as serious a crime as murder.

For the first quarter of the 19th century in the U.S., no federal or state laws addressed the issue of abortion. This situation gradually changed as the century progressed; physicians lobbied vigorously to outlaw abortion, motivated in part by a desire to put "quack" doctors out of business, by a belief that abortion was morally wrong, and by opposition to new social roles for women. By 1900 abortions were illegal everywhere in the U.S., a situation which prevailed until the 1960s when public attitudes toward abortion began to liberalize. Concerns about the "quality of life," as opposed to mere biological existence were voiced, as was the view that anti-abortion statutes discriminated against poor women, since the wealthy could, and did, travel abroad to obtain a desired abortion. At the recommendation of the American Law Institute, about one-third of the states by the late 1960s had amended their statutes to permit abortion in cases where 1) continuation of pregnancy would endanger the physical or mental health of the mother, 2) when the child might be born severely deformed or mentally retarded, or 3) when rape or incest resulted in pregnancy or when an unmarried girl under 16 became pregnant. By 1970 the states of Alaska, Hawaii, New York, and Washington had completely legalized first-trimester abortions.

In 1973 the U.S. Supreme Court invalidated all remaining state anti-abortion laws when, in the historic Roe vs. Wade decision, it ruled that states cannot place any restrictions on abortions during the first trimester other than to require that the procedure be performed by a physician. During the second trimester the state can regulate abortion only in ways to protect maternal health; only during the last trimester, said the Court, may the state prohibit abortion unless the life of the mother is in danger.[5]

Today Americans are among the 76% of the world's people who live in countries where induced abortion is legal. In such nations, where an abortion can be performed early in pregnancy by trained medical personnel, abortion is 11X less dangerous for the mother than is carrying a baby full-term (less than one woman in 100,000 in the U.S. dies of legal abortion, while 8 out of every 100,000 die from complications of pregnancy or childbirth). However, in societies where abortion is illegal or difficult to obtain due to cost or lack of facilities, many women resort to unskilled practitioners or try to self-abort. In such cases, lack of hygienic conditions and inexpert techniques entail a high risk of complications or even death. In fact, Planned Parenthood estimates the risk of death from illegal abortion as 30X higher than that of a legal abortion. While accurate figures on such a delicate subject are difficult to obtain, the World Health Organization estimates that approximately 200,000 women worldwide die of illegal abortions each year, most of them in Third World countries where access to legal abortion is still largely unavailable. In some Latin American nations, a large proportion of all maternal deaths result from botched illegal abortions, and complications due to such back-alley procedures are responsible for approximately half of all admissions to hospital obstetric units in that part of the world. The most clear-cut demonstration of the impact which abortion's legal status has on maternal health can be seen in the East European nation of Romania. After a restrictive abortion law was imposed in 1966 as a result of official concerns about a declining national birth rate, maternal deaths due to abortion jumped seven-fold. Quite obviously, prohibitions against abortion don't end the practice—they simply make it much more dangerous.[6]

From the perspective of slowing population growth, the legalization of abortion in itself does not greatly reduce birth rates because most legal abortions simply replace illegal operations. However, as a means of enhancing maternal health, access to legal abortion is an important part of a national health care program.

Control League and began publishing a monthly magazine, "The Woman Rebel", containing birth control information—which the Post Office therefore refused to distribute. The following year she circulated a more comprehensive birth control pamphlet, "Family Limitation", which also violated the Comstock Law. Sanger was indicted for this action, but the indictment was subsequently dropped. In 1916 Mrs. Sanger opened the first birth control clinic in America, in a section of Brooklyn, N.Y. For this offense she was arrested and served 30 days in prison, but the resulting public outcry led to a gradual easing of legal restrictions against the family planning movement. Mrs. Sanger traveled extensively throughout the country, seeking to persuade both the medical

Fig. 3–1

Abortion Incidence In Selected Countries

Country	Abortions/1000 women aged 15-44	% of all pregnancies ending in abortion
USSR	181	68
Romania	91	57
Yugoslavia	71	49
Bulgaria	62	48
China	62	43
Cuba	59	46
U.S.	27	29
Japan	22*	27
Italy	19	28
Sweden	18	25
Norway	16	22
England & Wales	13	17
Canada	13	14
Netherlands	6	10

*official government data; independent analysts suggest correct figure is much higher

Source: Henshaw, Stanley K., "Induced Abortion: A Worldwide Perspective", FAMILY PLANNING PERSPECTIVES, vol. 18, no. 6, Nov./Dec. 1986.

profession and the public at large of the importance of facilitating access to birth control. By 1932 the Birth Control League had established 80 clinics throughout the U.S.; in 1937 the American Medical Association officially endorsed birth control; and, finally, by 1938 two major court cases resulted in the overthrow of the Comstock Law and, in effect, made it possible for doctors to prescribe contraceptives to patients (except in Connecticut and Massachusetts where contraceptives remained illegal under state law until the 1960s).[7] In 1942 the National Birth Control League and the clinics became Planned Parenthood Federation, with Margaret Sanger as honorary chairman.

Birth Control—Its Health Impact

Over the years the services offered by Planned Parenthood have expanded to include pre-marital counseling and fertility assistance in addition to the original intent of providing birth control help to married women. However, the basic rationale of all family planning work in the U.S.—today as in 1916 when the first clinic opened its doors—is to promote the health and well-being of mothers and children by preventing unwanted births. Because of the threat which uncontrolled fertility poses, both to maternal health and to that of infants, it is generally accepted today that no community health program can be considered complete if it fails to provide ready access to birth control devices and information to all who desire them.

Enhancement of maternal and child health through family planning is largely related to one of three basic parameters: 1) age of the mother; 2) interval between births; and 3) total number of births during a woman's reproductive lifetime. A brief examination of each of these factors reveals how uncontrolled fertility has a major impact on mortality and morbidity rates among both women and infants involved.

Age of mother

Although the average woman is fertile from her early teens until her late 40s, the biologically optimum period for childbearing is much shorter, extending from approximately 20 years of age to age 30. From a safety standpoint, mothers either younger or older than this optimum group run an increased risk of difficulties or death during pregnancy and childbirth and their infants are statistically more likely to die than are babies of mothers in their twenties.

Teen-age mothers, whose reproductive organs are not yet fully developed, are more likely to die during childbirth than are women in their prime reproductive years. In addition, babies of young mothers have a tendency to be born premature or underweight, factors which greatly increase their susceptibility to infectious diseases and malnutrition. Studies have revealed consistently higher infant mortality rates among babies born to mothers under age 20 as compared to those born to mothers in their late twenties.

Among women over 35, pregnancy poses increasing risk of complications during childbirth; after age 45, statistics show a significant rise in maternal

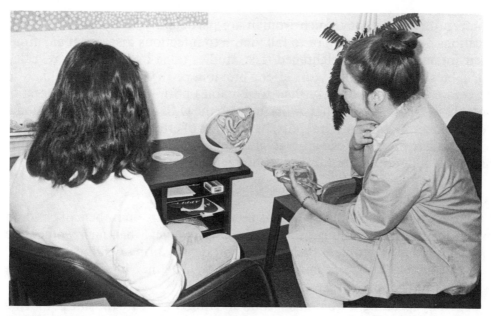

Family planning clinics provide a wide range of services to women seeking fertility or contraceptive assistance. Here a Planned Parenthood staff worker explains basic facts about the female reproductive system to a teenage client. [*Author's Photo*]

death rates. Mothers over 35 are more likely than younger women to bear a child with congenital disorders such as Down's Syndrome; recent research also indicates that the babies of women in this age group are twice as likely to be born underweight (less than 5.5 pounds) and that, in general, the older a woman is, the greater the potential for reduced fetal growth. Since there is a direct correlation between low birthweight and death during infancy, it is not surprising that these studies found that babies born to mothers aged 40 or older are at much higher risk of dying before their first birthday than are infants born to women in their 20s and 30s.[8]

Interval between births

Since a developing fetus draws on its mother's nutritional reserves, it should not be surprising that when the interval between successive pregnancies is short, time is insufficient for adequate replenishment of these reserves and serious health problems can be manifested in both woman and infant. Such effects are particularly noticeable among poorly-nourished individuals. While pregnant, a moderately active woman needs about 300 more calories per day than usual; if she is unable to secure this extra amount, her body draws upon its own reserves, with resulting harm both to herself and to her baby. A condition called "maternal depletion syndrome", characterized by premature aging, weakness, and anemia is frequently observed among undernourished women in poor societies, where teen-age marriage is typically followed by about 20 years of uninterrupted pregnancy. Such women are particularly likely to die of complications during childbirth or to fall victim to infectious diseases at any time. Their infants, too, face heightened risk. Studies done in rural India revealed that babies born less than 2 years after a previous birth were 50% more likely to die before their first birthday than were babies born after a birth interval of more than 2 years. Researchers working with the U.S. Agency for International Development in Bangladesh report that success of efforts to encourage women to space their pregnancies had a greater impact on reducing infant mortality than did childhood immunization campaigns or oral rehydration therapy.

Total number of births

Contrary to the popular notion that mothers with large numbers of children give birth "as easy as rolling off a log", statistics reveal that such women are especially prone to problem pregnancies and death during childbirth. Indeed, the total number of babies born to a woman during her lifetime can have a significant impact on her general state of health.

Generally speaking, a woman's second and third births are the safest; the first birth carries slightly greater risk statistically because it will reveal any physical or genetic abnormalities in the parents which could cause problems. With the fourth pregnancy, risk of maternal death, stillbirth, and infant death begins to rise, increasing sharply with the birth of the fifth and every succeeding child. Health workers in Bangladesh report triple the number of deaths among women giving birth to their eighth child as among those bearing their third. Degree of risk depends to a considerable extent on the socioeconomic status of the mother, the greatest hazards being faced by women from the lowest income groups. However, even among well-fed, affluent women, every birth after the fourth involves an increased degree of danger for both mother and child.

Significantly higher rates of infant and child mortality among higher-order births in poor families seem to be due primarily to poor nutrition, as the limited amount of food available must be divided among many mouths. Unlike their older siblings, the latest-born children must survive on reduced average portions during those early years when they are most susceptible to the effects of nutritional deficiency.[9]

Thus a family-planning program which provides contraceptive protection for teen-age women, women over 35, mothers who have already borne 3 or more children, and for women who have recently given birth can make a very positive contribution to improving public health.

Contraceptive Safety

In assessing the health impact of family planning, one must of course take into account possible risks posed by contraceptive use. There has been considerable controversy in recent years regarding the safety of the birth control pill and the intra-uterine device (IUD), raising public concerns and causing potential contraceptors to turn to less reliable methods or to abandon attempts at birth control altogether. What indeed are the risks vs. benefits of the most commonly used contraceptives? A brief summary of the most popular methods used in the U.S. indicates that although various adverse side effects may accompany the use of contraceptives for some women, all common means of contraception entail fewer risks than do pregnancy and childbirth.

Sterilization—In the United States today, the most widely-utilized method of family limitation is sterilization, relied upon by over one-third of all sexually active women and by more than half of all married couples, particularly by those who have already attained their desired family size. By far the safest method of birth control known, male sterilization, or vasectomy (a simple operation involving an incision in the scrotum to cut or block the vas deferens, tubes which carry semen from the testes to the penis), accounts for slightly under half of the sterilizations performed in this country each year. In the developed nations no problems with vasectomy have been reported, but in a few countries such as India a small number of deaths have occurred due to post-operative infections which developed as a result of inadequate medical facilities. Female tubal sterilizations also have a good safety record; in developed countries among women over 40, less than 0.03% die in undergoing a tubal sterilization, as compared to 0.12% of those who become pregnant. In underdeveloped nations the risks are slightly higher due to less adequate medical care, but the dangers of childbearing are also many times greater.

Oral Contraceptives—The second most popular method of birth control in the U.S., "The Pill" is used by approximately 32% of all women at risk of pregnancy. Long-term effects of prolonged pill use are still not known with certainty, since the pill was commercialized only in the early 1960s. Most concerns in recent years, however, have centered around the increased risk of such cardiovascular disorders as blood clots and heart attack due to pill use. Nevertheless, medical evidence supports the view that the pill is quite safe for younger women, with the exception of those who smoke or have a medical history of high blood pressure, high blood cholesterol, or diabetes; such women are advised to use methods other than the pill. Women over 40 are the only group for whom pill use poses a greater health threat than does childbearing; among this group increase in cardiovascular problems suggests the advisability of discontinuing pill use in favor of other contraceptive techniques. Interestingly, some doctors have suggested that oral contraceptives may be safer for women in poor countries than for those in more affluent societies because the former group has a much lower incidence of cardiovascular disease due to differences in diet and lifestyle. Within the past few years, medical researchers have found that oral contraceptives also confer some unanticipated health benefits to users: women who take the pill reduce their risk of both ovarian and endometrial cancer by at least 40%—an effect which persists for at least 15 years after pill use is discontinued.[10]

Intra-uterine device (IUD)—Once among the most popular forms of contraception in the U.S. and still widely relied upon by women in other countries (particularly in China where it is is the most common method of birth control), the IUD today is the method of choice for only 3% of contracepting American women. Indeed, by the mid-1980s, IUDs had nearly disappeared from the marketplace, withdrawn by manufacturers fearing legal liability for alleged harmful side effects of the device (a situation brought about by thousands of lawsuits against the A.H. Robins pharmaceutical firm, charging that the company's Dalkon Shield had caused numerous cases of bleeding, pelvic infections, and resultant infertility among users). Nevertheless, physicians and manufacturers consider most IUDs both safe and reliable and recently a new IUD, the Copper T 380 A, was introduced into the marketplace. Although among malnourished, anemic women IUD use has sometimes been correlated with increased blood loss during menstruation, for healthy, well-fed women IUDs are as safe as the pill and nearly as dependable. The major problem associated with IUD use is an increased risk of pelvic inflammatory disease (PID) which, if severe, can result in permanent infertility. IUDs are not recommended for women who have never been pregnant and in general are considered most suitable for young women who want no more children but are not yet ready for an irreversible surgical sterilization.

Fig. 3-2			
Preferred Contraceptive Methods by U.S. women aged 15-44 at risk of unwanted pregnancy			
Method	% Total	% Married	% Unmarried
All users	93	97	87
Sterilization	36	51	13
Female	22	28	12
Male	16	24	1
Pill	32	22	48
Condom	16	15	16
IUD	3	3	3
Diaphragm	4	4	4
Foam	1	3	1
Cream/jelly	*	*	*
Suppository	1	1	1
Sponge	3	1	4
Rhythm method	5	5	3
Withdrawal	5	5	6
Douche	1	1	1
Nonusers	7	3	13
*Less than 0.5%			
Source: 1987 Ortho Birth Control Study			

Box 3–2

Controversy Over the French Pill

The abortion controversy made front page news around the world for a few days in the fall of 1988 when the French pharmaceutical company Roussel-Uclaf announced that it was halting sales of its new fertility control drug, RU-486 (mifepristone) due to vehement protests by French and American Right-to-Life groups. Roussel-Uclaf's announcement provoked a storm of protest from French feminist groups, physicians, and family-planning organizations; two days later the government of France demanded that "out of concern for the public health and what this pill means for women" the company should resume sales. Roussel-Uclaf promptly complied with the government's wishes and French women today have access to what some observers consider the most important new class of contraceptive drugs to appear on the scene since introduction of "The Pill" in 1960.

Why the fuss over a birth control pill? Because RU-486, developed by a professor at the University of Paris, essentially acts as an abortifacient, blocking the action of progesterone, the hormone which prepares the lining of the uterus for implantation of the embryo. The embryo is then flushed from the uterus with the onset of menstruation, in effect terminating the pregnancy. Effective only through the 6th week of pregnancy, RU-486 is more reliable the earlier it is taken after conception. Researchers claim that RU-486 has an advantage over many other contraceptives in that it seems to have few side effects other than heavier-than-usual menstrual bleeding and possible cramps. However, because the drug sometimes results in incomplete abortions which can lead to dangerous infection, RU-486 should only be used under close medical supervision, a fact which some observers feel makes it unsuitable for use in Third World situations. Because it is impossible at present to know what the long-term effects of using RU-486 may be, the developer advises against using the contraceptive as a "once-a-month pill", recommending instead that it be utilized as a backup when conventional birth control methods fail.

Because RU-486 acts to prevent embryo implantation rather than to block conception, the same ethical concerns which surround the abortion issue surface in any discussion of RU-486. Pro-life forces fear that widespread availability of the French pill will make it possible for a woman desiring an abortion to induce fetal loss in the privacy of her own home without her doctor, friends, or abortion clinic protest marchers being any the wiser.

It is too early yet to say what the societal impact of RU-486 will be, but it appears safe to predict that American women will not have the opportunity for first-hand knowledge of the drug. Given the current political clout of the anti-abortion lobby in Washington and fears of legal liability on the part of pharmaceutical firms, there are no plans for introducing RU-486 onto the market in the U.S.

Vaginal Contraceptives—Diaphragms, cervical caps, suppositories, and sponges, used in conjunction with spermicidal creams, foams, or gels have few, if any, adverse physiological effects and are highly effective. While diaphragms and cervical caps must be fitted and require a prescription for purchase, the other types of vaginal contraceptives are available over the counter.

Condom—Like the vaginal contraceptives, condoms cause no adverse health effects other than an occasional allergic reaction to rubber among some individuals. Used alone, their reliability is significantly less than pills or IUDs, but in combination with vaginal contraceptives and in situations where legal, early abortion is available, they offer the safest means, other than sterilization, of totally effective fertility control.[11] The third most commonly used contraceptive method in the U.S. today, condoms are being actively promoted by health agencies not only for birth control reasons but also as an effective prophylactic against the spread of AIDS and other sexually transmitted diseases.

Natural Family Planning—Frequently referred to as the "rhythm method" or "periodic abstinence", this approach to birth control carries no health risk but has a consistently high failure rate. To utilize this method, a woman attempts to determine when she is ovulating by daily charting bodily functions such as basal temperature (i.e. temperature when the body is at its lowest level of metabolic activity, usually measured before getting out of bed in the morning) and by examining her cervical mucus. The problem is that many women experience monthly variations in their menstrual cycle, making accurate calculation of the fertile period problematic. In addition, the abstinence from sexual activity during fertile periods which must be rigorously observed by couples using natural family planning requires a high degree of motivation and cooperation between partners and can significantly limit the number of days each month when couples can have intercourse free from fear of unwanted pregnancy.

The success of the family planning movement in the U.S. is evident from surveys which reveal that among sexually active women at risk of an unwanted pregnancy, fully 93% are using some method of birth control. Among married women the figure is even higher—97%. In an age when sexual activity seems to be as popular a pastime as it ever was, an even more convincing indicator of contraceptive usage is the fact that the average number of children per U.S. couple is now 1.8, one of the lowest figures in our history. Apparently most Americans now agree with the family planning sloganeers who affirm that "A Small Family is a Happy Family".[12]

Box 3–3

Narrowing Options?

The perfect contraceptive—one which is 100% effective, safe, cheap, easy to use, reversible, and available without a prescription—is unlikely ever to be found, but until recently it was widely assumed that a host of new drugs and devices designed to meet the varying birth control needs of the world's women would soon become available. In the years after the pill ushered in the "Contraceptive Revolution", research and development of new birth control technologies was aggressively pursued by the pharmaceutical industry and by government-subsidized non-profit institutions. Due to shortcomings of existing methods, either in regard to side-effects, aesthetic concerns, inconvenience of use, etc., the need for a wider selection of improved contraceptives was universally acknowledged. Particularly urgent was the perceived demand for long-acting, inexpensive products appropriate for use in Third World settings where users were likely to be poor, uneducated, and living far from a regular source of supply. Even in developed countries, where birth control technologies today are indisputably better than they were just a few decades ago, the high rate of teenage pregnancies and the number of women using less reliable methods of contraception due to fears (often unfounded) about alleged side effects of the pill or IUD, confirm the need for an expanding array of birth control options to meet a broader range of needs.

Unfortunately, since the mid-1980s, hope for rapid breakthroughs in contraceptive development has dimmed and, in the U.S. at least, the range of choice is becoming narrower rather than wider. Most IUDs have been taken off the market by manufacturers worried about lawsuits and there are fears that spermicidal foams and gels are facing a similar threat. At the same time, the tempo of contraceptive research and development has markedly slowed throughout the industrialized world. Not that progress has halted altogether—several widely-hailed and initially promising new products are already in use in certain countries or are in an advanced developmental stage.

Most promising among the new generation of contraceptives are the hormonal implants and injectables. Like the birth control pill, these steroidal substances have a very low failure rate; unlike the pill, their effectiveness is long term and not dependent on the user's motivation to take them on a daily basis. NORPLANT, one of the best reversible contraceptives yet developed, consists of several 3 cm-long permeable rods containing a timed-release dose of progestin. These are surgically inserted under the skin of the upper arm and provide a high level of protection against pregnancy for 5 years. If the user should decide she wants to have a child, the rods can easily be removed and fertility quickly restored. NORPLANT has a safety advantage over the pill in that no estrogen component is present; thus the cardiovascular risk inherent to some extent with pill use is not a concern. NORPLANT is now being marketed in Finland and Sweden and may be introduced into several developing nations in the near future.

Depo-Provera, a steroid injectable, has been in use for more than a decade elsewhere in the world, approved for use in about 90 countries (but not in the U.S. where a conservative FDA has refused to give it the green light, in spite of endorsement by the World Health Organization, International Planned Parenthood Federation, and the medical safety agencies of more than 3 dozen governments). An injection of Depo-Provera prevents conception over a 3-month period; other injectable hormones now being used in Latin America and China provide one-month protection. In addition to NORPLANT and Depo-Provera, several biodegradable implants which don't require surgical removal and injectables which have fewer side effects and seem even more effective are now in the preliminary testing stage.

Efforts have been underway for more than a decade to develop a reversible male contraceptive which lowers sperm counts without reducing male sex drive. Considerable attention has been focused on gossypol, a cottonseed oil derivative, already tried on a limited basis in China but still far from market introduction elsewhere. Other long-awaited breakthroughs such as an anti-pregnancy vaccine or a female chemosterilant appear similarly unlikely anytime in the near future. The only radically new entry to the marketplace, RU-486, which acts essentially as an abortifacient, is highly unlikely to be approved for use in the U.S. unless the existing political climate changes drastically (see Box 3–2).

Why the gloomy outlook for potential new drugs which were once expected to usher in a second contraceptive revolution? Why are American couples in the 1990s likely to enjoy fewer birth control options than their counterparts in many other countries—indeed, perhaps fewer options than were available here in the 1980s? A number of factors can be cited to explain why the contraceptive boom has gone bust. Lack of funding has brought clinical research to a near-standstill. Neither governments nor private industry are supporting research at the level needed to achieve major new advances; at best, available funds are directed at modifications of existing methods. A slackening research effort by governments is to some extent a result of lessening concerns about population growth in the developed countries; thanks to falling birth rates and low infant and maternal mortality rates, developed nations' sense of alarm about a "population explosion" which motivated contraceptive research funding in the early 1970s is today lacking. Private industry, on the other hand, is less enthusiastic than formerly about pursuing contraceptive R & D efforts for various reasons of its own: the massive investment in time and money needed to carry out the rigorous safety testing demanded by FDA before a new drug can be approved for use; the modest profits to be made from the long-term, low-cost contraceptives needed by Third World women; the abortion controversy which has implications in the form of protests and threats of boycotts against pharmaceutical firms working on post-fertilization contraceptive methods such as vaccines or anti-implantation drugs; and, finally, fear of legal liability for potential user injury and the related near-impossibility of obtaining insurance for testing new birth control methods on human subjects.

Although a number of promising contraceptive technologies dance tantalizingly on the distant horizon, unless major changes occur in government funding decisions, FDA regulatory actions, and liability laws, these possibilities are unlikely to become reality. Without the removal of such barriers, it is entirely possible that the range of choice in tomorrow's contraceptive marketplace will be narrower than it is today.[13]

Family Planning in the Third World

Whereas the birth control movement in the United States and Europe grew out of the conviction that health and social considerations demanded that women receive help in regulating their fertility, the impetus for family planning in most Third World countries grew directly out of concerns regarding the very high rates of population growth experienced by such nations in the years following World War II and awareness that the "population explosion" which they were experiencing would impede their rate of economic development. Only after family planning programs had been launched did Third World governments attempt to justify their support for such efforts on the basis of protecting maternal and child health and of guaranteeing couples the means for regulating the spacing and number of their children. This superficial shift in emphasis constituted a publicly acceptable rationale for reconciling the interests of the nation with those of individuals.

In most cases, the initial promoters of family planning in the Third World were private organizations such as International Planned Parenthood Federation, the Ford and Rockefeller Foundations, and the Population Council; by 1989 there were Planned Parenthood affiliates in 125 countries. By the 1960s, however, even earlier in some countries, national governments were becoming increasingly active in establishing their own family planning programs, usually in conjunction with their ministries of health. Generally they were assisted by the private organizations mentioned above and, in later years, by the United States' Agency for International Development and various United Nations' agencies such as the World Bank and the United Nations Fund for Population·Activities (UNFPA). Funds, both governmental and private, allocated for family planning work increased sharply after the mid-1960s, but even today constitute a very small percentage of most national budgets. Today the vast majority of developing countries have some sort of family planning program in operation. How effective those programs are in achieving their goal of reducing national birthrates will in large part determine the success of such countries in raising living standards and ensuring a bright future for their people.

Spreading the Word

Since the main impetus for implementing family planning came from central governments or outside agencies rather than reflecting grassroots interest, as was the case in North America and Europe, success required intensive efforts to reach all elements of society, the majority of whom live at subsistence level in rural areas, often isolated from adequate medical care and frequently illiterate. Such people had to be made aware of the existence of fertility-regulating methods, provided with regular access to the same, and convinced that it was in their own best interest to use them.

In pursuing this goal, family planning workers in Third World countries have adopted methods radically different from those used in Western nations. Mobile units in the form of specially equipped vans or buses have been essential in carrying health workers and equipment into villages far from any hospital. Trained field workers actively attempt to recruit contraceptive acceptors,

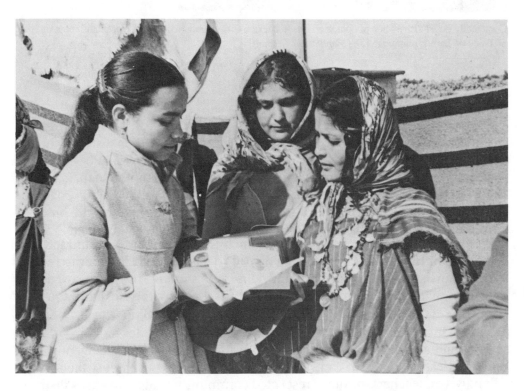

Female rural motivator in Tunisia encourages women to use family planning methods and makes follow-up visits to acceptors. [*The Population Council*]

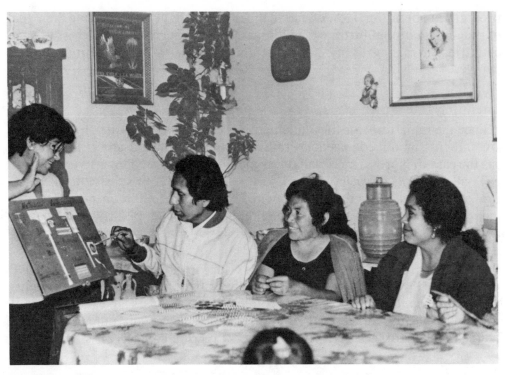

Community-based distribution of contraceptives in Mexico City—an outreach worker explains about different methods of family planning. [*The Population Council*]

meeting with women's groups, farmers, etc., to persuade their listeners of the advantages inherent in limiting family size. Considerable reliance has been placed on mass media communications; advertisements in newspapers, radio, and in cinemas regularly stress the benefits of small families while roadside billboards or posters on buses, in train stations—even painted on the hides of farm animals—proclaim such messages as "Two or Three—Enough!" Some governments have attracted participation by offering gifts to contraceptive acceptors. In India thousands of men agreed to vasectomies in order to receive a free transistor radio; in Thailand, the government has sponsored free distribution of condoms at sporting events or all-expense paid tours of Bangkok's temples for rural men agreeing to sterilization!

Most Third World programs, like those in the West, offer a choice of birth control methods and generally include information on child-spacing, nutrition, and child-care along with contraceptive services. Some also enlist the services of midwives, teachers, or other respected community leaders to act as distributors of contraceptives, particularly pills and condoms, thereby giving these influential individuals a vested interest in the success of such programs.

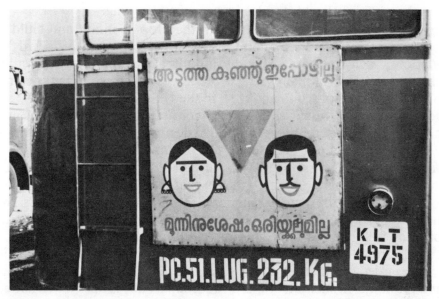

In many developing nations, prominent billboards and posters proclaim the virtues of family planning. This advertisement on the back of a bus in Kerala, a state of southern India, advises "Next baby not now; after three, not ever!" [*Author's Photo*]

Motivation—The Key to Success

Success in achieving a significant reduction in birth rates in the developing nations has been somewhat mixed. The recently conducted World Fertility Survey revealed that fertility has been declining in all major regions of the world except Africa, but that none of the Third World countries has yet achieved a birth rate under 20, the average for developed nations. The survey made it clear that the vast majority of women in such countries knew of the existence of at least one modern method of contraception, yet only 32% of such women, or their husbands, were using some form of birth control (as compared to 72% in developed countries).[14] To some extent, failure to use contraceptives is related to easy access; not surprisingly, contraceptive use was higher in communities where a family planning clinic or other source of contraceptive supplies was close by—a particularly important factor among people using either pills or condoms. A far more important determinant in contraceptive practice, however, is *motivation*—the desire of couples to limit family size. In many parts of the developing world economic and social factors interact to perpetuate the traditional attitudes toward child-bearing. For very practical reasons, many Third World couples have concluded that although 2 or 3 children per family might be in the best interest of society, they want and feel they need a significantly larger number themselves. In the absence of coercion, when individual and societal needs conflict, personal desires generally prevail.

Some of the facts of life accounting for this continued large-family preference among many Third World couples include the following.

High infant mortality rates—Although the drop in infant and child death rates was a major factor in fueling the explosive growth of Third World populations, such rates are still substantially above the levels prevailing in developed countries. In many parts of Africa, for example, infant death rates are over 100, as compared to about 10 in the U.S. The World Fertility Survey found that at the individual level, fertility consistently increased as the number of child deaths increased. Where childhood deaths are common, it is difficult to convince parents to limit themselves to 2 births.

Children as "social security"—In most Third World countries, lack of extensive social welfare programs means that most parents are dependent on their grown children for financial support in their post-retirement years. In such cultures, responsibility for elderly parents falls primarily on the sons; thus a couple may feel the need to produce at least 2 or 3 boys to ensure their being adequately provided for in old age. In addition, even during childhood, children may be regarded as financial assets, since their labor is needed on the farm or around the home. In such situations an additional baby is not viewed as another mouth to feed but rather as an additional pair of hands to gather wood, tend livestock, haul water, etc.

Desire for sons—Many family planning program administrators fear that the preference of many couples for sons rather than daughters will keep fertility rates high in many developing countries. Son preference is apparent in surveys of American couples, but is even more pronounced among parents in most Third World nations. In such cultures, doubt about whether they will have enough boys concerns parents who are asked to produce no more than 2 or 3 offspring. In such cultures, a woman's status, even the stability of her marriage, is dependent on her having sons. To some extent, such preferences are based on economic concerns: sons can support parents in old age, while daughters are a financial liability, often requiring an expensive dowry at time of marriage; in some societies daughters are considered expensive luxuries. Wherever such views are strongly held it is unlikely that couples will voluntarily limit their families to 2 children if the first two happen to be daughters. If a couple desires 2 or 3 boys, it is quite likely that they will ultimately have 4-6 children, since the male-female sex ratio at birth is almost equal.[15] The bias in favor of sons has taken a tragic twist in recent years, with a noticeable rise in female infanticide in several countries. After promulgation of the one-child policy in China (Box 3-4), numerous cases were reported of newborn girls being murdered by parents who hoped that perhaps a second try would produce a son. In a land where a preference for male children is traditional, some couples evidently decided that if they could only have one child, it had better be a boy. To its credit, the Chinese government has made vigorous efforts to prosecute such crimes and the incidence of these atrocities appears to have declined sharply in the past few years. In urban India, the overwhelming preference for sons is being expressed in another equally alarming manner. To a growing extent, amniocentesis is being employed to determine the sex of a fetus and, if results show that the baby will be a girl, it is promptly aborted. A survey conducted in Bombay hospitals revealed that of 8000 abortions performed, all but one were of female fetuses. While this trend has generated sharp criticism among commentators on the Indian scene, some defend the practice on the grounds that it is preferable for a woman to have abortions rather than produce 6 or 7 children in hopes of having one or two boys. Citing the abuse often directed at Indian wives who bear too many daughters, one physician defended the use of amniocentesis for sex selection by stating, "I practice amniocentesis as a lesser evil. It is better to have feticide than matricide."[16] In reaction to the adverse publicity regarding reports of tens of thousands of abortions performed for sex selection purposes, the government of the Indian state of Maharashtra, of which Bombay is the capital, recently outlawed the use of prenatal tests for sex determination.

Low educational and economic status of women — Birth rates today are highest in those parts of the world where women have little schooling and where opportunities for paid employment outside the home are few. In such societies, a woman's worth is measured in terms of her child-bearing abilities. Such women, striving to maintain favor with their husbands and in-laws, are unlikely to respond favorably to the idea of family limitation. In addition, illiterate women or women with only an elementary education are less likely than their better-educated sisters to have heard about modern contraceptive techniques or to know how to use them. Surveys indicate that providing women with at least a secondary school education is one of the most effective ways of reducing the birth rate in developing countries; in general, fertility drops noticeably as the level of female education increases, primarily because educated women tend to marry later, have greater opportunity for employment outside the home, are more aware of the advantages of smaller family size, and understand how to practice contraception more effectively.[17]

Such factors support the contention of many demographers that broad-based social and economic changes must precede or accompany population programs in developing countries if population growth is ever to be stabilized; simply making contraceptives more widely available will not be enough to overcome traditional biases which favor large families.

Box 3–4

Uncle Nicolae Wants You!

At a time when world population continues to grow at an alarming pace and national leaders struggle with programs to defuse the "population bomb," it seems somewhat anachronistic that a few countries are pursuing policies aimed at encouraging an increase in population size. Malaysia in 1984 decided to adopt childbearing incentives to forestall any further declines in its national birthrate, currently holding steady at 2.4%. Reasoning that a larger population would provide a strong domestic market for the country's burgeoning industrial output, Malaysian leaders are offering income tax deductions and maternity

---

benefits for women who bear up to 5 children. By so doing, they hope that Malaysia's present population of 70 million will more than quadruple by 2100. Similarly, in the French-speaking province of Quebec, Canada, the provincial government in the spring of 1988 instituted a new tax-exempt "birth bonus" to be paid automatically to qualified residents in 8 installments over a two year period (this is in addition to the monthly child allowance Ottawa remits to families throughout Canada). And this wasn't all—the provincial authorities also announced income tax cuts and interest-free home loans for parents. Why this desire to encourage a baby boom north of the border? Probably because this culturally distinct province, where separatist sentiment remains strong, currently has the lowest fertility rate in all of Canada (av. of 1.4 children per woman) and is experiencing a high rate of out-migration. Whether cash inducements for baby production are successful remains to be seen.

The policies described above represent positive incentives to encourage childbearing; couples are free to accept or reject the government's "carrot" as they choose and, in fact, experience has shown that in most countries where cash bonuses have been tried, a short-term upward jump in fertility has been followed by a return to pre-bonus levels.

A more draconian approach to stimulating population growth is being pursued today by the Communist government of Romania, where official concerns about a "birth dearth" prompted leaders in 1966 to declare that raising the Romanian birth rate and increasing population size by 30% were to be national goals. Since Romania's fiscal status would not permit generous monetary incentives to prospective parents, the government opted for the "stick" approach, adopting what must be the world's most repressive policies for promoting population growth.

For the first 18 years after adopting its pronatalist goals, the Romanian government limited itself to prohibiting most abortions, which had been unrestricted until that time, and to banning the manufacture or importation of all contraceptives. For a year or two following these actions, the birth rate surged sharply upward, but it then began to fall again and soon was as low as it had been before 1966. By 1984 Romanian dictator Nicolae Ceausescu decided to impose more drastic measures. He decreed that all employed women up to the age of 45 must submit to monthly pelvic examinations at their workplace. When a pregnancy is detected, it is carefully monitored to term; if a miscarriage should occur, it is up to the unlucky woman to convince her interrogators that the loss was spontaneous and not induced. To combat the more than 200,000 illegal abortions estimated to occur in Romania each year, the State Security Police have set up a special unit. Doctors performing an abortion can be imprisoned for 25 years and, in some cases, executed. To promote marriage and childbearing, Romania has lowered the minimum marriage age for women to 15; a special 30% income tax is levied against any unmarried citizen aged 25 or older and against childless married couples unless they can offer medical proof of infertility. That laws pertaining to confidentiality or rights of privacy are non-existent in Romania is obvious from the questions in a recent national demographic survey. Married Romanian women were queried about the number of times they had intercourse each week; they were then asked, "Why haven't you conceived?"[18]

The Romanian example makes it abundantly clear that population policies aimed at promoting growth can be every bit as destructive of human rights as efforts aimed at limiting fertility. Those who criticize China's leaders for insisting that "One is Enough!" might ponder the pro-growth pronouncements of Romania's President:

> *"The fetus is the socialist property of the whole Society. Giving birth is a patriotic duty, determining the fate of our country. Those who refuse to have children are deserters, escaping the laws of national continuity."*

> —Nicolae Ceausescu, 1986
> (quoted in *Der Spiegel*)

Family Planning vs. Population Control

With few exceptions, the family-limitation programs currently operating in most countries, the U.S. included, are aimed at helping couples to have the number of children they *want*. An implicit assumption in such programs is that most modern couples desire to control their fertility, but theoretically if a childless couple came to a clinic wanting assistance in producing 12 offspring, they would be helped to do so. The primary goal of such programs is to reduce birth rates by ensuring that "every child is a wanted child" through the prevention of unplanned pregnancies. Such a program, accurately designated as "family planning", makes no attempt to look at the implications of population growth from a societal standpoint, but rather from a purely individual one. In light of the impact which population growth has on depletion of natural resources and on environmental quality in general, many people today question whether reliance on family planning to curb population growth will be sufficient.

Obviously, the crucial consideration in family planning is the number of children the average couple says it wants. For population growth to stabilize (i.e. to attain ZPG), couples must just reproduce themselves. In developed countries, where infant mortality rates are relatively low, this means that an average of 2.1 children per family would result in maintenance of a stable population size. In the U.S. in recent years, average family size has been dropping steadily and currently stands at 1.8 children born to each woman during her reproductive lifetime. In this country, then, assuming that present trends continue (always a risky assumption!), family planning alone will provide the means to achieve ZPG.

In most of the developing world, by contrast, simply helping couples to prevent unwanted births cannot result in a levelling off of population growth because the majority of couples there *want* more than the number necessary to achieve stabilization. Since infant mortality rates are slightly higher in Third World countries than in the West, an average family size of 2.3 children (rather than 2.1) would be required to attain ZPG. However, in every one of these nations, the preferred number of children per family is greater than this, averaging 4.7 in the Third World as a whole, but as high as 7 or 8 in some African countries and 6 in parts of the Middle East.[19] A family planning program which assists a Kenyan woman in having "only" 7 babies when she probably would have had 10 without contraceptives is certainly of benefit to the woman involved, but it does little to help stabilize population growth in Kenya, currently the world's fastest-growing nation. In such cases, critics contend, what is needed is not family-planning, but rather programs aimed at *Population Control*. A true population control policy would represent a conscious decision on the part of society (or the government, a dictator, etc.) as to what the optimum population size of that society ought to be, given the availability of natural resources, carrying capacity of that society's environment, and other such considerations. Once such a decision is made, policies would be

Fig. 3-3

Birth Control Methods

	THE "PILL" (Oral contraceptives)	IUD (Intrauterine device)	DIAPHRAGM & CONTRACEPTIVE CREAM OR JELLY
What it is:	A series of pills made of substances similar to hormones which occur naturally in women's bodies.	A small piece of shaped plastic that is inserted into a woman's uterus.	A shallow rubber cup made to fit securely into the vagina to cover a woman's cervix.
How it works:	Raises the woman's hormone level so she will not ovulate. All pills must be taken to be effective.	Makes the uterus an unsuitable place for a fertilized egg to implant.	Used with contraceptive cream or jelly, it keeps sperm out of the uterus.
Advantages:	Highly effective and easy to use. Separate from the sex act.	Highly effective and separate from the sex act. No daily routine.	Does not change normal body functions.
Disadvantages:	Pills must be taken every day to be effective. Having certain health conditions, being over 35, or being a smoker may prohibit use.	Slightly higher chance of infections; brief pain on insertion. May cause heavier periods for the first few months.	Weight change or pregnancy may cause a change in size needed. May be messy. Must be inserted before intercourse.
Effectiveness:	Method failures: less than 1 (combination) and 2-3 (mini-pill—per 100 women. User failure: 2-3 per 100 women.	Method failures: 2-4 per 100 women. Device failures may be detected early by user.	Method failures: 2-4 per 100 women. User failures: 10-15 per 100 women.
How to get it:	See your doctor or clinic. Examination and prescription are needed. Periodic exams will be needed.	See your doctor or clinic. A qualified doctor or nurse practitioner must insert the IUD. Periodic exams will be needed.	See your doctor or clinic to be measured for a diaphragm. Cream or jelly requires no prescription.

Source: Planned Parenthood Federation

CONTRACEPTIVE FOAM	CONDOM (Prophylactics)	STERILIZATION	NATURAL FAMILY PLANNING (Rhythm methods)
A chemical substance that immobilizes sperm.	A thin rubber sheath made to fit over an erect penis.	Vasectomy for men; tubal ligation or laparoscopy for women. Permanent birth control.	Calendar, Temperature, and Cervical mucous methods determine the time of a woman's fertility.
Inserted in the vagina near the cervix to stop sperm from entering.	Worn during intercourse to keep sperm from entering the vagina.	Surgery prevents sperm from getting to the penis or eggs from getting to the uterus.	The couple abstains from sex during the woman's most fertile times.
Does not change normal body functions. Easy to get.	Male method. Easy to get. Helps prevent VD.	Highly effective. Does not alter any other body functions.	No artificial means. Couple oriented.
May be somewhat messy. Must be used for each act of intercourse.	Can burst or tear during sex. May decrease sensitivity. Must be used for each act of intercourse.	Relatively costly; permanent. Requires surgery.	Requires periodic abstinence; difficult for women with irregular cycles. Requires daily regimen.
Method failures: 2-4 per per 100 women. User failures: 13-16 per 100 women.

Foam & Condoms together = 99% safe | Method failures: 2-4 per 100. User failures: 6-13 per 100. | Method failures: less than 1 per 100 users. | Method failures: 5-10 per 100 women. User failures: 9-28 per 100 women. |
| Available at clinics or drug stores: no prescription needed. | Available at clinics or drug stores: no prescription needed. | See your doctor or clinic for information about the procedures available, costs, etc. | See your doctor or clinic for instructions about different methods. |

implemented to achieve that population size. For example, if a government decides that its population is too small, it might promote child-bearing by giving cash allowances or tax deductions for each additional child, special bonuses for "Hero Mothers," or by encouraging immigration. A population control policy to halt growth would undoubtedly involve less popular moves; the world's most ambitious and widely-discussed population control policy is the one currently being pursued in the People's Republic of China (see Box 3–5). The Chinese government has implemented a program aimed at rapidly stabilizing growth at a level only slightly higher than its present population size by urging couples to have no more than one child. Though such a program would be extremely controversial in a democratic nation (indeed, reports out of China indicate a certain amount of resistance even in that tightly-controlled society), the idea of striving to maintain human numbers at or below the carrying capacity of their environment makes eminently good sense. Demographers and environmentalists alike will be viewing the Chinese experiment with great interest to see what lessons it has to offer for an increasingly crowded world.

Box 3–5

China's One-Child Family Policy

With most recent census figures placing the population of China at more than one billion, Chinese leaders are understandably eager to reduce growth rates as rapidly as possible. Although some birth control clinics had been established in China in the 1950s and both abortion and sterilization legalized, not until the mid-1960s did the government launch serious efforts to encourage family limitation. Additional clinics were opened, improved contraceptive techniques developed (e.g. vacuum technique for abortions, simplified sterilization procedures, temporary male sterilants, and the "paper pill"—a water-soluble paper impregnated with oral contraceptives). Expansion of the health-care system throughout the vast countryside, aided by "barefoot doctors"—individuals trained to provide basic health care, including the distribution of contraceptives—made birth control easily accessible to rural peasants as well as to city-dwellers. Late marriage was promoted (mid-20s for women, late 20s for men) as a means of reducing births. All birth control services were provided free of charge and workers needing time off for abortions, sterilizations, or IUD insertions were given paid leave. During this period couples were urged to have no more than 2 children, with a 3 to 5-year interval between births. This effort appears to have been relatively successful, particularly in urban areas where having more than 2 offspring was viewed by one's peers almost as a form of anti-social behavior.

However, by the late 1970s it became apparent that the remarkable drop in Chinese birth rates (from 34 in 1970 to 17 in 1980) was still not sufficient to achieve stabilization.[20] Accordingly, in 1978 the Chinese leadership decided to make an unprecedented attempt to reduce total population size by urging that henceforth each Chinese couple should produce no more than one child (obviously the policy was not intended to be retroactive!). Because attitudinal surveys revealed that less than 20% of married couples would voluntarily restrict their number of offspring to one, the government established a system of rewards and penalties. Couples are urged to sign "Only Child Glory Certificates" which entitle them

---

to receive free medical care and school tuition for their child, monthly cash bonuses or, in rural areas, work points qualifying them for extra food and supplies. Certificate holders receive preferential treatment in obtaining housing, extra old age pensions in urban areas or a guaranteed standard of living for rural residents. When an adult, the only child is assured of preferential treatment in securing a job. However, if parents who sign such a contract violate its terms by having a second child, all benefits must be returned. Birth of a third child results in a 10% reduction of parents' wages, a charge for the extra child's rations, and restriction of access to housing designed for 2-child families. [21]

The results of China's vigorous fertility control effort have been impressive. In the 10-year period from 1974 to 1984, population growth rates plummeted from 3.3% to 1.0%; Chinese officials estimate that 86% of all couples are now practicing some form of birth control. Nevertheless, by the late 1980s, it was becoming apparent that growing resistance to the program was having an impact. In 1986 the birthrate jumped from 18 to 21 and has persisted at that level ever since. The growth rate rose to 1.4% and Chinese leaders expect it to remain high into the early 1990s. As a result, the target goal of a 1.2 billion population in the year 2000 will be exceeded by at least 84 million, and members of China's State Family Planning Commission agree that the situation is grim.

The reversal in what had been a steady downward trend in births can be blamed in part on simple demographics; the large cohort born during the last population surge from 1962-1975 is now entering its prime reproductive years and creating a mini-baby boom of its own.

Beyond that, however, not all Chinese couples have yet been persuaded that one child is sufficient. Although acceptance of current policy is high among urban Chinese, many of the 800 million peasants in China's countryside have ignored Beijing's appeals. Overall, only 15.2% of Chinese couples have signed the "Glory Certificates". Ironically, increasing prosperity encouraged by recent economic reforms has had a negative effect on promotion of one-child families: newly-affluent peasants, still adhering to the traditional view that "more sons mean more happiness", are willing to pay the fine levied against excess children.

Admitting that "China is once again facing a population crisis", Chinese officials are now imposing strict new policies to revitalize the program, making local officials accountable for the enforcement of population quotas. Efforts at convincing couples to sign one-child contracts are intensifying, and sex education classes in schools are being introduced throughout China. Demographers will continue to watch China's grand experiment with fascination for years to come. [22]

REFERENCES

[1]Lightbourne, Robert Jr., and Susheela Singh with Cynthia P. Green, "The World Fertility Survey: Charting Global Childbearing", *Population Bulletin*, vol. 37, no. 1, Population Reference Bureau, Inc., Washington, DC, 1982.

[2]Ehrlich, Paul R., Anne H. Ehrlich, and J.P. Holdren, *Ecoscience: Population, Resources, Environment*, W.H. Freeman and Co., 1977.

[3]Vietmeyer, Noel, "The Greening of the Future", *Quest*, Sept. 25, 1979.

[4]Stokes, Bruce, "Men and Family Planning", *Worldwatch Paper 41*, Worldwatch Institute, December 1980.

[5]League of Women Voters Education Fund, "*Public Policy on Reproductive Choices*", Pub. No. 286, July 1982.

[6]Henshaw, Stanley K., "Induced Abortion: A Worldwide Perspective", *Family Planning Perspectives*, vol. 18, no. 6, Nov./Dec. 1986.

[7]League of Women Voters Education Fund, op. cit.

[8]Lee, K.S. et al., "Maternal Age and Incidence of Low Birth Weight at Term: A Population Study", *American Journal of Obstetrics and Gynecology*, 158:84, 1988; A. Friede, et al., "Older Maternal Age and Infant Mortality in the United States", *Obstetrics and Gynecology*, 72:152, 1988.

[9]Eckholm, Erik, and Kathleen Newland, "Health: the Family Planning Factor:, *Worldwatch Paper 10*, The Worldwatch Institute, January 1977.

[10]"The Reduction in Risk of Ovarian Cancer Associated with Oral Contraceptive Use", *New England Journal of Medicine*, 316:650, 1987; "Combination Oral Contraceptive Use and the Risk of Endometrial Cancer", *Journal of the American Medical Association*, 257:796, 1987.

[11]Lincoln, Richard, and Lisa Kaeser, "Whatever Happened to the Contraceptive Revolution?", *Family Planning Perspectives*, vol. 20, no. 1, Jan./Feb. 1988; Atkinson, Linda E., Richard Lincoln, and Jacqueline Darroch Forrest, "The Next Contraceptive Revolution", *Family Planning Perspectives*, vol. 18, no. 1, Jan./Feb. 1986.

[12]Forrest, Jacqueline D., and Richard R. Fordyce, "U.S. Women's Contraceptive Attitudes and Practice: How Have They Changed in the 1980s?". *Family Planning Perspectives*, vol. 20, no. 3, May/June 1988.

[13]Lincoln et al., op. cit.

[14]Lightbourne, op. cit.

[15]Williamson, Nancy E., "Boys or Girls? Parents' Preferences and Sex Control", *Population Bulletin*, vol. 33, no. 1, Population Reference Bureau, Washington, DC, 1978.

[16]Green, Laura, "Amniocentesis as a Weapon?", *The Chicago Tribune*, Sept. 9, 1986.

[17]Lightbourne, op. cit.

[18]Haupt, Arthur, "How Romania Tries to Govern Fertility", *Population Today*, vol. 15, no. 2, February 1987.

[19]Ibid.

[20]David, Henry P., "China's Population Policy: Glimpses and a Minisurvey", *Intercom*, Population Reference Bureau, vol. 10, no. 9/10, September/October 1982.

[21]"The Population of China: One Billion, Eight Million People", *Interchange*, Population Reference Bureau, vol. 12, no. 2, May 1983.

[22]Cheng Gang, "China Faces Another Baby Boom", *Beijing Review*, July 4-10, 1988; Tyson, Ann Scott, "China adopts tough measures to curb population boom", *The Christian Science Monitor*, Feb. 16, 1988.

4

The People-Food Predicament

"Today we must proclaim a bold objective—that within a
decade no child will go to bed hungry, that no family will
fear for its next day's bread, and that no human being's
future and capacities will be stunted by malnutrition."
—Sec. of State Henry Kissinger

In the early post-War years, attainment of the lofty goals proclaimed by Sec.
of State Kissinger at the 1974 U.N.-sponsored World Food Conference
appeared within reach.

From 1950 until 1984 the world's farmers were successful in producing
increased quantities of food more rapidly than the world's parents were
producing babies. The global grain harvest more than doubled, rising from
624 million tons in 1950 to 1.6 billion tons in 1984. In spite of spiralling
population figures, per capita availability of food also increased steadily during
the period, resulting in impressive nutritional gains in many Third World
countries. This favorable over-all trend was somewhat deceptive, however, for
global food production averages were largely reflective of the massive increase
in North American crop yields during those years and masked the gloomier
statistics which showed that in many of the poorer nations per capita increase
in food production had halted by the late 1950s due to high rates of population
growth. A decade later, a reverse trend became evident in some Third World
regions, even while global averages conveyed the impression that all was well on
the food front. Since 1967 Africa's baby boom has resulted in a 15% drop in
food output per person on that continent; since 1981 Latin America has
experienced a similar decline.

General optimism about world food security was given a jolt in the early 1970s when a combination of factors caused an abrupt, though temporary, halt to the steady increase in per capita food supply which the world's people had come to take for granted. Several years of bad weather (floods in some areas, droughts in others) sharply reduced harvests in several of the world's major grain-growing areas. Huge purchases of American wheat by the Soviet Union in 1972, the largest food import deal in history up to that time, initiated the upward surge in food prices which has continued to the present. Food price stability which had characterized the preceding two decades suddenly vanished as the world price of grain doubled within a period of months. While sharply escalating farm prices undoubtedly had a devastating impact on nutritional levels among the world's poor, it provided agriculturalists with a financial incentive to expand production, which they promptly did. In the U.S., all the cropland idled under the Soil Bank program was returned to cultivation; elsewhere in the developing world, the resource-intensive technologies of the Green Revolution became profitable and once again overall production increased. Until as recently as the mid-1980s, news of huge crop surpluses dominated the farm pages of newspapers and laments of a worldwide "grain glut" were heard from Chicago to Melbourne. Even Western Europe, reliant on food imports for the past 200 years, became a major grain exporter during those golden years.

Behind the encouraging figures, however, some worrisome trends were becoming evident. After nearly 40 years of steady growth in world food output, a significant slowdown became apparent in many of the world's most populous countries. In India, grain production has been stagnant since 1983—at a time when India's population continues to increase by 17 million yearly; in China, agricultural output has dropped since 1984's peak harvest; Indonesia and Mexico have witnessed a levelling-off of their production, while in Japan, Taiwan, and South Korea grain output has been declining for years. Reports coming out of the USSR indicate that nation has had disappointing harvests several years in a row. Severe droughts which brought devastation to the grain belts of North America and China in the summer of 1988 caused a 76 million ton drop in world food output that year, following a 1987 decline of 85 million tons due to failure of the Indian monsoon. Within a brief two-year period the world "grain glut" had vanished, leaving reserves at their lowest level since the early post-World War II period.[1]

While many national leaders tend to blame adverse weather conditions for food shortfalls, the true causes are more complex: loss of good cropland to erosion and non-farm uses, inefficient agrarian structures, lack of investment in agriculture by city-oriented government officials, rising energy costs—and too many people.

Factors Influencing Food Demand

While it is obvious that the total yield of the world's croplands, pasturelands, and fisheries constitute the world's food supply, assessing food demand is slightly more complicated. **Population Growth**, not surprisingly, is the single largest factor in determining food demand. Since 90% of the world's population increase is occurring in the countries of Asia, Africa, and Latin America, food supply problems currently are most acute in these regions. An additional factor must be considered in assessing food demand, however. **Rising personal incomes** which have characterized the economic development of most industrialized countries since the Second World War have greatly added to world food demand. This is not because the typical American, Swede, or Japanese eats tremendously greater quantities than the average Peruvian, Pakistani, or Sudanese—obviously the human stomach can only hold so much!—but because higher incomes are generally translated into an increased demand for high-quality foods, particularly meat and dairy products. As you will recall from our discussion of trophic levels and energy transfer (Ch. 1), it requires approximately ten times as much grain to produce a pound of human flesh from beef as it would if that same grain were eaten directly, due to inescapable inefficiencies of energy conversion. Thus the shift to a greater reliance on animal products in the diets of citizens of high- and middle-income countries is having a marked impact on increasing food demand in those areas. Indeed, the present one-quarter of the world's people who live in the industrialized countries consume approximately *half* of the world's grain production each year, much of it in the form of meat. Taking both population increase and income growth into consideration, it has been calculated that for the foreseeable future, world food demand will increase at a 3% annual rate; to meet this demand, world food production will have to double in 24 years.[2]

Extent of Hunger

Determining the number of hungry people in the world today is a rather tricky business. Certainly there is a quantum difference between the teen-ager coming home from school complaining, "When's dinner, Mom? I'm starving!", and an Ethiopian child with stick-like limbs and protruding abdomen, dying of acute malnutrition. In an attempt to establish some basis for comparison, the Food and Agriculture Organization (FAO) of the United Nations has devised a concept called the Basal Metabolic Rate (BMR). The BMR is defined as the minimum amount of energy required to power human body maintenance, *not* including energy required for activity. On this basis, the FAO considers anyone receiving *less than 1.2 BMR* food intake daily to be undernourished. Using this rather conservative figure (some authorities feel the cut-off point should be raised to 1.5 BMR), the FAO estimates that today approximately 500 million people—one-tenth of humanity—are undernourished. Hunger, of course, is not equally shared among nations or even within nations. The vast majority of the world's hungry people inhabit the South Asian countries of India, Pakistan, and Bangladesh, parts of Southeast Asia, Africa south of the Sahara, and the Andean region of South America—all regions where rates of population growth

Fig. 4-1

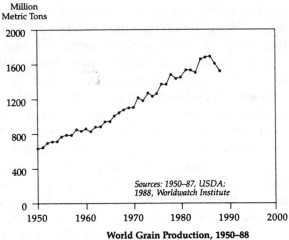

Million
Metric Tons

*Sources: 1950–87, USDA;
1988, Worldwatch Institute*

World Grain Production, 1950–88

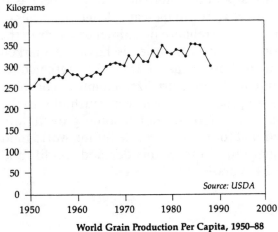

Kilograms

Source: USDA

World Grain Production Per Capita, 1950–88

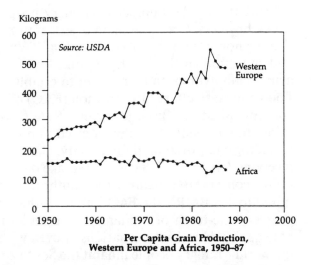

Kilograms

Source: USDA

Western
Europe

Africa

**Per Capita Grain Production,
Western Europe and Africa, 1950–87**

Impact of population growth on per capita grain production: slow-growing Europe has steadily rising food production/person, while rapidly-growing Africa is producing less food/person than it did 20 years ago.

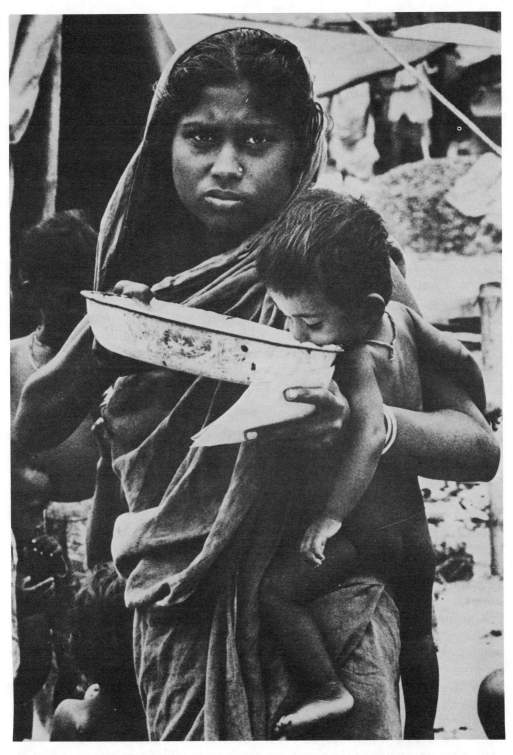

A child receives UNICEF-supplied milk at Salt Lake Camp, near Calcutta. [*UNICEF Photo 6390/Balcomb/Mullick/Nelson*]

The People-Food Predicament   **103**

continue to be high. Nevertheless, pockets of hunger can be found even within many affluent societies—in the U.S. malnutrition is distressingly common among the poor, the elderly, migrant farm workers, and American Indians. More than half of the world's undernourished people are children under the age of 5, and a significantly higher percentage of women than men are affected.[3] This situation exists because within households in many cultures men, being the primary workers and providers, are served the best food before the rest of the family eats. Children and women, including both pregnant and nursing mothers, whose nutritional needs in proportion to their size exceed those of men, subsist on whatever remains. In such situations, girl children frequently receive less than boys, since males are more highly regarded. While landless laborers are often fed on the job by their employers, their families are not, thus increasing the disparity in nutritional levels within families.[4]

The hunger issue most frequently impinges on the public consciousness during periods of severe famine, generally caused by prolonged droughts, floods, or wartime upheavals. During recent years, media coverage of starving children and anguished parents in Cambodia, Ethiopia, Bangladesh, and the Sahel have kept us grimly aware of human suffering during times of calamity elsewhere in the world. Such periodic episodes of famine, tragic though they are, do not represent the world's major hunger problem at present, however. Rather, the chronic, undramatic, day-after-day undernutrition of those who know that, good harvest or poor, their bellies will never be full constitutes today's most serious food supply dilemma.

Causes of Hunger

The existence of nearly half a billion undernourished people seems paradoxical when one considers the World Bank's report that if the global grain harvest were equally distributed, each person would receive 3000 calories and 65 grams of protein per day—more than enough for good health. The authors of the Global 2000 Report also conclude that resources exist to meet the food demands of the projected world population at the turn of the century. If this is so, why are so many people today suffering from inadequate diets? The current situation is caused largely by two factors: **uneven distribution** of food and **poverty.**

Although global averages suggest that there should be enough food for everyone, as was stated earlier many of the areas where hunger is endemic are regions where there is a widening gap between food production and population growth; only imports from food-surplus areas prevent the problem from worsening further. The most basic problem, however, is poverty. Even in chronically food-short countries, the rich eat quite well. By contrast, even in the wealthiest nations, where markets bulge with a veritable cornucopia of foods, people who lack money to purchase groceries go hungry. In Third World countries almost 40% of the people are too poor to afford a minimally adequate diet. For these hungry people, an increase in world food production will mean little unless corresponding social and economic changes increase their purchasing power.[5] Poverty's role as a determinant of hunger was clearly evident during the 1967 drought in Bihar, a state in eastern India threatened with severe famine due to near-total crop failure. Food aid rushed into the area by the U.S. and other donors was credited with averting large-scale loss of life and interviews with villagers after the crisis was over revealed that many of them ate better during this period of natural disaster than at any other time in their lives. Why? Because the donated wheat was distributed to the needy free of charge and all received a share. During normal times the poorer segments of society lacked money to buy sufficient food in the marketplace and so went hungry. As George Verghese, editor of the Hindustan Times and information advisor to Prime Minister Gandhi during the famine eloquently described:

> For the poorest sections of the society, 1967, the Year of the Famine, will long be remembered as a bonus year when millions of people, especially the children, probably for the first time were assured of a decent meal a day . . . in a 'normal year', these people hover on the bread line. They are beyond the pale, nobody's concern, they starve. In a famine year, they eat. Their health is better and the children are gaining weight. For them this is a year of great blessing. This is the deep irony, the grim tragedy of the situation.

Ironically, some of the improvements in agricultural technology much-heralded in recent years (i.e. "The Green Revolution") have actually worsened the nutritional status of landless laborers who found themselves displaced by machines, hence without any income to purchase food. The inflation of food prices which began with the Russian grain purchase of 1972 and has continued steadily in the years since has probably been more instrumental than any other single factor in reversing the nutritional gains witnessed during the 1950s and 1960s. The sharp increase in energy costs (e.g. gasoline to power farm machinery, natural gas for making nitrogen fertilizer and for drying grain), heightened demand for livestock feed in the developed countries, continued rapid increase in population size in the less-developed nations—all assure a continued escalation in food prices during the years ahead. Unless world economic conditions improve, with a more equitable distribution of resources and income, unless there are improvements in productivity and a slowing of population growth rates, it is unlikely that world poverty, which is the principal cause of hunger, can be substantially ameliorated.

Health Impact of Hunger

Stressing the national security aspect of world hunger issues, the Presidential Commission on World Hunger stated in its 1980 report that:

> Hunger has been internationalized and turned into a continuing global issue, transformed from a low-profile moral imperative to a divisive and disruptive factor in international relations. The most potentially explosive force in

Drought is ravaging the continent of Africa. Famine is a harsh reality for millions of people living there. Emergency food and water supplies are a first necessity. But for the long-term many complex problems—political as well as environmental—have to be solved.

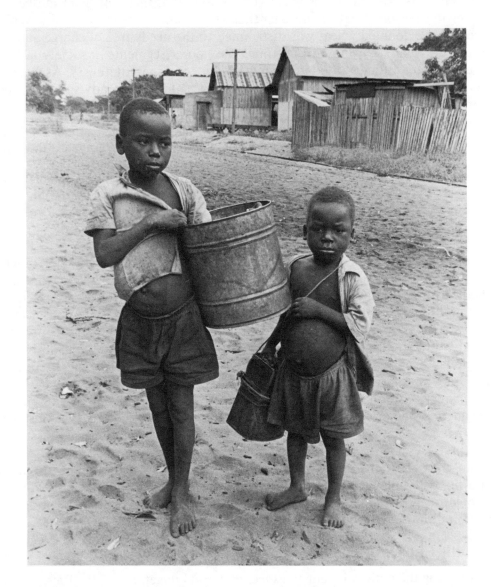

Displaced persons receiving food in Macuacua Camp in drought-stricken southern Mozambique. The Mozambican Red Cross is working with international relief agencies to prevent wide-spread starvation in the afflicted area. [*Un Photo 353609 / Kate Truscott*]

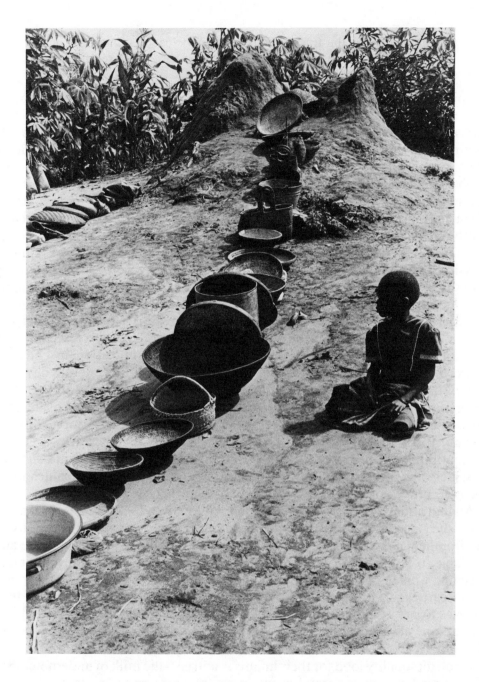

The empty baskets are lined up as displaced persons at a camp near Vilanculos wait for emergency food supplies. The Mozambican Red Cross together with several international relief agencies are trying to feed tens of thousands of people threatened by famine in the southern provinces of Mozambique. [*Un Photo 153645 / Paul Heath Hoeffel*]

the world today is the frustrated desire of poor people to attain a decent standard of living. The anger, despair, and often hatred that result represent a real and persistent threat to international order.

Political instability may be a worrisome consequence of hunger, true enough, but an even more fundamental reason for trying to eliminate hunger is its adverse impact on public health and well-being. Even during years when acute famine is absent, inadequate caloric intake has a significant impact on death rates. Among the poor in Third World countries, malnutrition is the #1 health problem and is the major factor responsible for the wide gap in infant mortality rates between developed and less-developed societies. Chronic undernourishment, harmful at any age, is particularly devastating to young children. If a child receives less than 70% of the daily standard food requirement, his growth and activity fall below normal levels; if food deprivation is prolonged, stunted physical development becomes irreversible and adult size is correspondingly reduced. As a result, the individual's work performance is affected, particularly if he is employed in manual labor (work performance in both agriculture and industry has shown a positive correlation with increased body size and height). Even more ominous than the link between malnutrition and decreased physical development, however, is the finding that severe malnutrition in children, especially very young infants, results in a permanent stunting of brain development, characterized by a decrease in the number of brain cells and an alteration of brain chemistry. Even milder cases of malnutrition can result in lowered performance on tests designed to measure learning and sensory abilities. Malnutrition, by reducing bodily defenses, also greatly increases a child's susceptibility to infectious diseases. Common childhood ailments such as dysentery and diarrhea, as well as a variety of parasitic diseases, are much more likely to prove fatal to an undernourished child than to a well-fed one.

Malnutrition takes its toll among older children and adults as well. Under-nourished people lose weight and become less able to combat infections or environmental stress. They thereby become less economically productive and less able to care for their families. At greatest risk, of course, are pregnant and lactating women. Such women, if malnourished, run a significantly higher risk of miscarriage or premature delivery than do adequately-fed mothers. If they manage to carry their babies full-term, the child is likely to suffer from low birth weight (one of the most frequent causes of infant mortality) or to be still-born.[6] The old myth that nursing mothers draw on their own nutritional reserves to provide top-quality food for their infants is untrue—the milk of undernourished mothers is lower than normal in vitamins, fat, and protein content.

Nutritional Deficiency Diseases

To be well-nourished implies not only an adequate caloric intake, but also a proper balance of carbohydrates, fats, proteins, vitamins and minerals. If amounts of any of these are insufficient, certain deficiency symptoms may become apparent even when all other vital nutrients are in adequate supply.

Some of the more common deficiency diseases include:

Kwashiorkor—the single largest contributor to high child mortality rates in Third World countries, kwashiorkor is a protein deficiency disease which affects millions of children in tropical areas, particularly in Africa. Kwashiorkor most frequently develops in babies who are weaned early and given only starchy, low-protein foods such as rice, cassava, or bananas to eat—common baby foods in many tropical regions. Symptoms of mild kwashiorkor include discoloration of the hair and skin (in dark-haired children, hair may assume a reddish cast), retardation of physical growth, development of a protruding abdomen due to accumulation of fluids, and a loss of appetite. In more severe cases the hair may pull out in tufts, digestive problems arise, fluid collects in the legs and feet, and the child becomes listless and apathetic. Once this stage of the disease is reached, the child is likely to die if he doesn't receive medical attention. In its milder forms, however, the effects of kwashiorkor are reversible and generally disappear as the child becomes older and is given a more varied diet.

Marasmus—the second of the two most commonly observed deficiency diseases among children, marasmus is an indication of over-all protein-calorie deprivation. Most frequently striking babies under 1 year of age, especially those no longer being breast-fed, marasmus often occurs after the child has been suffering from diarrhea or some other disease. Victims of

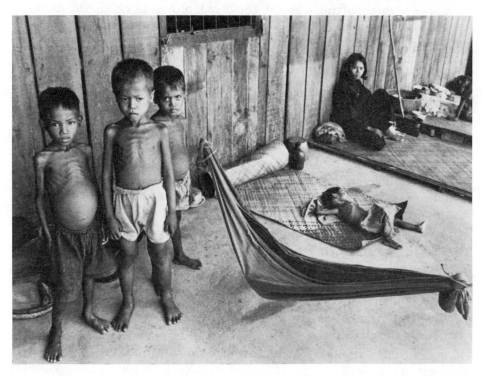

Children in Phnom Penh, Kampuchea, give evidence of the extent of malnutrition rampant in that war-ravaged country. The boy on the left is suffering from an advanced case of kwashiorkor; the child lying on the mat died soon after this photo was taken. [*Oxfam America*]

The People-Food Predicament **109**

marasmus can be distinguished by their thin, wasted appearance, with skin hanging in loose wrinkles around wrists and legs and eyes appearing unusually large and bright because of the shrunken aspect of the rest of the body.

Xerophthalmia (Blindness)—a deficiency in vitamin A, often associated with protein shortages, can result in a drying of the eye membranes or a softening of the cornea, leading to night-blindness and, if not treated, progressing to total blindness in its victims. Lack of sufficient vitamin A is common to the Western Pacific region, the Far East, semi-arid regions of Africa, and parts of Latin America. It is estimated that 250,000 children each year become blind due to vitamin A deficiency and that an additional 10 million develop clinical signs and symptoms of xerophthalmia. In recent years evidence has been growing that vitamin A deficiency not only can cause blindness, but that it is an important determinant of child mortality, even among children who are otherwise well-nourished and healthy. Studies conducted among Indonesian preschoolers suffering from night blindness showed that these children were 4-12 times more likely to die than their non-affected peers, apparently due to their greater susceptibility to respiratory and diarrheal infections (it is theorized that vitamin A deficiency interferes with proper functioning of the immune system). Additional data suggest that administration of supplementary doses of vitamin A to populations at risk could reduce overall childhood deaths within such groups by 20-30%. These findings have prompted demands that the World Health Organization and its member states act more vigorously to expand effective control programs to reduce the incidence of this deadly, but preventable, disease.[7]

Anemia—iron deficiency anemia is very common in the less-developed countries where 20-25% of children, 20-40% of women, and 10% of men may suffer from this disorder. Anemia is characterized by lack of energy and low levels of productive activity. It is especially dangerous—and especially common—in pregnant women, where anemia increases the likelihood of premature delivery or still-birth. Repeated pregnancies rapidly drain a woman's reserve supplies of iron, as do parasitic infections such as hookworm, common in areas where sanitation is poor.

Goiter—iodine deficiency, affecting about 200 million people world-wide, results in the swollen growth of the thyroid gland on the front or side of the neck known as goiter. Iodine deficiency in pregnant women can result in their babies being born dwarfed and mentally retarded. Goiter has largely been eliminated in the U.S. by the simple expedient of adding iodine to table salt.[8]

Other deficiency diseases which are much less common today than they were in the past due to fortification of dietary staples with the missing vitamin or mineral include: scurvy (vitamin C), beri-beri (thiamine—vitamin B_1), pellagra (niacin), and rickets (vitamin D).

Box 4–1

Bottle Babies

While plant breeders and farmers scramble to find ways of easing the population-food dilemma and nutritionists ponder ways of improving deficient diets, one of nature's finest—and cheapest—foods is being by-passed by a steadily increasing portion of humanity. Human breast milk, an excellent source of high quality protein containing all the essential amino acids, is the ideal food for babies, capable of satisfying all the infant's nutritional needs for the first 4-6 months of life (after 6 months supplemental feeding of solid foods is required to meet all the child's protein and caloric needs, but even then breast milk constitutes a valuable component of the diet). Unfortunately, in recent decades increasing numbers of mothers have curtailed or totally abandoned breast-feeding in favor of infant formulas, apparently regarding the former as too "old-fashioned" for the sophistication of the modern world (ironically, in Western countries there is a renewed interest in breast-feeding, particularly among the better-educated and more affluent segments of society!). Aside from the increased financial costs which this trend entails (e.g. expenditures for purchased milk or formula, bottles, nipples, sterilizing equipment, fuel for heating the water, etc.), the shift away from nursing to bottle feeding has some serious health implications.

Although commercial infant formulas can be a perfectly adequate food for babies when mixed in the proper concentrations, prepared under sanitary conditions with uncontaminated water, and placed in sterile bottles with clean nipples, such ideal conditions are frequently non-existent in many countries where the transition to bottle-feeding is occurring. As a result, in many Third World countries the abandonment of breast-feeding has been accompanied by a sharp rise in rates of infant malnutrition and death.

Although causes for the decline in maternal nursing include changing social values, rapid urbanization and modernization among formerly traditional societies (bottle feeding is largely an urban phenomenon in the developing world—most rural mothers continue to nurse their babies), and simple convenience, much of the blame in recent years has focused on the aggressive marketing techniques of multinational food companies. In both Africa and Latin America, corporations such as Nestle have conducted extensive radio advertising campaigns, supplemented by billboard and press advertisements, encouraging mothers to abandon breast-feeding in favor of "Lactogen," "Similac," or whatever product the company involved was promoting. In some areas, company representatives regularly visit maternity clinics or the homes of new mothers, distributing free formula samples, while in other places employment of nurses as sales girls conveys the impression that the formula is officially endorsed by the health profession. All too often, the women who are thus persuaded to give up nursing soon find that purchasing formula may consume 20-30% of the family budget. Often uneducated and unaware of the importance of proper dilution ratios, the mother may then water down the formula (often with impure water) to make it last longer. In some Latin American countries, mothers may add a popular brand of cornstarch to the diluted formula, assuming it has the food value of milk because it looks like milk; in Indonesia a rice fluid is a commonly-used milk substitute when formula supplies run low.[9] Little wonder, then, that infants fed on such a diet soon show signs of malnutrition or develop gastrointestinal ailments. The phenomenon is so common in some African cities that certain hospitals feature beds labelled "Lactogen Syndrome." At one time in Freetown, Sierra Leone, all but 4 of 717 babies hospitalized for malnutrition were bottle-fed; in parts of Chile death rates among infants under the age of 3 months was three times greater among those fed infant formula.[10]

In 1977 an international coalition of non-governmental, non-profit, voluntary organizations initiated a consumer boycott of Nestle products in the U.S. and 9 other countries in an effort to pressure the world's largest food manufacturer to cease promoting the use of infant formula in Third World countries. Boycott organizers contended it was immoral for manufacturers to push the use of powdered formulas in areas of the world where most families have neither the money, the education, nor the high levels of sanitation needed to prepare them safely. In response to political pressures and to growing concern about infant feeding practices, the World Health Organization in 1981 proposed an international code to limit the marketing of infant formula in developing countries. This code was subsequently endorsed by 118 nations (though not by the U.S.; to the acute embarrassment of American nutrition advocates, the Reagan Administration's delegates to the WHO assembly cast the only negative vote on adoption of the code, citing its "blatant interference with the free market system"). The WHO International Code of Marketing of Breast-Milk Substitutes prohibits distribution of free samples or supplies to hospitals or to mothers; it also forbids any form of direct promotion of infant formulas to consumers.

In 1984, after protracted negotiations between Nestle and boycott organizers, the giant corporation signed an agreement endorsing the WHO Code's key provisions and the boycott was officially terminated. Unfortunately, the story of "Bottle Babies" does not conclude with ". . . and they lived happily everafter." The Code's provisions are voluntary and evidence has been growing that formula "dumping" and extensive TV advertising promoting bottle feeding as chic and modern are as widespread as ever—and as misleading. In the Philippines Nestle brochures claim that their Nestrogen formula "is health-giving for baby . . . cost saving for mommy." Motivated by UNICEF estimates that over a million babies annually die of malnutrition and diarrheal diseases associated with bottle feeding, the Minneapolis-based Action for Corporate Accountability, a successor of the groups which organized the original anti-Nestle protest, in October of 1988 announced resumption of the boycott and its expansion to include American Home Products (the #2 marketer of infant formulas in the Third World). For those who wonder why the group deems another boycott necessary, organizers have a straightforward answer—"because babies are still dying."

Prospects for Reducing World Hunger

When confronted with stark pictures of starving babies or cold statistics on the growing prevalence of malnutrition, the typical reaction among most Americans is to say, "Let's do something about it!"—send a donation to CARE, eat a vegetarian meal once a week, write a letter to a Congressman urging a "yes" vote on the next food aid bill. Certainly there has been no shortage on suggestions as to what might be done to ease the population-food crunch. Newspapers and magazines regularly describe the latest "solution" to the problem of world hunger. Some of the approaches being tried have real merit, as well as limitations, while others are merely wishful thinking. It's important that the public have some understanding of the key elements in the ongoing debate as to how best to eradicate hunger, since this issue is certain to assume even greater urgency in the years ahead. Some of the most frequently mentioned ways of increasing world food supply include:

Expanding the amount of land under cultivation

From the beginning of the Agricultural Revolution right up to the early 1950s, increasing acreage put to the plow was the major, often the only, way of increasing food supply. Expanding the amount of cultivated land was accomplished by clearing forests, terracing mountainsides, or building irrigation systems—all of which permitted hitherto unproductive lands to be farmed. During the 1950s the Soviet Union vastly increased its agricultural acreage by opening up the "virgin lands" of Kazakhstan (the impact of this massive project on the total Soviet harvest varies widely from year to year, however, because the region is subject to periodic droughts); at the same time the Chinese completed some major irrigation networks and thus substantially expanded their cultivated acreage. Since that time, significant increases in highly-productive farmland have been quite limited. The hard truth is that the world's prime farmland is in finite supply, and after approximately 10,000 years of agricultural expansion most good land is already being cultivated. Since the 1950s most of the additional land cleared for farming has been so-called "marginal land"—land which, because of its poor soil, erodability, or steep slope is incapable of sustaining moderately good yields over any extended period of time. Farmers who today are moving onto marginal lands, desperately trying to eke out a living for their families, do so only because the better lands are already overcrowded. The additional food which such lands will contribute to world harvests is negligible and the long-term ecological damage caused by removing the natural vegetative cover from such lands may eventually have an adverse impact on better lands elsewhere.

Some optimists look hopefully to areas of the world such as the Gangetic Plain of northern India, the Mekong River basin of Southeast Asia, the Niger basin in Africa, or the Amazon region in Brazil, envisioning these lands as future world breadbaskets (or rice bowls, as the case may be) if large irrigation projects could be developed there. Such schemes may be technologically possible (though ecologists worry about large-scale environmental disruption and possible climatic changes if such visions should become reality, especially regarding development of Amazonia), but would require huge amounts of capital investment, far beyond the financial capabilities of the nations involved. Extensive grassy areas in the central African nation of Sudan also look promising for greatly increased livestock and crop production—but only if the tsetse fly can be brought under control. Thus even in parts of the world where potentially productive lands remain uncultivated, the prospects for their future agricultural development are uncertain. The long time period and enormous financial commitment required continue to be major obstacles to turning their potential into a reality.[11]

When assessing the contribution that additional farm acres could make to the total world harvest, commentators frequently overlook the other side of the coin, i.e. the substantial amounts of good crop land which are currently being lost every year to erosion, desertification, salinization and water-logging of irrigated fields, and to urban development. It is now being recognized that the increase in world food production witnessed during the 1970s and early 1980s was achieved in part through plowing of marginal lands unsuitable for sustained cultivation and by over-irrigation which has resulted in drastic drawing-down of groundwater reserves in many areas. Today in many of the major grain-producing areas of the world, the cropland base is beginning to shrink as highly erodable lands are abandoned. The U.S. is now taking 11% of its farmland out of production because of excessively high erosion rates and the USDA estimates that 25% of irrigated cropland is threatened with falling water tables, a trend which could lead to their eventual reversion to pastureage or less-productive dryland farming. The following chapter will examine these trends in more detail, but it is important to bear in mind that while most of the lands currently being added to our agricultural base are marginal acres, those being lost are, for the most part, prime crop lands which will never be returned to production.

Food from the Sea

When one considers that 71% of the earth's surface is water, it's understandable that many people, confronted with the prospect of impending food shortages, look to the oceans as the source of apparently limitless high-quality animal protein. Such optimism seemed justified during the years between 1950-1970 when total world fish catch tripled, from about 21 million tons to 70 million tons (60 million tons of marine species, 10 million of freshwater fish) during that 20 year period. By the early 1970s, however, total catch of sea fish slipped slightly and then stabilized around 60 million tons annually where it has remained up to the present. Many marine scientists today estimate that the current harvest figure of traditional fish species probably represents the maximum amount we can expect to obtain on a sustained-yield basis. Any further increase in harvest tonnage would have to depend on utilization of species not widely fished at the present time—squids, lantern fish, or Antarctic krill, for example. More efficient utilization of present fish catch could also be achieved by promoting direct human consumption of some of the lower-grade fish which are currently being processed into fish meal for feeding poultry and livestock or into fish oil (over ⅓ of present world fish catch is used for such purposes, with corresponding food-energy loss in the conversion process; most fish species used for fish meal and oil, however, are types widely regarded as undesirable for human consumption).

Several problems confront those who advocate intensified efforts to increase the catch of table-grade ocean fish. **Depletion of stocks** due to over-fishing has resulted in the near-collapse of several important fisheries during the last few decades. Since the late 1960s in the northwest Atlantic, herring catches have dropped by 40%, halibut by 90%. In the early 1970s, overfishing, plus a shift in the Humboldt Current off the western coast of South America, reduced the anchovy catch (which had earlier elevated Peru to the #1 position among fishing nations) from 12 million tons annually to a mere 2 million—a level which has not risen appreciably since then.[12] Increasingly efficient "floating factories" utilized particularly by the Eastern European Communist-bloc nations and by Japan have greatly increased those countries' share of total catch but threaten the long-term viability of the industry, since they harvest young and mature fish indiscriminately and thus prevent a replenishing of fish stocks. Recent moves by a number of maritime nations, the U.S. included, to extend their territorial waters to the 200 mile limit were prompted in part by a desire to gain greater control over the predatory activities of foreign fishing fleets which were driving local fishermen out of business.

A second major concern relating to long-term viability of world fisheries is the growing extent of *pollution of the seas.* It has not yet been possible to demonstrate a decline in the abundance of entire species in the open ocean due solely to pollution, but experiments have shown that toxic contaminants such as hydrocarbons, heavy metals, and synthetic organic compounds—all common water pollutants—can kill or injure aquatic organisms. In localized environments, bays and estuaries for example, pollution and/or development have already had a severe impact on commercial fisheries production. Shellfish and crustacean populations are particularly susceptible to pollution of near-shore areas; if not directly killed by toxic contaminants, they are often declared unmarketable because of their threat to the health of human consumers. Examples of pollution-degraded fisheries range from the oyster beds of Chesapeake Bay to the mackerel of Russia's Black and Azov Seas, where the original stock of 50,000-100,000 mackerel has vanished, the polluted waters being termed "almost lifeless".[13] In the U.S., approximately 1.2% of our shellfisheries are lost annually due to legal closure of such areas resulting from pollution.[14]

Although at present only about 2% of the world's calories are derived from fish or shellfish, about 14% of the world's protein comes directly from aquatic sources, more indirectly in the form of animal feed. Thus any decrease in fisheries production would have a significant impact on human nutrition, especially in countries like Japan which utilize marine products to a far greater extent than does the U.S. One bright ray of hope in an otherwise clouded outlook is the notable growth in aquaculture ("fish farming") during the past decade. Employed primarily with freshwater species, to a lesser degree with marine types, aquaculture yielded less than 10% of the total world fish harvest in 1975—but this figure was double that of 5 years earlier. Some countries, notably Israel, Japan, China, and the Philippines now obtain a significant portion of their fish products from aquaculture. Aquaculture in the U.S., while lagging considerably behind that of the above-mentioned countries, is steadily expanding and already accounts for most of our catfish and crayfish production, ¼ of the salmon harvest, and 40% of oyster production. Trout are also raised successfully by means of aquaculture.[15] A report issued a few years ago by the National Academy of Sciences concluded that while aquaculture in the

U.S. will have only a minimal impact on food production in the near-term, in the future it will be a significant means of increasing protein supplies—but only if research and development programs are expanded and better support and direction provided by the federal government.[16]

Reduction of Food Losses

Implementation of better methods of handling and protecting food between the time it is harvested and the time it appears on the consumer's plate may not sound particularly exciting—rat-proof grain bins are not the stuff of which poetry is made—but, in the short-run at least, such simple, well-understood measures could do more than anything else to increase the availability of food in the marketplace. Each year enormous amounts of harvested foods are lost to pests and spoilage, particularly in tropical countries. Rats, birds, insects, and molds all consume or render unfit for human use large amounts of stored foods which would otherwise have been available for people. Cultural practices are partially responsible for such losses. In many countries grains are stored in the open or in easily-penetrated sacks or bins. Lack of adequate refrigeration promotes spoilage, while poor transport facilities delay rapid movement of food from fields to consumers, thereby increasing chances of loss or spoilage. The FAO estimates that the development of improved storage and transport facilities alone could increase market availability of food by 20% or more in the Third World countries.[17]

Improving Yields per Acre

During the last 40 years, the biggest gains in world food supply were obtained not through adding more acres to our cropland base but by dramatically increasing per-acre yields on existing farmlands. In the U.S. during this time period, yields of wheat, rice, barley, and rye doubled, that of corn and peanuts increased 2½ times, and an acre of sorghum quadrupled its production.[18] These enormous gains were accomplished through the application of research and technological improvements gradually developed and perfected since the late 1800s, the major elements of which included new hybrid crop varieties, better farm machinery, tremendous expansion in the use of chemical fertilizers and pesticides, and increased use of irrigation.

The U.S. was not alone in realizing major gains in agricultural productivity during the past several decades. In the late 1960s, twenty years of plant breeding experiments to improve grain yields in tropical and semi-tropical regions resulted in the development of several strains of so-called "miracle wheat" and "miracle rice" which heralded the advent of what journalists dubbed "The Green Revolution". Within a few years after its introduction, the new hybrid wheat was giving farmers from Mexico to India yields 2 to 3 times greater than the best formerly obtained from traditional strains. Since the introduction of the first miracle wheat in India in 1968, that country has more than doubled its wheat production. Pakistan, Turkey, Tunisia, and Mexico also eagerly adopted the new technology and witnessed a corresponding surge in their wheat production statistics. Similarly, the miracle rice varieties developed at the International Rice Research Institute in the Philippines have approximately doubled the yields of this grain in situations where the hybrid seeds, along with proper fertilization and adequate irrigation were employed.

The spectacular gains of the Green Revolution led many political leaders during the early 1970s to relax on the population issue, assuming that continued dramatic increases in food production had erased the Malthusian image of starving millions. Agricultural experts, however, are less sanguine regarding the food-population crunch and warn that it would be a fatal mistake to assume that plant scientists will be able to achieve another doubling of the grain yield any time soon. Indeed, most food scientists agree there are no foreseeable "miracle technologies" lurking on the sidelines, ready to provide another quantum jump in world food production such as occurred during the 1950-1984 period. Norman Borlaug, often referred to as the "Father of the Green Revolution" for his key role in developing miracle wheat, estimates that between 75-85% of the maximum genetic yield potential of wheat has already been achieved. As supporting evidence he cites the fact that during the past 12 years or so, massive wheat-breeding programs have resulted in only marginal yield improvements; Borlaug foresees future gains coming in ever-smaller increments and being increasingly difficult to achieve.[19] Supporting this

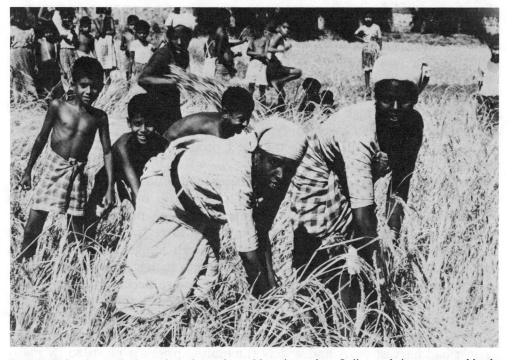

Traditional farming methods, such as those pictured here in southern India, are being augmented by the hybrid seeds of the "Green Revolution" which, along with increased use of agrichemicals and expanded irrigation systems, have substantially boosted yields per acre since the early 1970s. [*Author's Photo*]

outlook, Prof. Neal Jensen of Cornell University predicts that, in the U.S. at least, the increases in wheat yields which began in the mid-1930s will soon start to level off and we will encounter an absolute yield ceiling, resulting eventually in a widening gap between food production and people production.[20] Any absolute ceiling on crop production, assuming that such a concept is a valid one, would undoubtedly be reached sooner in the U.S. and other industrialized countries simply because improved varieties and modern farming techniques, the proper combinations of which have resulted in our record yields, have been in use longer here than elsewhere, leaving less margin for further improvement. As just one example of this, take the case of nitrogen fertilizer use in the American Midwest. Heavy applications of fertilizer have accounted for a substantial portion of the increase in corn yields witnessed since 1950, but in recent years the Law of Diminishing Returns appears to be making its presence felt. During the 1950s and 1960s, for every extra pound of nitrogen fertilizer applied a farmer could expect a yield increase of 15-20 extra bushels of corn. Today that increment is 5-7 bushels and falling. Such statistics imply that further increases in fertilizer application will produce only minimal boosts in yields per acre in the Corn Belt.

In many Third World nations prospects for significant increases in crop yields, even in the face of maximum *genetic* yield barriers, are good if the use of existing production technology becomes more widespread. Better utilization of pesticides and fertilizers, attention to proper land preparation and erosion control, wider use of improved seed varieties, more attention to efficient water use and proper planting dates, adoption of government financial policies which will encourage production of the new technologies and make it profitable for farmers to adopt them—all offer hope for increased crop yields in the developing countries. Such changes do not occur automatically, however. They require a continuing high level of government interest and financial support to assure that potential becomes reality; whether such support will be forthcoming will in large measure determine the food production outlook in the years immediately ahead.

Thus although the potential for increasing food production exists in many chronically food-short areas, continued rapid rates of population growth demand that Third World governments must give priority attention to modernizing their agricultural sectors in order to realize this potential. In addition, bountiful harvests alone will not eradicate hunger. By the late 1970s the Green Revolution had increased production to such an extent in countries such as India and Pakistan that those nations were declared as being self-sufficient in food grains; yet millions of their people still suffer the ravages of malnutrition because they are too poor to purchase the food they need. Finally, as population pressures mount, establishment of food reserves as a buffer against bad harvest years and widely fluctuating prices is regarded by many food experts as an urgent necessity. Yet despite much rhetoric, the bulk of world food reserves (calculated as carryover stocks plus cropland idled under

U.S. farm programs) consist of surpluses within the United States and in 1988 were equivalent to about 54 days of world consumption. This amount is regarded as adequate to maintain relatively stable prices in the world market, but could be depleted rapidly if there were a serious food emergency in any of the major grain-growing regions of the world.

As humanity moves into the 1990s, we are faced with demographic projections indicating that global population will continue to climb by more than 90 million each year—at a time when growth in per capita food supply has levelled off or even declined in some key areas of the world. With a shrinking cropland base, falling water tables, little promise for major new breakthroughs in yield-enhancing farm technologies, and the long-term specter of significant climatic change in some of the world's most productive agricultural regions (see Ch. 11—"Greenhouse Effect"), farmers may be hard-pressed to meet future food demands at prices hungry people can afford. More vigorous efforts at stabilizing population size and reversing land degradation are urgently needed if we are to prove Malthus wrong.[21]

Box 4–2

Supercorn And Supercows

With the 1980 Supreme Court ruling (Diamond vs. Chakrabarty) confirming patent rights for living organisms, what some commentators have dubbed the "Second Green Revolution" was off and running. During the 1970s significant advances in recombinant DNA techniques had made it possible to "genetically engineer" new forms of life—to insert hereditary material from one organism (most commonly a virus or bacterium) into another species, thereby producing a "designer" microbe, mouse—whatever. It was the landmark Court decision regarding patent rights that made such painstaking techniques profitable, however, and in the 1980s the new field of biotechnology began to grow by leaps and bounds. Comprising methods of manipulating living organisms for a specific purpose, biotechnology offers the potential for significant advances in crop and livestock production, as well as for controlling human genetic disorders—but at the same time raises fears of scientists' "playing God" by regarding life forms as mere commodities to be altered at will.

While controversy over the ethical aspects of biotechnology is likely to simmer on for years, corporate giants such as Monsanto, Ciba-Geigy, Unilever, Royal Dutch-Shell, and dozens of other chemical, pharmaceutical, and energy companies around the world are funding multi-billion dollar research and development efforts to commercialize the supercrops and supercows promised by the genetic engineers. While efforts are still in the preliminary stage, by 1988 more than 2 dozen field tests of genetically-engineered organisms had been conducted and it is widely believed that by the turn of the century biotechnology's impact on agriculture will be significant.

The most rapid progress to date has been with genetically-engineered plants and plant-bacteria combinations. Field experiments are now being carried out on corn plants within whose vascular tissues lurk genetically-altered bacteria, waiting to attack any luckless corn borer larva which decides to nibble on them; in Australia testing is underway on a high-protein strain of alfalfa; Dutch researchers have developed a potato variety which carries a foreign gene enabling the plant to fight off virus infections; and in Louisiana a scientist is striving to produce the "perfect potato"—one which, through gene transfer, could produce all 8 essential amino acids, giving it the nutritional value of meat. Many of the world's major food plants are now the subjects of intensive genetic research, with improvement efforts focused on goals such as improving their nutritional value, pest resistance, salt tolerance, or drought resistance. Some laboratories are striving for genetically-engineered corn plants with higher photosynthetic efficiency or cereals that could manufacture their own nitrogen, thereby reducing the need for chemical fertilizers.

Gene-tinkering with livestock lags behind that directed at crop plants, but researchers are excited about future possibilities. Since 1981 when a mouse with a rabbit gene attained fame as the first transgenic animal, the pace of genetic research on livestock has accelerated. Work is progressing on pigs which are 30% more efficient at converting feed into meat; mice have been given a sheep gene which allows them to produce higher protein milk (not that mice-breeders are intending to go into the dairy business—the experiment simply showed that transfer of genes into dairy animals represents real potential for producing milk with higher nutritional value). Genetic engineers envision custom-designed chickens which are disease-resistant and lay larger eggs, supercows which could double milk production, genetically improved salmon—perhaps even caterpillar farms for generating medically-useful human proteins!

Exciting as these developments sound, what hope do they provide for increasing world food supply at a time when the number of new mouths to be fed is inexorably escalating? Opinion seems divided among experts who anticipate super-high yielding crops guaranteed to satisfy the food demands of teeming millions and others who welcome a badly needed new weapon in humanity's war against hunger, but are convinced the fruits of biotechnology cannot fill the projected food gap. One of the most articulate spokesmen for the latter viewpoint, Lester Brown of the Worldwatch Institute points out that developing nitrogen-fixing grains, for example, would help farmers reduce their dependency on chemical fertilizers, but would not enhance yields, since the metabolic energy the plant expends in capturing nitrogen can no longer go into seed production. Public impressions to the contrary, genetic engineering is not magic, but simply represents a faster, more precise way of doing what plant breeders have been doing for thousands of years.

There is no doubt that biotechnology offers immense potential for helping farmers reduce dependence on costly, environmentally damaging agrochemicals; for alleviating nutritional deficiencies; for permitting use of lands too dry or waters too salty for cultivation of existing crop varieties. Whether the dream will become a reality, particularly for poor Third World farmers who most need the new technologies, is an open question. Because the lion's share of research is being conducted by giant multinational firms who have been rapidly acquiring seed companies and livestock genetics firms and claiming exclusive patent rights for the new species they create, there is a very real possibility that Third World countries will be barred access to the "Second Green Revolution". Throughout the industrialized world, gene power is bound to corporate power, and developing countries which lack the scientific and technical infrastructure to carry out their own research programs may find themselves growing ever more dependent on imported agricultural commodities and technologies they can ill afford. It is also possible that corporate goals of genetic research will differ from public goals. Companies, after all, are in business to make a profit and it might be too much to expect that a chemical company, for example, would deliberately develop a designer plant that no longer needs any agrochemical inputs. For this reason, it shouldn't come as a surprise that the first genetically-engineered plant to go commercial is one which is resistant to herbicides, permitting farmers to continue using chemical weed-killers without fear of damaging their crop.[22]

Nevertheless, whatever its potential pitfalls, biotechnology promises to revolutionize the future agricultural landscape. Whether it proves to be the panacea for solving world food problems remains to be seen.

REFERENCES

[1]U.S. Dept. of Agriculture (USDA), Foreign Agricultural Services (FAS), "World Grain *Situation and Outlook*", Washington, DC, August 1988; Brown, Lester, "The Changing World *Food Prospect: The Nineties and Beyond*", Worldwatch Paper 85, Worldwatch Institute, October 1988.

[2]Hopper, W. David, "Recent Trends in World Food and Population", *Future Dimensions of World Food and Population,* ed. Richard Woods, Westview Press, 1981.

[3]Report of the Presidential Commission on World Hunger, April 1980.

[4]Ehrlich, Paul R., Anne H. Ehrlich, and John P. Holdren, *Ecoscience,* W.H. Freeman and Company, 1977.

[5]Ibid.

[6]Berg, Alan, "A Strategy to Reduce Malnutrition", *Poverty and Basic Needs,* World Bank, September 1980.

[7]Sommer, Alfred, "Xerophthalmia, the Deadly Disease", *American Journal of Ophthalmology,* vol. 99, no. 2, Feb. 15, 1985.

[8]Pino, John A., and Andres Martinez, "The Contribution of Livestock to the World Protein Supply", *Future Dimensions of World Food and Population,* ed. Richard Woods, Westview Press, 1981.

[9]Berg, Alan, *The Nutrition Factor,* The Brookings Institution, 1973.

[10]"Kicking the Bottle", *The New Internationalist,* 1975.

[11]Borlaug, Norman, "Using Plants to Meet World Food Needs", *Future Dimensions of World Food and Population,* ed. Richard Woods, Westview Press, 1981.

[12]Brown, Lester, "World Food Resources and Population: the Narrowing Margin", *Population Bulletin,* vol. 36, no. 3, September 1981.

[13]Ibid.

[14]Sindermann, Carl J., "Aquatic Animal Protein Food Resources—Actual and Potential", *Future Dimensions of World Food and Population,* ed. Richard Woods, Westview Press, 1981.

[15]Ibid.

[16]National Academy of Sciences, "Aquaculture in the United States", U.S. Government Printing Office, Washington, DC, 1978.

[17]Food and Agriculture Organization, "State of Food and Agriculture", 1974.

[18]Borlaug, op. cit.

[19]Ibid.

[20]Jensen, Neal F., "Limits to Growth in World Food Production", *Science,* vol. 201, July 28, 1978.

[21]Brown, Lester, "The Growing Grain Gap", *World Watch,* vol. 1, no. 5, September/October 1988.

[22]Doyle, Jack, *Altered Harvest,* Viking Press, 1985; Cowen, Robert C., *"Biotechnology—Perfect Potatoes and Supercows",* The Christian Science Monitor, June 1, 2, and 3, 1988; Carey, John, "Brave New World of Super-Plants", *International Wildlife,* vol. 16, no. 6, November/December 1986.

5

Fall-Out From the "Population Bomb": Impacts on Human Resources and Ecosystems

"Man has lost the capacity to foresee and to forestall. He
will end by destroying the earth."
—Albert Schweitzer

Certainly the issue of how to feed a billion additional mouths in the year 2000, when close to half a billion of our present population is malnourished, looms as a monumental task for future world leaders. However, there are many other equally pressing problems inherent in a situation of rapid population growth—problems which are less dramatic and less publicized than famine, yet nearly as devastating in their impact on human well-being.

Some Consequences of Population Growth

Unemployment—Early on a July morning in 1987, the townspeople of Sierra Blanca, Texas, were horrified to discover in their midst a grim example of the personal risk some of their southern neighbors are willing to take in a desperate search for employment. That morning during a routine Border Patrol check of freight cars at the railway station, the inspector found 18 illegal aliens from

Mexico dead inside a locked steel-walled boxcar, killed by lack of oxygen and heatstroke as temperatures in the car soared to 120°F. A lone survivor described how the group had paid to be smuggled aboard the train at El Paso, destined for the bright lights of Dallas. The train had been delayed overnight in Sierra Blanca, the smuggler whose job it was to release them from the locked car never arrived, and thus ended the young men's dreams of a better life in the U.S. Since illegal border crossings all too frequently end in tragedy (this incident was unusual only in the number of people involved), why do individuals continue to expose themselves to such danger? Simply because, if successful, they can earn more money in a day in America than they could in a week in Mexico. They can find jobs in the restaurants of Dallas when none are available in their homeland. In spite of tough new immigration laws, similar, though usually less tragic, episodes occur daily as desperate Latin Americans pour into the U.S., legally or illegally, in search of employment.[1] News photos of poverty-stricken Haitians arriving in Florida in dangerously overloaded boats has in recent years dramatized the fact that provision of jobs for ever-growing populations is already a problem of crisis proportions, particularly in the underdeveloped countries. In the past 25 years the working age population of most such nations has doubled (in comparison with a 45% increase in the U.S.) and, since the creation of job opportunities has not kept pace, unemployment rates are climbing rapidly. Over the next two decades, the demand for jobs by new workers is projected to take a sharp upturn because of the very large number of children who will be of working age within a few more years. This rapid growth in the labor force also means that a large proportion of all workers are young and inexperienced. In Mexico, for example, 54% of all working-age people are under 30 years of age; in highly industrialized Japan the corresponding figure is 32%.[2] Since inexperienced workers are generally less productive, average productivity is lower with a youthful labor force. As a result, both per capita income and resources available for new investment are lower than they would otherwise be. According to Lester Brown of the Worldwatch Institute, for every 1% increase in the labor force, a 3% increase in the rate of economic growth is needed to generate jobs. Thus countries which are experiencing growth rates in the range of 3% annually need a 9% economic growth rate just to maintain the status quo. Unfortunately, with the world-wide business slump, economic growth rates have been falling rather than rising during recent years; consequently, fewer jobs are being created at a time when more than ever are needed. Large armies of unemployed and underemployed mean an increase in hunger and malnutrition, since people who have no income can't purchase food even when in plentiful supply. More ominous, unemployed youth—especially the educated unemployed—represent a serious and growing threat to the political stability of the global community.

Literacy—It seems paradoxical that after decades of intensive efforts at building schools and training teachers there are more illiterates in the world today than ever before (the *percentage* of illiteracy dropped from 44% to 34%

between 1950 and 1970, but total number of illiterates increased from 700 million to 800 million). Not surprisingly, illiteracy is most prevalent in the areas undergoing high rates of population increase. Although most developing countries spend about the same percentage of their GNP on primary education as do the industrialized nations (approximately 1.7% GNP), the fact that the developing countries have proportionally so many more children of primary school age (about 25% of the total population) than do the industrialized nations (15%) means that the poor countries must distribute their resources much more thinly. Spending on education per child is considerably less in the developing nations than in the developed ones both because their GNP is lower and because the amount they do spend has to be divided among so many more children. As a result, millions of children in poor countries never have a chance to attend school at all, while many others drop out of primary school without ever learning basic reading and writing skills.

Housing—The slums encircling Third World cities and rural shanties as well illustrate that the rising demand for building materials and the physical space on which to erect a dwelling have exceeded the financial capabilities of growing numbers to live in a decent home. In many cities it is not uncommon to see families living in packing crates, lean-tos, or other jerry-built structures assembled from whatever materials could be begged, borrowed, or stolen. Along the highway from Bombay's Santa Cruz International Airport into the city the author has observed an entire colony of pipe-dwellers—people who were living in large clay drainage pipes which had been set along the roadside prior to construction work, but were occupied by squatters before they could be put to their intended use. Families moved in, hung rags over the pipe openings for privacy, and doubtlessly considered themselves fortunate to have such a convenient shelter from the monsoon rains in a city where thousands are born, live, and die on the sidewalks. Housing shortages currently plague many industrialized countries as well and are currently causing considerable political turmoil in cities like West Berlin and Amsterdam where young anti-establishment squatters are defying municipal authorities by occupying abandoned buildings slated for demolition. Nor can the U.S. afford to be smug about other nations' housing shortages, as the crisis of the homeless in American cities has become a major national issue in recent years.

Poverty—High rates of population growth and poverty are mutually reinforcing; rapid population growth within a nation reduces the per capita availability of investment resources, thus slowing the creation of jobs, schools, and public health facilities. At the family level, large numbers of children reduce the amount of time and money parents can devote to each individual child. In many countries, rapid population growth has offset any economic growth and has prevented any gains in per capita income. In general, the higher a country's fertility is, the lower is its GNP and average life expectancy (obviously there are some exceptions to this pattern, oil-rich Kuwait being a notable example). At the same time, high infant mortality, high illiteracy rates, lack of women's

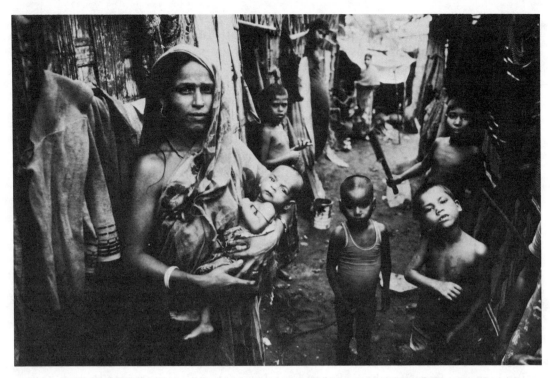

Women and children who live in a slum area of Dhaka. [*UN Photo 154361/Kevin Bubriski*]

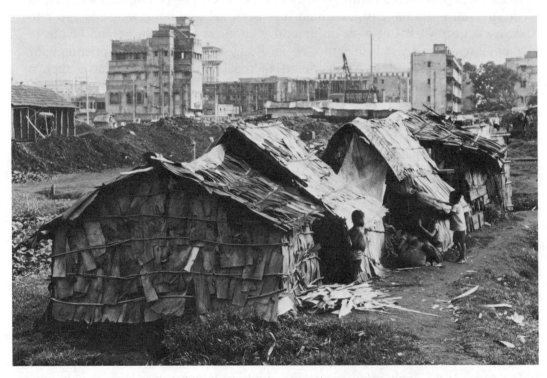

Slums of Calcutta. [*UN Photo 153,012/Oddbjorn Monsen*]

employment opportunities outside the home, lack of low-cost family planning services—all common among the poorest segments of society in developing nations—contribute to the likelihood that poor parents will continue to produce large numbers of children. Sociologists and government planners are still trying to devise a way of breaking this vicious cycle.

Political unrest—As more and more people exert increasing pressure on the world's finite amount of land, mineral resources, water, etc., conflict both among and within nations will result. As indicated earlier, many current world tensions are intimately related to problems of over-population. As human numbers continue to climb, it will be surprising indeed if civil turmoil and international conflict do not grow apace. In an age when both nuclear and chemical weapons are proliferating, nations may not be content to starve peacefully.[3]

Impacts of Growth on the Stability of Ecosystems

Commentators who optimistically predict that science and technology will somehow miraculously provide a way of producing ever-increasing amounts of food, fiber, and lumber to sustain the demands of additional billions of people ignore the growing evidence that in many parts of the world large human and livestock populations already have exceeded the carrying capacity of the land itself, resulting in a steady deterioration of that land's ability to support life. In effect, at a time when we are trying to produce more and more from a given land area to sustain growing human numbers, the activities of those populations are damaging natural ecosystems to the extent that they are becoming incapable of supporting present numbers, much less future additions.

Retrogression

Although under natural conditions succession, as we've seen, proceeds in a unidirectional pattern toward increasingly complex ecological relationships, under the pressure of human activities the normal pattern can be reversed. A good example of human impact on successional processes can be seen today in many parts of the world where over-grazing by livestock is gradually transforming pasture lands into desert-like conditions. Grassland communities are well-adapted to a moderate level of grazing by herbivores; herds of antelopes, bison, wild horses, etc., have for millennia been the dominant animals in the grassland biome, evolving and adapting in partnership with the native plants on which they are dependent. However, when human herdsmen increase the size of their herds and flocks beyond a certain size, or when they introduce types of grazing animals foreign to a particular plant community, the resulting pressure on that community often leads to degradation of the ecosystem. The effects of over-grazing are first seen in the declining populations of those plant species least able to tolerate the increased cropping. As these plants disappear, species more tolerant of heavy grazing pressures are then relieved of competition and expand to fill the niche vacated by the more vulnerable types. The loss of the latter, however, results in an over-all reduction in the height, biomass, and total coverage of the grassland. If over-grazing persists, even the more resistant native plants will be unable to withstand the pressure and give way to invader weed species which were not members of the original community. Such plants are generally much inferior to the native plants in nutritive qualities and as a result the vitality of the livestock causing the damage is adversely affected. Eventually, the weeds themselves may be trampled to such an extent that they, too, are reduced in coverage. The soil, thus exposed to the forces of wind and water erosion, may be worn away, leaving a barren mud flat or rocky hillside, devoid of any community.[4]

In such a series of events we can see the reversal of the trends which characterize succession. This sort of human-produced "backward succession" is called *Retrogression*, a term which doesn't necessarily imply a step-by-step retracing of the stages in a normal succession (since in some cases grassland invaders may not be herbaceous weeds but woody shrubs, resulting in transformation of pasture to a shrub community), but rather the reduction of the community in complexity, biomass, etc., as a result of stress. Unfortunately, as we shall see, retrogression is an increasingly common occurrence in many parts of the world today. While degradation of ecosystems potentially could occur anywhere, certain natural areas are more vulnerable to long-lasting destruction than others. Biomes such as tundra, desert, tropical rain forest, and arid grasslands are more easily damaged and take much longer to recover from disruption than does, for example, temperate deciduous forest. Because several of these areas today encompass the homelands of many millions of people whose well-being, and indeed survival, depends on the continued productivity of their land, it is important for us to take a closer look at some specific ways in which humans, consciously or not, are currently engaged in the radical altering of ecosystems.

Soil Erosion

Throughout much of the world, including the rich farmlands of the American Midwest, the fertile topsoil which is the basis of agricultural productivity is thinning at an alarming rate. Some degree of erosion is, of course, a natural process and occurs even in the absence of human intervention. Poor agricultural practices, however, greatly increase the rate of soil loss, and when that loss exceeds the rate at which new topsoil is formed (through the gradual decomposition of organic matter), then the layer of topsoil becomes thinner and thinner until it disappears completely, leaving only the unproductive subsoil or, in extreme cases, bare rock. Topsoil loss has a direct negative impact on cropland productivity, though in recent decades the relationship between soil erosion and diminishing yields has been largely masked, in North America at least, by the greatly expanded use of chemical fertilizers. We have, in a sense, been

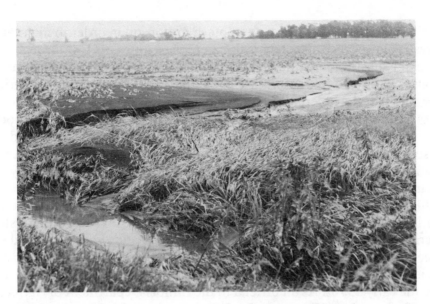

Sheet erosion after heavy rain robs farmland of valuable topsoil and causes water pollution and sedimentation problems in nearby streams and ditches. [*Gary Fak, Soil Conservation Service*]

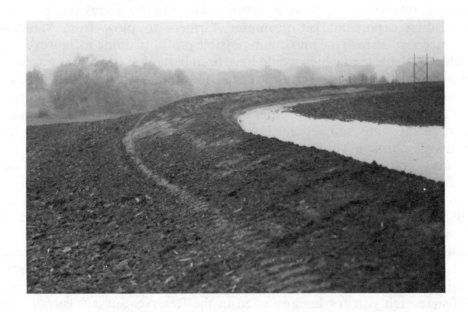

An effective erosion-control method is the construction of grass ridge terraces such as the one pictured here. A terrace reduces soil runoff by shortening the length of the slope and diverting water in a horizontal direction. When planted in perennial grasses, the approximately 10-foot-wide area has the additional benefit of providing valuable wildlife habitat. [*Gary Fak, Soil Conservation Service*]

Fall-Out From the ''Population Bomb'' **129**

substituting chemical nitrogen and potash for topsoil in order to maintain good harvests. However, while chemicals can replace nutrients lost through erosion, they can't substitute for the lost organic material necessary for maintaining a porous, healthy soil structure. In 1981 the U.S. Department of Agriculture estimated that the inherent productivity of 34% of the farmlands in the United States are decreasing because of high erosion rates.[5] Some scientists today are of the opinion that use of chemical pesticides and fertilizers has so damaged the soil that the degradation may be irreversible and further application of advanced technology can no longer compensate for topsoil loss. They predict we can expect a future drop in per acre yields if erosion trends aren't reversed.[6]

Although erosion-control methods such as contour plowing, terracing, planting of windbreaks, grass waterways, and the like are well-understood by American farmers, economic realities and the demands for agricultural exports to feed growing populations overseas and to ease U.S. balance-of-payments problems have combined to promote record levels of topsoil loss in the U.S. since the early 1970s. As an official in the Illinois Department of Agriculture is fond of remarking, "For every bushel of corn we ship overseas, we send 1.5 bushels of topsoil down the Mississippi River." In the push for expanded production, the traditional practice of crop rotation was abandoned in favor of continuous cropping of corn or soybeans, a practice which greatly increases erosion rates, since this leaves the soil surface without any plant cover during a considerable portion of the year. Termination of the Soil Bank program and an expanding export market prompted farmers to plow from "fencepost-to-fencepost" to reap the maximum possible profit. In doing so, however, much highly-erodable land which would have been better left in pasture was brought into production—and promptly began to wash away. In the Midwest fall plowing came into vogue and contributed to substantial amounts of erosion by both wind and water during winter and early spring. Efforts are now underway at both the state and federal level to reduce soil loss to tolerable levels, primarily through voluntary adoption of conservation tillage and no-till farming, practices which involve leaving large amounts of crop residue on the surface of the soil rather than plowing it under. Erosion control efforts in the U.S. were given a major boost when Congress passed the Food Security Act of 1985 which created the Conservation Reserve. Under this landmark program, both excessive production and soil loss are being curbed by taking at least 40 million acres (approximately 11% of all U.S. cropland) of highly erodable lands out of row crop production, converting them to pastures or woodlands. To implement the program, the USDA has agreed to compensate farmers roughly $50/acre each year for land enrolled in the Reserve. Surveys carried out on lands idled just one year after the program's initiation indicated a sharp decline in soil loss on such lands, from an average of 29 tons/acre to just 2 tons. On acres not enrolled in the Reserve but still experiencing unacceptably high erosion rates, the Act requires farmers to develop an approved soil conservation program by 1990 or risk losing their eligibility for farm program benefits such as crop insurance and price support programs.[7]

Currently the U.S. is the only major agricultural nation pursuing systematic efforts to reduce excessive soil erosion, yet outside this country the situation is equally serious. In both China and the USSR, soil erosion is endangering future gains in crop production. Indian agronomists estimate their country is losing 5 billion tons of topsoil annually, almost double the soil loss in the U.S. where the cropland area is about the same. The U.S. embassy in Ethiopia reports erosion is costing that nation's hard-pressed highland farmers 1 billion tons of topsoil every year.[8]

Between one-fifth and one-third of the world's cropland is estimated to be losing topsoil at a rate which will, over the long term, result in marked loss of productivity. In many Third World countries, population pressures on the land have forced farmers to forego the traditional practice of allowing the land to lie fallow every few years—short-term need for additional food has to take priority over good soil stewardship. As population mounts, many land-hungry farmers are forced to cultivate marginal lands, often on steep hillsides or semi-desert lands which are basically unsuitable for cultivation and erode rapidly. Eventually productivity of these fields falls to such an extent that the land has to be abandoned.[9]

Deforestation

For the last ten thousand years humans have been cutting and burning woodlands at an ever-increasing pace in their quest for additional farmland, fuel, and building material. Experts estimate world forests now cover somewhere between half and two-thirds their extent prior to *Homo sapiens'* arrival on the scene. As the rate of forest loss accelerates, so do pressures on ecosystems as soil erosion, species loss, even climate change become increasingly apparent. Nowhere is the threat more evident than in the world's tropical rain forests, lush laboratories of life, home to more than half of all the plant and animal species on earth. In the first comprehensive survey of tropical forests carried out by the United Nations Food and Agricultural Organization in 1981, researchers found that in country after country trees were being felled much faster than they were being replaced. In Third World tropics as a whole, the ratio was 10:1; in Asia, 5:1; and in Africa, 29:1. Recent satellite data indicate the picture is even more bleak than the 1981 survey's figures indicate. In India alone, remote sensing data reveal that forest loss is 9 times greater than previously estimated. A new FAO tropical forest inventory is just getting underway and within a few years should give a more accurate picture of deforestation rates. Current estimates suggest that fully 40 million acres of forests, a land area roughly equivalent to the state of Pennsylvania, are destroyed each year.[10] Indeed, Paul W. Richards, an expert on tropical rain forests, warns that if present trends continue, the tropical forest ecosystem world-wide will have virtually disappeared by the end of this century.[11] Elsewhere, in the semi-arid regions of Asia, Africa, and Latin America where forests have always been scanty, existing trees have almost entirely vanished. Only in Europe and, quite recently, in North America are forests being managed on a sustained-yield basis.

The largest single cause of deforestation today, as in the past, is the clearing of land for agriculture. The population pressures behind this trend and the ecological damage caused by exploitation of marginal lands not suited for sustained cultivation have already been described. A second major contributor to deforestation, also a direct result of human population growth, is the gathering of wood for fuel. For approximately 90% of the people in the world's less-developed nations, today's energy crisis is the scarcity of firewood. In most tropical countries wood is used largely for cooking, but in colder climates and mountainous regions it's used for heating as well. Spiralling population growth rates in such nations have boosted demand for firewood to such an extent that trees are being cut at a pace which far outraces nature's ability to grow new ones. As a result, treeless areas around towns and villages throughout Africa, Asia, and Latin America are expanding rapidly as desperate people gather every twig and sometimes even leaves and bark in their never-ending search for fuel. In once heavily-forested lands such as Nepal, whole mountainsides are being stripped by villagers who now spend most of the day searching for a supply of firewood which two decades ago could have been gathered in an hour. The investment in time and physical energy required just to obtain enough fuel to cook the family meal has thus increased tremendously in just one generation. Of greater concern to Nepali officials, however, and to their counterparts in the vast Indian subcontinent to the south is the fact that the progressive denudation of the Himalayan slopes is resulting in a massive increase in soil erosion in this ecologically fragile mountain region. As a result, not only is the productive capacity of the land rapidly decreasing, but also much more frequent and severe flooding, with corresponding heavy loss of life, is occurring downstream in the river valleys of northern India, Pakistan, and Bangladesh due to greatly increased amounts of runoff in the headwaters area of the Ganges, Indus, and Brahmaputra Rivers. The devastating floods which left 25 million Bengalis homeless and killed 1200 during the 1988 monsoon season in Bangladesh represented an "unnatural disaster" caused by increased runoff from the denuded Himalayan watershed upstream and increased rates of siltation in lowland deltas, diminishing their water-holding capacity. While flooding of such severity used to occur perhaps twice in a century, five "50-year floods" occurred during the 1980s and threaten to become a regular occurrence if deforestation in the Himalayas is not reversed. As the supply of fuelwood continues to diminish, prices rise accordingly, imposing additional burdens on already impoverished populations. In the West African nation of Niger, for example, an average laborer's family must spend close to 25% of its income for firewood; in neighboring Burkina Faso the figure may approach 30%. Where people can't afford such sums, women and children spend much of their time scrounging the countryside for anything burnable—dry grass, fallen leaves,

Box 5-1

Inferno in the Amazon

Fires are raging across Brazil, both literally and figuratively. In the western Amazonian province of Rondonia, where Brazil rubs elbows with Bolivia, 30,000 square miles of virgin forest was burned during one summer season. Brazilian scientists at the country's Space Research Center counted 170,000 separate fires in the province—as many as 5,000 on a single day. Rondonia, which faces the real possibility of losing all its tree cover before the turn of the century, has already experienced deforestation over 23% of its area. While an influx of landless peasant farmers from the impoverished Northeast are a part of the problem, 80% of the devastation is being caused by large cattle ranchers who receive generous tax breaks from the government to clear the forest. When the fragile tropical soils wear out within a few years, the ranchers simply burn down more trees.

The situation in Rondonia is finally beginning to provoke criticism of government policies both within Brazil and abroad. Not only is there profound concern about the effect of tree loss on species preservation—the Amazonian rain forest is one of the world's richest ecosystems—but expressions of alarm are also being voiced about the impact of Rondonia's fires on global warming trends, the so-called "Greenhouse Effect" (see Ch. 11). In 1988 the New York Times editorialized that the burnings in the Amazon now contribute fully one-tenth of the planet's CO_2 emissions.

Not surprisingly, when one country encourages an activity that endangers global climatic stability, the world community is not likely to remain silent. Outcries of protest from the U.S. and European nations have bolstered the hopes of Brazilian environmentalists who have watched the pace of forest destruction with anguish. They have also prompted reforms at the World Bank, where a newly-created department now must pass on the environmental merits of all its projects before loan funds are disbursed. Several international lending institutions are now in the process of devising positive alternatives to deforestation. Such concepts as "extractive reserves"—forest areas permanently set aside for production of tree crops such as Brazilnuts or rubber—are being tested on a trial basis. The U.S. Congress has advanced a proposal for "debt for nature" swaps, whereby the Brazilian government would set aside selected areas as nature reserves in return for cancellation of a portion of Brazil's multi-billion dollar foreign debt.

While such proposals superficially appear to indicate movement in the right direction, irritable rumblings emanating from Brasilia, the nation's capital, suggest that the international attention being focused on the Amazon is increasingly viewed in some political and military circles as blatant interference in Brazil's domestic affairs and may produce a xenophobic backlash. At the same time as the "little people" of the Amazon—the rubber tappers and Indians who depend on the forest for their livelihood—were appealing for help from abroad, influential businessmen from Sao Paulo told a Congressional fact-finding delegation that Brazil's rapid population growth and development needs made the settlement of Amazonia necessary. President Sarney was even more blunt: implying his resentment of foreign involvement in Brazil's affairs, Sarney stated his opposition to linking environmental aims with debt reduction, saying "We don't want the Amazon to become a green Persian Gulf". Nevertheless, by early 1989, with the government's own environmental protection program stagnating because of sharp budget cuts, the Brazilian Foreign Ministry indicated its willingness to use foreign funds, channeled through international organizations, to protect forest resources. Qualifying the extent to which outside assistance would be welcomed, a government spokesman declared that "There is room for international cooperation as long as conservation projects stay in Brazilian hands and are in some way supervised by the government." To forestall over-zealous actions from abroad, however, the Brazilians warned they would not tolerate "any solutions where outsiders think they can take over a piece of the Amazon."[12]

animal dung, garbage. In the industrialized nations, which until about 100 years ago had been just as dependent on wood for fuel as the underdeveloped countries are today, the substitution of coal, petroleum products, and natural gas for wood forestalled a growing pressure on their forests for fuel. Until recently it was widely hoped that increasing use of kerosene or bottled gas stoves in Third World countries would ease the burden on those nations' timber resources. The virtual overnight quadrupling of world oil prices which OPEC imposed on the world economy in 1973 and further escalation in the price of petroleum products since then have placed wood substitutes such as kerosene out of reach of millions of the world's poorest people and guaranteed continued over-exploitation of forest products. Thus can economic decisions in Riyadh or Tripoli upset the ecological stability of a mountain hamlet in Peru or a dusty village in Ethiopia.

While the clearing of land for subsistence farming and the increasing demand for fuelwood are the two most prominent factors resulting in destruction of forests on a world-wide basis, in some areas, most notably in southeast Asia, commercial lumbering is decimating valuable tropical hardwood reserves in order to supply the increased demands of industrial nations for furniture, plywood, and paper pulp. In Indonesia alone, the amounts of timber cut for export by American and Japanese logging companies soared twenty-fold between 1966 and 1970 and have been accelerating since that time as mechanization makes possible ever more rapid felling of the rain forests. Such wholesale destruction is particularly wasteful in the rain forest where the more valuable trees are scattered over a wide area and the less desirable species are frequently burned or left to decay in wide expanses of clear-cut forest land.

In Latin America, cattle-ranching has imposed additional pressures on threatened forests. Millions of acres have been cleared in Central America and Brazil to meet increasing demands for cheap beef to supply fast-food chains in the U.S. In the last few years the "hamburger connection" with Central America has largely been disrupted by a decline in American beef consumption and by political instability in the region, but in Brazil ranching continues to take a heavy toll on forests.[13]

That destruction of the earth's forest cover will have a serious and adverse impact on terrestrial ecosystems—and on their human inhabitants as well—is undisputed. Past history should have taught us that heedless deforestation can lead to excessive erosion rates, decrease the soil's water-absorbing capacity, increase the amount of run-off and flooding, and lead to the transformation of once-productive environments into desert-like conditions. Today we have growing evidence to indicate that loss of forest cover can also lead to local climatic changes, with an increase in temperature and drop in annual rainfall when large expanses of woodland are cleared.

One might suppose that since the consequences of deforestation are well understood, a serious attempt to reverse current trends would be well underway.

Unfortunately, in many of the countries most seriously affected reforestation efforts are negligible. Even where the political will exists and funds are available, large-scale tree-planting programs encounter serious difficulties which are inextricably related to the cultural, political, and economic facts of life in rural societies. In many areas saplings planted with high hopes are promptly devoured by over-abundant and freely-roaming goats, sheep, and cattle. In some places nomads passing through an area may decimate a village's efforts at reforestation, while in still other areas villagers themselves may uproot young trees because they simply have no other source of fuel. Successful reforestation efforts require extensive administrative efforts to protect the plants for years—efforts which may be politically unrewarding to officials trying to win voters' approval for next year's election rather than a "good job well done" 20 years in the future. There have been some reforestation success stories, most notably in the People's Republic of China where efforts by the Communist regime to mobilize millions of rural laborers to plant and maintain trees during the off-season between harvest and planting time have resulted in the gradual reversal of a 5000-year trend of forest loss. Ultimately the most serious obstacle to curbing forest loss is the continued rapid growth of human populations in the countries most affected.[14] As a Costa Rican squatter on a partially forested ranch poignantly stated, "By subsisting today I know I can destroy the future of the forest and the people. But I have to eat today."[15]

Box 5-2

Tragedy in the Sahel

Throughout the broad belt of sub-Saharan Africa which stretches from Mauritania and Senegal in the west to Chad in the east—an area larger than the continental U.S.—a human tragedy of massive proportions unfolded during the early 1970s. It was a tragedy largely of human making, though Nature did her part in hastening the inevitable disaster.

The Sahel, a term derived from the Arabic word for "border", in reference to its position at the southern edge of the Sahara, refers collectively to the six West African nations of Mauritania, Senegal, Mali, Burkina Faso, Niger, and Chad. These are semi-arid lands with a combined population of about 35 million, six million of whom are nomadic tribesmen of such legendary fame as the Tuareg and Fulani. During the period between 1968-1973 a severe drought struck the Sahelian countries, a drought which for several years was little noticed by the West until TV newsreels and front-page photos began shocking the world with pathetic scenes of emaciated mothers and dying babies, dusty refugee camps, and once-proud independent nomads standing in bread lines. A belated relief effort eventually eliminated most outright starvation, but even so estimates indicate that hundreds of thousands of people, mostly nomads, perished before aid could reach them. Equally devastating for those who survived was the loss of the herds on which they depended for their livelihood. In Mauritania, for example, 80% of the total livestock herd perished. Herdsmen who knew no other way of life were forced to live on handouts in refugee-swollen cities—or to starve.

Aid-givers were hopeful that the catastrophe was the result of a freakish stretch of weather and that the return of the rains in 1974 marked the end of Sahelian suffering.

Scientists analyzing the drought and its effects were less sanguine, however. Climatologists pointed out that the Sahelian region had always experienced recurring cycles of drought and asserted that the 1968-1973 period was not any more severe than several others which occurred during this century. Why, then, were its effects so much more ruinous than those of other dry spells? Kai-Curry Lindahl, a scientist with the United Nation's Environmental Programme based in Nairobi, Kenya, insists that the true villain in the Sahelian disaster was not nature but man. Thanks to a decline in intertribal warfare and increasing access to modern medicines, human populations in the Sahel, as elsewhere in Africa, have been growing rapidly for several generations. Even in years of normal rainfall, agricultural production has been rising less than 1% annually, while the population growth rate stands close to 3%. Perhaps even more significant than the growth of human numbers, however, has been the expansion of livestock herds. Just as modern medical technology brought about sharp declines in human death rates, so access to veterinary medicines permitted pastoralists to enlarge greatly the size of their herds. A history of overgrazing in the region resulted in the replacement of nutritious forage with shrubs of little value, thus reducing the vitality of the animals and increasing mortality rates when conditions deteriorated. As the drought worsened and many water holes dried up, livestock became so concentrated around the few remaining sources of water that the surrounding area became completely trampled and stripped of vegetation; thus land which was once good pasture turned to desert.

Unfortunately, after a few relatively good years during the late 1970s and early 1980s, drought has again returned to the Sahel as well as to lands farther east. In 1984 and 1985 severe famine extended from the Sahel to Ethiopia, Somalia, and the Sudan; once again media coverage of mass starvation and suffering prompted an outpouring of food aid from abroad. African leaders and outside experts alike agree that the long-term solution for the problems of the region lies not in food shipments from overseas nor in mass infusions of aid money, foreign technology and expertise, but in the adoption of a radically new lifestyle by the Sahelian nomads and reduction of excess rates of population growth. Whether the habits of a thousand years can be changed quickly enough to avert further calamity remains to be seen. Events now unfolding in the Sahel provide a graphic example of how excessive human pressures on fragile environments can overwhelm the carrying capacity of a region and bring ruin not only to the land but to the human societies whose activities precipitated the crisis.

Desertification

That man can create desert-like conditions on once-productive land has been known, though largely ignored, since the time 2300 years ago when Plato bewailed the ecological fate of his native Attica, writing that "our land, compared with what it was, is like the skeleton of a body wasted by disease. The soft, plump parts have vanished and all that remains is the bare carcass." This sorry situation was brought about by the cutting of forests and over-grazing of livestock which in that semi-arid climate inevitably resulted in erosion of topsoil and the drying up of springs which were no longer being recharged, since rainwater quickly ran off the bare ground rather than percolating through the soil. The formation of cultural deserts which occurred over two millenia ago in Greece and the lands around the eastern Mediterranean is a process which has so increased in extent during the 20th century that it has been graced with the somewhat unwieldy, though descriptive term "desertification"—the enlargement of deserts by human pressures.

Desertification to many people evokes images of sand dunes relentlessly sweeping over green fields and pastures, and in some cases this is indeed what is happening. More commonly, however, the process is one of the desert being pulled into once-productive land as a result of human actions. Desertification seldom involves the steady influx of sands along a uniform front; rather, climatic fluctuations and land-use patterns interact to extend desert-like conditions irregularly over susceptible land. Spots of extreme degradation are especially likely to grow around water holes when nearby pastures are heavily grazed and trampled and around towns when people denude adjacent lands in their search for fuelwood. In arid and semi-arid regions year-to-year fluctuations of rainfall can be moderately destructive even under natural conditions, but in the long run natural processes can correct the imbalance. However, when the hazard of erratic rainfall is coupled with pressure brought to bear on the land by people, then the damage may be irreversible.

Desertification is a process occurring today on an unprecedented scale. The human tragedy embodied in the great dust storms which blackened the skies in

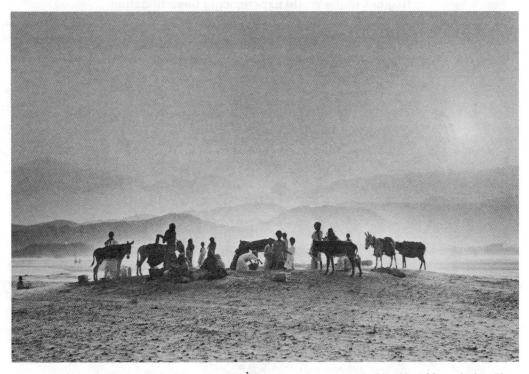

Poverty, climate and population pressures are forcing more and more marginal land in Africa to be brought under cultivation. The result, according to the 1988 'State of World Population' Report from UNFPA is "erosion and ultimately desert conditions." [*UNFPA/Sebastiao/Salgado/Magnum*]

Fall-Out From the "Population Bomb"   137

the American prairie states during the 1930s is being repeated today in sub-Saharan African where the nomadic herdsmen and their over-sized flocks seem to have pushed the carrying capacity of the land beyond the point of no return; in northwest India, the world's most densely populated arid zone and, thanks to the large herds of cattle, camels, goats, etc., also perhaps the world's dustiest area; in North Africa, where the Sahara Desert is gradually encroaching northward onto lands that were once the granary of the Roman Empire; and in the American Southwest where over-grazing during the past several hundred years may be largely responsible for the formation of Arizona's Sonoran Desert. Many of these areas still have the potential to reestablish their former grassland ecosystems if the constant pressure of over-grazing and over-plowing could be removed, but some have been irreversibly degraded by complete loss of topsoil. If human pressures continue to mount, retrogression of arid land ecosystems will result in the permanent destabilization of existing ecosystems and a continuing impoverishment of both ecological and cultural conditions. Ecosystems, like civilizations, can decline and fall if pushed too far.

Fig. 5-1   Regions of the World Experiencing Desertification

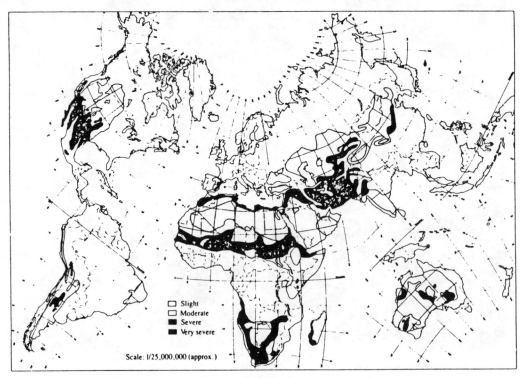

Source: *Global 2000 Report*

Wetlands Destruction

Swamps, bogs, tidal marshlands, estuaries, ponds, river bottoms, flood plains, prairie potholes—all fall under the designation of "wetlands". Until very recently most people viewed wetlands as a nuisance, useful only to frogs and mosquitoes, and thus prime candidates for draining or filling to convert them into more "profitable" areas for farming, mining, or urban development. As a result, nearly half the wetlands which existed in this country when European settlers first arrived have now disappeared and an additional 458,000 acres continue to be lost each year.[16] The significance of this loss is just beginning to be recognized and belated efforts to control wetlands conversion are now underway at both the federal and state level.

Today the importance of wetlands in both ecological and economic terms is unquestioned. Their ability to retain large amounts of water makes them extremely valuable as nature's own method of preventing devastating floods. Not surprisingly, as wetlands along the Mississippi River Valley have been destroyed, the severity and frequency of floods in that region has escalated. Wetlands provide the major recharge areas for groundwater reserves and also serve as "living filters" for purifying contaminated surface waters as these percolate into the ground. Indeed, some communities are currently utilizing nearby wetlands as a method of tertiary sewage treatment, allowing wastewater to flow through a swamp or marsh to remove unwanted nutrients and then

Fig. 5-2

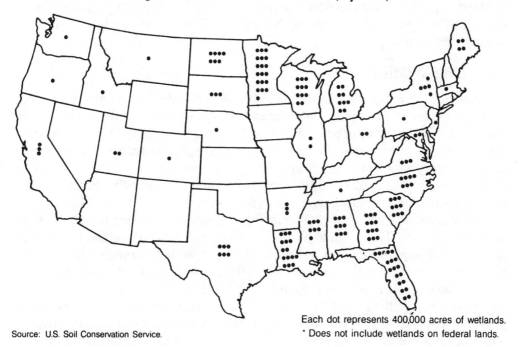

Wetland Acreage in the Coterminous United States, by State, 1982*

Each dot represents 400,000 acres of wetlands.
* Does not include wetlands on federal lands.

Source: U.S. Soil Conservation Service.

Fall-Out From the "Population Bomb"   **139**

drawing water out from the other side. The sustained productivity of commercial fisheries is also heavily dependent on the existence of wetlands. Between 60-90% of fish caught along the Atlantic and Gulf coasts spend at least some portion of their life cycle, usually the vulnerable early stages, in coastal marshes or estuaries. Further inland in the Midwest the system of lakes, marshes, and prairie potholes extending from the Gulf of Mexico north into Canada provides the major life-support system for millions of migratory waterfowl (half of all ducklings in North America are hatched in the prairie potholes of the Dakotas and Canada). A $1 billion recreational hunting industry, attracting 2.5 million duck hunters each year, is thus totally dependent on preservation of these vital wetlands breeding areas. Wetlands also provide a habitat not only for ducks and geese but for many other bird and mammal species—whooping cranes, river otters, black bears, etc. Fully ⅓ of all American wildlife species listed as "endangered" inhabit wetlands.

Although some wetlands are lost due to natural causes such as erosion, land subsidence, storms, or salt water intrusion, human activities account for by far the greatest amount of loss. Draining of swamps or bottomlands for agricultural purposes is the leading cause of wetlands destruction (87% of the total loss between the mid-1960s and mid-1970s), but dredging for canals and port construction, flood control projects, road construction, and urban development have also taken a significant toll. In spite of increased awareness, the losses continue today, particularly along the inland waterways of the Mississippi.[17] Reflecting the growing national demand to protect our remaining wetlands resource, Congress included a section in the 1985 farm bill referred to as the "Swampbuster Provision", aimed at discouraging draining of wetlands for agriculture by stating that farmers who do so will lose their farm program benefits.

Vanishing Wildlife

Extinction of a species, like the death of an individual, is a natural process. As fossil evidence clearly indicates, many groups of plants and animals which dominated life on earth in past millennia have died out, only to be replaced by newly-evolving organisms. The rise and fall of species throughout the course of earth's history was determined largely by a population's ability to adapt to changing environmental conditions or to become increasingly specialized for life in a particular ecological niche. As evolution proceeded, the number of plant and animal species proliferated, increasing at a more or less steady pace right up to historic times. Today biologists have classified approximately 1½ million species of living things, but estimate that the actual number currently in existence, many yet undiscovered, ranges from 3 to 10 million, the majority of these in the tropics. Unfortunately, it is widely feared that many of these species will vanish before their existence is ever noted or recorded. The sad truth of the present situation is that human actions have greatly accelerated the rate at which species are becoming extinct; indeed, for the first time in many millions

Fig. 5-3 Listed Endangered and Threatened Species, by Taxonomic Group, 1973–1985

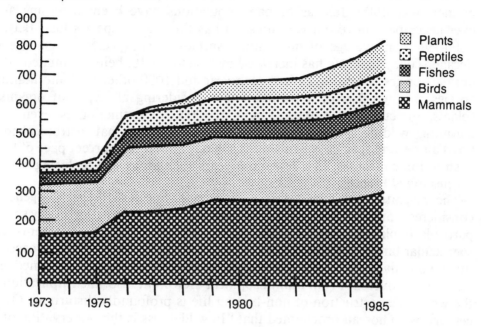

Number of species

Plants
Reptiles
Fishes
Birds
Mammals

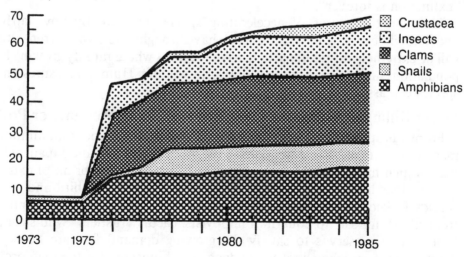

Number of species

Crustacea
Insects
Clams
Snails
Amphibians

Source: U.S. Fish and Wildlife Service.

of years species are vanishing more rapidly than new ones are evolving, resulting in a diminishing diversity of life forms. The first recorded animal extinction—that of the European lion—was documented in 80 A.D.; more than half of the animal species which have disappeared since that time have become extinct since 1900. Just as human populations have been increasing at an ever-faster pace in recent centuries, so has the rate of species loss. Between 1600-1950, an average of one animal species or subspecies vanished every decade. Today that rate has increased by a factor of 10, being estimated at one animal species becoming extinct each year and 1000 other bird and mammal species threatened with a similar fate. Considering all types of organisms (plants, insects, fish, molluscs, etc.), the rate of extinction is even more alarming; wildlife specialist Norman Myers estimates that in tropical forest areas alone, one species is vanishing each day and, if the current pace of forest destruction continues, in a few more years such areas will be losing another species every hour.[18]

The magnitude of such a loss is staggering. Species diversity is generally considered a prime determinant of ecological stability; extinction of key species, particularly plant species, may lead to the collapse of whole ecosystems. Less spectacular but equally distressing from a human viewpoint is the prospect of many potentially useful plant species being lost before their food or medicinal value is discovered. From a philosophical viewpoint also, the implications of the wholesale destruction of non-human life is profoundly disturbing. Over a century ago Thoreau proclaimed that "In wilderness is the preservation of the world". Much ethical discussion in recent years has centered around the question of whether man has the moral right to exterminate another form of life, to abruptly terminate the product of millions of years of evolution. Undeniably, "extinction is forever".

Although the causes of accelerating species loss are by now fairly well understood, reversing the trends which have brought about the current situation will be extremely difficult, particularly in regions where rapidly growing human populations are in direct competition with wildlife. Human pressures on other species can assume a variety of forms.

Direct Killing or Collecting of Wildlife for Food, Pleasure, or Profit

From European Stone Age man who decimated the wooly mammoths and mastodons with primitive weapons to the modern Russian and Japanese fishing fleets which have brought several species of whale to the brink of extinction, over-zealous hunters have totally eliminated a number of bird and mammal species. Collectors who dynamite reefs to obtain chunks of coral or capture rare tropical fish for sale to aquarium hobbyists; cactus "rustlers" who steal plants from nature preserves to satisfy the growing demand for rare houseplants; African poachers who shoot the endangered rhinoceros for the high profits its powdered horn will bring in the markets of the Orient (rhinoceros horn has long been considered an aphrodisiac in China and the Far East)—all contribute to the demise of species, as do the consumers whose purchases of these items provide the incentive for such actions.

Environment and the Law:
The National Environmental Policy Act (NEPA)

Recognizing that to maintain ecological stability the integrity of ecosystems must be carefully preserved, the U.S. Congress passed one of our most far-reaching pieces of environmental legislation, the National Environmental Policy Act (Public Law 91-190). This law, signed on January 1, 1970, made the protection and restoration of the environment a matter of national policy. It does this by requiring all federal agencies to take environmental considerations into account in their decision-making processes and implementation of programs. In the years since NEPA has been in effect it has had a major impact on a wide variety of programs, including the siting of oil-drilling facilities, highway and other public works construction, river channelization projects, dam building, and many others.

The key provision of NEPA is Section 102(2)(c) which mandates that all federal agencies prepare environmental impact statements (EIS) for any of their major activities which could substantially affect the environment. The purpose of this provision is to guarantee that all federal policies, regulations, and actions include the goals of environmental protection.

Every environmental impact statement must include 1) the positive impact of a proposed action; 2) any possible adverse impact; 3) alternatives to the proposal; 4) a comparison of short-term use of natural resources versus the maintenance and enhancement of long-range productivity; and 5) any irreversible commitment of resources if the proposal is implemented. Although no federal activities are strictly prohibited, NEPA forces public officials to consider and publicly discuss the environmental consequences of proposed projects. As a result of the EIS requirement, a number of poorly-conceived projects were either altered extensively (e.g. Alaskan oil pipeline) or dropped entirely (some bridge projects, airport construction, etc.). Impact assessments have led the U.S. Army Corps of Engineers to modify almost one-third of their active projects. Although some government agencies regard impact statements as mere paperwork exercises, supporting decisions already reached rather than as a basic part of planning, most now make an honest effort to integrate ecological considerations into their decision-making processes.

Compliance with NEPA's requirements is monitored by the Council on Environmental Quality, a 5-member group created by NEPA to advise the President on environmental issues and to work with Congress and executive agencies to solve them. CEQ regulations concerning preparation of environmental impact statements require that a draft statement must be circulated among other federal agencies and made public for both official and citizen comment at least 90 days before a decision is made on the proposed action. When comments are received, these must be considered in the final statement which likewise must be circulated for at least 30 days before action is taken. Opening of the decision-making process to public, as well as official input, has resulted in the filing of hundreds of court cases by groups and individuals demanding that projects be abandoned or postponed until adequate impact analyses were made. This element of public participation in environmental decision-making has been one of the most important changes brought about by NEPA.

Federal agencies themselves report both fiscal savings and economic and environmental benefits from NEPA. Construction project modifications resulting from the EIS process frequently result in cost reductions (in one case $438.4 million was saved because a plant was redesigned on a smaller, more appropriate scale than the one originally proposed); public and official comments on federal highway EISs have resulted in the provision of

Pollution of Air and Water with Toxic Chemicals

The death of entire aquatic ecosystems due to acid rainfall is but the latest well-publicized example of the effect man-made toxic pollutants are having on other forms of life. Particularly since the introduction of the synthetic organic pesticides after World War II, numerous wildlife species, especially carnivorous birds, have suffered sharp population declines and contamination of rivers, lakes, and estuaries with poisonous industrial effluents threaten the sustained productivity of those ecosystems. The impact of pollution on wildlife was a major topic of international discussion in the summer of 1988 when beaches along Europe's North Sea and the U.S. East Coast were littered with the bodies of dead and dying seals and porpoises. Though the cause of the marine mammals' demise was ultimately determined to be a type of pneumonia, it was theorized that swimming in highly polluted coastal waters weakened the animals' resistance to disease and thereby contributed to their death.

Habitat Destruction

By far the most significant cause of species loss, and the most difficult to control, is the destruction of those natural areas which wildlife require for breeding, feeding, or migrating. As the pressures of expanding populations and economies increase, forests are chopped down, swamps are drained, prairie-lands are put to the plow, rivers are dammed. Some wildlife species can thrive in close proximity to man—most cannot and perish when their natural habitat is destroyed or reduced in size below a critical minimum. Today problems of habitat loss are most acute in tropical countries where land-hungry peasant farmers carve garden plots out of the forest or governments desperate for foreign exchange grant timber concessions to multinational corporations. Short-term material considerations in such cases are far more pressing than the realization that in the long term such policies have disastrous ecological implications. In countries where poverty is rampant and population growth rates are high, even national leaders with a strong commitment to conservation find it politically impossible to give wildlife preservation high priority. As Chief

Gatsha Buthelezi, leader of the KwaZulu "homeland" in South Africa stated some years ago, "More and more of my people see my enthusiasm for the wilderness getting less and less relevant to the major issue of their survival".[19] Sadly, unless population growth rates drop quickly and the status of the poor is improved, concern for vanishing wildlife, however legitimate, will continue to be overshadowed by the more urgent demands of human survival.

REFERENCES

[1]"18 Aliens, Trapped in a Boxcar, Die in Bungled Smuggling Attempt", *The New York Times,* July 3, 1987.

[2]Birdsall, Nancy, "Population Growth and Poverty in the Developing World", *Population Bulletin,* vol. 35, no. 5, December 1980.

[3]Brown, Lester, Patricia L. McGrath, and Bruce Stokes, "The Population Problem in 22 Dimensions", *The Futurist,* Oct. 1976.

[4]Whittaker, Robert H., *Communities and Ecosystems,* MacMillan Publishing Company, 1975.

[5]Brown, Lester, "World Food Resources and Population: the Narrowing Margin", *Population Bulletin,* vol. 36, no. 3, Sept. 1981.

[6]1981 Yearbook of Agriculture, "Will There be Enough Food?", United States Department of Agriculture, 1981.

[7]Berg, Norman A., "Making the Most of the New Soil Conservation Initiatives", *Journal of Soil and Water Conservation,* Jan./Feb. 1987; USDA, Economic Research Service, *Agricultural Resources: Cropland, Water, and Conservation Situation and Outlook Report,* Washington, DC, 1987.

[8]Brown, Lester, "The Changing World Food Prospect: the Nineties and Beyond", *Worldwatch paper 85,* Oct. 1988.

[9]Eckholm, Erik, *Losing Ground,* W.W. Norton and Co., 1976.

[10]Postel, Sandra, "Global View of a Tropical Disaster", *American Forests,* vol. 94, nos. 11 and 12, Nov./Dec. 1988.

[11]Richards, Paul W., "The Tropical Rain Forest", *Scientific American,* December 1973.

[12]Pasca, T.M., "The Politics of Tropical Deforestation", *American Forests,* vol. 94, nos. 11 and 12, Nov./Dec. 1988; Lenssen, Nicholas, "Reprieve for the Rain Forest?", *World Watch,* vol. 2, no. 1, Jan./Feb. 1989; Simons, Marlise, "Brazil Tells Americans Their Rain-Forest Fears", *The New York Times,* Jan. 25, 1989; Simons, Marlise, "Brazil Agrees to Accept Aid to Save Rain Forests", *The New York Times,* Feb. 5, 1989.

[13]Postel, op. cit.

[14]Eckholm, op. cit.

[15]Hamilton, John Maxwell, "Rescuing the Bounty of Rain Forests", *The Christian Science Monitor,* Jan. 26, 1989.

[16]Savoye, Crain, "Disappearing Wetlands", *The Christian Science Monitor,* July 13, 1983.

[17]Wakefield, Penny, "Reducing the Federal Role in Wetlands Protection", *Environment,* vol. 24, no. 10, Dec. 1982.

[18]Myers, Norman, *The Sinking Ark,* 1979.

[19]Eckholm, Erik, "Disappearing Species: The Social Challenge", *Worldwatch Paper 22,* July 1978.

PART II

PART II

Our Toxic Environment
Does *everything* cause cancer?

Newspaper headlines screaming "Ozone Alert!"; a $1 million damage settlement to an asbestos worker's widow; public protests over a leaking hazardous waste dump; migrant workers hospitalized for pesticide poisoning; accidental sewage discharge forcing closure of public beaches—such situations represent but a handful of the issues daily facing modern society in which some aspect of environmental quality has a direct impact on human health.

From primitive times up until the mid-19th century the idea that health and disease were determined, at least in part, by environmental factors was widely accepted (witness the belief that night air precipitated fever and chills). The middle 1800s, however, marked a period of rapid progress in research relating to disease causation. The discovery of the anthrax bacterium by the German Robert Koch and his demonstration in 1877 that this organism was responsible for an important human disease revolutionized society's view of health. For the next 70 years virtually all the ailments of mankind were blamed on pathogenic organisms such as bacteria, viruses, and protozoans. It was widely assumed that the development of preventative vaccines or curative antibiotics should be our main focus in protecting public health.

More recently, however, recognition of the role which deprivation or stress can play in initiating serious health problems and the sharp increase, particularly in more affluent societies, of the so-called "degenerative diseases" (cardiovascular disease, cancer, hypertension) have led to the realization that good health depends on more than just the absence of disease-causing microorganisms. Some of today's most prevalent ills are increasingly blamed on toxic environmental contaminants—synthetic chemical wastes carelessly dumped in waterways or landfills, products of combustion spewed into the air, pesticide residues and chemical additives in the food we eat; others are associated with personal habits which in the broad sense can be considered aspects of environmental quality—smoking, drinking, high-fat diets, lack of regular exercise. Perception of the threat which such factors pose to human well-being provided the main thrust behind the environmental movement of the last two decades. Preservation—or restoration—of environmental quality means far more than protecting bald eagles or ensuring that the last coastal redwood isn't converted into a picnic table; the prime emphasis among environmental advocates has always been the protection of human health, with the implicit recognition that human well-being is inextricably intertwined with the health and stability of the natural ecosystems of which we form an integral part.

149

While not a perfect standard, the health status of societies is often measured in terms of life expectancy—the number of years an average individual in that society can expect to live. In terms of longevity, health conditions in the Western world have improved markedly in recent centuries. Whereas in the days of Roman emperors average lifespan was about 30 years, today in most industrialized countries it has reached 72-74 years, up from 50 years at the turn of the century. In the less developed nations average lifespan today is somewhat less, ranging from the low 40s in some African and Asian nations to 70 in some parts of Latin America, but nevertheless is sharply higher than it was just a few generations ago. Many people, looking at such statistics, assume that the major factor accounting for increased longevity world-wide was the introduction of modern medicines and pesticides which provided the first really effective weapons against many of the infectious epidemic diseases. While medical science undoubtedly played a part in reducing mortality rates, many observers feel that a more fundamental reason accounting for this change was the general improvement in living conditions brought about by the better nutritional levels made possible by increased agricultural productivity and through the upgrading of sanitary conditions which accompanied the construction of sewer systems and the provision of safe drinking water supplies, refuse collection, sewage treatment, the enforcement of housing codes, and so forth. Rising incomes, increasing levels of education, mass communications, and improved standards of personal hygiene have also been extremely important determinants in furthering the health advances observed in most parts of the world.

However, we seem to have now reached a longevity plateau and are no longer observing a continued rapid drop in death rates such as characterized the years between 1950-1960. There appears to be general agreement that future gains will come, not so much through new medical discoveries, but when—and only when—currently unmet essential preconditions of better health are everywhere available. These essential preconditions relate largely to environmental considerations: sufficient quantities of uncontaminated water, elimination of malnutrition, proper handling and disposal of human wastes, control of toxic pollutants, adoption of healthier personal lifestyles. The environmentally-induced diseases currently plaguing much of humanity can best be controlled through a strategy of prevention, rather than cure, requiring not only application of technology but also social, political, and behavioral changes. Adopting such a strategy and enlisting the public support necessary to attain the goal of a healthful society require a thorough understanding of the issues and dilemmas involved. The following chapters will delineate the major concerns regarding our increasingly toxic environment and the health implications inherent in our present life-style; they also attempt to show that improving human health and enhancing environmental quality are but two sides of the same coin.

6

Environmental Disease

"The most important pathological effects of pollution are
extremely delayed and indirect."
—Rene Dubos

Polluted air and water, excessive levels of noise, sunshine, nuclear weapons
fall-out, over-crowded slums, toxic waste dumps, inadequate or overly-
adequate diet, stress, food contaminants, medical X-rays, drugs, cigarettes,
unsafe working conditions—these comprise but a partial listing of the many
environmental factors which, through their adverse impact on human health,
can be regarded as causative agents of environmental disease. In recent years
public concern about rising levels of pollution and environmental degradation
has increasingly focused on the question of whether such trends may be
influencing disease rates, particularly ailments such as heart disease, cancer,
stroke and other ills which have assumed major importance following the
conquest of the microbial killers of yesteryear. If such a connection exists, as
virtually all authorities agree it does, then society's response should be clear:
most environmentally-induced diseases, unlike those caused by bacteria or
other pathogens, are difficult to cure but theoretically simple to prevent—
remove the adverse environmental influence and the ailment will disappear. In
other words, by preventing the discharge of poisons into our air, water, and
food, by avoiding exposure to radiation, by refusing to fill our lungs with
cigarette smoke or our stomachs with synthetic food colorings we can protect
our health far more effectively and cheaply than we can by desperately searching
for an often non-existent cure after our bodies succumb to a malignancy or
degeneration of vital organs or when our children are born deformed. The old

adage, "Prevention is the best cure" has never been more true than when applied to environmentally-induced diseases.

Historically the environmental health profession has concentrated primarily on reducing the incidence of epidemic diseases spread through contaminated

---

Box 6-1

General Disease Classification

Human disease conditions can be categorized in various ways: infectious or non-infectious; endemic or epidemic; acute or chronic. It is important to have an understanding of the basic nature of any particular disease state in order to know how to respond to the problem in an appropriate manner.

Infectious vs. Non-infectious

Infectious diseases are those caused by pathogenic organisms such as bacteria, viruses, protozoans, parasitic worms, etc. Infectious diseases can be spread from one person to another by inhalation of airborne pathogens released when an infected person coughs, sneezes, or talks; by direct contact with food, water, soil or clothing which has been contaminated with fecal matter or saliva from an infected person; through sexual intercourse or other close physical contact with a diseased individual; or as a result of activities of a non-pathogenic disease-carrier, or *Vector*, such as mosquitoes or body lice which transfer the disease agent from an infected person to a healthy one. Many of the leading killers of the past included such infectious diseases as malaria, smallpox, cholera, typhoid, measles, and tuberculosis.

Non-infectious diseases, currently the major causes of mortality in industrialized societies, are those which are not caused by pathogenic organisms and are not transmitted from one person to another (except in the case of hereditary conditions). Non-infectious diseases frequently have multiple causes, often related to adverse environmental conditions, and may develop slowly over a number of years. Unlike many infectious diseases which, if survived, are of short duration, most non-infectious diseases are irreversible. Although many can be kept under control with proper medical treatment, few such conditions can be permanently cured. Examples of some of the leading non-infectious diseases include cardiovascular disease, cancer, diabetes, emphysema, sickle-cell anemia, asthma, and cerebral palsy.

Endemic vs. Epidemic

When the causative agent of an infectious disease such as typhoid is carried by many individuals within a population without leading to a rapid and widespread outbreak of illness and a high death rate, the disease is said to be endemic within that population. An epidemic disease, by contrast, involves a sudden severe outbreak of an infectious disease affecting a large number of people. The term "pandemic" refers to an epidemic which is world-wide in extent.

Acute vs. Chronic

Generally used in reference to certain infectious diseases such as smallpox, plague, or cholera which can be quite severe but are of short duration, an acute illness can also be caused by a short-term, high-dose exposure to a toxic substance. In most cases, if the victim survives the initial attack, the effects of the illness are reversible. With chronic conditions (e.g. malaria, tuberculosis, heart disease, cancer, emphysema) the illness is of long duration, often lasting a lifetime, occasionally flaring up, sometimes going into remission, or, in some cases, growing progressively worse as the years pass.

---

food and water. Their success, through implementation of such now taken-for-granted procedures as drinking water purification, sewage treatment, and vector control can be seen in a comparison of present and past statistics of mortality rates for diseases such as cholera and typhoid fever. These filth-related killers are now extremely rare in the U.S., though the causative organisms are still present and would undoubtedly return with a vengeance if we were to relax the environmental controls which hold them at bay. The threat posed by these water- and food-borne diseases, as well as the hazards related to air contaminants, radiation, pesticides, and noise—all features of the modern environment—will be discussed in greater detail in the chapters dealing with those topics.

In spite of the fact that environmental factors can affect human health in many ways, the focus of most environmental health concern today in this age of toxic pollutants is on those substances which, in ways not yet completely understood, act at the cellular level to initiate often irreversible changes which can kill or damage the cell in question. Although health damage due to environmental pollutants may be manifested by outward symptoms, research has shown that the action of such contaminants in fact occurs at the level of an individual cell or cells. In spite of its small size, the cell is an exceptionally complex structure—the end product of billions of years of evolution and natural selection in response to existing environmental conditions. Thus it should not be surprising to find that a sudden change in the environment to which a cell has become so finely adapted (e.g. exposure to X-rays, synthetic organic chemicals, heavy metals, etc.) can kill or injure the cell. Cell death, in many respects, is a lesser concern than cell injury because it has no further implications—the cell is dead. Cell *damage*, on the other hand, has more ominous implications. The subject of extensive scientific and medical research for the past half century, cell damage can be manifested in one of three ways: mutation, birth defects, or cancer.

Mutation

Mutation, defined as ***any change in the genetic material***, is perhaps the most worrisome type of cell damage because of its potential for harming not only the person or organism harboring the mutant cell but, if the mutation occurs in an egg or sperm, unborn generations as well. To understand the significance of mutation, it is necessary to examine the nature of the hereditary material itself.

The most conspicuous organelle in most cells is the nucleus, readily visible under an ordinary light microscope. The nucleus contains thread-like structures called ***Chromosomes***; each species of plant or animal has its own characteristic number of chromosomes per cell—in humans the chromosome number is 46. When cells undergo mitosis (cell division), each chromosome splits longitudin-ally into 2 daughter ***Chromatids***, one of which goes into each of the two

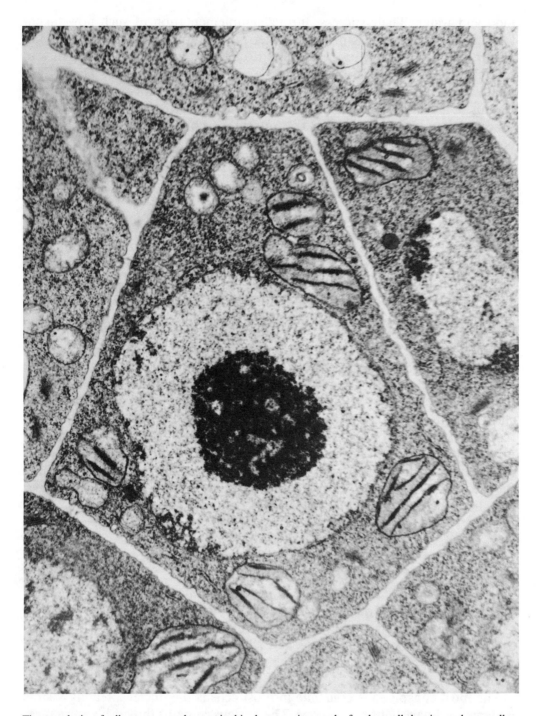

The complexity of cell structure can be seen in this electron micrograph of a plant cell showing such organelles as nucleus, chloroplasts, ribosomes, endoplasmic reticulum, mitochondria, and vacuoles. Environmental toxins act here at the cellular level within organisms. [*Mathew Nadakavukaren*]

newly-forming cells. Thus the number of chromosomes per nucleus remains constant and the hereditary material contained within the chromosomes is equally shared.

Chemically, chromosomes consist of a single giant molecule of **DNA** (deoxyribonucleic acid) and associated histone and non-histone proteins. The DNA molecule itself is composed of two parallel strands of alternating units of a 5-carbon sugar and phosphate molecules, cross-linked by one of four different nitrogenous bases (adenine, guanine, thymine, and cytosine), and twisted into a helical configuration. The pairing of the nitrogenous bases is quite specific: adenine can pair only with thymine and guanine with cytosine. Along any one strand bases can occur in any sequence, but once the order on one side is given, the sequence on the parallel strand is automatically determined. The adenine-thymine (A-T) or guanine-cytosine (G-C) combination making up each cross-connection is referred to as a **Base Pair.**

DNA is vitally important to cellular function and is often referred to as the "Master Molecule" because (1) it passes genetic information from one generation to the next and (2) it controls cellular metabolism by giving the instructions for protein synthesis.

The hereditary characteristics are controlled by **Genes** along the length of the chromosome. In essence, a gene is a section of chromosome consisting of approximately 1500 base pairs. Each gene is responsible for the production of a particular protein necessary for proper cell function. It is absolutely essential that the integrity of the DNA molecule be maintained if the correct information for protein synthesis is to be passed from one generation to the next. Any change within the gene, resulting in production of the wrong protein, constitutes a mutation. There are 3 basic types of mutations recognized.

1. *"Point" Mutation* (gene mutation)—By far the most common type of mutation, point mutations involve a change at the molecular level within a gene. Such a change usually consists of the deletion or substitution of a base pair, resulting in the "misreading" of the genetic code (the sequence of bases along a DNA strand is all-important; any change can result in the wrong protein being formed). Depending on precisely where within a gene the change occurs, severity of a point mutation can range all the way from being lethal to causing an almost imperceptible loss of vigor. Point mutations are now known to be responsible for several serious human ailments. These include sickle-cell anemia, hemophilia, diabetes, and achondroplastic dwarfism. Though such ailments are tragic for the victim (prior to modern forms of treatment, which are only partially effective, these diseases invariably resulted in death at a fairly early age), many geneticists are more concerned about the accumulation of sub-lethal mutations in populations. Such sub-lethal mutations don't kill their victims outright, but render the individual less fit than he would otherwise be. Examples of the types of impairment which could result from a sub-lethal mutation include reduced physical or mental vigor, shortened life span, increased susceptibility to disease, or varying degrees of malformation of some organ. Such changes, though possibly debilitating, nevertheless permit the

Fig. 6-1

DNA Double Helix

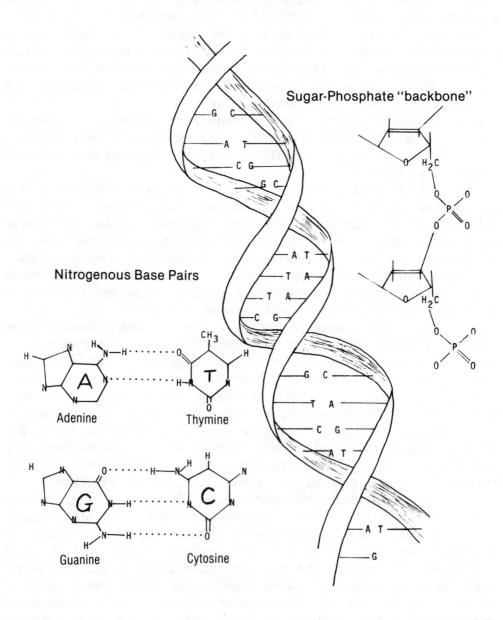

Sugar-Phosphate "backbone"

Nitrogenous Base Pairs

Adenine   Thymine

Guanine   Cytosine

afflicted individual to survive, reproduce, and pass his defective genes on to succeeding generations, resulting in what some researchers refer to as the "contamination of the human gene pool."

Box 6-2

Sickle-Cell Anemia

A single base pair substitution, resulting in the production of the amino acid valine instead of glutamic acid along one polypeptide chain of the hemoglobin molecule, has been identified as the cause of the disabling and usually fatal disease, sickle-cell anemia. The most common long-term illness among black children, sickle-cell is characterized by misshapen red blood cells which clump and block the smaller blood vessels, impeding circulation and eventually leading to the death of affected tissues. Sickle-cell can be quite painful and can lead to pneumonia due to lung damage, rheumatism as a result of muscle and joint deterioration, and damage to heart and kidneys. Victims suffering from sickle-cell usually die before reaching reproductive age. Many healthy adults, however, carry the sickle-cell trait (a victim must have 2 defective genes, one from each parent, to develop the disease). Efforts are now being made to persuade potential carriers to have a simple diagnostic blood test prior to having children in order to determine the risk of producing a baby with this genetic disorder.

---

2. *Chromosomal Aberrations*—These represent gross structural changes in the chromosome, usually caused by the loss or addition of sizeable pieces of a chromosome or the reversing of chromosome parts which frequently occurs during a stage of meiosis (reduction division) when the homologous chromosomes are in synapsis and crossing-over occurs. Although some types of chromosomal aberration seem to have little outward effect, the loss of part of a chromosome usually is fatal to the cell—i.e. represents a lethal mutation.

3. *Change in Chromosome Number*—Caused by the non-disjunction (failure to separate) of paired homologous chromosomes during meiosis, this type of mutation features some cells with more than the normal chromosome number, others with less. The best known human ailment resulting from a change in chromosome number is Down's Syndrome (sometimes called "mongolism" because the flattened facial features give a superficial Oriental appearance to victims). Afflicting about 14 out of every 10,000 babies born in the U.S. and inevitably resulting in mental retardation, Down's Syndrome occurs due to the presence in the victim's cells of 47 chromosomes instead of the normal 46 (to be more precise, three #21 chromosomes rather than two). Interestingly, the likelihood of a woman's giving birth to a mongoloid child increases as the mother gets older. Whereas on the average only 13.5% of all pregnancies occur among women over 35, these older mothers produce more than half of the children with Down's Syndrome. Prevailing theory is that since each female child is born with all the egg cells she will ever have, these eggs are subject to

deterioration with aging or with exposure to toxic substances. The older the woman, the greater the possibility that her egg cells could sustain damage resulting in a mutation. It is common medical procedure today for pregnant women over 35 to undergo a process called amniocentesis. Usually performed in the 4th month of pregnancy, amniocentesis involves inserting a needle through the woman's abdomen into the uterus and withdrawing about 20 ml of amniotic fluid. An analysis of the fetal cells that have sloughed off into this fluid can reveal the presence of Down's Syndrome as well as approximately 100 other genetic diseases. If tests for such disorders are positive, the parents then have the option of terminating the pregnancy.[1] Two other human abnormalities resulting from a change in chromosome number are Klinefelter's Syndrome, found only in males, and Turner's Syndrome, restricted to females. Whereas a normal man has an X and a Y sex chromosome, victims of Klinefelter's Syndrome have an extra X, or 47 chromosomes altogether. This condition causes severe mental retardation, sterility, a failure to develop male secondary sexual characteristics and, in some cases, enlarged breasts. The frequency of Klinefelter's births is relatively high—1 in 800—and, as is the case with Down's Syndrome, is more common among children of older mothers. Turner's Syndrome, by contrast, occurs when one X chromosome is missing; i.e., the victim has only one sex chromosome, for a total of 45 instead of the normal 46. This malady is outwardly expressed by retarded sexual development (no breast development, failure to menstruate or ovulate), unusually short stature, and lower-than-average intelligence in some Turner's females. Treatment methods developed within recent years have made it possible for an increasing number of Turner's Syndrome women to live near-normal lives. Interestingly, the incidence of Turner's Syndrome is far lower than that of Klinefelter's—only 1 in 3500. This discrepancy appears to be due to a very high rate of intrauterine deaths among fetuses with only one sex chromosome. Indeed, examinations of spontaneously aborted fetuses reveal that fully 10% were afflicted with this chromosomal condition.[2]

Cause of Mutations

That mutations occur is not in question; their underlying cause is less well understood. A great many mutations occur spontaneously due to natural causes. Some of these spontaneous mutations have been attributed to radiation exposure from cosmic rays and radioactive minerals in the earth's crust. However, it is thought that such relatively low levels of background radiation are insufficient to account for the majority of spontaneous mutations, the cause of which remains a mystery.

During the 20th century a number of man-made substances capable of inducing mutations have been introduced into the human environment and have raised serious concerns within the scientific community regarding their potential for increasing mutation rates. Such substances capable of inducing a mutation are known as *Mutagens*. X-rays were the first mutagens to be recognized, their mutagenic effect on fruit flies being described in 1927 by the great geneticist H. J. Muller at Indiana University. Subsequently a number of chemical compounds have been found to possess mutagenic properties, among them formaldehyde, mustard gas, nitrous acid, colchicine, and vinyl chloride. Many other candidates are now under suspicion as being possible mutagens; in fact, it is now widely assumed that most, if not all, of the substances which cause cancer also cause mutations.

Mutation Rates

The probability of any given human gene undergoing a spontaneous mutation has been calculated as 1 per 100,000 gametes (eggs or sperm). While this ratio may sound quite low, one must keep in mind that each person has perhaps 2 million genes. The chances of a gene mutation occurring in at least one of those genes is thus quite large. In fact, the English geneticist Harry Harris asserts that, on the average, every newborn child may be "expected, as the result of a new mutation in either of its parents, to synthesize at least one structurally variant enzyme or protein". [NOTE: Since only those mutations which occur in an egg or sperm have the potential to be passed on to subsequent generations, studies of mutation frequency have focused on these so-called "genetic mutations". Typically mutations occuring in a person's sex cells have no effect upon him/her but present a risk to succeeding generations of offspring. On the other hand, a mutation occurring in any cell other than an egg or sperm (somatic mutation) can adversely affect the person who sustained the mutation, but such injury will not be inherited by his/her children and thus represents no threat to the human gene pool.]

In this context it is of interest to note that 10-15% of all human conceptions spontaneously abort within the first month of pregnancy; 12-15% more are miscarried before the 27th week; and 2% terminate as stillbirths. Thus approximately 30% of all human conceptions fail to survive until birth.[3] Much of this reproductive failure is thought to be due to mutations. Chromosomal studies of miscarried fetuses reveal that fully half have gross chromosomal abnormalities, while lethal point mutations are suspected in many of the others.

The great concern among geneticists today is that exposure of populations to the artificial mutagens so common in the modern environment could further increase mutation rates. Since most mutations are harmful to some degree, it is in humanity's long-term interest to keep mutation rates as low as possible.

Birth Defects

As we have seen in the previous section, mutations in parents' sex cells can result in their children being born with structural or functional abnormalities, but by no means are all birth defects due to mutations (approximately 25% of all birth defects are attributed to mutation).[4] Living things are far more sensitive to adverse environmental influences during their early stages of fetal development than they are at any other time in their lives. Embryos which are perfectly normal genetically can be seriously or fatally damaged if exposed to extraneous hazards. Investigations over the past several decades have revealed the sad truth that the womb is not the safe haven it was once assumed to be.

The likelihood that all abnormal development is triggered by some aspect of the environment (even hereditary disorders were at some point initiated by a mutation caused by some mutagenic influence) has given rise to the science of *Teratology*—the study of the adverse effects of environment on developing systems—and to the search for *Teratogens*—substances which cause birth defects.

Fig. 6-2   **SOME KNOWN HUMAN TERATOGENS**

TERATOGEN	EFFECT
Ionizing Radiation	
X-rays	central nervous system disorders, microcephaly, eye problems, mental retardation
nuclear fall-out	
Pathogenic Infections	
German measles	congenital heart defect, deafness, cataracts
syphilis and herpes simplex type 2	mental retardation, microcephaly
cytomegalovirus	kidney and liver disorders, pneumonia, brain damage
toxoplasmosis	fatal lesions in the central nervous system
Drugs and Chemicals	
thalidomide	phocomelia
methyl mercury	mental retardation, sensory and motor problems
DES	vaginal cancer in girls, genital abnormalities in boys
dioxin	structural deformities, miscarriages
anesthesia	miscarriages, structural deformities
alcohol	mental retardation, growth deficiencies, microcephaly, facial irregularities
cigarette smoke	low birth weight, miscarriage, stillbirth
dilantin	heart malformations, cleft palate, hare lip, mental retardation, microcephaly
valproic acid	same as dilantin
Accutane	cardiovascular abnormalities, deformation of the ear, hydrocephaly, microcephaly
Tegison	same effect as for Accutane

Interest in birth abnormalities is undoubtedly as old as humanity itself, although prior to the present century most ideas regarding birth defects involved considerably more fantasy than fact. From ancient times until fairly recently, some societies believed that the emotional state and visual impressions of an expectant mother could influence the physical development of her child. For this reason women in ancient Greece were encouraged to gaze at statuary representing the ideal human form, while Norwegian mothers-to-be were cautioned against looking at rabbits, for fear their babies would be born with hare-lip! The Babylonians and Sumerians regarded certain types of malformations as portents of coming events; medieval Europeans regarded them as evidence that the mother had indulged in intercourse with Satan or other demons and occasionally used this event as an excuse to execute the unfortunate mother and child. The so-called "Theory of Divine Retribution", also prevalent in Europe during the Middle Ages, viewed the birth of a defective child as God's punishment on the parents for past sins. With the rebirth of scientific inquiry in the Western World following the Renaissance, less mythical interpretations of teratogenesis were sought. In the 17th century birth defects were attributed to such factors as the narrowness of the mother's uterus, poor posture of the pregnant woman, or to a fall or blow on the abdomen during pregnancy. Though inaccurate, these explanations at least were an attempt to find a rational explanation for what remained a mysterious phenomenon. Discovery by Gregor Mendel of the laws of genetics, followed by an explosion of research into the mechanism of heredity led in the early 20th century to acceptance of the idea that all developmental errors could be attributed to faulty genes. This view prevailed for the first 40 years of this century, but a series of significant discoveries and observations since that time has once again altered our perception regarding teratogenesis and has given new impetus and urgency to the field of teratology.

The first key discovery to change the prevailing view that heredity is all-important emerged from animal studies investigating the influence of maternal diet on the outcome of pregnancy. In 1940 a report was published showing that specific types of nutritional deficiencies in pregnant rats caused predictable types and percentages of malformations in their offspring.[5] Old ideas about the over-riding importance of genes and the conviction that the fetus could parasitize the mother if necessary to ensure normal development were effectively shattered. Continued research into the influence of maternal diet on fetal development has confirmed and broadened these original findings. It is now known that a wide range of nutrients, from proteins to trace minerals to specific amino acids are essential for normal development. Conversely, an *excess* of some of these necessary substances (e.g. phenylalanine, vitamin A) can exert teratogenic effects.

In 1941 an unusually large number of babies in both the United States and Australia were born suffering from congenital heart defects or deafness. Epidemiological studies launched to try to determine the cause for such an outbreak found that the only common thread linking all the victims was the fact that during the first trimester of pregnancy, their mothers had contracted German measles (*Rubella*) which had reached epidemic proportions that year. The fact that a virus could cross the placental barrier and damage the fetus was thus established.

While these two developments demonstrated that mammalian embryos are vulnerable to such commonplace environmental influences as inadequate diet and infections, the most dramatic confirmation that certain environmental factors (in this case a man-made drug) must be regarded as a potential risk to the unborn came only in the early 1960s with revelation of what has since come to be referred to as the Thalidomide Tragedy.

Thalidomide was a drug first synthesized by a pharmaceutical company in Germany in 1953 and subsequently developed and widely marketed in Western Europe as a mild sedative. Preliminary testing on laboratory animals indicated that thalidomide had little injurious effect even when taken in quantity (in fact, humans who attempted to commit suicide using the drug survived extremely large doses). With evidence of its safety regarding overdosing, but with virtually no testing for other side effects, the German manufacturer put thalidomide on the market as a non-prescription sleeping pill and, thanks to an aggressive advertising campaign stressing its safety, thalidomide (sold under the trade name "Cantergan") became the most widely used sedative in Germany and was extensively sold in Great Britain and several other European countries as well. Two American drug companies initially showed interest in acquiring thalidomide but concluded from their own tests that the drug was less effective than the brands they were already marketing. Somewhat later another American firm, impressed by the growing popularity of thalidomide in Europe, began another series of tests and released the drug for prescription use in Canada. In the U.S., however, a doctor with the Food and Drug Administration had nagging doubts about some unexplained neurological results among long-term thalidomide users and restricted use of the drug in this country to a small clinical human trial. At about this time (1960) the European medical community was becoming increasingly puzzled at the sudden increase in what had formerly been an extremely rare type of birth abnormality. In near-epidemic proportions children were being born with a condition known as phocomelia ("seal-limb"), in which there is typically a hand or foot attached directly to the torso without an arm or leg. In some cases, however, even the hands and feet were absent, the babies being born with only a head and torso. The presence of large numbers of babies with such an obvious deformity couldn't be overlooked, but intense questioning of the parents regarding their hereditary background, blood type, radiation exposure, or chromosomal aberrations in other children failed to reveal a common link. Finally two alert physicians made the connection between thalidomide use early in pregnancy to the birth of limbless babies. Subsequent studies revealed that 40% of the women who had taken thalidomide during their first trimester of pregnancy delivered babies afflicted with phocomelia. As proof of thalidomide's teratogenic properties gained acceptance, use of the drug was gradually discontinued in country after country, but not before nearly 10,000 children had been permanently disabled.[6]

The thalidomide saga not only emphasized the importance of testing new drugs for their teratogenic effects, but also raised the profoundly disturbing question of what other drugs and medicines widely used by pregnant women might be doing to their unborn babies. Thalidomide produced such a distinctive type of abnormality that it could scarcely go unnoticed. Conceivably, however, other teratogens which result in slight impairment of mental abilities, slight physical abnormalities, or diminished vigor, might never be suspected as harmful. The thalidomide episode, tragic though it was, stimulated research, still ongoing, into what other substances present a threat to the unborn. Though much remains to be learned, investigations over the past two decades have implicated an increasing number of drugs and chemicals as proven or suspected teratogens. Among them, in addition to thalidomide: dioxin, organic mercury, diethylstilbestrol (DES), lead, cadmium, anesthesia, alcohol, and—responsible for by far the largest number of birth abnormalities and miscarriages—cigarette smoke. In spite of the gruesome lessons of past tragedies, pregnant women continue using various drugs (e.g. aspirin, antacids, barbiturates, tranquilizers, cough medicines), drinking, and smoking, even though it is generally accepted that excess use of any substance carries some risk of fetal damage.

While some progress in elucidating the mechanism of teratogenesis has been made in recent years, much more research is needed. Nevertheless, some broad generalizations about the causation of birth defects can be made. Perhaps most critical is the finding that fetal vulnerability to teratogens depends on the stage of development at the time of exposure. By far the most sensitive period is the time of tissue and organ formation (organogenesis), a period lasting from about the 18th day after conception to approximately the 60th day, with the peak of sensitivity around the 30th day. During this time interference with development can result in gross structural defects. In the case of the thalidomide episode, it was found that virtually all of the thalidomide mothers had taken the drug precisely during those few days when the limb buds were forming. Those women who used thalidomide before or after this critical time gave birth to normal babies. During the first week after conception, when the embryo is a relatively undifferentiated mass of cells, any damage caused by teratogenic exposure will be lethal to the developing embryo. After the 8th week, though the fetus is barely an inch long, its organs are already basically formed. Exposure to teratogens after this time can cause such harm as mental retardation, blindness, or damage to the external sex organs, but the time for major structural deformation has passed.

A second widely-accepted generalization about teratogenesis is that as the dosage of a teratogen increases, the degree of damage increases. Basing their assumptions on the results of animal studies, teratologists thus presume the existence of a threshold below which no injury of any kind can be demonstrated.

Box 6-3

Accutane—Boon or Bane?

Severe, recalcitrant cystic acne is neither infectious, fatal, nor even debilitating, but for those young men and women suffering its ravages it can leave both physical and psychological scars. The scourge of adolescents since time immemorial, cystic acne has been treated with an untold number of home remedies or bona fide pharmaceutical formulations, but until recently nothing provided any significant, long-term relief. Thus when a highly effective new drug, Accutane (isotretinoin), received FDA approval in 1983, it encountered an enthusiastic reception.

Accutane is the first—indeed, the only—medication that can totally cure this particularly severe type of acne. While other forms of treatment are lengthy and only effective in holding the condition at bay as long as medication continues, after a few months of taking Accutane drug use can be stopped and, in most cases, the skin remains clear. For males, who comprise by far the largest number of cystic acne sufferers, this is unmitigated good news—they now have access to a cure for their problem. For females, however, (and 40% of all Accutane prescriptions are for young women), deciding whether or not to use Accutane may entail choosing between a beautiful face or a healthy baby. For Accutane is a known teratogen; of women using the drug during pregnancy, one out of four has given birth to a defective child. Since Accutane is a Vitamin A derivative and large doses of Vitamin A also are known to be teratogenic, Accutane received FDA approval with the stipulation that its use during pregnancy be forbidden. Nevertheless, it is now apparent that such use contrary to label requirements has occurred, with predictable results—malformed infants, miscarriages, and induced abortions by women wishing to avoid the birth of a defective child.

Alarmed by what was happening, representatives of such prestigious groups as the Centers for Disease Control and the American Academy of Pediatrics urged the FDA to pull the drug from the market. Equally concerned dermatologists and pharmaceutical company representatives pleaded for the rights of acne sufferers, the majority of whom are *not* pregnant, to have continued access to the only medication which can help them. After lengthy consultations among the various concerned parties, a compromise agreement was reached whereby the FDA will continue to allow marketing of Accutane under very stringent conditions. Henceforth labeling information for the patient will provide explicit descriptions and warnings of Accutane's teratogenic potential. The patient will be told not to use the drug unless she is protected by an effective form of contraception; to safeguard against the possibility that she may already be pregnant but not yet realize it, the patient is told not to begin using the drug until the second or third day of her normal menstrual cycle.

Instructions to physicians have also been drastically revised under the new agreements. Doctors are being told not to prescribe Accutane to any woman of child-bearing age unless she: 1) has severe, disfiguring cystic acne which won't respond to any other type of treatment; 2) can be relied upon to follow instructions; 3) is using an effective method of contraception; 4) has had a negative pregnancy test within 2 weeks of the beginning of Accutane use; and 5) has received verbal and written warnings of Accutane's teratogenic potential, as well as the risks of contraceptive failure, and has signed a statement saying she understands these. Hoffmann-LaRoche, the manufacturer of Accutane, has agreed to undertake extensive professional educational efforts and to conduct follow-up studies on drug use.

Officials are hopeful that with these increased efforts to inform women about the inherent danger of Accutane use and to prohibit access by pregnant or potentially pregnant women, an otherwise valuable drug can continue to be available to those for whom nothing else is effective.[7]

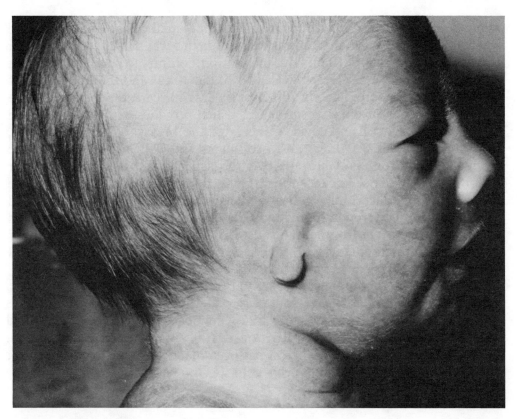

This infant has obvious defects which were caused by the mother taking Accutane during pregnancy. [*Dr. Reba Michels Hill, St. Luke's Episcopal Hospital*]

Determining exactly where that threshold is for any particular substance is, however, uncertain at best and expectant mothers are well advised to limit their exposure to potential teratogens to the greatest extent possible.

CANCER

Few words arouse such emotions of sheer terror and hopelessness today as does the term "cancer". As the second-leading cause of death in the U.S. at the present time (heart disease ranks #1), cancer appears to have assumed epidemic proportions. Cancer now accounts for slightly over 20% of all deaths each year; it is estimated that one out of every 4 Americans will develop cancer eventually and that 6 out of 10 in this group will die of the disease. Although cancer rates rise with increasing age, half of all cancer deaths occur before the age of 65. Among women between 30-40 and children between 3-14, cancer is the leading killer; next to accidents, it is the most frequent cause of death among Americans under the age of 35.[8] Yet in spite of these grim statistics, the future outlook for reducing cancer deaths is good. Unlike most forms of heart disease and stroke, many cancerous conditions are curable. Treatment methods are improving and whereas in the 1930s less than one cancer victim in 5 was still alive 5 years after treatment, today 4 out of 10 survive. In addition, contrary to popular belief, not all forms of cancer are increasing. Cancer of the uterus and the stomach have both declined by approximately 70% over the last 40 years, the former because of widespread use of the Pap smear test which provides early diagnosis, the latter for reasons still unknown. Cancers of the breast, colon and rectum, prostate, pancreas, bladder, and esophagus, as well as leukemia, have maintained more or less stable rates over the last half century. By far the major factor to which the rise in cancer death rates can be attributed is the explosive increase in lung cancer. Lung cancer alone accounts for about one-third of all cancer deaths.[9] The growing conviction that approximately 85% of all cancers can be traced to environmental causes provides the greatest reason for optimism: eliminate contact with cancer-causing agents (or "carcinogens") and one can drastically reduce the incidence of this dreaded disease.

Unfortunately, eliminating exposure to carcinogens is easier said than done, not only because it involves, in some cases, altering long-established lifestyles and personal habits, but also because many carcinogens have yet to be identified and the mechanism of cancer-causation is still but imperfectly understood. Nevertheless, a great deal of progress has been made in recent years and major break-throughs in explaining why cells become cancerous appear to be tantalizingly close.

What is Cancer?

"Cancer" is a collective term used to describe a number of diseases which may differ in origin, prognosis, and treatment, but which share the common characteristic of uncontrolled proliferation of cells. No longer subject to the regulating forces governing normal cells, cancer cells continue to divide and spread, invading other tissues where they interfere with vital bodily functions and eventually lead to death. Although the precise manner in which certain cells become cancerous is not yet know, evidence suggests that the basic problem involves an alteration in the DNA such as could be caused by a point mutation or chromosome breakage (abnormal chromosomes or an extra chromosome are frequently observed in cancerous cells) or through the activation of genes that are normally repressed, such changes then leading to a loss of control over cell growth.

Causes of Cancer

The search for agents responsible for initiating cancer has implicated a wide variety of factors, including viruses, hereditary characteristics, and environmental agents such as chemicals and radiation, the latter group being thought responsible for about 85% of all cases.

Viruses are definitely known to cause some forms of cancer in animals (e.g. viral leukemia in cats, Rous sarcoma in chickens) and are suspected of being involved in the type of human cancer known as Burkitt's lymphoma, though definitive proof is lacking. Similarly, there is suspicion that a herpes-type virus may play a part in the development of some cases of cervical cancer, since this disease is most common in women who have had intercourse with various partners. Again, however, evidence is only circumstantial.

Heredity as a major factor leading to the development of cancer was largely discounted by studies carried out earlier in this century by researchers who compared the incidence of specific types of cancer among the descendants of immigrants to this country and members of the same ethnic group remaining in the homeland. For example, a 1944 study of the incidence of liver cancer showed that black Americans have much lower rates of this disease than do blacks in Africa; similarly, Japanese-Americans exhibited low rates of stomach cancer—comparable to those of the general population—while stomach cancer remained very common in Japan. By contrast, these Japanese-Americans exhibited typically high incidence of colon cancer, a disease quite rare in Japan. Such results indicate that environmental factors (probably diet) rather than genetic predisposition account for the development of these types of cancer.

Nevertheless, it is now know that a few types of cancer *are* hereditary; one of the best known hereditary cancers is retinoblastoma, a cancer of the eye, resulting from a single dominant gene which is passed on from parents to children according to well-understood genetic principles. If diagnosed early, this disease can be cured by surgically removing the eyes. Some hereditary cancers have been traced to recessive genes and are thus less frequent because both of the victim's parents would have had to be carriers in order for the genetic defect to be expressed. In some cases a genetic *predisposition* to cancer exists but will not result in development of the disease unless exposure to a carcinogenic agent occurs. For example, among people with a disorder called xeroderma pigmentosum, the cells are unable to produce an enzyme that in normal cells repairs DNA molecules damaged by ultraviolet light. If individuals with this inherited condition are then exposed to U-V light, multiple skin cancers will develop. In such a situation, the disease itself is not inherited, but a predisposition to contracting the ailment if the necessary environmental stimulant is present does exist and is hereditary.[10] Similarly, a recent study of colon and rectal cancers found that an inherited predisposition contributed to approximately 50% of all cases. In situations such as these, where both genetic and environmental factors are involved in disease causation, relatives of a cancer patient are advised to begin having periodic checkups at an earlier age than would generally be recommended for the public at large and to be careful to avoid the types of environmental exposure suspected of leading to that type of malignancy (e.g. the high fat, low fiber diet thought to contribute to colon or rectal cancer).[11]

A great many *environmental agents* such as synthetic chemicals, sunlight, air

Box 6-4

"Too Much of Anything Will Cause Cancer!"
True?—False!

In 1977 a Canadian study documenting an excess rate of bladder cancer among male rats fed a 5% diet of saccharin created a furor among an American public unconvinced that the food additive posed a real health threat and dismayed at the possible banning of the only non-caloric sweetener on the market at that time. Intelligent assessment of the implications of the saccharin research was not helped by the statement by a top FDA official that humans would have to drink 800 cans of diet soda daily to consume an amount of saccharin equivalent to that fed the experimental rats. The issue was widely aired in outraged letters to Congressmen and newspaper opinion pages, laughed about on late-night talk shows, and used as the butt of many a cartoonist's jokes. The public was given the impression that the tests were meaningless as far as human health was concerned, an attitude most aptly expressed by Congressman Andrew Jacobs of Indiana who proposed that his colleagues pass a bill requiring that products containing saccharin bear the label: "Warning: the Canadians have determined that saccharin is dangerous to your rat's health."

Unfortunately, the Congressman's remarks, echoed by millions of his countrymen, reveal a profound lack of understanding regarding the methods routinely used for determining the safety of new chemicals. The objections raised to the Canadian saccharin tests—and to animal testing procedures in general—focus primarily on the following 2 points:

1) Animals aren't humans—do the substances which cause cancer in mice, monkeys, or rats (Canadian or otherwise!) predict cancer causation in humans? The prevailing assumption among researchers is that the basic biological processes in all mammals are fundamentally the same. For ethical reasons it is impossible to prove the thesis that any chemical which causes cancer in animals also causes the disease in man—to do so would require deliberately exposing humans to a known animal carcinogen and waiting to see if cancer develops! However, numerous tests have been successfully carried out to prove the reverse: every substance known to induce human cancer causes cancer in animals as well. Thus it seems logical to assume that the opposite is true also and that animal testing is a valid method for determining which chemicals are carcinogenic. What animal testing cannot tell us, however, is how strong or weak a given carcinogen will be in humans. This is because different species show varying degrees of sensitivity to the same substance, some developing cancer only at high levels of exposure while others are vulnerable to relatively low doses. Unfortunately it is not possible to calculate the level of human risk to a carcinogen based on the risk level in animals. We may be more vulnerable or less vulnerable; the tests indicate only *which* substances are a threat, not *how much* of the substance can be expected to result in a given number of human cancer cases.

2) The question of dosage—does *everything* cause cancer when present in excess? Contrary to popular belief, only carcinogens cause cancer. A test animal might be fed a mountain of sugar or salt and die of toxemia, but it will *not* develop a malignancy because neither substance is a carcinogen. Feeding or exposing test animals to extremely high doses of a suspected chemical is a universally-accepted procedure necessary for obtaining meaningful results within a reasonable time period, given the constraints of such experiments. In a typical study, for reasons of expense and space considerations, only 50 to 100 experimental animals are used in each test group. Such animals have a relatively short life span in comparison with humans, so in order to compensate for the long latency period involved in cancer initiation and to increase the chances for a weak carcinogen to be revealed in in the small study population, massive doses are used. This method does not alter the final result but simply facilitates the collection of data in a much shorter time period and at considerably less expense than would be possible using larger test populations

and lower dosages. That such tests are valid and that administration of large doses does not guarantee that cancer will develop is indicated by the results of past experimentation. A researcher at the National Cancer Institute a few years ago reported that of 3,500 suspected carcinogens tested in the routine manner, only 750 proved, in fact, to be carcinogenic—hardly support for the thesis that large doses in themselves are cancer-causing.

pollutants, heavy metals, X-rays, high-fat diet, chemical pesticides, and cigarette smoking are known to be carcinogenic and are widely believed responsible for the vast majority of human cancers. The exact mechanism by which such agents induce cancer is still not completely understood, but it is thought that in most cases a 2-step process is involved, often with a time gap of many years between the two. The first step, termed **"initiation"**, involves a permanent, irreversible change in the genetic material (i.e. an induced mutation), caused by a brief interaction between the target organ or tissue and a carcinogenic substance. Cells which have undergone initiation do not inevitably give rise to malignant growth unless they are subsequently acted upon by another group of agents called **"promoters"**. Promoters by themselves are neither mutagenic nor carcinogenic, but after prolonged contact, promoters can cause initiated cells to commence uncontrolled (i.e. cancerous) growth. A number of environmental agents have now been identified as initiators, others as promoters, while a few act as both. Other environmental factors known as **"anti-promoters"** seem to counter the effect of promoters. The characteristic latency or **"lag"** period between the initial exposure to a carcinogenic substance and the development of a malignancy after a period typically ranging from 10-20 years is more understandable in light of the findings regarding initiation and promotion of cancer. A number of researchers now theorize that the most effective way of reducing cancer incidence would be to reduce exposure to promoting agents or increase exposure to anti-promoters. Since long-term exposure to a promoting agent is necessary to trigger malignant growth, eliminating or reducing such exposure will result in initiated cells remaining permanently in the latent phase—"all dressed up, but no place to go".

The fact that an environmental agent can cause cancer was first reported over 200 years ago when, in 1775, an English physician, Sir Percival Pott, recognized an association between cancer of the scrotum and exposure to soot. Every patient he examined with this relatively rare ailment had, as a child, worked as a chimney sweep, being lowered naked into chimneys to clean out the soot which accumulated there. In the process, the boys were covered with soot and grime themselves and with the low standards of personal hygiene which characterized those times, some of this soot remained in the folds of the scrotum for long periods, eventually resulting in the development of scrotal cancer years later (more recently the active ingredient in this soot was identified as benzopyrene, known as a very potent carcinogen). Not until the present century, however, was much research directed toward detecting environmental carcinogens. Work during the early 1900s revealed the cancer-causing properties of a number of coal tar products and of X-rays, but not until mid-century as cancer rates began to soar did the search for cancer causation acquire new urgency. Since that time the public has been bombarded with so many dire warnings that the average citizen may be excused for thinking that indeed *everything* causes cancer. This of course is untrue, but the very large number of new chemicals and products that have been coming into widespread use each year, many without adequate testing for harmful side-effects, justifies concern. Surveys carried out on the "geography of cancer" indicate that the incidence of certain types of cancer are much higher in heavily industrialized areas (New Jersey, site of approximately 1200 chemical plants and related industries, is notorious as "Cancer Alley", having the highest overall cancer rate in the U.S.).[12]

Debate currently rages over the extent to which present cancer rates reflect exposure to chemical pollutants as opposed to personal habits such as smoking or diet. The outcome of this controversy is obviously of political and economic importance, since extensive regulation would be required to control the former, while education and persuasion represent the practical limits to reducing the latter. Several of the most prominent public concerns in relation to cancer causation include the following.

Smoking—Tobacco use, particularly the smoking of cigarettes, is now recognized as far and away the leading contributor to cancer mortality in the U.S. Rates of lung cancer are most reflective of the impact of smoking on health and the drastic rise in this disease neatly parallels the increase in the smoking habit in American society. Today about ⅓ of all cancer deaths are due to lung cancer and of the 130,000 new lung cancer victims diagnosed each year, 80% are cigarette smokers (most of the remaining 20% are individuals industrially exposed to carcinogens such as asbestos fibers). Death rates among lung cancer victims, as opposed to victims of some other types of cancer, are quite high largely because they are seldom diagnosed before they have reached a size of about 1 cm in diameter. By that time they have been growing for about 10 years and have usually spread to other parts of the body. Lung cancer rates began their steady rise in the mid-1930s, approximately 20 years or so after cigarette smoking became popular. Interestingly, until the mid-1950s it was widely assumed that women were resistant to the disease because the incidence of lung cancer among females was negligible compared to that among men. Since the mid-'50s, however, lung cancer mortality among women has been rising rapidly in a fashion parallel to that of males several decades earlier, reflecting social pressures which inhibited women's smoking prior to the "female emancipation" of the 1920s and '30s. By the late 1980s, lung cancer had surpassed breast cancer as the leading cause of cancer mortality among women, making it for the first time the #1 cancer killer among both sexes. As the advertisement for Virginia Slims puts it, "You've come a long way, Baby"—all the way from virtually no lung cancer to approximately 51,000 new cases

Box 6-5
Public Outcast #1

Pity the poor smoker. Once a national symbol of success and sophistication, he is now rapidly becoming a social outcast, banished to the hallways at professional meetings, passed over for promotions, excluded from some restaurants and many public places, and nagged unmercifully by his spouse and children. "Nonsmokers' Rights" has become a battle-cry across the nation, relegating the once-admired Marlboro Man to the status of second class citizen. Why this sudden evaporation of public tolerance for a habit still prevalent among more than a quarter of American adults? Why do 41 states now restrict smoking in public places? Why has the U.S. government banned smoking on all flights under 2 hours duration? Nonsmokers have always suffered physical discomfort when forced to breathe air polluted with tobacco smoke, yet as long as the belief persisted that smokers were only endangering their own health, they felt they had no right to complain. Personal grumbling turned to open militancy only with medical evidence proving that not only are cigarette smokers killing themselves in record numbers (approximately 350,000 Americans die from tobacco-related diseases each year), but they're damaging the health of family members, friends, and co-workers as well. With growing public awareness of the impact of "passive smoking" (i.e. exposure of nonsmokers to indoor air pollution from tobacco smoke), the three-fourths of Americans who don't smoke have resolved to remain the silent majority no longer.

Tobacco smoke inhaled by a nonsmoker can originate either from the "mainstream" smoke exhaled by a smoker or from the "sidestream" smoke emanating from the burning end of the cigarette. The latter accounts for approximately 85% of the pollution in the proverbial "smoke-filled room" and contains higher concentrations of carcinogens per unit weight than does mainstream smoke. While the sidestream smoke is significantly diluted by the volume of air in the room, two of its major components—carbon monoxide and nicotine—nevertheless have been measured at concentrations exceeding the ambient air quality standards in public places and meeting rooms. For nonsmokers who frequent these smoky environments, blood levels of carboxyhemoglobin are as high as if they had just smoked 5 cigarettes; their nicotine levels also are equivalent to those of a light smoker.

Much of the health research on passive smoking has focused on a possible association with enhanced lung cancer rates among nonsmokers. Numerous studies have been conducted in several different countries, and while the evidence is not yet universally accepted, EPA researchers estimate an average of 5000 nonsmoking Americans die annually due to working or living in an atmosphere contaminated with tobacco smoke. Studies in Japan and Greece likewise support a link between passive smoking and lung cancer mortality.

Far more prevalent, however, are the more mundane health complaints by nonsmokers forced to inhale someone else's smoke. While the following problems may not be life-threatening, they seriously diminish the nonsmoker's sense of well-being: 1) eye irritations—experienced by 69% of those reporting problems; 2) headaches—33%; 3) nasal symptoms—33%; 4) cough—33%. While these represent the most common problems reported, a sizeable number also mention allergic reactions, wheezing, or sore throats. Angina patients report more frequent attacks when exposed to passive smoke and bronchial asthma sufferers show sharp declines in pulmonary function when in a smoky environment.

The most tragic victims of passive smoking, however, are those members of society least able to speak out in their own defense—infants, children, and the unborn. That parental smoking could be considered another form of child abuse has been amply documented in numerous studies. Respiratory illnesses such as pneumonia and bronchitis are more frequent among children whose parents smoke, as are asthma and wheezing. A significantly greater number of children whose mothers smoke are hospitalized for respiratory conditions than are children of nonsmoking mothers. Children suffering from asthma have been shown to experience marked improvement when their parents quit smoking.

Even more vulnerable to tobacco's insidious effects are children in the womb. When a pregnant woman smokes (and 19% of pregnant Americans *do* smoke), she is exposing her fetus to nicotine, carbon monoxide, radioactive polonium, and numerous other toxic chemicals. Carbon monoxide appears to be the most fetotoxic of these, causing a rise in carboxyhemoglobin in the blood of both mother and child and resulting in retarded fetal growth rates. Infants born to smoking mothers weigh on the average about 10% less at birth than do babies of nonsmokers. Since low birth weight is a major risk factor for infant mortality, it is not surprising that approximately 10% of all U.S. neonatal deaths each year are blamed on maternal smoking. Smoking during pregnancy is also blamed for an estimated 50,000 miscarriages annually and for somewhere between 11-14% of all premature births, the risk of which rises the more heavily the mother smokes.

Considering the extent to which a smoker's habit can adversely affect those around him/her, it's no wonder that smoking is increasingly viewed as anti-social behavior. With the proliferation of clean indoor air regulations in cities and states across the country sharply curtailing smokers' freedom to light up in public, the possibility of the Surgeon General's dream of a "smoke-free America" becoming a reality by the turn of the century seems ever more likely.[13]

among women each year.[14] Unfortunately, while smoking among Americans in general is declining, the habit is gaining in popularity among teen-age girls, the only segment of our society in which smoking is on the increase. This trend is particularly disturbing in view of the now well-documented adverse impact of smoking in relation to problem pregnancies and birth defects.

Cigarette smoke is now known to contain at least 29 different carcinogens, including benzopyrene, arsenic, cadmium, benzene, and radioactive polonium. Since these substances are inhaled, it is not suprising that the lungs are the tissue most directly affected. However, smoking has also been documented as a major cause of cancer of the mouth, esophagus, and larynx and is thought to contribute to the development of bladder, kidney, and pancreatic cancer (and is a major factor in the development of heart disease as well). Thus a report from the United States Surgeon General categorically states:

> "There is no single action an individual can take to reduce the risk of cancer more effectively than to stop smoking—particularly smoking cigarettes".

Dietary Factors—Recent scares about everything from coffee to charcoal broiled meat to peanut butter having the potential to cause cancer have prompted consumers to fear that many food additives and contaminants are

Synergism: 1 + 1 = 5

Virtually all laboratory tests to determine carcinogenicity of suspected substances are based on responses to single-source exposures. Results of such testing methods may significantly underestimate risks in the real world because it is now well known that certain substances in combination are far more hazardous than either one would be if acting independently. For example, people who smoke cigarettes are 10 times more likely to develop lung cancer than are non-smokers; asbestos workers incur significantly higher risk of lung cancer than do people not exposed to asbestos. However, a person who both smokes cigarettes *and* works with asbestos is *90* times more likely to get lung cancer than is a person exposed neither to cigarette smoke nor to asbestos—far higher than the risk factor for either type of exposure separately. This phenomenon, where the interaction of 2 or more substances produces an effect greater than the sum of their independent effects, is know as **synergism** and can perhaps be most easily thought of as a situation where 1 + 1 = 5.

Synergistic effects are well-documented in relation to interactions between various air pollutants, water pollutants, etc., and will be mentioned again in the chapters dealing with those topics. Synergism has been most studied, however, in the context of cancer and smoking in an effort to demonstrate the degree of risk inherent in various types of smokers' lifestyles. In addition to the smoking-asbestos connection, other synergistic associations with smoking include:

Smoking and Alcohol Consumption—much higher rates of cancer of the mouth, larynx, and esophagus
Smoking and Living in Areas of High Air Pollution—elevated risk of lung cancer
Smoking and Working with Chemicals or in Uranium Mines—high lung cancer risk

Fig. 6-3

Relative Risk of Dying of Lung Cancer due to Smoking and Occupational Asbestos Exposure*

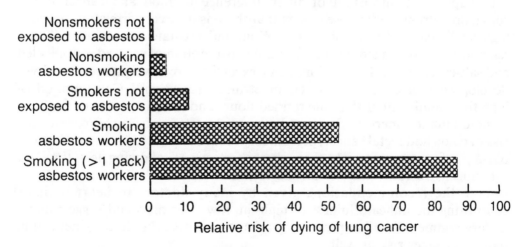

* Includes asbestos workers, but not other workers exposed to asbestos.

Source: Surgeon General of the United States.

potential carcinogens—a concern that is reflected in the growing popularity of so-called "natural" or "organic" foods. This topic will be discussed at greater length in the chapter on Food Quality. Suffice it to say here that although some food additives—particularly the coal tar dyes used for artificial coloring—are known to be carcinogenic in tests on laboratory animals, no solid evidence yet exists to indicate that human cancer rates are rising because of these substances in food. The stable rates of breast, liver, bladder, prostate, colon, and pancreatic cancer—forms of the disease which would be expected to rise if chemicals in food were a major problem—indicate no serious cause for alarm at present. However, bearing in mind the long latency period of many forms of cancer and the fact that many additives have been widely used for only a few decades, it may yet be too early to say that such chemicals won't cause future problems.

Ironically, while many people worry, perhaps unjustifiably, about synthetic food additives, they pay little attention to findings regarding naturally-occurring carcinogens in food. Substances called *Aflatoxins,* potent carcinogens produced by the fungus *Aspergillus flavus,* are known to cause liver cancer in animals and are suspected of being responsible for the high rates of human liver cancer observed in parts of Africa and Southeast Asia (although lung cancer accounts for the majority of cancer deaths in the U.S., liver cancer is the leading cancer killer in the world as a whole). The toxin-producing mold grows on peanuts, pistachios, corn, rice, and certain other grains and nuts when temperatures and humidity are high. If large quantities of aflatoxin are present in the food, liver damage and death may occur very quickly; in small amounts, consumed over a period of time, aflatoxins are among the strongest carcinogens known. Other natural carcinogens in food include safrole, an extract of sassafras long used to flavor root-beer until banned by the FDA in 1960, and oil of calamus, used until 1968 to flavor vermouth.

Perhaps most important of all in reference to food and cancer is the conviction among many researchers that there is a direct correlation between high fat intake and rates of breast, colon, and prostate cancer, as well as a relationship between stomach cancer and consumption of smoked, salt-pickled and salt-cured foods. In addition, being excessively overweight seems to favor development of cancer of the endometrium in women.[15] Consumption of high-fiber foods rather than the refined flours and heavily processed foods so common in the American diet has also been suggested as a way of reducing the risk of colon and rectal cancer, presumably because a high fiber content hastens passage of waste materials through the intestines, allowing less time for carcinogens to form and act on the intestinal surfaces.[16] These findings reinforce the recommendations given by many doctors to heart patients concerning the unhealthfulness of high-fat, low fiber diets and suggest that a dietary regimen aimed at preventing coronary disease should be beneficial in reducing cancer risk as well.

Air Pollution—It is well known that urban air contains a number of carcinogenic substances, benzopyrene included. It has not been possible, however, to prove conclusively that breathing polluted air, by itself, induces cancer. The fact that many cancer victims living in polluted areas are also smokers makes it difficult to say which factor was the decisive one and the fact that even non-smokers are simultaneously exposed to a variety of potentially carcinogenic substances further clouds the picture. Although the "gut feeling" of many researchers is that air pollution is probably, at the least, a contributing factor to the development of some cancers, the impossibility of carrying out a controlled scientifically valid experiment on humans makes the obtaining of conclusive evidence unlikely. Nevertheless, it is an observed fact that people living in cities larger than 50,000 population run a 33% higher risk of developing lung cancer than do people living in small towns or rural areas. The reasons behind this phenomenon, referred to as the *Urban Factor,* have never been conclusively determined.

Box 6-7

How Much of a Carcinogen is Too Much?
The Threshold Controversy

In regulating any hazardous substance an attempt is made to determine at what minimum level of exposure adverse health effects occur and then to set standards at or below that level. The assumption in such standard-setting is that risk of health damage is directly proportional to dosage or degree of exposure; the lower the dosage, the less chance of an individual suffering harm (or the fewer the number of people in the population who will be adversely affected). Below a certain point, termed the "threshold" level of exposure, no damage whatsoever will occur. The concept of thresholds rests on the fact that the body's defense mechanisms are able to detoxify many hazardous substances when these are present in small amounts, but can be overwhelmed when assaulted by doses in excess of a certain critical level.

Whether the threshold concept has validity in reference to carcinogens, however, is hotly disputed at the present time. Many cancer researchers argue that because carcinogens do their damage at the gene level, altering the hereditary material itself, then even one molecule of a cancer-causing agent could react with a molecule of DNA to derange the genetic code, thus leading to a malignancy. If this is true, then obviously there could be no threshold for carcinogens—no level of exposure, no matter how low, that could be considered absolutely safe for everyone.

From a regulatory point of view, there are other objections to the existence of thresholds; these center around the fact that cancer is actually a number of different diseases and that, even if thresholds do exist, it is highly unlikely that each type of cancer would have the same threshold even when caused by the same carcinogen. There are also wide variations in susceptibility to cancer, as to other diseases, among various individuals, further complicating attempts to establish an all-purpose threshold level. Finally, because many cancers are caused by the interaction of numerous carcinogens, it makes little sense to set a threshold for exposure to one carcinogen when simultaneous contact with other toxins may overwhelm the natural defenses on which the threshold level was based.

Definitive proof for or against the existence of a threshold for cancer causation is still lacking, but on the conviction that it is preferable to err on the side of public health protection, regulation of carcinogenic substances at present is based on the assumption that there is *no safe level of exposure to a carcinogen.*

Occupational Exposure—Since the days of Sir Percival Potts' observations on scrotal cancer among chimney sweeps, it has been recognized that certain occupations entail heightened risk of specific diseases. In recent decades the proliferation of new synthetic chemicals in industry, as well as the continued use of older substances only recently recognized as hazardous, has been reflected in cancer rates among certain segments of the work force far higher than in the general public. Today over 6 million American workers are exposed to substances known to be carcinogenic; many others work with materials suspected to be carcinogens but on which the necessary testing has not yet been done. Although there has been considerable difference of opinion between industry and labor regarding the health impact of exposure to carcinogens in the workplace, researchers estimate that occupational exposure accounts for 2-8% of U.S. cancer incidence.[17] Until passage of the Toxic Substances Control Act in 1976, giving the federal government the power to require testing of potentially hazardous substances before they go on the market, hundreds of new chemicals with unknown side effects came into industrial use each year. Unfortunately, workers, rather than laboratory animals, have been the "guinea pigs" who, by falling sick or dying, have discovered many substances now known to be carcinogenic. Some of the most significant industrial carcinogens thus discovered include: *asbestos,* one of the best known occupational hazards which is expected to cause the death of between 30-40% of all asbestos workers; *vinyl chloride,* a basic ingredient in the manufacture of plastics, found in 1974 to induce a rare form of liver cancer among exposed workers; *anaesthetic gases* used in operating rooms have been traced as the reason nurse anesthetists develop leukemia and lymphoma at 3 times the normal rate—and also have higher rates of miscarriage and birth defects among their children; *benzene,* long known to be a powerful bone marrow poison, capable of causing aplastic anemia, has now been shown to cause leukemia as well; *radioactive mine dusts* have been a particular problem in uranium mines, resulting in lung cancer rates among miners 4 times higher than the national average. Although pressure from labor unions and adoption of protective government legislation have resulted in some improvements in reducing occupational hazards, standards set for protecting workers are far less stringent than those set for protecting society at large.[18] In addition, until a few years ago workers often lacked basic information about the nature of the materials with which they worked and were thus unable to take precautionary action even if they desired to do so. A major step forward in this regard was promulgation by the Occupational Safety and Health Administration (OSHA) in 1983 of its Hazard Communication Standard, intended to provide employees in manufacturing industries access to information concerning the hazards of chemicals which they encounter in the workplace. Essentially a federal "Employee Right-to-Know" law, this ruling requires that manufacturers inform their employees of any workplace hazards and how they can minimize risk of harm. Manufacturers must also ensure that all chemicals are properly labeled and that Material Safety Data Sheets for each chemical are available for any employee who requests them.

Preventing Cancer

The preceding discussion should make it apparent that while we still have much to learn about the nature of carcinogenesis, we have already discovered enough to suggest a variety of personal actions which individuals can take to reduce substantially their own risk of contracting cancer. Cancer biologist S.B. Oppenheimer lists the following guidelines, based on current medical research, which if generally followed could result in a significant reduction in cancer rates through prevention of this dreaded, but certainly not inevitable, disease:[18]

1. stop smoking
2. avoid excessive exposure to sun
3. avoid exposure to known carcinogens
4. avoid heavy alcohol consumption
5. reduce consumption of fats and increase consumption of high-fiber foods
6. reduce consumption of salt-cured, salt-pickled, smoked, and charred foods
7. maintain lifestyle that prevents obesity
8. avoid unnecessary exposure to radiation
9. eat foods rich in vitamins A, C, and E
10. avoid or try to limit psychosocial stress

REFERENCES

[1]Norwood, Christopher, *At Highest Risk,* Penguin Books, 1980.

[2]Volpe, E. Peter, *Man, Nature, and Society,* Wm. C. Brown Co., 1975.

[3]Ibid.

[4]Wilson, J. G., *The Environment and Birth Defects,* Academic Press, 1973.

[5]Warkany, J., "Trends in Teratologic Research", *Pathobiology of Development,* E. Perrin and M. Finegold, eds., Williams and Wilkins, 1972.

[6]Glasser, Ronald J., *The Greatest Battle,* Random House, 1976.

[7]Willis, Judith, "New Warning About Accutane and Birth Defects", *FDA Consumer,* vol. 22, no. 8, October 1988.

[8]*Cancer Facts and Figures,* American Cancer Society, 1987.

[9]Oppenheimer, S. B., *Cancer: A Biological and Clinical Introduction,* Allyn and Bacon, Inc., 1982.

[10]Ibid.

[11]Schmeck, Harold M. Jr., "50% of Colon-Rectal Cancers Tied to Genetic Predisposition", *The New York Times,* Sept. 1, 1988.

[12]Environmental Defense Fund and Robert H. Boyle, *Malignant Neglect,* Random House, 1979.

[13]*Cancer Facts and Figures,* op. cit.

[14]Fielding, Jonathan E., "Smoking: Health Effects and Control", *New England Journal of Medicine,* vol. 313, no. 8, Aug. 22, 1985.

[15]National Research Council, National Academy of Sciences, *Report on Diet, Nutrition, and Cancer,* 1982.

[16]Oppenheimer, op. cit.

[17]Doll, R., and R. Peto, "The Causes of Cancer: Quantitative Estimates of Avoidable Risks of Cancer in the United States Today", *Journal of the National Cancer Institute,* vol. 66, 1981.

[18]Oppenheimer, S.B., "Prevention of Cancer", *American Laboratory,* February 1983.

7

Toxic Substances

"Being born a human being, but not being able to live as
a human being, is the most painful thing to me."
—Tsuginori Hamamoto,
Minamata Disease victim

Human illness or death due to contact with toxic materials in the environment is certainly not unique to the modern age. Hippocrates described the symptoms of lead poisoning as early as 370 B.C.; mercury fumes in Roman mines in Spain made work there the equivalent of a death sentence to the unfortunate slaves receiving such an assignment; for centuries Turkish peasants living in homes built of asbestos-containing volcanic rock have been dying of lung disease. Yet for the most part, such examples of disease caused by direct contact with toxic substances have been confined to certain occupational groups or to people who, by chance, happened to be living in an area where there was an unnaturally high concentration of some toxic material. By and large, in the past large populations seldom, if ever, were exposed to significant amounts of poisonous substances on a sustained basis. Today, however, that situation is changing, thanks in part to the tremendous increase in industrial production during the present century, as well as to the "chemical revolution" which has witnessed the introduction of thousands of new man-made compounds into widespread use in recent decades. Some of these substances, several of which were briefly mentioned in the preceding chapter, are largely confined to an occupational setting and pose little threat to the general public, although of course they are a major concern to workers and their families. Others, however, are now virtually omnipresent throughout the human environment and are

179

generating considerable controversy as to the degree of public health threat they present. In this chapter we will take a closer look at several of these substances— some naturally-occurring, others man-made—to which human exposure is nearly universal and which are known to cause serious health damage.

Polychlorinated Biphenyls (PCBs)

In 1964 Dr. Soren Jensen, a Swedish chemist at the University of Stockholm, began a project to determine DDT levels in human fat and wildlife samples; instead he discovered that the tissues he was examining contained large amounts of synthetic organic chemicals called PCBs. His findings, published in 1966, were greeted with widespread surprise and disbelief because PCBs, unlike DDT and other chlorinated hydrocarbon pesticides, were not being deliberately released into the environment but were restricted to use in an industrial setting. Despite the initial skepticism, subsequent studies by researchers in many countries confirmed Dr. Jensen's findings. Virtually every tissue sample tested, from fish to birds to polar bears to animals living in deep sea trenches, contained detectable levels of PCBs. Humans also were shown to have accumulated large amounts of the chemical. The U.S. Environmental Protection Agency calculated that 91% of all Americans have detectable levels of PCBs in their fatty tissues and human breast milk contains significant amounts, the average level being 7 times higher than the amount legally permissible in cow's milk![1] As the evidence continued to mount, it became generally accepted that PCBs, whose toxic properties were already well-documented, are *the most widespread chemical contaminant known.*

How could this situation come about?

Polychlorinated biphenyls were first synthesized in 1929, their production being taken over in 1930 by Monsanto which sold the chemical under the trade name "Arochlor". PCBs, which range in consistency from oily liquids to waxy solids, are extremely stable substances with a high boiling point, high solubility in fat but low solubility in water, low electrical conductivity, and high resistance to heat—all qualities which made them valuable for a wide variety of industrial uses. Primarily employed as cooling liquids in electrical transformers and capacitors, PCBs have also been used in hydraulic fluids, in carbonless carbon paper, insulating tapes, adhesives, paints, caulking compounds, sealants, and as road coverings to control dust.

The chemical stability which made PCBs so attractive to industry, however, is the very characteristic which has made them such an environmental and health hazard. Although designed for industrial use, there are many ways in which PCBs can inadvertently escape and contaminate the environment: 1) *discharge of PCB-laden wastes from factories into waterways* have resulted in mammoth pollution problems, the most notorious episodes being Outboard Marine Corp.'s dumping of PCBs into Waukegan Harbor, which currently holds the dubious distinction of containing the highest PCB concentrations documented in the U.S., and a similar situation in the Hudson River, traced to two General Electric plants; 2) *vaporization* from paints or landfills or *burning of PCB-containing material* can result in the chemical becoming airborne and then re-entering the ecosystem with precipitation. It's estimated that 11,000 pounds of PCBs enter Lake Michigan with rain and snow each year.[2] A classic example of fire causing extensive PCB contamination occurred early in 1981 in Binghamton, NY, where PCB-containing electrical equipment in the basement of the newly-built 17-floor State Office Building caught fire. Although the blaze was quickly extinguished, inspectors subsequently discovered that contaminated soot had been carried through the air conditioning system and deposited throughout the entire building. Air sampling indicated that this soot contained 10%-20% PCBs, as well as lesser amounts of dioxin and dibenzofurans formed during the combustion process. The ensuing cleanup operation took 7 years to complete and cost New York taxpayers $37 million;[3] 3) *leaks in industrial equipment* have resulted in numerous instances of PCB contamination, such as the case during the summer of 1979 when 200 gallons of PCBs leaked from an electrical transformer at a feed processing plant in Billings, Montana, contaminating about a million pounds of meal used in chicken feed. Subsequently, $2.7 million worth of chickens and eggs had to be destroyed because the birds had eaten the contaminated meal before the leak was discovered;[4] 4) *accidental spills* or *illegal dumping* are a source of increasing concern because the high cost of legally disposing of PCB wastes has tempted some haulers to dump such materials along roadsides, in ditches, or other out-of-the-way places. In August of 1978 such "midnight dumpers" opened the discharge pipe while driving along 210 miles of back roads in North Carolina, releasing 31,000 gallons of PCB-laden waste oil along the roadside where most of it remains to this day.

Whatever the route, once PCBs enter the environment they persist there for decades, resisting break-down. Contamination of living organisms with PCBs generally occurs via the food chain, the concentration of the chemical increasing as it moves from lower to higher trophic levels ("biomagnification"—see Ch. 1). Within an individual organism, especially among higher-level consumers such as carnivorous birds, fish, and humans, PCBs accumulate in fatty tissues such as liver, kidneys, heart, lungs, brain, and breast milk, and increase over a period of time, a process known as **Bioaccumulation.** Though ingestion of PCBs with food is the primary route of human exposure to these chemicals, PCBs can also be inhaled or absorbed through the skin.

PCB Threat to Health

Widespread human exposure to PCBs has concerned health and regulatory officials because laboratory testing has shown the chemicals to be toxic to several animal species even at very low concentrations. In experiments with rodents, minks, and Rhesus monkeys, PCB exposure has resulted in the development of a number of adverse health effects: liver disorders, miscarriage, low birthweight, abnormal multiplication of cells, and (in rats only) liver cancer. Researchers presumed that chemicals which could produce such effects in some mammalian species were likely to have similar effects on humans, and the knowledge that virtually everyone on the planet has been exposed to at least trace amounts of PCBs was considered cause for alarm. Evidence that many foods, especially freshwater fish, were contaminated with PCBs prompted the U.S. government to take regulatory action. In 1973 the FDA established tolerance levels for PCBs in food; passage of the Toxic Substances Control Act in 1976 specifically banned the production, sale, distribution, and use of PCBs in open systems, and in 1977 Monsanto, the sole U.S. manufacturer of the chemicals, terminated PCB production.

In the meantime, research on the human health impact of PCBs continued. Evidence documenting adverse health effects among workers occupationally exposed to the chemicals began accumulating in the early 1930s, soon after production of PCBs began. The most frequent complaint among these individuals was the appearance of an acne-like skin disorder now referred to

---

Box 7-1

Beware of Lake Michigan Trout!

The presence of PCBs in Lake Michigan would have generated little public attention were it not for the fact that these toxins bioaccumulate in fish and can be passed along the food chain to humans, becoming increasingly concentrated as they move from one trophic level to the next. High PCB readings in Great Lakes fish have dealt a serious blow to the commercial fisheries of the area, particularly to the Green Bay region of Lake Michigan, where the alewife fishery has been virtually wiped out. The FDA has set 5 ppm as the maximum allowable level of PCBs in fish sold for human consumption. While the catch of sports fishermen cannot be regulated, they too are warned by state and federal agencies to avoid frequent consumption of fish species known to exhibit high PCB concentrations. Since PCBs are stored in fatty tissues and increase in concentration as the fish ages, fish with the highest PCB levels tend to be the larger individuals among such fatty species as lake trout, brown and steelhead trout, Chinook and coho salmon, chubs, and carp. By contrast, lean fish species such as perch, sunfish, pike, bluegills, bass, and brook trout seldom contain dangerous levels of toxins.

Health advisories issued by Illinois and Michigan regarding fish from Lake Michigan recommend that pregnant and nursing mothers, as well as small children, avoid eating lake trout and other fatty fish such as those mentioned above. They also advise everyone to restrict consumption of such species to less than ½ pound per week.

Certain methods of preparing Great Lakes fish can help to limit PCB consumption for those who can't resist a tempting lake trout or salmon. As much fat as possible should be removed during the cleaning and filleting process; significant amounts of PCB are eliminated by cutting off the fatty belly flap and the dorsal back flap. Rather than frying the fish, baking, broiling, or charcoal grilling are advised to allow additional fat to drip off during cooking.

Fortunately, with the curbs on PCB production and use, there is evidence that PCB levels in Lake Michigan fish are now beginning to fall. If the decline continues, certain Great Lakes fisheries may become economically viable once again—good news for fishermen and consumers alike!

---

as "chloracne" and regarded as the most characteristic symptom of PCB-poisoning (or poisoning with any of the related group of chemicals known as chlorinated hydrocarbons). Some workers complained of a burning sensation in their eyes, nose, and throat; others experienced liver ailments. Additional problems reported during the early years of PCB use included a range of vague symptoms such as general tiredness, loss of appetite, diminished sex drive—all now recognized as classic signs of PCB intoxication.

All of these cases, however, involved acute health effects resulting from relatively high levels of workplace exposure and left unanswered the question of whether the public at large need fear chronic health damage (liver cancer being a major worry) due to long-term, low-level PCB exposure in food, air, and water. A large outbreak of what was thought at the time to be PCB poisoning occurred in Japan in 1968 when 1300 Japanese developed chloracne, swelling and pain in the joints, eye discharges, weakness, headaches, and a host of other acute symptoms after consuming rice oil which had been contaminated when a PCB-containing heat exchanger fluid leaked from a pipe into the vat of oil during processing. Referred to as "Yusho (rice oil) disease", this incident provoked alarm around the world as an example of how easily food supplies can inadvertently be contaminated with toxic chemicals. In 1978-79 a similar accident occurred in Taiwan, where it was dubbed "Yu-cheng disease". While most of the adverse health effects reported by victims of these two episodes were short-term (i.e. acute effects), consumption of the contaminated cooking oil by pregnant women resulted in some babies being born with dark skin discoloration and low birthweight; in other cases, infants were born with erupted teeth and followup studies in later years showed that among these children, dentition of the permanent teeth was affected. For years following the Yusho incident, close medical monitoring of the affected population was carried out in hopes of gaining information on chronic health effects of PCB exposure. Eventually, however, it was concluded that the troubles experienced by both Japanese and Taiwanese victims of contaminated rice oil were not due to PCBs at all, but rather to a related, more toxic group of chemicals called dibenzofurans which were also present in the heat exchanger fluid. As a result, investigators are left without a single convincing case of chronic human health damage caused by low-level environmental PCB exposure. In fact, even among those occupationally exposed to the chemical, there is no convincing evidence that PCBs cause cancer—or any other chronic health problems—in humans.

Although PCB production in the U.S. halted in 1977, the chemicals remain very much a part of the American scene. During the years between 1929-1977, 1.4 billion pounds of PCBs were produced in the United States. Hundreds of millions of pounds are still in use in closed systems, especially by the utility industry as coolants in high voltage capacitors (common on ordinary utility poles) and in electrical transformers. In addition, approximately 500 million pounds of PCBs have been dumped into landfills and waterways where they continue to pose an environmental threat. As existing PCB-containing equipment becomes obsolete and is replaced, safe methods for disposing of this material must be found. Many such wastes are currently being held in barrels in temporary storage facilities, subject to accidents, fires, or spills because there is at present no legal way to discard them. High-temperature (2200° F or more) incineration is the only EPA-approved method for destroying high-level PCBs at present but, due to high cost and public opposition to siting of such facilities, is not yet very common. Also, although production of PCBs is now banned in the U.S. and Western Europe, they are still being manufactured in Czechoslovakia and East Germany and hence continue to enter the environment.

Dioxin (TCDD)

In the wet spring of 1983 public apprehension about the dangers of dioxin soared when the U.S. Environmental Protection Agency announced that inhabitants of the tiny riverside community of Times Beach, Missouri, should abandon their homes and evacuate the town. Soil analyses had revealed high levels of dioxin contamination due to oiling of roads for dust control in the early 1970s; the oil had been scavenged from a trichlorophenol factory by a waste hauler and was heavily laced with the toxic chemical.

Times Beach is but one of numerous places around the world where industrial accidents, deliberate dumping, or inadvertent use of dioxin-tainted pesticides have resulted in environmental contamination which has provoked alarm, sometimes panic, among local residents. Public concerns, in turn, have been generated by debatable statements by some researchers that "dioxin is the most toxic substance ever created by man", and by allegations of a wide range of health problems and genetic disorders among American servicemen exposed to dioxin during their tour of duty in Vietnam (see Box 8-3, "The Dioxin Dilemma"). Widespread fears that serious human health damage can be caused by infinitesimally small amounts of the chemical have led to such controversial regulatory actions as the evacuation of Times Beach and the suspension of the selective herbicides 2, 4, 5-T and silvex, yet the results of numerous followup studies on exposed populations fail to show a single case where human death has resulted from dioxin exposure. What are the facts about this chemical whose very name seems to generate hysteria?

Chemically related to PCBs and other chlorinated hydrocarbons, dioxins form a large group of chemicals of widely varying levels of toxicity. The most dangerous dioxin is 2, 3, 7, 8-tetrachlorodibenzo-p-dioxin, generally referred to as TCDD or, simply, "dioxin". TCDD, unlike its chemical cousin PCB, has no industrial usefulness and has never been intentionally manufactured; it is formed as an unwanted by-product in the manufacture of certain herbicides and the germ-killer hexacholorophene. Dioxin may also be produced when PCB-containing trash is burned—a fact which is mobilizing popular opinion in many communities against the construction of waste-to-energy municipal incinerators. TCDD in minute quantities is now very widespread throughout the environment, present in soil, dust, chimneys of wood furnaces, in eggs, fish tissues, and human fat. The chemical binds tightly to soil particles and, where protected from light exposure, breaks down very slowly—experimental evidence suggests that its half-life in soil may exceed 10 years.

Statements that dioxin is the "most deadly of all man-made chemicals" are somewhat misleading because they are based on evidence of TCDD's extreme toxicity to guinea pigs, by far the most sensitive species to dioxin. Hamsters, by contrast, can tolerate doses of dioxin up to 1900X the amount that will kill a guinea pig. For other test species, dioxin's toxicity ranges somewhere between the extremes represented by guinea pigs and hamsters (nevertheless, whether or not it is accurate to label dioxin as the *most* poisonous synthetic chemical, there is no dispute that the substance is indeed highly toxic to all experimental animals). Studies carried out with a variety of laboratory species (rabbits, monkeys, rats, mice, etc.) to ascertain dioxin's long-term health effects have shown it to cause liver cancer in both rats and mice when large doses were consumed over an extended time period. Reproductive effects were also observed, including developmental defects such as cleft palate and kidney abnormalities, as well as a high incidence of fetal loss. Dry, scaly skin, hair loss, loss of fingernails and toenails, as well as chloracne, are some of the acute reactions to dioxin poisoning recorded in laboratory experiments with certain animal species.

The implications of all this so far as human exposure is concerned remains somewhat problematic. Over the years thousands of people, particularly chemical industry workers, have had extensive exposure to the chemical at relatively high levels (e.g. a 1949 incident in a Monsanto plant in Nitro, WV, exposed over 200 workers to dioxin; more spectacularly, a 1976 explosion at a trichlorophenol factory near Milan, Italy, released a toxic cloud which settled on the nearby suburb of Seveso, exposing 37,000 people of all ages to considerable amounts of dioxin). It is estimated that additional millions have been exposed to low concentrations (e.g. the farmers and ranchers using dioxin-contaminated herbicides, military personnel exposed to Agent Orange, residents of Times Beach and other communities where dioxin-laced waste oils were sprayed on dirt roads, consumers of TCDD-tainted fish, etc., etc.). Nevertheless, the only confirmed dioxin-related health problems in humans have been relatively short-term acute symptoms such as chloracne, muscle aches and pains, nervous system disorders, digestive upsets, and some psychiatric effects. Allegations that dioxin has caused soft tissue sarcoma (a type of cancer) or birth abnormalities have not been substantiated.

For those charged with protecting the public health and setting regulatory requirements regarding TCDD exposure, the dioxin issue presents some difficult decisions. The chemical is acutely toxic to laboratory animals and has been shown to produce severe chronic problems in many species as well. However, in spite of extensive human exposure to TCDD, only a handful of transitory acute effects have been confirmed in people. This leads investigators to conclude that dioxin is less toxic to humans than it is to experimental animals and that extrapolation of animal results to humans is fraught with uncertainties.

One problem hampering better understanding of dioxin's impact on human health is the difficulty of establishing the amount of dioxin exposure needed to produce a given health effect. This can only be done by actually measuring the levels of dioxin in the body tissues of exposed individuals, but doing so requires surgery to obtain liver and fat samples—a contribution which the human subject of inquiry is generally unwilling to make! USEPA's response to the public's dioxin fears has been the promulgation of regulations aimed at controlling the formation, release, and disposal of TCDD-containing materials. Some critics charge that the Agency is indulging in overkill, pointing out that the low environmental concentrations of dioxin don't appear to have had any serious chronic effects on humans. Nevertheless, politics guides policy, and as long as the public perceives dioxin as a menace to be controlled at all costs, the Agency is unlikely to relax existing restrictions.[5]

Asbestos

Probably no other hazardous substance has resulted in so many deaths and cases of disabling disease as has asbestos, the collective term for a group of fibrous silicate minerals found almost world-wide. Utilized by humans ever since Stone Age potters employed the substance to reinforce their clay, asbestos was woven into cloth during Greek and Roman times and was regarded as having magical properties because of its invulnerability to fire.

In modern times asbestos has acquired great economic value as an essential component in thousands of commercial products and processes. By the late 1970s, over 6 million tons of asbestos were being produced worldwide. About $2/3$ of the asbestos used in the U.S. is employed in building materials, brake linings, textiles, and insulation, while the remaining $1/3$ is consumed in such diverse products as paints, plastics, caulking compounds, floor tiles, cement, roofing paper, radiator covers, filters in gas masks, conveyor belts, pot holders, ironing board covers, theater curtains, fake fireplace ash, etc., etc.

Unfortunately, in addition to being very useful, asbestos also represents an occupational hazard of major proportions. It is now estimated that of the 8-11 million of current and retired workers exposed to large amounts of asbestos on the job, 30-40% can be expected to die of cancer. Several different types of asbestos-related diseases are known, the most significant being:

Asbestosis—a chronic disease characterized by a scarring of the lung tissue, asbestosis most commonly occurs among workers who have been exposed to very high levels of asbestos dust (once inhaled, asbestos fibers remain in lifelong contact with the lung tissue). It is an irreversible, progressively worsening disease, the first symptom of which is shortness of breath following exertion. Lung function is adversely affected, the maximum volume of air a victim can inhale being reduced. In most cases, it takes 20 years or more of exposure to asbestos before symptoms of the disease appear; unfortunately, by this time asbestosis has usually reached an advanced state.

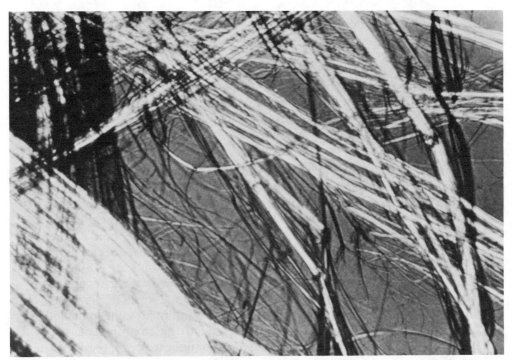

Asbestos fibers magnified to show the needle-like configuration of these hydrated silicate minerals. [*Illinois Dept. of Public Health*]

The severity of asbestosis is influenced not only by the duration of exposure, but also by the type of asbestos fibers inhaled and by the synergistic effects of cigarette smoking. Until about 40 years ago when concerns about workers' health led to regulations regarding dust levels in asbestos factories, asbestosis was the leading cause of death among asbestos workers. Since the 1940s, however, rates of severe asbestosis have been substantially lowered. Nevertheless, even today standards for permissible levels of asbestos exposure are based on those amounts deemed low enough to protect workers from asbestosis, in spite of the fact that this disease is no longer the most significant asbestos-related health threat.

Lung Cancer—with the gradual reduction in dust levels in asbestos factories, deaths due to asbestosis have been decreasing, allowing workers to live long enough to develop today's #1 cause of asbestos-related mortality, lung cancer. Compared to the 4-5% of the general population who die of lung cancer, as many as 20-25% of asbestos workers now succumb to this disease. The risk is especially great when exposure to asbestos fibers is accompanied by exposure to cigarette smoke. Studies have shown that while asbestos exposure alone increases an individual's risk of lung cancer death by a factor of 7, exposure to both asbestos *and* cigarette smoke entails a 60X greater risk of lung cancer than that experienced by persons who are not exposed to asbestos and don't smoke.

Gastrointestinal Cancer—cancer of the GI tract, which includes cancer of the colon, rectum, esophagus, and stomach, strikes asbestos workers with greater frequency than it does the general public, although a direct causative link is still not conclusively established. It is known that inhaled asbestos fibers can pass from the lungs to the stomach, colon, or intestines and cell culture studies have demonstrated that the epithelial cells of the human intestine are particularly sensitive to damage by asbestos. With the exception of esophageal cancer, the risk of gastrointestinal cancer is not enhanced by smoking.

Mesothelioma—this previously rare cancer of the lung or stomach lining today kills more than 5% of all asbestos workers. Like many other forms of cancer, mesothelioma is characterized by a long latency period, onset of disease symptoms occurring 25-40 years after initial exposure. Mesothelioma is of special interest to researchers because, unlike other forms of cancer, the only known causative agent for this disease is asbestos. Thus mesothelioma is considered a "marker disease" indicating asbestos exposure.[6] Since no effective treatment exists, mesothelioma is an invariably fatal ailment, with death generally occurring within 2 years of diagnosis. Even very low levels of asbestos exposure can result in mesothelioma and since asbestos is now so widespread throughout the environment, it is expected that the incidence of this disease will continue to rise for the next 20 years.

Although research has not yet been able to establish conclusively the degree of asbestos exposure necessary to initiate cancer, evidence suggests that some individuals who were exposed to high levels of asbestos for only *one day* developed cancer years later as a result. For this reason the current presumption is that there is *No Safe Level For Asbestos Exposure.*

While asbestos workers constitute by far the largest percentage of victims to asbestos-related disease, others may be affected through indirect exposure. Mesothelioma has claimed casualties among people living in the vicinity of asbestos factories and among children of asbestos workers whose only exposure to the fibers was from their fathers' work clothes when they returned from the factory. When asbestos is brought into the home, it becomes a permanent part of the domestic environment, embedded in carpets and draperies and suspended in the air where it constitutes a 24-hour/day source of exposure not only to the less vulnerable healthy adults of the household but also to the very young, the sick, and the elderly who are the groups most susceptible to any type of environmental irritant. For this reason, asbestos workers today are cautioned to shower and change clothes at the workplace in order to avoid inadvertent contamination of their homes with asbestos fibers.

Asbestos Problems in Public Buildings

Until fairly recently, most asbestos-related health concerns were focused on the millions of American workers who had experienced significant levels of occupational exposure to the hazardous fibers. It thus came as an unwelcome

Water Woes in Woodstock

Residents of Woodstock, NY, were angry—and a bit frightened. In November, 1985, people all over town began noticing mysterious clumps of blue fibers clogging drains, faucets, and shower heads. Quick analysis yielded an alarming answer to the "what is it?" question: asbestos. The source?—corroding cement asbestos pipe which Woodstock, like so many other communities, used to transport drinking water from municipal supplies to private residences. Though safe in most situations, when asbestos-cement pipe is laid in acid soils or where the water itself is slightly corrosive, the cement gradually deteriorates and, as in Woodstock, asbestos fibers can be released into the water. Asbestos levels as high as 300 million fibers per liter forced residents of Woodstock to drink bottled water for 18 months while the town replaced its old water distribution system with new iron pipes. In the meantime, citizens were left with unanswered questions about possible health risks associated with drinking asbestos-contaminated water.

While the Woodstock situation was particularly dramatic, many municipal water supplies are known to have measureable levels of asbestos. Asbestos concentrations ranging from 1 million to 2400 million fibers/liter have been detected in city waters in places such as San Francisco, Philadelphia, Seattle, New York, Atlanta, and Boston. In most cases the source of these fibers is the serpentine rock (serpentine contains a type of asbestos known as chrysotile) underlying the waterways or aquifers from which the water is drawn. It is possible also that some of the asbestos may be washed off city streets and enter adjacent waterways during storm episodes.

Fortunately for the peace of mind of Woodstock residents and citizens of other communities where asbestos is present in municipal water supplies, *drinking* asbestos, as opposed to *inhaling* the fibers, does not appear to increase disease risk. Studies conducted among inhabitants of Canadian mining towns where asbestos concentrations in drinking water ranged from 22 million-1200 million fibers/liter failed to show any elevated incidence of asbestos disease among non-miners. However, Woodstock residents are not entirely mollified; preliminary investigations carried out by New York State health officials revealed that townspeoples' exposure consisted of more than simple ingestion—when showers were used, a surprisingly high level of asbestos fibers were released into the air and were, presumably, inhaled. Thus did Woodstock's citizenry discover how easily the fine distinction between water pollutants and air pollutants can be blurred.

surprise when the EPA announced several years ago that the general public has been receiving asbestos exposure for years simply by working or living in any of the estimated 700,000 commercial, governmental, or residential buildings which contain friable asbestos ("friable" refers to asbestos material which, when dry, can be crumbled to a powder by hand pressure). Of greatest concern was the revelation that as many as 2–6 million school children and 300,000 teachers in 31,000 primary and secondary schools across the nation might be inhaling asbestos fibers on a daily basis. During the years from 1946-1973, asbestos-containing fireproofing materials were extensively used in constructing or renovating schools throughout the country. By 1973 increasing documentation of the health threats posed by asbestos had caused the EPA to ban all spray applications of asbestos in insulating and fireproofing materials and in 1977 new restrictions totally halted the spray application of asbestos. Such regulation had no effect, however, on existing asbestos-containing materials which, by this time, were beginning to deteriorate in many schools, releasing potentially dangerous asbestos fibers into the classroom environment. When asbestos-containing dust is swept up by janitors or disturbed by students' coming and going, it becomes resuspended and can remain in the air—at breathing level—for as long as 80 hours. The high levels of asbestos fibers measured in the indoor air of many schools have prompted concerns for elevated rates of lung cancer and mesothelioma among today's schoolchildren 20–40 years hence. The initial EPA response to this perceived threat was to issue an advisory to school districts throughout the country, informing them of the situation and requiring that they inspect their buildings for the presence of asbestos-containing materials (ACM). If friable asbestos was found, the districts were to notify parents or the PTA of that fact. The federal authorities apparently assumed that if an asbestos hazard was identified, parental concerns about their children's safety would be sufficient to ensure prompt remediation of the problem. Such did not prove to be the case, however, as financially-strapped school districts, in the absence of a firm federal mandate, postponed expensive remediation projects. By 1983, 66% of the nation's school districts had not yet even inspected for asbestos or had failed to report doing so to the USEPA.

Consequently, in the fall of 1986, President Reagan signed into law the far-reaching **Asbestos Hazard Emergency Response Act (AHERA)**, requiring that all primary and secondary schools be inspected for the presence of asbestos; if such materials are found, the school district must file *and carry out* an asbestos abatement plan. EPA was charged with promulgating rules detailing correct inspection procedures, establishing asbestos abatement standards, certification programs for contractors, and standards for the transportation and disposal of asbestos. Although AHERA created a $50 million revolving fund to be used for grants and no-interest loans to needy school districts, the amount available represents a tiny fraction of the total cost. In spite of the maximum $5000 fine that can be imposed on school districts which violate AHERA's mandate, it is expected that many school districts simply do not have the financial resources to comply with the law.

Asbestos Abatement

When an asbestos hazard is identified, those charged with remedying the situation have several options from which to choose:

1. **encapsulation**—a technique in which exposed asbestos is heavily coated with a polymer sealant to prevent further release of fibers.
2. **enclosure**—feasible when the area affected is relatively small, this process involves building a non-permeable barrier between the source of exposure and surrounding open areas.
3. **removal**—a labor-intensive process whereby all asbestos-containing materials are physically removed from the structure.

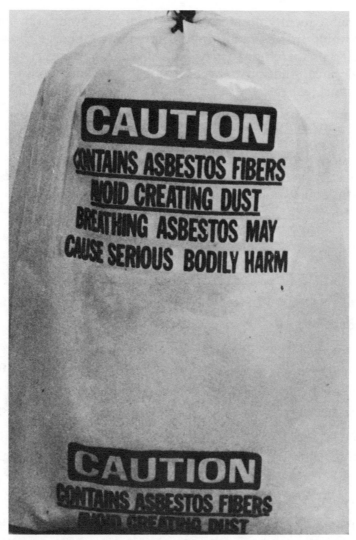

Asbestos disposal: after removal, damp asbestos-containing material should be placed in labelled, 6 mm thick plastic bags, and buried in a landfill. [*USEPA*]

Of the various abatement alternatives, complete removal is the most expensive and time-consuming. It also entails the risk of worker exposure to asbestos fibers and, if carelessly done, could endanger the public as well. However, since removal absolves a building's owner of future liability and because encapsulated asbestos requires periodic reinspection, removal may, in the long run, be cheaper than encapsulation. In addition, federal laws require that any buildings which are going to be demolished or renovated, other than private homes or apartments with 4 or less dwelling units, must have all asbestos-containing materials removed before work can commence. Essentially this means that if a school district chose encapsulation as its asbestos abatement option and subsequently decided to tear down or substantially renovate that building, it would first have to hire a contractor to remove all encapsulated asbestos materials, thereby paying twice to have the job done. For these reasons, even though encapsulation is an acceptable method of reducing asbestos exposure, most asbestos abatement projects today involve complete removal.

Asbestos removal projects must adhere to strict federal and state regulations to protect both workers and the general public. EPA has set a standard of "no visible emissions" for any asbestos removal activities. Asbestos-containing materials must be wet down before work commences and must be kept damp throughout the course of the project, right up to final disposal. Damp asbestos

Fig. 7-1   Summary of Asbestos-Containing Products

Product	Average percent asbestos	Binder	Dates used
Friction products	50	Various polymers	1910-present
Plastic products			
Floor tile and sheet	20	PVC, asphalt	1950-present
Coatings and sealants	10	Asphalt	1900-present
Rigid plastics	<50	Phenolic resin	?-present
Cement pipe and sheet	20	Portland cement	1930-present
Paper products			
Roofing felt	15	Asphalt	1910-present
Gaskets	80	Various polymers	?-present
Corrugated paper pipe wrap	80	Starches, sodium silicate	1910-present
Other paper	80	Polymers, starches, silicates	1910-present
Textile products	90	Cotton, wool	1910-present
Insulating and decorative products			
Sprayed coating	50	Portland cement, silicates, organic binders	1935-1978
Trowelled coating	70	Portland cement, silicates	1935-1978
Preformed pipe wrap	50	Magnesium carbonate, calcium silicate	1926-1975
Insulation board	30	Silicates	Unknown
Boiler insulation	10	Magnesium carbonate, calcium silicate	1890-1978
Other uses	<50	Many types	1900-present

Source: U.S. Environmental Protection Agency

wastes must be containerized in thick plastic bags or plastic lined containers, tagged with a warning label, and transported in a covered vehicle to a sanitary landfill. Since asbestos is not classified as a hazardous waste, the EPA-approved method of asbestos disposal is to bury the material in an area of the landfill separate from other household wastes, covering the containers with at least 6 inches of soil or other non-asbestos materials before compacting. Final cover of an additional 30 inches of non-asbestos material is required.

Legal Status of Asbestos

The mass of evidence documenting asbestos' adverse health impact has led to passage of legislation in several countries restricting the use of this otherwise valuable material. The United Kingdom, West Germany, and Sweden have all banned some uses of asbestos and are searching for acceptable substitutes. Japan is similarly discouraging imports of the material. In the United States, action against asbestos is proceeding on several fronts. Occupational exposure, which in the 1970s was lowered first to 5 and subsequently to 2 fibers/cm^3 of air, has now been reduced to 0.2 fibers/cm^3 over an 8-hour time-weighted average. Employers are required to sample at factory sites every 6 months and daily at construction sites unless employees are wearing respirators. In situations where fiber levels exceed 0.1/cm^3, employers must install exhaust ventilation and dust control systems and air vacuuming methods to reduce worker exposure to asbestos dust. Medical surveillance of workers, provision and laundering of protective clothing, maintenance of respirators, provision of showering and changing facilities—all are employer responsibilities to enhance the health and safety of asbestos workers.

An asbestos-free American environment is a longer-term goal. In 1986 USEPA proposed a total phase-out of all asbestos uses over a 10-year period, starting with 5 groups of products for which the Agency feels there are already substitutes available: roofing felt, vinyl asbestos floor tile, clothing, flooring felts, and asbestos cement pipes and fittings. Under this proposal, imports of asbestos into the U.S. would be restricted and other uses of the material would gradually be phased out over the period (exemptions would be made for specific products for which an appropriate substitute had not yet been developed, but such products would be required to bear a warning label). The EPA proposal was intended to spur development of non-hazardous asbestos substitutes, but it has met with strong opposition from asbestos product manufacturers, from the federal Office of Management and Budget, and from the government of Canada (largest single exporter of asbestos to the U.S.).[7] In the summer of 1989, the EPA Administrator cut short this debate by announcing the Agency's decision to phase out all uses of asbestos by 1997.

Lead

Human contact with lead, a naturally-occurring mineral element widespread throughout the environment, dates back thousands of years. The metal was first smelted about 4000 B.C. as a by-product of silver processing and soon found use as an ingredient in paints, glazes, and as an alloy. Among those who worked with the metal, it early became apparent that in addition to being commercially valuable, lead is a potent human poison. Over the millennia, evidence of the multi-faceted aspects of lead's toxicity has continued to mount. Lead poisoning is even thought to have made an impact on the course of history; a Canadian geochemist, J.O. Nriagu, recently reported in the New England Journal of Medicine that a review of records left by Roman writers and doctors document-ed a high incidence of gout—a symptom of chronic lead poisoning—among the Roman ruling classes. He speculates that a number of Roman emperors, such as Caligula, Claudius, and Nero, suffered from chronic lead poisoning which contributed to their erratic personalities. Lead poisoning may also have contributed to the low birth rate and high incidence of mental retardation among the Roman aristocracy. Wealthy Romans used lead extensively for both cooking and drinking vessels, but the major source of their exposure to the metal is thought to have been a grape juice syrup which was brewed in lead pots and subsequently used to sweeten foods and wine. Nriagu asserts that even one teaspoonful of such syrup would have been more than enough to cause chronic lead poisoning. Thus the degeneration of the Roman ruling class and the subsequent fall of the Empire may have been due, at least in part, to lead poisoning.

Sources of lead

Today lead is used in a wide range of industrial products, most notably for storage batteries and as an anti-knock additive in gasoline. It is produced in larger quantities than any other toxic heavy metal (world lead production is now estimated at 3 million tons per year) and is found in greater or lesser concentration throughout the environment—in soils, water, air, and food. Since 1940, lead levels in the general environment have increased sharply, pri-marily due to lead-containing auto emissions. Other sources of environmental contamination include emissions from metal smelters (the largest source prior to the introduction of leaded gasoline) and lead-containing paints and glazes.

Route of entry into body

With the exception of those persons occupationally exposed to lead, the major source of lead intake is through drinking water; USEPA estimates that as many as 40 million Americans live in homes where tap water contains elevated levels of lead due to the presence of lead pipes or lead solder in household plumbing (see Ch. 15). Food, especially leafy vegetables, may be another significant source of lead exposure. Plants absorb lead largely through their leaves, to a lesser extent from the soil. Vegetables or fruits growing near busy highways generally show the highest lead loads, sometimes as much as 3000 ppm.[8] Canned foods may also represent a significant lead hazard if contained in lead-soldered cans (one study of lead contamination in canned tuna showed that while the fresh fish contained but 0.3 ppm lead, tuna from the supermarket shelf in a lead-soldered can measured *1400* ppm lead!).[9] Housepaint remains an important source of lead poisoning problems, even though the use of lead in paints was halted years ago. In structures built prior to the 1950s, deterioration or renovation activities may expose older layers of paint, providing access to toddlers who may inadvertently consume the poison chips or paint dust. Similarly, soil or dust adjacent to housing once painted with lead-base paints may contain high lead levels; children playing in such locations and subsequently putting dirty fingers in their mouths can swallow prodigious amounts of lead. Vegetables grown in home gardens near structures once painted with lead paint can also prove hazardous: one group of researchers demonstrated that a child who ate 1 ounce of leaf lettuce grown in lead-contaminated garden soil consumed 200 micrograms of lead along with the greens. The fact that lead may remain in soils as long as 2000 years indicates that where dirt contains high lead levels, homeowners would be well advised to restrict their gardening efforts to growing flowers. Since bans on lead-based paint are not universal, another potential source of lead poisoning includes painted toys from overseas, especially Asia.

Interestingly, **ingested** lead poses a much greater hazard for small children than it does for adults. Whereas only 10% of lead swallowed by adults passes from the intestine into the bloodstream, 50% of the lead ingested by preschoolers remains within their bodies, making such youngsters the highest risk group for lead poisoning within our population. **Inhaled** lead from gasoline emissions, paint fumes, soldering activities, burning of lead-containing materials, etc., poses a more serious health threat to adults than does ingested lead because although it comprises a smaller portion of total lead intake for the average person, 30-50% of inhaled lead reaches the bloodstream. Much of the lead taken into the body is excreted, mainly through the feces but also in urine and sweat. The remainder is absorbed into the bloodstream and circulates throughout the body. Over a period of time, lead is slowly deposited and stored in the bones, particularly in the long arm and leg bones where it replaces calcium. Lead may also accumulate in children's baby teeth, which have been used in research to indicate a child's lead burden. In the bones, lead is usually harmless, but under certain conditions such as old age, high fever, or cortisone therapy, accumulated lead may dissolve out into the bloodstream in dangerously high amounts.

Biological effects

Lead can adversely affect human health in a number of ways. It interferes with blood cell formation, often resulting in anemia; lead can cause kidney damage, sterility, miscarriage, and birth defects. Because lead has a strong affinity for nerve tissue, injury to the central nervous system is perhaps the most serious manifestation of lead poisoning. Depending on the degree of exposure, lead poisoning can be reflected by hyperirritability, poor memory, or sluggishness at lower levels all the way to mental retardation, epileptic

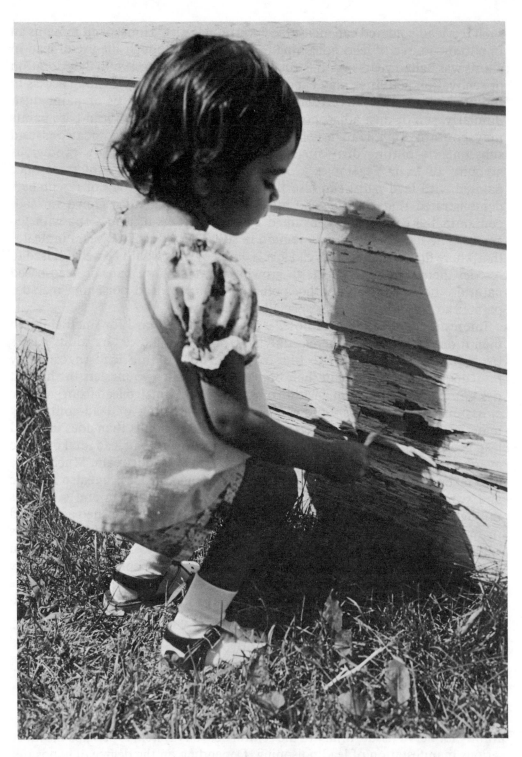

Children aged 1-5 are the group most at risk of lead poisoning because of their tendecy to ingest lead-containing materials such as paint chips. [*Illinois Dept. of Public Health*]

convulsions, coma, and death at high levels. A recent report to Congress from the Agency for Toxic Substances and Disease Registry stated that between 3-4 million American children, most of them living in inner city areas, are exposed to health-threatening levels of lead. The report also stated that an additional 400,000 fetuses each year are at risk because their mothers are suffering from elevated lead levels.

The public is most aware of the lead poisoning menace in relation to cases among young children who had consumed chips of lead-base paints. Although such paints have not been used for interior purposes since 1940, children living in older houses, especially those in deteriorating condition, not uncommonly developed lead poisoning by chewing on windowsills or eating flaking paint or dirt that had accumulated on floors (similar problems have been documented among zoo animals who contracted lead poisoning by gnawing on painted cage bars). This condition frequently is fatal among small children (the majority of victims range in age from 1 to 3 years of age); those receiving treatment in time generally survive but commonly suffer from mental retardation, recurrent seizures, cerebral palsy, or atrophy of the optic nerve, leading to blindness.

Fortunately, a very successful public education effort aimed at warning parents about lead hazards, plus the sharp reduction in exterior paint lead levels since 1971, has greatly reduced overt cases of lead poisoning in recent years.

However, new and disturbing evidence has been reported recently, indicating that even at levels previously considered safe, chronic low-level exposure to lead can inhibit the normal development of children's intellectual abilities. A

Box 7-3

The Case of the Poisonous Pitcher

The McDevitt family in Pocatello, Idaho, presented their physician with a major diagnostic challenge several years ago when both parents and 3 out of 4 of their children developed a strange complex of gradually worsening health conditions. They complained of stomach pains, constant fatigue, and vomiting. They noticed personality changes in each other and an increasing tendency to quarrel. Most of their meals were left unfinished. Only the youngest child, a baby still on formula, retained a normal appetite and disposition. A slight accident involving a blow to the head caused one of the children to commence vomiting and produced a paralysis of the left arm and leg, resulting in hospitalization. As the child underwent tests, doctors detected signs of serious anemia. Other family members were then examined and found to display the same symptoms. Noting the characteristic stippling of red blood cells, the physicians diagnosed the family's problem as lead poisoning. This solved only half the mystery, however. The question remained as to where the lead exposure could have occurred. The family was an affluent one, not in the habit of eating paint chips or chewing on toothpaste tubes. After an extensive investigation the source of the poisoning was finally discovered—an earthenware pitcher whose lead glaze had not been fired sufficiently long was being used daily to pour the family's breakfast orange juice. The acidity of the juice had resulted in enough leaching of lead from the glaze to poison the entire family—with the exception of the baby who drank only milk. Once the cause of the problem was removed, all of the poisoning victims recovered.[10]

study carried out in the Boston area among 2nd-grade students revealed that those whose baby teeth (which they had willingly witheld from the Tooth Fairy to contribute to Science!) had a relatively higher lead level also exhibited a greater incidence of unruly classroom behavior, a lesser ability to follow instructions, and lower scores on IQ tests than did students with low lead levels in their teeth.[11] Yet none of these children would have been categorized as lead-poisoning victims based on prevailing views regarding "safe" levels. There is increasing concern that as many as 18% of all inner city children today are being adversely affected in terms of learning ability and behavior by sub-clinical levels of lead in their systems.

Mercury

This liquid metal, the "quicksilver" of ancient times, has been used for a wide variety of purposes for at least 2500 years—and has been contributing to illness and death among those exposed to it for an equal period of time. Although at very low levels of exposure mercury does not appear to be damaging, the margin of safety is small. Mercury is a valuable constituent of many industrial products and processes. It is used as a catalyst in the manufacture of plastics, as a slime-retardant in paper-making, as a fungicide in paints, as an alloy in dental fillings, in the manufacture of scientific instruments, and for many other purposes.

While mercury has always been present in the environment in trace amounts, concentrations have been increasing during the modern era thanks to such human activities as coal-burning (combustion releases many of the impurities found in coal deposits, mercury included) and the dumping of mercury-laden wastes into waterways. Evaporation of mercury from paints as they dry adds significant quantities of this substance to the air, as does incineration of mercury-containing paper products. Large amounts of mercury also enter the atmosphere and oceans through vaporization of mercury compounds naturally-occurring in the earth's crust.

Health effects of mercury exposure

Inorganic Mercury—The action of mercury on the human system depends primarily on the form of mercury to which the victim is exposed. Inorganic metallic mercury frequently attacks the liver and kidneys; it also can diffuse through the alveolar membranes of the lungs and travel to the brain where it can cause such neurological problems as lack of coordination. Inorganic mercury can enter the system either by inhalation of mercury vapors or by absorption of mercury compounds through the skin after prolonged contact. Examples of human poisoning with inorganic mercury include the malady prevalent among hatmakers in 17th century France called the "Mad Hatters' Disease" (immortalized by a character of the same name in Lewis Carroll's "Alice in Wonderland"). This neurological disorder, manifested as tremors and mental aberrations, resulted from the practice at that time of soaking animal hides in a solution of mercuric nitrate for purposes of softening the hairs. Since the hatmakers' bare arms and hands were in frequent contact with the solution as they manipulated the hides, skin absorption of mercury led to development of the disease symptoms. Poisoning by inhalation is more common than skin absorption, however, and represents the most common form of occupational exposure to mercury. Dentists and dental hygienists have experienced high rates of inorganic mercury poisoning caused by inhalation of fumes released when filling amalgams are prepared. Mercury miners are another group at risk, especially if they smoke. Many people have become ill and some deaths have been reported among persons and animals exposed to mercury fumes when large amounts of mercury were accidentally spilled within a confined area where ventilation was poor. One case involved a schoolboy who brought home about half a pound of liquid mercury and, while playing with it, spilled the entire amount on the living room carpet. His mother's attempts to vacuum it up only resulted in spreading the contamination. As the mercury vaporized, every member of the family contracted mercury poisoning, experiencing generalized tremors, skin eruptions, and, in one case, hallucinations.[12] Contrary to common fears, however, swallowing inorganic mercury, such as could occur if an oral thermometer were to break while in the mouth, poses virtually no health threat. Such mercury simply passes through the gastrointestinal tract and is excreted through the kidneys within a few days.

Organic Mercury—Far more toxic than elemental mercury are the organic mercury compounds such as methyl mercury which, being extremely soluble, can readily penetrate living membranes. Organic mercury circulates in the bloodstream bound to red blood cells and gradually diffuses into the brain, destroying the cells which control coordination. Symptoms of organic mercury poisoning generally don't appear until a month or two after exposure, showing up initially as numbness in the lips, tongue, and fingertips. Gradually speech becomes slurred and difficulty in swallowing and walking becomes apparent. As mercury levels rise, deafness and vision problems may develop and the victim tends to lose contact with his surroundings. Before the nature of mercury poisoning was understood, such people were often thought to be neurotic or mentally ill and were occasionally placed in insane asylums.

Several tragic episodes involving methyl mercury poisoning have been documented in recent decades. In 1972 over 6500 Iraqi villagers became seriously ill and 459 died after eating bread which had been made from seed wheat coated with an organic mercury fungicide. A similar situation, fortunately on a much smaller scale, occurred in the U.S. three years earlier when several members of a family in Alamagordo, N.M., suffered permanent neurological impairment after they butchered and ate a hog which had been fed fungicide-treated seed corn. Undoubtedly the most famous episode of mass poisoning with methyl mercury occurred during the years from 1953–1961 in the coastal town of Minamata on the Japanese island of Kyushu. A plastics factory, Chisso Corp., had for a number of years been discharging inorganic mercury wastes into the waters of Minamata Bay where many of the local residents earned their livelihood as fishermen. In the anaerobic conditions among the sediments at the bottom of the bay, the inorganic mercury was converted into highly toxic methyl mercury by the bacterium *Methanobacterium amelanskis.* Readily soluble, the methyl mercury thus began moving through the aquatic food chain, being passively absorbed by microscopic algae which were subsequently eaten by zooplankton, which were eaten by small fish, etc., the methyl mercury becoming increasingly concentrated at each higher trophic level.

Trouble first became apparent in Minamata when the town cats developed what residents first thought must be a strange viral disease, yowling continuously and sometimes leaping into the sea to drown. When the townspeople themselves started to complain of vague maladies such as extreme fatigue, headaches, numbness in their extremities and difficulty in swallowing, it was first suspected that they were contracting some sort of illness from the sick cats. Eventually the true nature of their mutual problem was discovered—methyl mercury poisoning derived from a diet composed primarily of mercury-contaminated fish. By this time over 100 people had been stricken with such symptoms as mental derangement, inability to walk or use chopsticks, visual disturbances, and convulsions. Forty-four of the Minamata victims died during this period and many others were permanently disabled. As this sad episode unfolded, the teratogenic properties of methyl mercury became apparent. Twenty-two brain-damaged babies were born during this period to mothers who themselves exhibited no outward signs of mercury poisoning, though several mentioned experiencing a slight numbness of the fingers during pregnancy and analysis showed a high level of mercury in their hair. Subsequent studies have revealed that methyl mercury has a special affinity for fetal tissue, easily crossing the placental barrier where it severely damages the developing child while leaving the mother unharmed. The ultimate human toll of Chisso's poisoning of Minamata Bay included 700 deaths and 9000 individuals left with varying degrees of paralysis and brain damage. Estimates are that as many as 50,000 persons living within 35 miles of the bay who consumed its fish have suffered at least mild symptoms of mercury poisoning.[13] Follow-up studies on the people of Minamata have indicated that in some areas of the town as many as 25% of the children are regarded as "mentally deficient", though outwardly they appear normal, suggesting that even low levels of methyl mercury in the maternal diet have left their subtle imprint.[14]

Cadmium

This soft, silver-white toxic metal plays no beneficial role in the metabolism of living things. Used primarily in the electroplating industry, cadmium is also an important constituent of nickel-cadmium batteries, engine parts for automobiles and aircraft, in the manufacture of plastics, radios, and television sets. Particles of the metal can become airborne during the manufacture of

A Brazilian Minamata?

Across the vast expanse of Brazil's Amazon River Basin, the lessons of Minamata are today being relearned the hard way. Amazonia is in the throes of a modern-day gold rush, with an estimated half-million prospectors roaming the region, searching along riverbeds for traces of the precious metal. Watching gold production steadily climbing, Brazilian geologists affirm that "the future of Amazonia is mineral exploration" and are convinced the region's potential yield is 2-3X greater than the 100 tons now being extracted each year. While the bonanza promises to make Brazil one of the world's leading gold producers, it is also wreaking havoc on the natural environment and on the health of local populations in the areas beset with gold fever. If present trends are any indication, entire ecosystems may be irrevocably poisoned before the eventual depletion of reserves brings a halt to mining operations.

Amazonia's toxic troubles can be traced to the technique used for extracting the region's treasures. Brazil's gold rush is dominated by hundreds of thousands of individual entrepreneurs employing methods which would have looked entirely familiar to California's "Forty-niners" over a century ago. Digging or pumping mud from riverbeds, the miners scrutinize the muck for a glimpse of tell-tale glitter. If gold is present, the prospector pours liquid mercury into the mixture, causing the formation of a gold/mercury alloy which is easily separated from the mud. This amalgam is then subjected to treatment with a blowtorch to burn off the mercury, leaving purified gold behind. Unfortunately, this procedure pollutes the surrounding air with mercury vapors, presenting a distinct health hazard to anyone within breathing distance. To make matters worse, prospectors frequently pour mercury into the water where—just as happened at Minamata—it enters the aquatic food chain, poisoning fish and, ultimately, people who have no way of knowing if the fish on their dinner plate contains mercury or not. It is estimated that miners are dumping anywhere from 200-1000 tons of mercury into the Amazon every year. An American biologist currently working in Brazil has reported finding fish with mercury concentrations 5X higher than the safety limits recommended by the World Health Organization. Bewailing the extent of the problem, the biologist observed that, "Wherever there's gold mining the fish are contaminated, and there's gold mining now across an area half as big as the United States."

The lethal legacy of this situation is already becoming tragically evident. While there is no way of knowing how many have already died, a leading citizen of Itaituba, near the center of Brazil's gold rush, claims that hundreds in his home region are sick; he should know—doctors in Sao Paulo told him that he too was suffering from mercury poisoning at levels well in excess of those causing violent disorders.

The Brazilian government has finally begun to respond to the situation; in 1988 an edict was issued, banning the use of mercury by miners. Observers doubt that the prohibition will have much, if any, impact, however, because there aren't enough inspectors to enforce the law. The area is simply too vast for effective policing and the miners themselves remain unconvinced that they are a part of the problem. Unfortunately, it appears that until a major health disaster becomes too obvious to ignore, the poisoning of the Amazon will continue—but by that time the damage may well be irreversible.[15]

pesticides and fertilizers (phosphate rock often contains cadmium), when cadmium-containing products are incinerated, and can contaminate waterways when industrial wastes are flushed into rivers and streams. This cadmium can then enter human systems in food, water, or polluted air.

The largest outbreak of cadmium poisoning documented thus far involved a number of people living near the Jintsu River basin in Japan who, during the 1950s and 1960s, experienced severe bone pains and kidney malfunctions. As their condition worsened, victims developed a condition known as osteomalacia, suffering multiple bone fractures and excruciating pain (hence the villagers' name for the condition: itai-itai, or "ouch-ouch" disease). The whole skeleton became abnormally soft and death generally followed, usually due to kidney failure. Most frequently the victims were persons who were malnourished or middle-aged women under physiological stress due to numerous pregnancies or menopause. Eventually it was discovered that the mysterious itai-itai disease resulted from cadmium discharges from a lead and zinc mine upstream from the affected farming community. Cadmium fumes and particles from the mining operation, as well as cadmium-laden wastewaters, had contaminated farmland and irrigation water with the toxic metal. Plants readily absorb cadmium from soil and water, and it was found that both rice and soybeans grown in the area contained high levels of the metal; consumption of cadmium-contaminated foods thus proved to be the cause of the disease outbreak.[16]

Although most Americans exhibit some body accumulation of cadmium, most of it in the kidneys, instances of acute poisoning in recent times are rare. Occasionally outbreaks of food poisoning due to cadmium intoxication are traced to the consumption of acidic drinks (e.g. lemonade) or foods served in galvanized metal containers which contained a cadmium alloy.

Today one of the main concerns regarding cadmium focuses on the possible adverse effects of using cadmium-tainted sewage sludge as a soil conditioner for vegetable gardens or sewage treatment plant effluent containing cadmium for irrigation purposes. Since plants can absorb and accumulate cadmium, using such materials on crops may pose a threat to the health of those consuming the vegetables. Obviously this is only a problem when the particular sewage treatment plant in question receives discharges from industries using cadmium; it would not be a concern in those systems where only domestic wastes are received for treatment.

In addition to the toxic materials discussed above, there are many other substances capable of causing health damage in humans when present in more than trace amounts or when exposure to even very low levels persists over an extended time period. Fluorides, selenium, copper, nickel, chromium, and arsenic are but a few of the naturally-occurring toxins which are known, under certain conditions, to affect human health adversely. Unfortunately, because the symptoms of exposure to toxic substances are often so vague or so similar to those of other more common ailments, they are frequently either ignored or misdiagnosed. Thus it would not be surprising to find that health damage due to such toxins is more prevalent than commonly assumed at present.

REFERENCES

[1]Environmental Defense Fund and Robert H. Boyle, *Malignant Neglect,* Random House, 1979.

[2]Great Lakes Basin Commission, "PCBs: You can store them up, but can you throw them out?", *Great Lakes Communicator,* vol. 11, no. 3, December 1980.

[3]Fawcett, Howard H., *"Hazardous and Toxic Materials: Safe Handling and Disposal",* John Wiley & Sons, 1988.

[4]Regenstein, Lewis, *"The Poisoning of America",* Acropolis Books Ltd., 1982.

[5]Tschirley, Fred, H., "Dioxin", *Scientific American,* vol. 254, no. 2, February 1986.

[6]Brodeur, Paul, *The Asbestos Hazard,* New York Academy of Sciences, 1980.

[7]"Asbestos: A Review of its Properties, Uses, Hazards, and Regulation", Staff Report to the Chairman, New York State Joint Legislative Commission on Toxic Substances and Hazardous Wastes, June 1988.

[8]Waldbott, George L., *Health Effects of Environmental Pollutants,* The C. V. Mosby Company, 1978.

[9]Settle, D. M., and C. C. Patterson, "Lead in albacore: Guide to lead pollution in Americans", *Science,* vol. 207, 1980.

[10]Block, J. L., "The Accident That Saved Five Lives", *Good Housekeeping,* Nov. 1969.

[11]Needleman, H. L., et al., "Deficits in Psychologic and Classroom Performance of Children with Elevated Dentine Lead Levels", *New England Journal of Medicine,* 300 (1979):689–695.

[12]Howie, R. A. and H. Smite, "Mercury in Human Tissue", *Forensic Science,* 7:90–96, 1967.

[13]Weisskopf, Michael, "Japanese Town Still Staggered by Legacy of Ecological Disaster", *The Washington Post,* April 18, 1987.

[14]Smith, A., "Congenital Minamata Disease", *Proceedings of a Conference on Women and the Workplace,* Washington, DC, The Society for Occupational and Environmental Health, 1977.

[15]Gillam, Martin, "Amazon gold rush takes its toll as mercury poisons fish—and people", *The Christian Science Monitor,* December 19, 1988; Margolis, Mac, "Amazon Ablaze", *World Monitor,* vol. 2, no. 2, February 1989.

[16]Waldbott, G. L., op. cit.

8

Pests and Pesticides

"And the locusts came up over all the land of Egypt, and settled on the whole country of Egypt... they covered the face of the whole land, so that the land was darkened, and they ate all the plants in the land and all the fruit of the trees... not a green thing remained, neither tree nor plant of the field, through all the land of Egypt."

Exodus 10:14–15 RSV

What is a Pest?

The infestation of locusts which caused Pharoah and his people such distress was but one of countless incidents recorded throughout history of the harmful, sometimes disastrous, impact which certain insects, fungi, rodents, etc., can have on human health and well-being. Such organisms are typically referred to as "pests"—a term derived from the Latin word *pestis* ("plague"), which was applied to a number of deadly epidemic diseases which periodically swept through the ancient world.

Biologically speaking, there is, of course, no such thing as a "pest"; no classification system divides living things into categories labelled "good species" and "bad species". The term "pest", then, is a purely human concept and refers broadly to any organism—animal, plant, or microbe—which adversely affects human interests. Pest species comprise only a small percentage of the total number of organisms on earth, the vast majority being either beneficial or, more commonly, neutral so far as their impact on humans is concerned. Pests are not restricted to any one taxonomic group; representative

205

species can be found among such invertebrates as the insects, mites, ticks, and nematodes. Several bird species such as starlings, pigeons, and English sparrows can be considered pests, as can some mammals—rats, mice, moles, rabbits, and, in some situations, deer, coyotes, or even elephants! Many types of microorganisms, such as disease-causing bacteria, viruses, rickettsia, and fungi, are pests, as are weeds—plants which happen to be growing where they're not wanted (i.e. the proverbial petunia in the onion patch could justifiably be considered a pest).

Conflict between people and pests has existed since time immemorial and is generated primarily when such organisms compete with humans for the same resources, cause us discomfort, or are vectors of disease. The need to protect human interests by limiting pest damage as much as possible has created a demand for better methods of combatting such problems and constitutes the chief justification for the development and use of chemical pesticides. Although the use of such toxic compounds has, for a variety of reasons, come under increasing scrutiny and criticism in recent years, it is important to review the types of problems caused by pests in order to understand why suggestions to limit or abolish the use of chemical pesticides generates such controversy.

Resource Competition: Insects, weeds, and plant pathogens (fungi, nematodes) are responsible for the loss of an estimated 33% of all agricultural crops in the U.S. each year, in spite of the use of about 1 billion pounds of pesticides annually and the widespread utilization of other non-chemical means of control. Insect problems are particularly severe on corn and cotton (60% of all insecticides in the U.S. are used on these two crops), soybeans, rice, wheat, fruits, and vegetables. Fungal diseases cause significant losses primarily to fruits and some vegetables, while yield reductions due to weed infestations are most pronounced on acreage devoted to corn and soybean production. In addition to such losses in the field, about 6% of our annual harvest is lost to pests while in storage or transit.

A reduction in current pesticide use would undoubtedly result in a further increase in crop loss due to pest depradation—a cause for concern both to farmers and to humanitarians worried about feeding a hungry world. The extent of such loss is hotly disputed, however. The U.S. Department of Agriculture estimates that without pesticides, American agricultural production would drop by at least 25% and food prices would rise by 50%. Some agriculturalists, such as Norman Borlaug ("Father of the Green Revolution") and former Agriculture Secretary Earl Butz predict crop losses as great as 50% if all pesticide use were banned. Others, however, calculate that preharvest losses of all crops resulting from a ban on pesticides would be only 9% greater than at present; if only food crops were considered, losses above current levels would be only 5% and no significant food shortages in the U.S. would develop (certain crops such as apples, peaches, onions, and tomatoes would be greatly reduced, however).[1]

Although loss in farm production is the major example of resource competition between humans and pests, many other instances of conflict can be cited: termites cause millions of dollars worth of property damage annually; clothes

Fig. 8–1

SOME SERIOUS PEST-BORNE DISEASES OF HUMANS

DISEASE	CAUSATIVE AGENT	VECTOR	METHOD OF INFECTION
African sleeping sickness	trypanosome	tsetse fly	bite
Cholera	bacterium, Vibrio cholerae	house fly	contamination of foods
Dengue fever	virus	Aedes mosquito	bite
Dysentery, amoebic	protozoan	housefly	contamination of foods
Dysentery, bacillary	bacterium, Shigella sp.	house fly	contamination of foods
Encephalitis	virus	Culex mosquito	bite
Lyme Disease	spirochete bacterium Borrelia burgdorferi	deer tick	bite
Malaria	protozoan, Plasmodium vivax	Anopheles mosquito	bite
Onchocerciasis (River blindness)	parasitic worm, Onchocerca volvulus	black flies	invasion of bite
Plague	bacterium, Pasteurella pestis	Oriental rat flea and other fleas	bite or contact with infected rodents
Rocky Mt spotted fever	rickettsia Rickettsia rickettsi	American dog tick	bite
Typhoid fever	bacterium, Salmonella typhi	house fly	contamination of food and water
Typhus	rickettsia, Rickettsia prowazeki	human body louse	contamination of bite and abrasions
Yellow fever	virus	Aedes mosquito	bite

moths have destroyed many a fine winter coat or woolen blanket; prairie dogs and fire ants construct burrows and mounds, respectively, on pasture lands, significantly reducing their value; rats and mice cause enormous economic loss, both by consuming vast amounts of food and by damaging property (between 5–25% of the fires of unknown origin on farms are suspected of being caused by rats gnawing the insulation from electric wires).[2]

Sources of discomfort: Itching, buzzing, creeping, and crawling may not seem like serious concerns, but the creatures responsible have been driving mankind to distraction for millennia and have been the targets of a great deal of pesticide use in recent decades. Some of the major villains involved in producing acute human discomfort, if not illness, include:

LICE—head lice, body lice, and crab lice are all human parasites which can cause severe itching, secondary infections, and scarred or hardened skin. Lice are typically associated with people living in crowded conditions where opportunities for bathing and laundering clothes are limited. With the introduction of DDT following World War II, the incidence of lice infestations dropped to low levels. As the use of this insecticide became restricted, however, cases of head lice among school children have been increasing.

FLEAS—aside from the flea species which transmit the deadly plague bacterium (see next section), fleas commonly found on domestic animals can cause severe irritation, loss of blood, and discomfort. Although most fleas prefer to feed on their animal host, they frequently bite humans if the normal host is absent. Such bites can be extremely painful and may cause swelling and a reddening of the skin.

MITES—these tiny insect relatives are responsible for the serious skin condition known as scabies, as well as a number of other forms of dermatitis such as "grocers' itch", acquired by handling mite-infested grain products, cheese, dried fruits, etc. Mites that normally live as ectoparasites on birds may become very serious pests of humans when they migrate in large numbers into homes after starlings or sparrows leave their nests. For this reason, householders should discourage birds from nesting on eaves or windowsills or other locations in close proximity to homes. Chiggers, a type of mite inhabiting many parts of the southern or midwestern U.S., can cause extreme skin irritation lasting for a week or more when they attach themselves to a human host, usually around the waist or armpits.

BEDBUGS—hiding during the day in mattresses, bedsprings, cracks in the wall, etc., bedbugs cause many a sleepless night and produce large, intensely itchy welts on sensitive victims. Fortunately they are not known to transmit any disease.

SPIDERS—although many people harbor an irrational antipathy and fear of spiders; the vast majority of these 8-legged insect relatives present no threat to humans. Only two U.S. species are poisonous: the black widow (female only) and the brown recluse (both sexes). Black widow venom acts as a nerve poison and a bite may be fatal if the victim doesn't receive medical treatment. The bite of a brown recluse spider, while not life-threatening, is very painful and generally leaves a large, ugly scar.

In addition to the above, the buzzing of flies, mosquitoes, gnats, June bugs, or wasps—even when these insects are not carrying disease organisms—can provoke extreme annoyance. Ants marching across the floor, crickets chirping in a corner, or spiders spinning their webs on the chandelier often sufficiently arouse the householder into reaching for a can of pesticide spray. Certain plant species also, particularly poison ivy and its relatives, have been prime targets of chemical herbicides because of the intensely irritating rash which contact with these plants can produce.

Vectors of disease: Public health practitioners, along with farmers, were among the first to greet the introduction of synthetic chemical pesticides with great enthusiasm. Compounds such as DDT were viewed as perhaps the ultimate weapon in freeing humanity from the threat of a number of insect- or rodent-borne diseases responsible for millions of deaths and illnesses each year. Quite appropriately, the first use to which DDT was put involved the wartime spraying of refugees in Italy to curb an outbreak of typhus fever. The success of this effort led to extensive spraying campaigns in many parts of the world against the vectors of such dreaded killers as malaria, yellow fever, river blindness, bubonic plague, and encephalitis. Although the medical community's high hopes for complete eradication of the carriers of these diseases have proven overly optimistic, pesticide use has played a significant role in lowering death rates and improving public health in many parts of the world. Some pests of particular public health importance include:

> *Mosquitoes*—mosquitoes have probably been responsible for more human deaths than any other insect, though their role as disease-carriers was not recognized until late in the 19th century. Worldwide, even today millions of people become ill each year due to such mosquito-borne ailments as malaria, yellow fever, dengue, filariasis, and encephalitis. In the past, there have been major outbreaks of all these diseases, particularly malaria and yellow fever, in parts of the U.S.

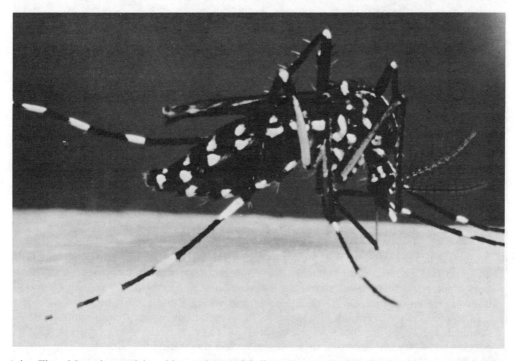

Asian Tiger Mosquito: a vicious biter and potential disease vector, Aedes albopictus has spread rapidly through the southern and midwestern states since its accidental introduction to the U.S. in 1985. [*American Mosquito Control Association/L. Munstermann*]

In recent years, entry of large numbers of infected immigrants from tropical regions where malaria is still endemic has been primarily responsible for the several hundred new cases of malaria being reported in the U.S. each year. In addition, some cases of so-called "airport malaria" have been diagnosed among Americans returning from trips abroad as a result of visiting countries where malaria is still a problem. One traveler, en route home after a business trip to Australia, was bitten by an infected mosquito during a one-hour refueling stop in Liberia and several weeks later died of malaria when his personal physician in Connecticut misdiagnosed his fever and chills as a bad case of influenza. As malaria rates continue to rise in Africa and southern Asia, such cases prompt warnings to travelers not to neglect taking prophylactics for this very serious disease before visiting affected areas.

Box 8–1

This is No Paper Tiger!

Scare stories which embellish the truth about the pest fad of the moment flourish and fade on a regular basis—there hasn't been much talk lately about the "super rats" in New York subways; the flying Asian cockroaches recently touted as sounding the death knell for evening patio parties after making their debut in Florida have yet to make much of an impact in the heartland; "killer bees" continue their slow migration north through Mexico, but remain a distant threat to Americans. By contrast, the Asian Tiger Mosquito (*Aedes albopictus*) has already arrived, is spreading rapidly throughout the South and Midwest, and public health officials are worried.

The unwelcome immigrant was first spotted in August, 1985, in Houston, Texas, arriving as a stowaway in a shipment of used tires sent from northern Japan for reprocessing. Tiger mosquitoes lay their eggs just above the water line in treeholes or manmade containers such as flowerpots, roof gutters, tin cans—or tires. It didn't take the mosquitoes long to decide they liked their new home; they rapidly spread throughout Houston, and moved on to New Orleans. Within a year they were found throughout the South and had traveled as far north as St. Louis and east to Ohio, presumably hitchhiking on the truckloads of used tires which ply the interstate highway system to facilitate their journey. By 1988 *A. albopictus* had been reported in 17 states, taking up residence in cities from Chicago to Baltimore. Because tiger mosquito eggs can overwinter, *A. albopictus* is already becoming established in the northern states; unlike many other mosquitoes, it can also live inside houses year-around, breeding in pet water dishes, in the standing water around sump pumps, and in the saucers under flowerpots.

More than just an interesting novelty, *A. albopictus* has set public health alarm bells ringing because of its potential to become the most important carrier of mosquito-borne diseases in this country. The tiger mosquito is a vicious biter and, in its Asian homeland, is an important disease vector. Although as yet no outbreaks have been attributed to the newcomer, researchers have determined that *A. albopictus* has the ability to pick up and transmit the viral pathogens for dengue fever and encephalitis.

In response to the tiger mosquito invasion, new regulations require that tire imports be disinfected and open used tire storage areas are now receiving much closer scrutiny by local public health officials. Such action, however, is akin to shutting the barn door after the horse has bolted. The Asian Tiger Mosquito is here to stay, but a comprehensive control strategy has yet to be devised.

Of mosquito-borne disease outbreaks within the U.S. today, only encephalitis continues to occur with some frequency. During times when mosquito populations are high and when the viral pathogen of the disease has been detected in birds or small mammals (the virus is generally carried to humans by a mosquito which has previously bitten an infected bird), chemical spraying may be carried out by local authorities to prevent the possibility of encephalitis, a disease which in severe cases can permanently damage the central nervous system or even kill its victim.

Flies—many species of flies, particularly the common housefly, are important carriers of serious gastrointestinal diseases such as typhoid fever, cholera, dysentery, and parasitic worm infections due to their habit of feeding on human and animal wastes. If such wastes contain pathogenic organisms, the fly can pick these up either on the sticky pads of its feet, on its body hairs or mouthparts and mechanically transmit them to humans when it alights on food materials. Fly vomitus and feces also frequently contain pathogenic bacteria which can inoculate human food, multiply rapidly in the food medium, and subsequently result in outbreaks of intestinal diseases when the food is consumed by people.

Body Lice—as mentioned in the previous section, body lice can be a source of intense discomfort, but they are of special public health concern because of several serious epidemic diseases of which they are the vectors. Typhus fever, characterized by elevated temperature, severe headache, and a rash, has been a major killer in past centuries, particularly during wartime when perhaps as many soldiers died from typhus as from swords or bullets. The rickettsial pathogen responsible for the disease is passed from louse to human by the feces of the insect, not its bite. When a person infested with lice scratches himself, minor abrasions on the skin permit entry to the rickettsia. Other lice subsequently feeding on a person infected with typhus ingest the pathogen and spread it as they move from person to person. This method of transmission explains why typhus outbreaks are most prevalent when people are living together in crowded, unsanitary conditions. Insecticidal dusting of louse-infested persons has proven to be an effective method for controlling the spread of typhus fever. Two other louse-borne diseases, also most common during wartime but with much lower fatality rates than typhus, are trench fever and relapsing fever.

Rat Fleas—aside from the enormous economic damage caused by rats, these pests are of great public health concern because they are vectors of a number of diseases, the most deadly of which is plague (the "Black Death" of medieval times). The plague bacterium actually is carried by fleas on rats, not by the rats themselves. When infected fleas feed on their rat hosts, the rats too sicken and die. If rats are living in close proximity to humans, a flea whose host has died may then hop onto a person for a blood meal and thus spread the plague organism to human populations. Because of the tendency of fleas to substitute hosts when necessary, rat poisoning campaigns should always be preceded by insecticidal spraying of rat-infested areas to kill the fleas first. If this in not done, one runs the risk of transferring rodent diseases to humans.

Ticks—among our most common parasites, ticks are a source of profound annoyance to campers, hunters, dog owners, and livestock raisers who frequently discover themselves or their pets providing a blood meal to these tiny pests. Ticks are far more than a nuisance, however. They are vectors of several serious human diseases such as Rocky Mountain spotted fever, a condition that frequently results in death within 2 weeks and which, contrary to its name, is not restricted to mountainous areas but is found throughout the continental U.S., with the largest number of cases being reported from North and South Carolina; Lyme disease, an ailment scarcely heard of by most Americans until a few years ago, has now been reported from 33 states and is currently the most commonly diagnosed tick-borne disease in the nation (see Box 8–2); Q-fever, relapsing fever, tularemia, and tick paralysis are just a few of many ailments which can be transmitted by ticks. Species which most commonly feed on humans generally are found in areas of wild vegetation such as woods, high grass, parks, and along paths frequented by wild animals. Here they lie in wait for a potential human or animal host, clinging to bushes or tall weeds, ready to latch onto an unwary passer-by (contrary to popular belief, they don't drop onto victims from trees). People planning outdoor activities in tick-infested areas should take such precautions as applying tick repellent to exposed areas of skin, wearing socks and long trousers, and avoiding sitting on the ground or on logs. They should also be diligent about checking their bodies for the presence of ticks at least twice a day and immediately removing them, since most tick-borne diseases are transmitted only after the creature has been feeding for several hours.

Box 8–2

"The woods are lovely, dark, and deep . . . " but beware of Lyme Disease!

It was late in the fall of 1975 when the small town of Lyme in southeastern Connecticut became the unlikely setting for the opening chapter of a modern-day medical mystery and ultimately bestowed its name on the vector-borne scourge of the late 20th century, Lyme Disease. In November of that year, the Connecticut State Health Department was notified of an abnormally-high incidence of juvenile rheumatoid arthritis, normally a very rare ailment, in Lyme and several neighboring communities. Suspecting that something was amiss, Department officials summoned a team of epidemiologists from Yale to investigate the situation. The geographic distribution and timing of disease outbreaks (most of the victims lived in wooded areas and developed disease symptoms between June and late September) suggested that some sort of vector-borne pathogen was involved, but it took several years of extensive investigation by researchers at a number of institutions to solve the baffling puzzles posed by this new ailment.

It is now known that the villain responsible for the wide array of unpleasant symptoms which make life miserable for Lyme disease victims is a spirochete bacterium, *Borrelia burgdorferi*, transmitted to humans (as well as to dogs and horses which are also susceptible) by the bite of an infected deer tick, *Ixodes dammini* (on the West Coast the main vector is the closely related species, *I. pacificus*).

That the tiny arthropod should first surface as a troublemaker in the well-to-do

---

residential developments spreading into New England woodlands is, in retrospect, not surprising; deer ticks are most abundant in the transitional vegetation characteristic of woody suburban areas where clearings have been cut in the forest or lawns established amidst woods—the type of habitat attractive to deer and a variety of small mammals and birds which provide the main source of sustenance for *I. dammini.* Similarly, conservation efforts which have resulted in a population explosion among deer herds have also contributed to a corresponding increase in the prevalence of deer ticks.

The tick's life cycle extends over a 2-year period; after hatching from eggs laid early in the spring, deer ticks spend their first year as tiny 6-legged larvae which feed just once on the blood of a small mammal or bird, then overwinter and molt the following spring into a slightly larger 8-legged nymph. Nymphs also must take a blood meal before molting to the adult stage at the end of their second summer. Although the white-footed mouse is the most frequent host for tick nymphs, an unwary human is also fair game, and it is at this stage of the tick's life cycle that people are most likely to be bitten. Adult deer ticks, about the size of a match-head, climb onto shrubs or vegetation about 3 feet off the ground and lie in wait for a deer, human, or other large animal upon which they climb, feed once, drop to the ground, and then mate. Because the tick is so small and inconspicuous, a human victim may not even realize he/she has been bitten until disease symptoms appear, generally several days to a month later.

Three distinct phases of the disease have been described, though not all victims experience each stage. The first and most characteristic feature of Lyme disease is a spreading red rash ("erythema chronica migrans") which begins as a small red bump but expands outward in a circular pattern, 4-20 inches in diameter, resembling a rosy "bull's eye" because of the pale area of skin in the center. Most often occurring on the back, buttocks, chest, or stomach, this rash is frequently accompanied by a splitting headache, fever, chills, backache, and a feeling of extreme fatigue. The second stage manifests itself primarily as nervous system dysfunction and muscular pains. Some sufferers experience heart problems which may require temporary use of cardiac pacemakers, while others occasionally develop such serious neurological disorders as meningitis or Bell's palsy. The onset of arthritis, usually in the knees or other large joints, typifies the third stage of the disease; attacks generally persist for a few days to several weeks at a time and can be extremely painful.

Luckily, since the pathogen causing Lyme disease is a bacterium, once diagnosed the ailment can be treated by oral administration of an antibiotic such as penicillin or tetracycline. When given early during the rash stage of the disease, such medication generally leads to a quick and complete cure. When used to treat later stages of the disease, antibiotics may or may not be effective—perhaps as many as 50% of patients who have developed chronic symptoms don't respond. The major problem in treating Lyme disease is accurate diagnosis; because not all patients develop the tell-tale rash and because so many of the symptoms mimic other diseases, physicians may fail to identify the true cause of this relatively new health problem. Urgent efforts are currently underway to alert both the medical community and the general public to the facts regarding Lyme disease as the number of reported cases steadily escalates and the geographic area affected expands. Cases of Lyme disease, which only a few years ago were restricted to southern New England, New York, and New Jersey, have now been reported from 33 states in the U.S. (the theory is that birds are carrying *I. dammini* from one region of the country to another); the disease also occurs throughout Europe and in parts of Africa, Asia, and Australia.

Currently there is no vaccine available against Lyme disease, so for hikers, campers, or suburbanites visiting or living in tick-infested areas the advice is be wary, wear protective clothing, promptly remove any ticks discovered on the body, and contact a physician immediately if mysterious problems arise after a walk in the woods.[3]

Although the above is by no means a complete listing of the human health problems caused by various pest species, it should convey some realization of the need for pest control and an understanding of why many public health officials feel that the abandonment of chemical pesticides would entail the risk of increased mortality and morbidity rates due to vector-borne disease.

Pest Control

Early attempts at pest control—Human efforts to control pest outbreaks date back to the development of agriculture approximately 10,000 years ago, when relatively large expanses of a single crop and sizeable numbers of people living close together in none-too-sanitary conditions favored an increase in pest populations which wouldn't have been possible among small, scattered societies living a nomadic, hunter-gatherer type of lifestyle. Early attempts to reduce pest damage included purely physical efforts—stomping, flailing, burning—as well as the offering of prayers, sacrifices, and ritual dances to the local gods. A few effective measures were discovered even at such early dates, however. The Sumerians, in what now is Iraq, successfully employed sulfur compounds against insects and mites more than 5000 years ago; over 3000 years ago the Chinese were treating seeds with insecticides derived from plant extracts, using wood ashes and chalk to ward off insect pests in the home, and applying mercury and arsenic compounds to their bodies to control lice. Among the Chinese is found the earliest example of using a pest's natural enemies to control it: by 300 A.D. the Chinese were introducing colonies of predatory ants into their citrus groves to control caterpillars and certain beetles.

During the peak of Greek civilization, records indicate that some of the wealthier citizens used mosquito nets and built high sleeping towers to evade mosquitoes. They also used oil sprays and sulfur bitumen ointments to deter insects. The Romans designed ratproof granaries, but relied largely on superstitious practices such as nailing up crayfish in different parts of the garden to keep away caterpillars.

In medieval Europe people increasingly relied on religious faith to protect them from pest depredations; as late as 1476, during an outbreak of cutworms in Switzerland, several of the offending insects were hauled into court, proclaimed guilty, excommunicated by the archbishop, and banished from the land!

Not until the 18th and 19th centuries did efforts at pest control make any meaningful progress. This was a time when European farming practices were becoming more productive and scientific and help in combatting agricultural pests was eagerly sought. Botanical insecticides such as pyrethrum, derris (rotenone), and nicotine were introduced at this time. Heightened interest in improved pest control methods was generated during the mid-19th century by several of the worst agricultural disasters ever recorded—the potato late blight in Ireland, England, and Belgium in 1848, caused by a fungal disease; the fungus leaf spot disease of coffee in Ceylon which completely wiped out coffee cultivation on the island; and the outbreak of both powdery mildew and an insect pest, grape phylloxera, which nearly destroyed the wine industry in Europe. Such problems led to the development of new chemical pesticides and ushered in a whole new era of pest control. Two of the first such compounds, Bordeaux mixture (copper sulfate and lime) and Paris Green (copper acetoarsenite), were originally employed as fungicides but were subsequently found to be effective insecticides as well. Paris Green became one of the most widely used insecticides in the late 19th century and Bordeaux mixture even today is the most widely used fungicide in the world. Early in the 1900s arsenic-containing compounds such as lead arsenate, highly toxic to both insects and humans, became the most widely sold insecticides in the U.S. and retained their leading position until the advent of DDT after World War II.[4]

In 1939, Paul Müller, a Swiss chemist working for the Geigy corporation, discovered that the synthetic compound dichlorodiphenyltrichloroethane (referred to as DDT for obvious reasons!) was extremely effective in killing insects on contact and retained its lethal character for a long time after application. Müller had simply been looking for a better product to be used against clothes moths, but the outbreak of war in Europe which coincided with Müller's discovery gave far wider significance to the new chemical. Military authorities, recognizing that extensive campaigns would be carried out in the tropics where insect-borne disease threatened high troop losses, made the search for better insecticides a top priority. DDT, highly lethal to every kind of insect yet harmless to humans when applied as a powder, was just what the military needed. Initially, production of DDT was exclusively for use in the armed forces where it was employed first as a louse powder and later for mosquito control. At the end of the war DDT was released for civilian use, both in agriculture and for public health purposes. Its use quickly spread world-wide, amidst high expectations of complete eradication of many diseases and greatly reduced crop losses due to insects. Müller was awarded the 1948 Nobel Prize in Physiology and Medicine in recognition of his contribution. The enthusiastic reception given to DDT encouraged chemical companies in their search for new and even more effective synthetic pesticides. By the mid-1950s at least 25 new products which would revolutionize insect control practices were put on the market, among the more important of which were chlordane, heptachlor, toxaphene, aldrin, endrin, dieldrin, and parathion.[5] The age of chemical warfare against pests had begun.

Types of Pesticides

Pesticides, substances which kill pests, are subdivided into groups according to target organism. For example, insecticides kill insects, herbicides kill weeds, rodenticides kill rats and mice, nematicides kill nematodes, and so forth. Within each of these groups there may be further subdivisions based on such characteristics as route of intake of the poison or physiological effect on the target organism. A brief survey of some of the most common groups of pesticides currently in use would include the following.

Insecticides—the largest number of pesticides are employed against a wide variety of insects and include *stomach poisons* (taken into the body through the mouth; effective against insects with biting or chewing mouthparts, such as caterpillars); *contact poisons* (penetrate through the body wall); and *fumigants* (enter insect through its breathing pores). Representative types include:

Inorganic insecticides—most of these compounds, such as lead arsenate, Paris Green, and a number of other products containing copper, zinc, mercury, chlorine, or sulfur, act as stomach poisons and were the most commonly used insecticides until after World War II. Many of these products are quite toxic to man as well as to insects and their heavy use left significant concentrations of toxic metals in some fields and orchards. In addition to these compounds, some petroleum derivatives such as kerosene, diesel oil, and #2 fuel oil have been sprayed on water surfaces to suffocate mosquito larvae.

Botanicals—certain plant extracts such as pyrethrum, an extract from chrysanthemum flowers, and rotenone, derived from a tropical legume, are very effective contact poisons, providing quick knock-down of insects. Because it is non-toxic to humans and domestic pets, pyrethrum is one of the very few insecticides that can be safely used indoors, even in the kitchen. Rotenone also is harmless to humans and most mammals (except pigs!) and is commonly the active ingredient in home garden dusts because it can be safely used on produce right up to the time of harvest. Pyrethrum and rotenone also are recommended for use on young puppies and kittens for flea control.

In recent years synthetic chemical analogs of pyrethrum such as allethrin, resmethrin, and permethrin have taken over a major share of the market for botanical insecticides. Like natural pyrethrum, these compounds are both effective and have very low acute human toxicity. While these products are considerably more expensive than other insecticides, they can be used effectively at much lower rates of application and their good safety record is promoting their widespread adoption for both structural and agricultural pest control purposes.

Chlorinated hydrocarbons—DDT and its chemical relatives (chlordane, heptachlor, lindane, BHC, endrin, aldrin, mirex, kepone, toxaphene, etc.) are all contact poisons. They act primarily on the central nervous system, causing the insect to go through a series of convulsions prior to death. Members of this group are *broad-spectrum* insecticides, meaning that they kill a wide range of insects and other arthropods, and are also *persistent* in the environment, breaking down very slowly and therefore retaining their effectiveness for a relatively long period after application. Because the chlorinated hydrocarbons are not water-soluble, they tend to accumulate in fatty tissues when taken up by living organisms and may remain in the body indefinitely. In recent years many of the chlorinated hydrocarbons have been banned for most uses in the U.S. because animal testing has shown them to be carcinogenic.

Fig. 8-2

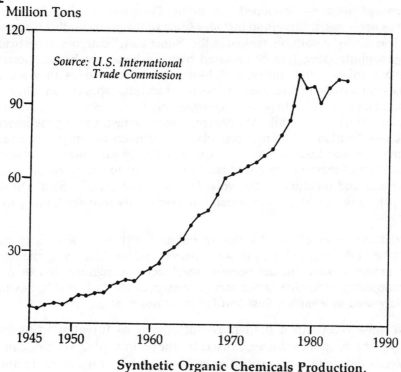

Million Tons

Source: U.S. International
Trade Commission

**Synthetic Organic Chemicals Production,
United States, 1945-85**

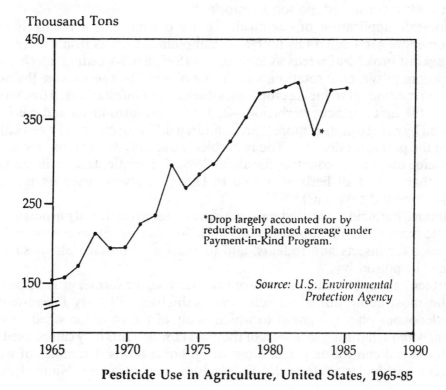

Thousand Tons

*Drop largely accounted for by
reduction in planted acreage under
Payment-in-Kind Program.

Source: U.S. Environmental
Protection Agency

Pesticide Use in Agriculture, United States, 1965-85

Pests and Pesticides   **217**

Organophosphates—developed first by the Germans for possible wartime use as nerve gases, this group includes some of the most deadly insecticides such as methyl parathion, ranked in the "super toxic" category of pesticides. Organophosphates, like chlorinated hydrocarbons, are broad-spectrum contact poisons, but unlike the chlorinated hydrocarbons they are not persistent, usually breaking down 2 weeks or less after application. Thus they present far less danger to non-target organisms. Organophosphates are nerve poisons which act to inhibit the enzyme cholinesterase, causing the insect to lose coordination and go into convulsions. Members of this group range in terms of human toxicity from the extremely deadly parathion and phosdrin (one drop of these in the eye is fatal to an adult) to the moderately toxic diazinon and dichlorvos (the volatile compound used in Shell Oil pest strips), to the slightly toxic malathion, commonly sold for home garden use.

Carbamates—widely used today in public health work and agriculture because of their rapid knock-down of insects and low toxicity to mammals, carbamates too are contact poisons which act in a manner similar to the organophosphates. One of the most common of the carbamates, Sevin, is widely used as a garden dust and for mosquito control.

Herbicides—Weeds in a field may not appear as threatening as hordes of insects, yet the economic losses caused by these unwanted species can be very high. Weeds compete with crop plants for vital mineral nutrients and water, thus reducing crop yields; they make harvesting more difficult and some species, when consumed, poison livestock.

Widescale application of chemicals for weed control is a relatively new phenomenon. Although a few inorganic compounds such as iron sulfate were used against broad-leaf weeds as long ago as 1896, hand-weeding, mechanical cultivation, tillage, crop rotation, and the use of weed-free seeds were the most common methods of reducing crop losses due to weed infestations. After World War II, the first synthetic herbicide—2, 4, D—was introduced and has been followed by a succession of more than a hundred different chemical weed killers during the past three decades. Today herbicide use has considerably surpassed insecticide use, now accounting for about 85% of all pesticide sales in the U.S. (more than 2/3 of all herbicides sold to U.S. farmers are used on just two crops—corn and soybeans).[6]

Although herbicides are used most extensively for agricultural purposes, they are also important in public health work for control of weeds to reduce harborage for insects and rodents, and to eradicate nuisance plants such as ragweed or poison ivy.

Herbicides may be either **selective** or **non-selective,** the former group being by far the most common. Most selective herbicides kill only broad-leafed dicotyledonous plants, a group to which many of the common weed species belong, without harming members of the grass family. Thus they can be used for effective weed control on cereal crops or on home lawns. Examples of some selective herbicides include 2,4-D, alachlor, and atrazine. Non-selective

Fig. 8-3   **U.S. Production of Pesticides, by Type,
1960–1984**

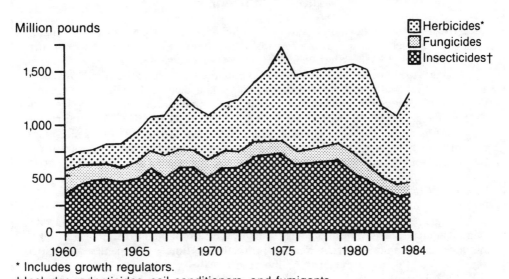

* Includes growth regulators.
† Includes rodenticides, soil conditioners, and fumigants.

Source: U.S. International Trade Commission.

herbicides kill any plant with which they come into contact and thus have much more limited use, such as spraying railroad and highway right-of-ways. Sulfuric acid, glyphosate (Roundup, Kleenup), and paraquat are examples of non-selective herbicides.

Although most herbicides are thought to be only slightly toxic to humans, in recent years there have been several studies suggesting that herbicide exposure can cause genetic mutations, cancer, and birth defects. Farm workers occasionally blame health problems such as weight loss, nausea, vomiting, and loss of appetite to contact with herbicides. In 1986 researchers reported that Kansas farmers who used 2,4-D for more than 20 days per year had a 6X greater risk of lymphatic cancer than did a control group with no exposure to herbicides.[7] Recognition that some of the most widely used herbicides are known or suspected carcinogens has prompted concerns among some federal regulators that residues of these chemicals on food or in well water may be exposing the American consumer to long-term health risks. By far the greatest public controversy surrounding herbicide use in recent years concerns the alleged health effects of exposure to Agent Orange (see Box 8–3), a selective herbicide widely used by the U.S. military for defoliation purposes during the Vietnam War. There has also been considerable outcry by anti-pesticide activists in some communities about dangers posed to people, pets, and the environment by chemicals used by the rapidly growing commercial lawn care

Box 8–3

The Dioxin Dilemma

Regarded by many as the most deadly of all man-made chemicals, dioxin is a chlorinated hydrocarbon which is formed as an unavoidable contaminant in the manufacture of such organic compounds as the selective herbicides, 2,4,5-T and silvex.

The danger to public health which these dioxin-tainted herbicides pose first was alleged during the Vietnam War. Reports of miscarriages and deformed babies among South Vietnamese villagers were linked to repeated aerial sprayings of the countryside with "Agent Orange," a 50–50 mixture of the weed-killers, 2,4-D and 2,4,5-T, during the defoliation campaign pursued by the U.S. military between 1961 and 1970. Agent Orange contained relatively high levels of dioxin and it is roughly estimated that between 350 and 1000 pounds of this toxin rained down upon South Vietnam during the course of the war (to put this amount in perspective, only 3 *ounces,* evenly distributed, could kill everyone in New York City).

After American forces left Vietnam in 1973, little more was heard about Agent Orange until the late 1970s, when increasing numbers of Vietnam veterans began to report a wide range of ailments, ranging from acne-like skin disorders to emotional disturbances, weight loss, birth defects among their children, and cancer (by this time the Vietnamese authorities were also reporting a sharp increase in liver cancer cases).[8]

The possibility that these problems were caused by wartime exposure to Agent Orange gained increasing acceptance with the belated revelation that in the course of duty many thousands of U.S. military personnel came into direct contact with the herbicide. The Veterans' Administration continues to deny that Agent Orange exposure is responsible for any ill health effects among former servicemen, but other veterans' groups continue to press for further studies on this issue and seek to obtain medical and financial assistance for suspected victims. In the late spring of 1984, seven chemical companies agreed to an out-of-court settlement for $180 million with a group of veterans claiming health damage due to Agent Orange exposure. While many observers interpreted the settlement as an admission of guilt on the part of the industry, the federal judge hearing the case told the attorneys for the plaintiffs that "in no case have you shown causality for the health effects alleged."

Additional controversy surrounding the impact of herbicide spraying made headlines in 1979 when the EPA suspended the use of 2,4,5-T and silvex on forests, pastures, and rights-of-way. This action was prompted by reports of an unusually high incidence of miscarriage among women near Alsea, Oregon—lumber country where herbicide spraying to eliminate brushy undergrowth among the Douglas fir saplings was a regular occurrence. The fact that all the reported miscarriages followed sprayings and that at other times of the year women had normal pregnancies appeared to EPA officials to be more than coincidental. Buttressed by laboratory tests which showed that 500 parts per trillion (ppt) of dioxin caused female monkeys to abort and die and that as little as 5 ppt dioxin in the diet induced tumors in rats, EPA imposed the suspension, even though direct evidence of a causal relationship in the case of the Alsea women had not been established. This so-called Alsea II study subsequently came in for severe criticism by an interdisciplinary group of researchers at Oregon State University and is now widely regarded as discredited because the purported link between herbicide spraying and miscarriage couldn't be established from the data used by the Agency. Faulty science notwithstanding, suspension of the two herbicides continued and eventually Dow Chemical gave up the battle for their reinstatement and announced it would no longer manufacture the chemicals.

industry. Making the point that "Dandelions don't kill you, pesticides do!", concerned citizens' groups have been vociferously demanding that lawn care companies post warning signs on treated lawns, inform residents of what pesticides are being used, and provide health and safety data on those chemicals.

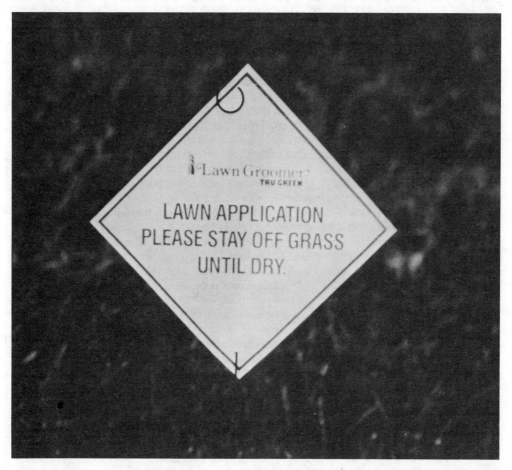

Fears of health or environmental damage resulting from herbicidal applications by commercial lawn-care firms have given rise to demands that warning signs be posted on freshly-treated yards. [*Author's Photo*]

Rodenticides—Although good sanitation and rat-proofing of buildings and food storage facilities provides the only effective long-term control of domestic rodents, use of poisons is an important additional tool in keeping rat populations low. Because some rodenticides used in public health work are extremely toxic to humans as well as to rodents, their use is restricted to certified applicators. General-use rodenticides, chemicals which should not present a serious hazard either to the user or to the environment when used in accordance with instructions, can be purchased by the general public. The rodenticides most commonly recommended for use by householders act as anticoagulants.

Such poisons as warfarin, fumarin, PMP, Pival, diphacinone, and chloropha-cinone are all multiple-dose poisons which must be consumed over a period of several consecutive days before the rat dies. Thus a child or pet would not be ser-iously endangered by eating a single portion of bait. Anti-coagulants cause internal hemorrhaging, causing the rodents to bleed to death painlessly. These poisons provide excellent control of both rats and mice, although up to 2 weeks may be required to get an effective kill.[9]

Box 8–4

To Catch a Mouse

To eliminate the occasional mouse in the pantry, there is probably no more effective device than the old-fashioned snap trap. To use the trap most efficiently, however, one should take the rodent's behavior patterns into consideration. The male mouse, unlike his sociable cousin the rat, is a loner, establishing his own territory with one or more females and seldom venturing beyond its borders. If food is present and the population density of mice in the general area is high, these individual territories may be quite small; it is not uncommon under such circumstances for mice to venture no further than 6-10 feet from their nests. For this reason, effective control requires the use of multiple traps, placed no more than 10-20 feet apart. Mice are most active at night and tend to travel close to walls, between objects, or in runways where they can feel their whiskers in contact with vertical surfaces. For this reason, a trap placed in the middle of a room or at some distance from a wall is unlikely to catch a mouse. For optimum results, a trap should be baited with any type of fresh food (mice like the same types of food people do—peanut butter makes a fine bait since, due to its stickiness, it cannot be easily removed) and placed at a right angle to the side wall across the runway with the baited end of the trap closest to the wall. Concerns that handling the trap could leave a human odor that might frighten the mouse away are unwarranted; mice live in such close association with people that they are constantly surrounded by human smells and pay no heed to such odors.

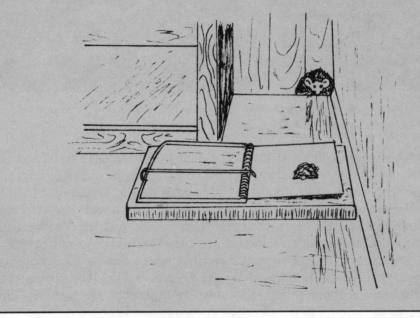

Environmental Impact of Pesticide Use

In the early 1950s, bird-watchers in both the U.S. and Western Europe were confronted with a baffling mystery—a sudden, inexplicable decline in the populations of bald eagles, pelicans, and peregrine falcons appeared to threaten the very survival of these well-loved species. Investigations into the reasons behind such an unanticipated population "crash" ultimately revealed that the villain in the piece was not a disease, nor over-killing, nor a scarcity of food, but rather was the presence in the tissues of these birds of startlingly high concentrations of the new insecticide DDT. Although DDT did not appear to have a direct lethal effect on the adult birds, it interfered with their ability to metabolize calcium, thereby resulting in the production of eggs with shells so thin that they broke when the nesting parents sat on them. Thus pesticide-induced reproductive failure—the inability of the birds to produce viable offspring—was ultimately shown to be the factor responsible for the ornithologists' distress.

This episode represented one of the first glimmerings of awareness on the part of the scientific community at least, that the advent of the new wonder chemicals was not an unmitigated blessing. The public at large, however, remained largely unaware and unconcerned about such matters until the publication in 1962 of Rachel Carson's literary bombshell, "*Silent Spring*". This best-seller represented a scathing indictment of pesticide misuse and for the first time made the average American aware of the havoc which indiscriminate reliance on chemicals could wreak on the environment and on human well-being. In retrospect, the publication of Silent Spring made "ecology" a household word and was probably the most important single event in launching what became the environmental movement of the 1970s. Miss Carson and many subsequent researchers clearly demonstrated that extensive use and near-total reliance on chemicals for pest control have been accompanied by unanticipated and undesired side effects, many of which have raised problems serious enough to threaten the continued usefulness of these products. The major environmental effects of pesticide use causing concern today are:

Development of Resistance

Those who dreamed that the new pesticides held promise of complete eradication of certain insect or other pest species were obviously ignorant of the principles which govern how the forces of natural selection act upon chance variations occurring within any population—particularly insect populations whose long evolutionary history demonstrates the remarkable ability of these organisms to evolve and adapt rapidly to changing environmental conditions. The widespread, frequent, and intensive application of chemicals such as DDT in the years following the war created a new environmental challenge which was initially successful in drastically reducing pest populations but which eventually was responsible for providing the selective forces which would produce new strains of "super bugs", rendering the original poisons worthless. The mechanism by which this occurs can be visualized by considering a hypothetical population of, say, boll weevils ravaging a field of cotton. Aerial insecticide spraying may kill perhaps 99% of the weevils, but a few will survive, either by chance (perhaps an overhanging leaf shielded them from the spray) or because something in the genetic make-up of a particular individual somehow made it less vulnerable to the poison than were its fellow weevils who promptly died. Such a hereditary trait might be the possession of a particular enzyme capable of detoxifying the pesticide, a less permeable type of epidermis which prevented penetration of the contact poison, a behavioral characteristic which allowed the individual to avoid fatal exposure, or some other factor of this nature. In a pesticide-free environment (the type of situation prevailing prior to the introduction of DDT) such a genetic trait would confer no special advantage to the individual carrying it, so the frequency of such a gene within that population would remain low. Once DDT came into widespread use, however, the boll weevils' environment was radically altered and those few individuals possessing the gene for immunity suddenly enjoyed a tremendous selective advantage. As the accompanying diagram indicates, successive sprayings largely eliminated boll weevils susceptible to the insecticide, but promoted the build-up of a population in which the vast majority of individuals now carry the gene (or genes) conferring resistance to the chemical. In order to combat this new situation, those seeking to control pest outbreaks turn to newer and more powerful chemicals, only to witness the same cycle of events repeat itself. This "pesticide treadmill" is of benefit only to the firms which manufacture and sell pesticides; it is becoming increasingly obvious that the war against pests can never be won by chemicals alone.[10]

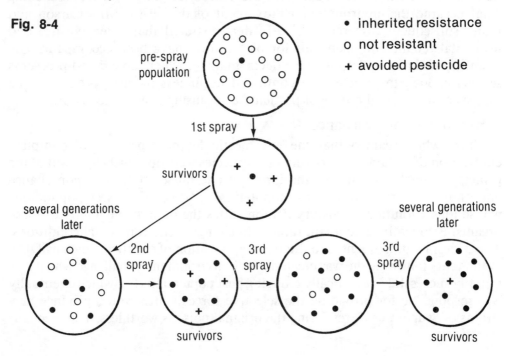

Fig. 8-4

• inherited resistance
o not resistant
+ avoided pesticide

pre-spray population

1st spray

survivors

several generations later

2nd spray

survivors

3rd spray

several generations later

3rd spray

survivors

Since pesticide resistance had appeared as a localized problem even with the old-fashioned insecticides, it shouldn't have come as a total surprise when development of resistance to DDT began to appear in the late 1940s and early '50s. Among the first species to display immunity were certain populations of houseflies and mosquitoes which, as early as 1946, could no longer be controlled with DDT. In 1951, during the Korean War, military officials were alarmed to discover that human lice, vectors of typhus, had become resistant to DDT. Among agricultural pests, spider mites, cabbage loopers, codling moths, and tomato hornworms developed resistance to several of the common insecticides; by the mid-'50s when the boll weevil became resistant to many of the chlorinated hydrocarbons, the need for alternative control methods became obvious.[11] At present, over 445 species of insects and mites are resistant to common pesticides—more than double the number that were resistant just 20 years ago. Largely due to problems of pesticide resistance, crop losses due to insects are twice as high now as they were when DDT was first brought onto the market—in spite of the fact that American farmers are using ten times more pesticides now than they did in 1945. In the public health field, as in agriculture, growing pesticide resistance is causing serious concern. Worldwide, incidence of malaria is now on a sharp upswing as approximately 64 species of mosquitoes have become resistant to insecticides, according to World Health Organization officials. Problems of pesticide resistance are not restricted to species of arthropods (i.e. insects, mites, ticks, spiders, etc.). Approximately 50 weed species are now herbicide-resistant, as are more than 150 species of plant pathogens (fungi and bacteria), and some rodent populations.

Killing of Beneficial Species

Only a small percentage of insect species are considered pests, yet the most widely-used synthetic insecticides are broad-spectrum poisons, killing both friend and foe alike. The destruction of many beneficial predator insect species as well as the target pest has led to two related types of problems.

The first of these, referred to as *Target Pest Resurgence,* occurs when insecticide application which initially resulted in a drastic reduction in the pest population is quickly followed by a sudden increase in pest numbers to a level higher than that which existed prior to the spraying. This occurs because the natural enemies of the pest, which formerly kept its numbers under control, were also heavily decimated by the spraying. Since any predators which survived the pesticide would subsequently starve or migrate elsewhere due to lack of food, the few remaining target insects would then confront ideal conditions—no natural enemies and an abundance of their favorite food (i.e. the crop which had been sprayed). As a result, their populations can increase in size very rapidly, above and beyond the original level.

A second situation, known as *Secondary Pest Outbreak,* involves the rise to prominence of certain plant-eating species which, prior to the spraying, were unimportant as pests because natural enemies kept their populations below the level at which they could cause significant economic damage. After pesticides eliminated most of their predators, such insects suddenly experience a population explosion and become major pests in their own right. A classic example of this phenomenon was the outbreak of cottony cushion scale in the citrus groves of California after the trees had been sprayed with DDT for control of other citrus pests. The spraying proved devastating to a predator insect, the vedalia beetle, which had been doing such a good job of keeping the scale populations low that the presence of this pest had been largely forgotten. With its natural enemy removed, however, the cottony cushion scale suddenly assumed major importance, causing great economic loss. Only after the adjustment of spraying schedules permitted reestablishment of the beetle population did the scale insect cease to be a problem.

Environmental Contamination

Liberal use of pesticides on a world-wide basis has resulted in a more thorough contamination of the biosphere than anyone in 1945 would have dreamed possible. Today pesticide residues, especially those of the chlorinated hydrocarbons, are found virtually everywhere in the tissues of creatures as diverse as Antarctic penguins, fish in deep ocean trenches, decomposer bacteria, and every human being. Since no one deliberately sprayed pesticides in Antarctica or in the middle of the Pacific, how could this have happened? Because the chlorinated hydrocarbons are persistent pesticides (meaning that they break down very slowly), they can circulate through the ecosystem for a long time, often traveling long distances from their point of origin. When such chemicals are aerially sprayed on forest, field, or pastureland, less than 50% of the pesticide actually hits the target; the remainder is carried off by air currents and is subsequently deposited miles away where it will eventually be washed into waterways or taken up by living organisms in the food they eat. The results of this unintended contamination include:

> *direct killing of organisms exposed to chemicals*—Many species of fish, some birds and small mammals, and a number of plants, including phytoplankton, as well as beneficial insect species, are extremely sensitive to chemical pesticides and die immediately after coming into contact with such substances. A dramatic example of this occurred a few years ago when 700 Brant geese died after walking and feeding on a New York golf course which had been treated with the widely-used organophosphate insecticide diazinon. As a result of this and numerous other bird kills linked to the insecticide, EPA cancelled the use of diazinon on golf courses and sod farms, but this decision was subsequently voided by the courts.

> *groundwater contamination*—in the spring of 1988 the Environmental Protection Agency launched a nationwide survey to determine levels of pesticide contamination in rural wellwater supplies. This action was undertaken in response to results of state-initiated monitoring efforts which revealed that routine farming practices, particularly in areas where shallow

sand and gravel aquifers were overlain by coarse-textured soils, have polluted drinking water with pesticides in at least 23 states. While the levels of farm chemicals found in groundwater supplies are too low to cause acute poisoning, they raise concerns about chronic health effects among rural residents. Alachlor (LASSO) and atrazine (Aatrex), two of the most widely used farm herbicides, were the pesticides most frequently detected in wellwater samples. The presence of alachlor is of some concern since this chemical is regarded as a probable human carcinogen.[12]

indirect contamination via food chains—Since the chlorinated hydrocarbons are not water-soluble they are not excreted from the body when ingested but instead are stored in fatty tissues such as liver, kidneys, and fat around the intestines. Toxic substances present in minute amounts in the general environment can thus become quite concentrated as they move along a food chain, sometimes reaching lethal doses in organisms at the highest trophic levels. This process, known as ***Biomagnification,*** was the phenomenon responsible for the reproductive failure in the various birds of prey referred to earlier in this chapter. Eagles, pelicans, and falcons are all top carnivores, fish-eaters, at the end of relatively long food chains. As such, they had accumulated amounts of DDT sufficiently high to interfere with important bodily processes, with the results already described.

The classic example of biomagnification can be seen in the case of Clear Lake, California—a favorite fishing spot about 90 miles north of San Francisco. Recreational fishermen had long been annoyed by the swarms of non-biting gnats which were frequently present at Clear Lake. The new synthetic pesticides offered what appeared to be an easy way of getting rid of a nuisance, so in 1949 it was decided to spray Clear Lake with a dilute solution of DDD (a chemical cousin of DDT which is less toxic to fish). After the first spraying, gnat populations dropped to barely detectable levels, but by 1951 the pesky insects were back in bothersome numbers, so the spraying was repeated. Several more sprayings followed in succeeding years as the gnat populations displayed increasing resistance to the poison. Then some strange side-effects became apparent. By 1954 visitors to Clear Lake began reporting significant numbers of carcasses of the Western grebe, a type of water fowl, around the lake. By the early 1960s, the grebe population at Clear Lake had plummeted from 1000 nesting pairs to almost none. Suspecting that the repeated pesticide applications might somehow be related to the birds' demise, biologists began to measure DDD concentrations in various components of the lake ecosystem. Although the lake water itself contained traces of DDD in barely detectable amounts (0.02 ppm), concentrations of the pesticide increased dramatically when the tissues of living organisms were examined. The facts they uncovered are entirely consistent with the basic principles of a food chain:

ORGANISM	DDD CONC. IN TISSUES (ppm)
Phytoplankton (producers)	5
Herbivorous fish (primary consumers)	40 - 300
Carnivorous fish (secondary consumers)	up to 2500
Western grebes (secondary consumers)	1600

The pesticide which had been sprayed on the lake in what everybody at the time assumed was a safely dilute amount was absorbed and concentrated by the plankton which were the producer organisms of Clear Lake. When these were consumed by the herbivorous fish (primary consumers), the DDD became more concentrated. By the time these fish were eaten by grebes or by bullheads, the DDD had become sufficiently concentrated to cause the death of the birds.

By the late 1960s the futility of spraying to control the now-resistant gnats became obvious and a gnat-eating fish was introduced into the lake in what subsequently proved to be a very successful method of biological control. As pesticide levels gradually dropped, the grebes returned to Clear Lake and today are once again thriving at approximately their pre-1954 population levels. Numerous other examples of biomagnification involving other chlorinated hydrocarbons and heavy metals (e.g. methyl mercury at Minamata) have since been described and illustrate the unanticipated effects which toxic substances can have as they move through ecosystems.

Hazards to Human Health

Although pesticides are used specifically to kill pests, many of them are quite toxic to humans as well. In the world as a whole, it is estimated that somewhere between 400,000-2 million pesticide poisonings occur each year, 10,000 of them fatal.[13] Deaths due to pesticide poisoning have been decreasing as knowledge of safe handling practices has spread, but several thousands of cases of pesticide-induced illnesses are reported annually, while many more go unreported. The segments of the population which account for the largest number of pesticide poisonings are children under 10 (half of all deaths due to pesticides occur within this group) and pesticide applicators. One factor accounting for the high rate of accidental poisoning among the latter group is the fact that many agricultural workers in the U.S. are either illiterate or read only Spanish and thus cannot follow the safety precautions printed on pesticide labels.

To cause harm, a pesticide must be taken internally through the mouth, skin, or respiratory system. Most oral exposure is due to carelessness—e.g. leaving poisons within reach of young children, smoking or eating without washing hands after handling pesticides, using the mouth to start siphoning liquid pesticide concentrates, eating unwashed fruit that was recently sprayed, or accidentally drinking pesticides which were poured into an unlabelled container. Exposure through the skin can occur when pesticides are spilled on the body or when wind-blown sprays or dusts come into contact with skin.

Fig. 8-5   Dermal absorption rates as compared with the forearm.

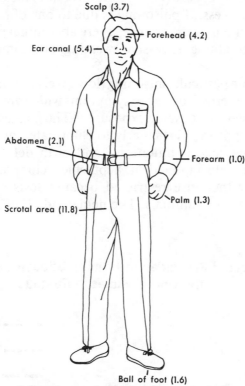

The seriousness of absorbing pesticide through the skin depends on the dermal toxicity of the chemical, the size of the contaminated skin area, the length of time the material is in contact with the skin, and the rate of absorption through the skin. As the diagram indicates, different parts of the body have very different rates of skin absorption.

Source: *Illinois Pesticide Applicator Study Guide,* University of Illinois Cooperative Extension Service.

Re-entering a field too soon after pesticide application or careless handling of discarded containers can also result in absorption of pesticides through the skin. The larger the skin area contaminated and the longer the duration of contact, the more serious the results of such exposure will be. Theoretically, dermal exposure could be reduced significantly through the use of protective clothing and equipment. In practice, however, such precautions are frequently ignored. Such gear is often expensive, cumbersome, and uncomfortable, especially during hot weather. All too often, applicators who know better fail to comply with safety recommendations and have been observed, in some instances, to ply their trade wearing little more than bathing suits! Poisoning due to inhalation is most common in enclosed areas such as greenhouses but can also occur outside when pesticide mists or fumes are inhaled during application or if the applicator is smoking.

Symptoms of acute exposure (i.e. "one-time" cases) include headache, weakness, fatigue, or dizzyness. If poisoning is due to one of the organophosphate insecticides, the victim may experience severe abdominal pain, vomiting, diarrhea, difficulty in breathing, excessive sweating, and sometimes convulsions, coma, and death.

In contrast, chronic pesticide poisoning (low-level exposure over an extended time period) is characterized by vague symptoms which are difficult to pinpoint as having been caused by pesticide exposure.[14] The greatest concern regarding chronic pesticide exposure, particularly to chlorinated hydrocarbons, is their potential for causing cancer, mutations, and birth defects. Within the past decade DDT, endrin, aldrin, dieldrin, heptachlor, chlordane, and mirex have all been banned or their use restricted because tests showed them to be carcinogenic to laboratory animals. The nematicide DBCP is known to have

Fig. 8-6   **Selected Pesticides in Human Adipose Tissue in the United States, 1970–1983**

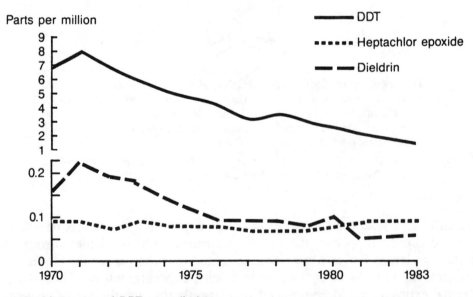

1972—Most uses of DDT cancelled.
1974—Most uses of Dieldrin cancelled.
1983—Most uses of heptachlor cancelled or registrations denied.

Source: U.S. Environmental Protection Agency.

230   Chapter Eight

Box 8–5
Read That Label!

While most of the controversy regarding pesticidal applications has focused on agricultural use of these chemicals, a substantial portion of total U.S. sales of insecticides, herbicides, and fungicides is to homeowners who use prodigious amounts of these toxic products to zap dandelions in their lawns, banish aphids from their rose bushes, or annihilate roaches in the cupboard. Acre for acre, city dwellers apply considerably larger amounts of pesticides to their lawns and gardens, or inside their homes, than do farmers—and they frequently do so with far less knowledge of safe storage, handling, and application practices. Thus it should not be too surprising when horror stories of chemical-related illnesses and environmental damage surface in local newspapers.

In some cases, reported problems are simply due to unknown inherent hazards of certain pesticidal products. Unfortunately, the fact that a chemical is EPA-registered and legally available to the general public does not necessarily guarantee its safety. Many older chemicals already on the market before passage of the 1972 federal law requiring safety data on new pesticides submitted for registration have still not been tested for their chronic health effects and have been liberally used by unsuspecting consumers for years. Just recently, for example, the EPA issued a strong warning regarding the carcinogenicity of the organophosphate insecticide, dichlorvos—one of the most commonly used household pesticides. Known by the trade name DDVP or Vapona, this chemical, on the market since 1948, is the active ingredient in the "NO PEST" strips used to deter flying insects in homes, restaurants, and offices, and is also widely used in pet flea collars. After allowing use of these products for decades without any suggestion of possible risk, EPA now warns that people inhabiting areas where pest strips are in use have a 1 in 100 risk of developing cancer, as do cats or dogs wearing flea collars containing DDVP. EPA is now conducting a risk-benefit analysis of dichlorvos to determine whether the product's uses should be cancelled, but the review process can drag on for years and provides small comfort to the millions who have lived in close association with the chemical for years.[15]

Nevertheless, the majority of pesticide-related health problems experienced by non-professionals, particularly cases of acute poisonings, are due to careless or ignorant *misuse* of these products. Take, for example, the case of an Illinois couple who became quite ill from inhalation of chlordane vapors after dousing their living room carpet with the undiluted concentrate in order to eliminate a flea problem! Not only were they acting foolishly—they were breaking the law, since at the time of the incident chlordane was registered solely for termite control, had to be properly diluted, and could only be applied by rodding or trenching into the soil. Examples such as this, multiplied by the thousands, constitute our most serious pesticide poisoning threat.

Some rules of safe pesticide use are plain common-sensical: keep pesticides in their original containers, keep them out of reach of children and pets, always wear protective clothing when applying chemicals, avoid spraying when conditions are windy. However, for all users of these explicitly toxic chemicals (obviously we wouldn't be using them if they weren't poisonous), the #1 safety rule—and the one most often ignored—is: **READ THE LABEL!** The label on a pesticide container, along with any accompanying fliers or brochures, constitutes a legal document; anyone using the product in a manner contrary to label directions is in violation of the law. Simply from the standpoint of concern about one's own personal welfare and getting optimum use out of the product, careful reading of the label directions makes good sense, for the information it contains cost millions of dollars to acquire and represents the most extensive data available for that chemical. The label tells the concentration at which the pesticide should be used (contrary to popular myth, mixing a solution stronger than recommended does not enhance the killing power of a pesticide; at best it is a waste of money, at worst it can be environmentally damaging and diminish the effectiveness of the chemical), lists the pests which the product may be used to control, recommends frequency of spraying and the appropriate interval between applications, gives directions for safe use, supplies antidote information in case of accidental poisoning, classifies the chemical as to its degree of toxicity, describes any special environmental hazards the product may present, lists the names and amounts of active ingredients, etc. Since the so-called "general use" pesticides available to the public are those considered safe when used according to directions, the incidence of pesticide poisonings could be sharply reduced if all users would conscientiously read all label information prior to hauling out the spray equipment or grabbing that aerosol "bug bomb"!

caused sterility among men who worked in the factory where it was manufactured, while dioxin in the herbicide 2,4,5-T has been implicated in cases of birth defects, miscarriages, and cancer. Dietary exposure to pesticides via residues on food has attracted intense public scrutiny since the 1987 publication of a study by the National Academy of Sciences, estimating that traces of carcinogenic fungicides, insecticides, and herbicides on the nation's fruits, vegetables, and meat could result in an additional 20,000 cancer deaths per year in the U.S. These findings, hotly disputed by agrichemical interests, have generated intense public concern with how pesticides are regulated and are spurring demands for reform. Much more research on the long-term effects of pesticide exposure is needed, but mounting evidence suggests that low-level, chronic exposure to these substances which are now virtually ubiquitous throughout the environment may represent a significantly greater threat to public health than the occasional accident involving acute pesticide poisoning.

Alternatives to Chemical Pest Control

As increasing numbers of pest species become resistant to available chemicals and as doubts concerning the long-range effects of pesticide exposure on human health and the environment continue to grow, many have begun to question the advisability of continuing to rely exclusively on chemicals for pest control.

In recent years a different philosophy of pest control has gained support, a strategy known as *Integrated Pest Management* (IPM). After ascertaining that a pest problem does indeed exist, IPM practitioners combine various compatible methods to obtain the best control with the least possible environmental disruption. While the emphasis in IPM is on utilizing natural controls such as predators, food deprivation, or weather to increase pest mortality, it can include pesticide application also, but only after careful monitoring of pest populations indicate a need. Unlike the total chemical control approach, IPM recognizes the extraordinary adaptability of insects and does not attempt to eradicate a particular pest entirely, but rather is aimed at keeping pest populations below the level at which they can cause significant economic loss.

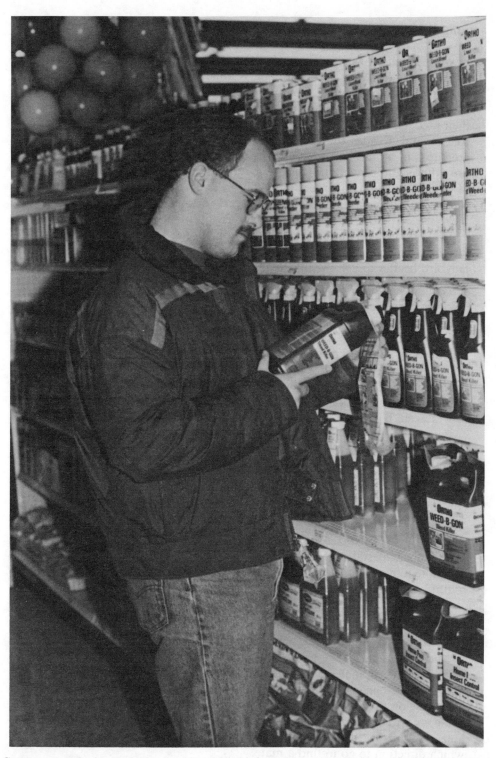

Consumers purchasing pesticides should read label information carefully before using the product. Many human health and environmental problems have been caused by over-use or misuse of these toxic chemicals. [*Author's Photo*]

Among the methods which could be included in an IPM strategy are:

natural enemies—Many of our most serious insect and weed pests (e.g. Japanese beetle, gypsy moth, fire ant, Klamath weed, water hyacinth, etc.) are foreign imports which rapidly multiplied here in the absence of their natural enemies. Other native pests have caused serious problems only after their predators were eliminated by indiscriminate use of pesticides. Over the past several decades the government has imported more than 500 insect predators in an attempt to control alien pests; about 20 of these are now providing significant control of several important pests. Laboratory breeding of large populations of insect predators in hopes of overwhelming certain pests is also being attempted. Great success in controlling scale insects and mealybugs in citrus orchards was obtained by massrearing and release of vedalia beetles and certain parasitic wasps. Home gardeners and organic farmers are urged to purchase praying mantis egg cases or containers full of ladybird beetles to achieve effective non-chemical insect control.

pathogens and parasites—A further step in biological warfare against insects involves introduction of various disease agents into a pest population. About a dozen such microbial pathogens are now being commercially developed or produced in various parts of the world. Two kinds of bacteria have been approved for commercial pest-control in the U.S.—*Bacillus popilliae*, which causes the milky spore disease of Japanese beetles, and the widely used *Bacillus thuringiensis* (BT), which can be used effectively against more than 100 species of caterpillars, including gypsy moth larvae, currently the target of widescale BT applications.[16]

Pathogenic viruses are also being viewed as offering a promising method of pest control, since viral diseases in nature are frequently devastating to pest populations. A commercial preparation of polyhedrosis virus which kills the cotton bollworm is being tried on a limited scale and field experiments on control of corn earworm by one of the baculoviruses have been so encouraging that commercial preparations are now available.

A protozoan, *Nosema locustae,* has been successfully employed to control grasshopper infestations. *Nosema* spores sprayed on a wheat-bran bait are consumed by the grasshoppers, germinate inside the insect's stomach, multiply rapidly, and devour the grasshopper from inside.

sex attractants—Certain chemical stimulants (pheromones) control many aspects of insect behavior, including mating. Sex pheromones may be excreted by the female to attract the male, or vice-versa. Some of these female pheromones have been synthesized in the lab and used to bait traps which can attract males from miles around. When the males enter the trap, expecting to encounter a receptive female, they are caught by a sticky substance on the bottom or sides of the trap. A variation on this method of using sex attractants involves the "confusion technique" in which an infested area is sprayed with so much female hormone that the males don't know in which direction to go to find a mate.

juvenile hormones (JH)—Just as pheromones control insect behavior, juvenile hormones keep an insect in the larval, or immature, stage. Only when the supply of JH is switched off at the time of metamorphosis can the insect become an adult. By synthesizing JH and applying it to larval insect populations, reproduction of the target pest can be prevented. One type of synthetic JH has been registered for use against floodwater mosquitoes. A compound already in widespread use among structural pest control operators, advertised as "birth control for cockroaches", is used to render German cockroaches sterile. Applied in combination with another insecticide, this chemical helps to provide long-term control of this troublesome household pest. An obvious limitation on the use of JH is that they are only useful against insects which cause damage as adults; many of the worst agricultural pests are larvae (e.g. caterpillars, grubs, etc.) against which JH is totally ineffective.

sterile male technique—This method relies on the mass-rearing and release of huge numbers of male insects which have been sterilized by X-rays or chemicals. Mating of a normal female with a sterile male naturally results in the production of infertile eggs. If the ratio of sterilized to normal males is sufficiently large, most matings will be unsuccessful and pest populations will fall rapidly. This method, which was very successful in eliminating the screw-worm fly from the island of Curacao and from Florida, is most effective when the pest population is geographically isolated, making re-invasion of the area with normal males unlikely.

development of resistant host plants—Probably the most ecologically sound method of reducing crop damage due to microbial pathogens and nematodes, host resistance has also been successfully employed against such insect pests as the Hessian fly, grape phyloxera, spotted alfalfa aphid, rice stem borer, and corn earworm.

crop rotation—Well-known but often neglected, crop rotation is an effective way of controlling pests which can't survive prolonged periods without contact with the preferred host. In the midwestern Corn Belt, corn rootworm populations were formerly kept at low levels by rotating corn, oats, and clover. As the price of corn relative to other crops has increased, farmers have largely abandoned crop rotation and are now growing corn year after year on the same land. As a result, the corn rootworm has spread from a small area in southern Nebraska to assume major pest status in 18 western and midwestern states.

sanitation—For control of insect and rodent pests in residential areas or business establishments, the most effective way of reducing pest numbers and keeping them low is to apply the basic principles of sanitation. To survive and multiply, pests need a source of food, water, and harborage. If these are in short supply, large pest populations cannot be maintained. Strict observance of the rules of good housekeeping—promptly cleaning up spilled food, storing foods in tightly-sealed containers, keeping garbage cans covered, regularly collecting and disposing of animal feces—will be far more effective in eliminating flies, rats, and roaches over the long term than is the temporary palliative of pesticidal spraying. Similarly, structural alterations such as screens, metal or cement barriers, and caulk applied to cracks and crevices can assist in "building out" certain household pests. Habitat

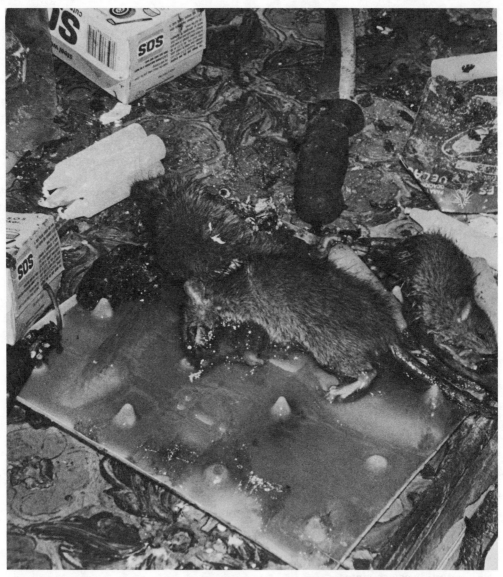

Alternative to chemical rodenticides: in situations where use of rat poison is ineffective or hazardous, glue boards provide an alternative method of rodent control. [*Chicago Bureau of Rodent Control*]

modification such as changing water in birdbaths frequently, keeping roof gutters free of twigs and leaves to permit complete drainage of rainwater, and maintaining premises free of discarded articles which could collect water can be very effective in reducing mosquito breeding. Pesticide use can provide a "quick fix", but without adherence to good sanitary practices, control will be temporary at best.

None of the above methods alone is the total answer to effective pest management. However, in the proper combination after an accurate assessment of a specific pest situation, IPM techniques promise a safer, more ecologically sound, and ultimately more successful approach to limiting pest damage than does the total reliance on chemicals which has characterized U.S. pest control efforts during the past 40 years.

REFERENCES

[1]Pimental, et. al, *Bioscience,* vol. 28, no. 12, 1977.

[2]Pratt, Harry, B.F. Gjornson, and K.S. Littig, *Control of Domestic Rats & Mice,* Centers for Disease Control, HEW Pub. No. 77-8141, 1977.

[3]Habicht, Gail, Gregory Beck, and Jorge L. Benach, "Lyme Disease", *Scientific American,* vol. 257, July 1987.

[4]Flint, M.L., and R. vanden Bosch, *Introduction to Integrated Pest Management,* Plenum Press, 1981.

[5]Perkins, John H., *Insects, Experts, and the Insecticide Crisis,* Plenum Press, 1982.

[6]"A Look at World Pesticide Markets", *Farm Chemicals,* September, 1981.

[7] Blair, Aaron, et al., "Cancer and Pesticides Among Farmers", *Pesticides and Groundwater: A Health Concern for the Midwest,* The Freshwater Foundation, 1987.

[8]Miller, Alan S., "2,4,5-T: Chemical Time Bomb", *Environment,* vol. 21, no. 5, June 1979.

[9]Koren, Herman, *Handbook of Environmental Health and Safety: Principles and Practices,* vol. 1, Pergamon Press, 1980.

[10]Flint and vanden Bosch, op. cit.

[11]Perkins, op. cit.

[12]Postel, Sandra, "Defusing the Toxics Threat: Controlling Pesticides and Industrial Wastes", *Worldwatch Paper 79,* September 1987.

[13]Dover, Michael J., "*A Better Mousetrap: Improving Pest Management for Agriculture*", World Resources Institute, Center for Policy Research, Study 4, September 1985.

[14]Bever, Wayne, et al., *Illinois Pesticide Applicator Study Guide,* Cooperative Extension Service, University of Illinois College of Agriculture, Special Publication 39, 1975.

[15]Mueller, David, "Dichlorvos in Danger?", *Pest Control,* April 1988.

[16]Dotto, Sydia, "Battling the Bugs", *Science Forum,* March/April, 1979.

9
Food Quality

"There was never the least attention paid to what was cut up for sausage; there would come all the way back from Europe old sausage that had been rejected, and that was moldy and white—it would be dosed with borax and glycerine, and dumped into the hoppers, and made over again for home consumption. There would be meat that had tumbled out on the floor, in the dirt and sawdust, where the workers had tramped and spit uncounted billions of consumption germs. There would be meat stored in great piles in rooms; and the water from leaky roofs would drip over it, and thousands of rats would race about on it . . . These rats were nuisances, and the packers would put poisoned bread out for them; they would die, and then rats, bread, and meat would go into the hoppers together . . . the meat would be shoveled into carts, and the man who did the shoveling would not trouble to lift out a rat even when he saw one—there were things that went into the sausage in comparison with which a poisoned rat was a tidbit."

—*The Jungle* by Upton Sinclair (1904)

The overwhelming sense of revulsion experienced by the American public upon reading Upton Sinclair's blockbusting expose of conditions in Chicago's meat-packing industry at the turn of the century was a major factor leading to the passage in 1906 of this nation's first Food and Drug Act (Wiley Act). Although Sinclair's stated purpose in writing the novel was to obtain social justice for the downtrodden workingman of the day, the most immediate impact of *The Jungle* was the introduction of new regulations to protect the quality of food consumed by Americans. Sinclair himself made the wry observation that "I aimed at the public's heart and by accident I hit it in the stomach".

From colonial days until the mid-1800s, problems relating to unknown quality of food were relatively rare, since most Americans raised their food at home or at least knew from whence it came. Consumers carefully inspected purchased items for signs of insect infestation, sniffed meat and fish to detect spoilage, and in general served as their own food inspectors. Government regulation of food quality prior to the 20th century was extremely limited, focusing primarily on commercially baked bread. Early bread laws were designed to standardize the weight of loaves in relation to the price of wheat; i.e. they were essentially price-fixing laws. Other regulations prohibited adding foreign substances such as ground chalk or powdered beans to flour. Subsequent laws provided for inspection of weights and flour quality.[1]

The growth of cities and the expansion of transportation networks which characterized the years immediately following the Civil War gave birth to an organized food industry whose rapid development was marred by unhygienic conditions (such as those described in *The Jungle*) and frequently unethical practices. The biggest scandal of 19th century food establishments involved the widespread practice of **Adulteration**—the deliberate addition of inferior or cheaper material to a supposedly pure food product in order to stretch out supplies and increase profits. Adulteration has undoubtedly been practiced on a small scale for millennia by unscrupulous merchants when they thought they could get away with it, but the anonymity of large, unregulated corporations selling foodstuffs to faceless consumers hundreds of miles away gave great impetus to the proliferation of this age-old practice. Substances used as adulterants in some cases were harmless ingredients, cheating consumers only in a financial sense; in other instances, the adulterants consisted of toxic substances which posed a serious health threat to those consuming the adulterated products. Some foods commonly adulterated during the 18th and 19th centuries included: 1) *black pepper,* commonly mixed with such materials as mustard seed husks, pea flour, juniper berries, or floor sweepings; 2) *tea,* adulterated on a large scale with leaves of the ash tree which were dried, curled, and sold to tea merchants for a few cents per pound. Green China tea was often adulterated with dried thorn leaves, tinted green with a toxic dye; black Indian tea was more easily adulterated by collecting used tea leaves from restaurants, drying and stiffening them with gum and then tinting them with black lead, also toxic, to make them look fresh; 3) *cocoa powder* "enriched" with brick dust; 4) *milk* supplies extended with water; 5) *coffee* blended with ground acorns or chicory.

Perhaps even more alarming were revelations in the mid-19th century that many of the food colors and flavorings in widespread use were poisonous, e.g. pickles colored bright green with copper, candies and sweets brightly tinted with lead and copper salts, commercially-baked bread whitened with alum, beer froth produced by iron sulfate.[2]

The 1906 Federal Food and Drug Act referred to previously reflected growing awareness of such problems and dealt largely with consumer protection against adulteration, mis-labeling of foods, and harmful ingredients in foods. As a result of this Act and of subsequent food quality legislation, instances of adulteration in the United States are now much rarer than they were in former years, though regulations have had to be instituted from time to time to prevent the gradual degradation of foods, such as the increase in fat or ground bone content of hot dogs or the decrease in fruit content of jams or fruit pies. However, occasionally flagrant abuses still do occur. In 1988, two top executives of Beech-Nut Nutrition Corporation, the nation's second largest manufacturer of baby food, were given jail sentences and the company fined in excess of $2 million for knowingly marketing over a 5-year period millions of containers of flavored sugar water fraudulently labelled as "100% apple juice".

Within recent years the focus of public attention regarding food quality has shifted from adulteration to a concern over the presence of contaminants and additives in our modern food supply. The fact that few Americans today produce their own foods at home means that almost all of us, to a greater or lesser degree, have no choice but to rely on foodstuffs produced by a massive food industry—foods which contain many kinds of additives and, in some cases, contaminants over which we have very little control. The rising interest in "health foods" is due, in no small measure, to the feeling of many people that industrially-produced food is somehow less safe and less nutritious than the "natural" foods of yesteryear. Representatives of the food industry and, indeed, many scientists, counter that chemical additives are both safe and essential to ensure an abundant supply of food at affordable prices to a still-growing population. In an attempt to understand the nature of the debate and the rationale behind existing or proposed regulations, it is helpful to distinguish between those substances accidentally introduced into foods and those deliberately added to prevent deterioration or to enhance taste or attractiveness.

Food Contaminants—*substances accidentally incorporated into foods*, contaminants include dirt, hairs, animal feces, fungal growths, insect fragments, pesticide residues, traces of growth hormones or antibiotics, etc., which are introduced into food during the harvesting, processing, or packaging stage. They serve no useful purpose in the finished product and are presumed to be harmful unless proven otherwise (in many cases, however, common food contaminants constitute an aesthetic affront to consumers rather than an actual health threat; for example, the thought of eating a fly wing hidden among the oregano leaves on a frozen pizza may be repugnant, but it won't make you sick—at least not if you don't see it!). Certainly every effort should be made to keep our foods as free from contamination as possible; however, it has never been, and probably never will be, possible to grow, harvest, and process crops that are totally free of natural defects. In order to ensure that foods are *never* contaminated by even a few insects, rodent hairs or droppings, etc., we would have to use much larger amounts of chemical pesticides and would thus risk exposing consumers to the potentially greater hazard of increased levels of toxic residues. Current philosophy holds that it is wiser to permit aesthetically unpleasant but harmless natural defects rather than pouring on more synthetic chemicals. For this reason, the Food and Drug Administration (FDA) has established what it terms "Defect Action Levels", specifying the maximum limit of contamination at or above which the agency will take legal action to remove the product from the market. It is important to understand that such defect action levels are not *average* levels of contamination—the averages are considerably lower—but represent the upper limit of allowable contamination. Defect Action Levels are set at that point where it is assumed there is no danger to human health. Some examples of existing defect action levels are shown in Fig. 9-1.

Fig. 9-1

EXAMPLES OF FOOD DEFECT ACTION LEVELS

Product	Defect	Action Level
Apricots, canned	Insect filth	Average of 2% or more by count insect-infested or insect-damaged
Beets, canned	Rot	Exceeds average of 5% by weight of pieces with dry rot
Broccoli, frozen	Insects and mites	Average of 60 aphids, thrips, and/or mites per 100 grams
Cherries, maraschino	Insect filth	Average of over 5% rejects due to maggots
Corn, canned	Insect larvae (corn ear worms, corn borers)	Two or more 3 mm or longer larvae, cast skins or cast skin fragments of corn ear worm or corn borer, the aggregate length exceeding 12 mm in 24 pounds
Curry powder	Insect filth	Average of more than 100 insect fragments per 25 grams
	Rodent filth	Average of more than 4 rodent hairs per 25 grams
Olives, pitted	Pits	Average of more than 1.3% by count of olives with whole pits and/or pit fragments 2 mm or longer measured in the longest dimension
Peanut butter	Insect filth	Average of 30 or more insect fragments per 100 grams
	Rodent filth	Average of 1 or more rodent hairs per 100 grams
	Grit	Gritty taste and water insoluble inorganic residue is more than 25 mg per 100 grams
Tomatoes, canned	Drosophila fly	Average 10 fly eggs per 500 grams; or 5 fly eggs and 1 maggot per 500 grams; or 2 maggots per 500 grams

Several groups of food contaminants which are less visible but more worrisome are the traces of antibiotics and growth hormones in meat products and toxic pesticide residues on fruits and vegetables. Subtherapeutic amounts (i.e. levels lower than those used to treat disease) of antibiotics such as penicillin and tetracycline, both of which are extensively used to treat human illnesses as well, have been incorporated into livestock and poultry feed to an increasing extent since the early 1950s. While the livestock industry contends that this practice helps to prevent disease, promotes growth, and results in greater weight gain per unit of feed consumed, critics point out that beneficial effects are most pronounced when animals are raised under crowded, unsanitary conditions and are, in effect, germ-killers which would scarcely be necessary in situations where high standards of hygiene existed. Concern about the use of antibiotics centers around the fact that widespread use of these drugs could promote the development of bacterial strains resistant to penicillin, tetracycline, etc.,—resistance which it is now known can be genetically transferred from one strain of bacteria to another, human pathogens included. In recent decades an increasing number of bacteria which cause such human ailments as salmonellosis, gonorrhea, and pneumonia have become resistant to one or more kinds of antibiotics and it is suspected that the use of such drugs in animal feed, as well as the overprescription of antibiotics for human use, has played a significant role in the resistance problem. Although it hadn't been conclusively shown that subtherapeutic use of antibiotics in livestock fodder threatens public health, a corresponding lack of proof that their use was safe prompted the FDA in 1977 to propose banning such uses of both penicillin and tetracycline, making feeds containing these drugs available only upon a veterinarian's order—a procedure instituted in Great Britain as early as 1969. Immediate protests from a livestock industry whose economic interests were threatened caused Congress to intercede, halting regulatory action and insisting on further studies.[3] Concerns about acquired antibiotic resistance gained new credibility in the spring of 1985 when the most serious outbreak of salmonellosis on record afflicted more than 16,000 in six Midwestern states and left two people dead. Transmitted through contaminated milk, the strain of bacteria which caused this outbreak demonstrated resistance to tetracycline and all forms of penicillin and was believed to have arisen from the animal population.

Chicken producers initiated use of the sex hormone DES as a feed additive to promote weight gain in poultry in 1947, with cattle raisers following their lead a few years later. Before long, poultry farmers found it more efficient to implant pellets of DES into the necks of chickens, a practice which led to the country's first DES-inspired lawsuit when, in the early 1950s, irate mink farmers went to court after their animals became sterile from eating heads and necks of hormone-treated chickens. When it was discovered that the average DES content of chicken skin fat was higher than the level which induced breast cancer in mice, the FDA suspended the use of this hormone in poultry. Because subsequent testing of beef revealed consistent low-level residues of DES in meat also, the government in 1971 ordered that DES feeding be halted at least one week prior to slaughter, assuming this would be sufficient time for the hormone to be eliminated from the animal's system. Either the original assumption was incorrect or beef producers ignored the mandate, because DES residues continued to be found in beef throughout the 1970s. The link between DES "pregnancy supports" and the development of vaginal cancer in DES daughters generated further concerns about the use of the hormone in cattle feed and by mid-1977 the FDA finally was able to impose a ban against its use. Ironically, the growth promotion aspects of DES use highly touted by the livestock industry bring increased risks but no benefits to the consumer, since the weight gained is almost entirely fat and water, not protein.[4]

Pesticide residues in food can result from direct spraying of crops or from the consumption by livestock of pesticide-contaminated fodder, traces of which can then be translocated into meat, eggs, or milk. The EPA has established so-called "tolerance levels" for all pesticides used on food crops, such levels being based on toxicological testing of laboratory animals. In many cases, unfortunately, tolerance levels are set on the basis of little more than educated guesswork and not uncommonly must be revised downward as more complete information is obtained. In 1987 the National Research Council of the National Academy of Sciences published an alarming report estimating a significant increase in cancer mortality among American consumers due to ingestion of certain pesticide residues on food, even when the amounts of such chemicals are within the established tolerance levels (see Box 9–1). Of far greater concern than chemical residues on U.S. agricultural commodities, however, is the health threat posed by toxins on imported foods. Since the mid-1970s when the Environmental Protection Agency banned such pesticides as DDT, endrin, dieldrin, aldrin, heptachlor, and Kepone due to test results showing them to be carcinogenic, many consumers have assumed their exposure to the toxins has ceased. Recent revelations, however, indicate that the food Americans eat still contains potentially dangerous pesticide residues because of pesticide use overseas. Many of the chemicals now banned in the U.S. are sold to developing nations who use them extensively in producing crops for export to the American market. Government estimates indicate that at least 10% of all imported food is contaminated, mostly with pesticides no longer permitted for use in this country. For example, a 1977 FDA study revealed that 45% of unroasted coffee beans tested contained illegal pesticide residues;[5] tea and sugar from India as well as cocoa from Ecuador are imported bearing residues of highly toxic chlorinated hydrocarbon pesticides. Bananas are repeatedly sprayed with dieldrin, Kepone, and DDT—all banned in the U.S. (fortunately such residues are largely discarded with the banana peel).[6]

Such facts and figures may represent but the tip of the iceberg, since the General Accounting Office (GAO) found that the methods used by the FDA for testing food imports for pesticide contamination are highly ineffective, capable at best of detecting only 90 of the 268 pesticides for which the government has set tolerance levels. Even these are seldom found, since less than 1% of all the food shipments entering the U.S. are tested at all. When illegal pesticide residues *are* detected, it is usually too late to prevent marketing and consumption of the product because the shipment isn't detained at the port of entry while a sample is being analyzed.[7] Indeed, the GAO reports that during one 15-month period, half of all the food identified by the FDA as being contaminated was subsequently marketed to consumers without any warning announcements, nor

---

Box 9–1

Toxic Tomatoes

What do tomatoes, beef, potatoes, oranges, and lettuce have in common? According to a controversial 1987 report by the National Research Council, these 5 foods are at the top of a list of major dietary sources of public exposure to cancer-causing pesticide residues. Grappling with issues of pesticide regulatory reform, the NRC focused its study on a selected group of widely used farm chemicals which EPA has identified as carcinogens or possible carcinogens and attempted to estimate the impact which residues of these pesticides in the American food supply might have in terms of increasing cancer risks. A public which has taken the basic safety and wholesomeness of the food it eats for granted was somewhat disturbed at the conclusions of the study: the Council estimates an additional 20,000 cancer deaths per year in the United States (1 million over a 70-year lifetime) due to consumption of carcinogenic pesticide residues on meat and produce. Although the EPA considers 60% of herbicides, 30% of insecticides, and 90% of fungicides applied to be carcinogens, most of the dietary cancer risk from agrichemicals is posed by just 7 fungicides, 2 insecticides, and 1 herbicide on 15 foods: the five listed above, plus apples, peaches, pork, wheat, soybeans, beans, carrots, chicken, corn, and grapes (listed in decreasing order of risk).[8]

Agribusiness interests vigorously contest these estimates, arguing that what the NRC itself admits is a "worst-case scenario" is based on faulty assumptions which greatly overstate the risk: e.g. that every acre of cropland receives pesticidal applications and that the maximum allowable amount of residue is present on all foods—neither of which is the case. On the other hand, advocates of reduced pesticide use insist the NRC report underestimates the problem, pointing out that only 28 out of the 53 known or suspected carcinogenic pesticides used on food crops were included in the study. They are also concerned that the so-called "inert" ingredients used as carriers or fillers in pesticidal formulations are not considered when tolerance levels are set, even though some inerts are now recognized as carcinogens themselves. Critics complain that the dietary risks postulated in the report were established on the basis of debatable assumptions regarding the amount of certain foods an average American eats and they emphasize that tolerance levels themselves are set on the basis of incomplete or non-existent health and safety data.

As bewildered consumers weigh these conflicting viewpoints and as EPA administrators struggle to reform the existing system for regulating pesticides on food, individuals wishing to minimize their own exposure can choose to be diligent about washing and peeling fruits and vegetables (not all poisons can be removed in this way, but many can); they may preferentially purchase in-season, domestically-grown produce or may patronize markets selling organically-grown foods. Best of all, they may begin to raise at least some of their own fruits and vegetables; by doing so they can then decide whether to use chemical pesticides on those tomatoes or not and, if so, can choose those posing the fewest health and safety risks.[9]

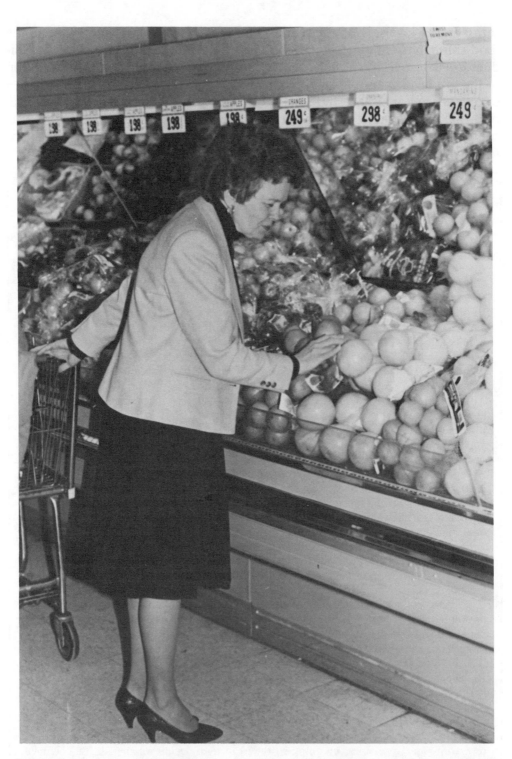

Consumer concerns about pesticide residues on food have been heightened by reports from such groups as the National Academy of Sciences and the Natural Resources Defense Council, warning that many fruits and vegetables in the marketplace bear traces of cancer-causing agrichemicals. [*Author's Photo*]

were the importers penalized in any way.[10] In light of the extent to which pesticide residues are commonly present as contaminants on fresh produce, the oft-ignored motherly admonition to wash fruits and vegetables well, or to peel them, before eating takes on new significance.

Food Additives—More controversial than the accidental, often unavoidable, food contaminants are the approximately 2800 food additives, *substances intentionally added to food to modify its taste, color, texture, nutritive value, appearance, resistance to deterioration, etc.* The years since the end of World War II have witnessed explosive growth of the food chemical industry, as food processors responded to public demand (or occasionally created public demand) by promoting a host of new products—convenience foods, frozen foods, dehydrated foods, ethnic foods, low-calorie foods, etc. Many of these products could not exist in a world free of additives. Nevertheless, a great many people are automatically suspicious of additives with long, unfamiliar, often unpronounceable names; reading the list of ingredients on virtually any supermarket package, can, or bottle seems a bit like a quick tour of a chemical factory. However, there's nothing inherently evil about using additives, provided that the chemical in question has no adverse effect on human health and performs a useful function. Many substances that can technically be termed "additives" have been in use for thousands of years—sugar, salt, and spices constitute just a few examples. Some additives come from natural sources: lecithin, derived from soybeans or corn, exemplifies a natural additive used as an emulsifier to achieve the desired consistency in products such as cake mixes, non-dairy creamers, salad dressings, ice cream, and chocolate milk. Other food additives are factory-made but are chemically the same as their natural analogs. The synthetic vitamins and minerals added to foods to improve nutritive value are examples of these; identical in chemical composition to natural vitamins and minerals found in food, they are preferentially used because they are less expensive and more readily available. Such man-made additives frequently are more concentrated, more pure, and of a more consistent quality than some of their counterparts in the natural world. The use of synthetic vitamins and minerals in food over the past half century has had a profound impact on public health in the U.S., virtually eliminating certain deficiency diseases which in former years afflicted large numbers of Americans. The addition of vitamin D to milk, iodine to table salt, and niacin to bread has relegated rickets, goiter, and pellagra, respectively, to nearly non-existent status in this country. Other additives perform such useful functions as retarding spoilage, preventing fats from turning rancid, retaining moisture in some foods and keeping it out of others.

Most people don't quarrel about additives used for these purposes. What *does* concern many scientists and laypersons alike is that a not-insignificant number of chemicals are used as food additives for purely cosmetic purposes—and many of these have been shown to be toxic, carcinogenic, or both.

Until 1958, food processors wishing to use a new additive were free to do so unless the FDA could prove that the additive in question was harmful to human health. With the passage of the Food Additives Amendment to the Food, Drug, and Cosmetic Act in that year, the situation was reversed: the manufacturer of any proposed food additive now has to satisfy the FDA that the product is safe before it can be approved for use; such approval can be rescinded at any time if new information indicates that the additive is unsafe. Undoubtedly the section of the Food Additives Amendment which has generated the most

---

Box 9-2

Sulfites and Salad Bars

Until an FDA-imposed ban on the addition of sulfiting compounds to raw fruits and vegetables took effect in 1986, the trendy salad bar posed a temptation best avoided by up to 1 million Americans whose reactions to the chemicals can range from the unpleasant to the deadly: nausea, flushing, fainting, diarrhea, hives, difficulty in swallowing, shortness of breath, anaphylactic shock, even death. At greatest risk are the 10 million asthma sufferers, 5-10% of whom experts estimate are sensitive to sulfites.

Sulfites, a general term used to describe a number of sulfur-containing compounds such as sodium sulfite, sodium and potassium bisulfite, potassium metabisulfite, and sulfur dioxide, have been used for many years in foods, wines, and drugs to prevent discoloration and spoilage. Long considered safe, sulfites seemed a logical choice for food service managers who sprayed or dipped cut foods in sulfite solutions to keep salad greens crisp, mushrooms light, and fruits unbrowned while sitting for hours on display. Unfortunately, although sulfiting compounds pose no hazard to most people, a not-insignificant minority of the population lacks the enzyme to metabolize sulfites and hence may experience a severe allergic response to the chemical. After receiving over 700 reports of adverse sulfite reactions, including several deaths, the FDA banned use of the additive on raw cut fruits and vegetables—a move aimed primarily at salad bars and supermarkets which were the sources of most reported illnesses.

While restaurants can turn to alternatives such as citric acid and lemon juice to maintain an attractive buffet, other sectors of the food and drug industry have few replacement options. Winemakers, who use sulfites to halt bacterial growth in wine, have no substitute for the chemical. In spite of complaints from some consumer groups, the FDA has refused to restrict the use of sulfites in packaged and canned foods, pickles, dried fruits, and potato and shrimp salad, arguing that few illnesses have been related to these sources and that the use of sulfites in such foods confers benefits far out of proportion to the risks. Instead, the agency now requires that if these foods contain at least 10 ppm sulfites, this information must be specifically included among the ingredients listed on the label. Certain medications present a more troublesome situation; over 1000 commonly used prescription drugs rely on sulfites to maintain their stability and potency. Many of these products are used by potentially-sensitive asthmatics, but at present there is no effective substitute for sulfur compounds in pharmaceuticals. The best the FDA can do in this case is to require that sulfite-containing prescription drugs carry a warning to advise sensitive persons of the possibility of serious allergic reaction to the medication. It is hoped that the current regulatory approach, combining a selective ban, warning labels, and efforts at consumer education will permit the continued use of an additive which, though hazardous to some, presents no health threat to the majority of consumers and performs a valuable role in a wide variety of products.[11]

---

heated controversy in recent years, particularly in reference to the proposed saccharin ban (see Ch. 6), is the **Delaney Clause,** which flatly prohibits the use *in food* of any ingredient shown to cause cancer in animals or humans (people who question why the FDA bans certain moderately carcinogenic food dyes yet takes no action against cigarettes have to be reminded that the Delaney Clause pertains solely to carcinogenic food additives, not to carcinogens in general; if a food processor should propose to add cigarette smoke as a flavoring to, say, cured meats, this would undoubtedly be prohibited under the Delaney Clause).

Fig. 9-2

COMMON TYPES OF FOOD ADDITIVES

Group	Purpose	Examples
Antioxidants	prevent fats from turning rancid and fresh fruits from darkening during processing	BHA, BHT, propylgallate
Bleaching agents	whiten and age flour	benzoyl peroxide, chlorine, nitrosyl chloride
Emulsifiers	to disperse one liquid in another to improve quality and uniformity of texture	lecithin, mono-and diglycerides, sorbitan monostearate, polysorbates
Acidulants	maintain acid-alkali balance in jams, soft drinks, vegetables, etc., to keep them from being too sour	sodium bicarbonate, citric acid, lactic acid, phosphoric acid
Humectants	maintain moisture in foods such as shredded coconut, marshmallows, and candies	sorbitol, glycerol, propylene glycol
Anti-caking compounds	keep salts and powdered foods free-flowing	calcium or magnesium silicate, magnesium carbonate, tricalcium phosphate, sodium aluminosilicate
Preservatives	control growth of spoilage organisms	sodium propionate, sodium benzoate, propionic acid
Stabilizers	provide proper texture and consistence to ice cream, cheese spreads, salad dressings, syrups	gum arabic, guar gum, carrageenan, methyl cellulose, agar-agar

Since many hundreds of food additives were already in widespread use at the time the 1958 amendment was passed, a portion of this legislation exempted such substances from the rigorous safety testing demanded for new additives. Instead, additives already in common usage were designated "generally regarded as safe" and placed on what is referred to as the *GRAS* list. In order to remove a food additive from the *GRAS* list, the FDA must demonstrate that the substance in question is harmful. Original screening of existing food additives to determine whether they should be placed on the *GRAS* list was done rather haphazardly, and by the 1970s it was recognized that long-time usage is no firm guarantee of safety. Recently more thorough studies of certain substances included on the *GRAS* list have resulted in withdrawal of approval for their use. Some of the once-common food additives subsequently removed from the *GRAS* list include:

Box 9-3

Why All the Fuss About Sodium Nitrite?

Nitrosamines are well recognized as powerful carcinogens. No one is deliberately adding these substances to food products—the Delaney Clause would prevent any such attempt—but many authorities fear that widescale exposure of the population to nitrosamines is occurring, regardless, in the form of sodium nitrite preservatives used in bacon, hot dogs, ham, lunch meats, smoked fish, and imported cheeses. Sodium nitrite can react with amines in the human stomach to form the hazardous nitrosamines (nitrosamines can also form in sodium nitrite-treated meats, especially bacon, during cooking), thus theoretically increasing an individual's cancer risk. This being so, why hasn't the use of sodium nitrite in meats been banned? Mainly because the chemical has a useful function which to many outweighs its drawbacks. Sodium nitrite is used primarily as a preservative, intended to deter both spoilage and botulism; it is also added to "fix" the red color of fresh meats, thereby masking discoloration and rejection by consumers. While the latter reason, at least, might seem a less than compelling reason for continuing use of a potentially dangerous substance, scientific evidence to date casts doubt on the thesis that removing sodium nitrite from meats would lower cancer rates. Researchers point out that the large amounts of natural nitrates ingested by humans in many vegetables (e.g. spinach, celery, lettuce) are readily converted first to nitrites and then to nitrosamines. These, added to other nitrites in water and air, constitute a much larger share of total body load than do the nitrites in cured meats. Natural body processes also contribute to nitrite exposure. Reduction of nitrate in the saliva contributes 10 times more nitrite than do hot dogs or bacon; thousands of times more nitrite is formed in the intestine than is consumed through nitrite-containing meats. Thus based on current evidence, it appears that the risk involved from nitrite preservatives is minimal compared with nitrites from bodily metabolism. Though future investigations may reveal a connection, there is no indication at present that sodium nitrite in cured meats has contributed to human cancer rates. Nevertheless, inasmuch as the foods containing this additive are also high in fats, cholesterol, salt, food colorings, and calories, concerned consumers might choose to avoid these items altogether in favor of more nutritious fare.[12]

- *cyclamates*—artificial sweeteners banned in 1970 because animal testing indicated they could induce bladder cancer and birth defects.
- *cobaltous salts*—used from 1963-1966 to improve the stability of beer foam; associated with fatal heart attacks among heavy beer drinkers in the U.S. and Canada.
- *polyvinyl chloride*—in plastic liquor bottles, banned in 1973 when carcinogenic vinyl chloride was detected in liquor.
- *safrole*—carcinogenic, mutagenic extract of sassafras root, formerly used to give root beer its characteristic flavor.
- *food colors*—a number of coal-tar dyes such as Red Dye No. 2, Orange No. 1 and 2, Violet No. 1, Yellow No. 1, 2, and 4 have been delisted because they were shown to be carcinogenic or to cause organ damage.

Box 9-4
Benefit/Risk Analyses: Who Benefits, Who Takes the Risk?

Is a pretty orange worth the threat of cancer? Should diet soda devotees be more worried about obesity or malignancy? Such controversial questions regarding the pros and cons of food additives are part of a wider debate over the extent to which government regulation can, or ought, to protect the public from environmental contaminants.

Desirable though it might be, elimination of all hazards faced by mankind is an impossibility—there is no such thing as absolute safety. Many, if not most, of the hazardous substances discussed in this book are either intrinsically useful themselves or are the unintended by-products of desirable goods or manufacturing processes. Rather than completely doing away with such substances, thereby losing the benefits they confer, society has attempted to reduce the risk by lowering exposure levels, at the same time permitting the chemical to remain in use. The difficulty in this approach, of course—and perhaps the key problem in environmental health—is to determine what level of risk is acceptable.

In recent years it has become fashionable in government circles, particularly among those wishing to undercut environmental protection laws, to resort to a procedure called risk (or cost)/benefit analysis—an effort that attempts to assign a monetary figure to all costs and benefits of a project or product (e.g. dam on a river, mosquito abatement program, installation of filters to reduce dust in an asbestos factory, etc.). The figures are then tallied and, depending on which side of the balance sheet the total is larger, the project is either killed or given the go-ahead. Of course the accuracy of original risk/benefit assumptions is crucial in arriving at a correct decision, as became quite obvious during the debate over whether the use of saccharin as a food additive should be revoked, per Delaney Clause mandate. Opponents of the ban belittled the cancer threat, citing the unreliability of animal testing and warning that millions of diabetics and overweight persons would, in the absence of diet colas, drink sugared beverages and thereby suffer even greater health risk. Supporters of the ban countered with evidence that consumption of saccharin has no positive effect on dieting but rather makes it harder to lose weight. They also cited diabetic experts who felt that victims of this condition have no intrinsic need for saccharin. Obviously there was no consensus on risks and benefits in this case.

Risk/benefit critics have long pointed out an obvious drawback to this exercise: it is virtually impossible to attribute monetary value to a human life or to abstract concepts such as scenic beauty, peace of mind, happiness, quality of life, and so forth. Thus many such studies undervalue risks, giving a false impression of the magnitude of benefits in undertaking environmentally questionable projects. Less discussed but equally relevant are the questions, "Benefits to whom?" "Risks to whom?" Although it's a common assumption that risks vs. benefits are but opposite sides of the same coin, this is not always true. The case of food colorings is a prime example of the frequent divergence in risks and benefits. Few dispute the fact that this class of food additives serves no beneficial purpose in terms of making the food more nutritious, extending its shelf life, etc. Food colors are used solely for cosmetic purposes—to make the food more attractive to the buyer, thereby promoting sales. Consumers have come to expect bright orange oranges (the natural color is slightly greenish), reddish hot dogs, and tinted dog food (obviously for the sake of the owner, since dogs are color-blind), even though the natural articles, while less eye-appealing to some, are just as tasty. In fact, the use of colors has aided manufacturers in subtly degrading the quality of their products. Dyes which make devil's food cake mix a dark, appetizing brown permit the producer to add less chocolate; yellow dye in "egg" bread makes it possible for the baker to reduce egg content—but not the price, of course; bright pink in strawberry or cherry-flavored ice cream substitutes for the lighter pink which use of the real, and more expensive, fruit would confer.

Thus the consumer obtains no real benefit from the use of food colors but does incur a certain degree of risk; a number of leading food colors have recently been removed from the *GRAS* list due to their proven carcinogenicity, while many others still in use are similarly suspect. For industry, however, the situation is the reverse. Eye-appealing products boost sales and tinting with synthetic chemicals is far cheaper than using real fruits, vegetables, and chocolate. The end result—enormous profits—make the use of artificial food colors extremely beneficial to industry with few, if any, risks. Risks and no benefits to the consumer, huge benefits and no risk to the food industry—this dichotomy exemplifies one of the most serious limitations in making equitable risk/benefit analyses.

Numerous other additives still on the *GRAS* list are considered of dubious safety by many researchers, yet remain in use due to lack of conclusive evidence or because of industry pressure on FDA regulators. Critics of current policy insist that food additives require a higher standard of care than other environmental chemicals and shouldn't be used if they present a health risk. They base this judgment on the fact that everyone is exposed to chemicals in food, not only those who voluntarily assume the risk. Varying levels of susceptibility among individuals and the effects of simultaneous exposure to other chemicals, including synergistic effects, have to be taken into consideration. Both MSG (monosodium glutamate), a flavor enhancer which can cause the headache, dizziness, nausea, and facial flushing sometimes referred to as "Chinese Restaurant Syndrome", and a group of sulfur-containing compounds known collectively as "sulfites" or "sulfiting agents" (see Box 9–2) are examples of food additives which serve a useful purpose and pose no danger to the majority of consumers but which can provoke severe allergic reactions among a sizeable minority of sensitive individuals. Because of the vast processed food market, any miscalculation of risk can have far-reaching implications on a public which assumes and expects that special care is being taken with the nation's food supply. Nevertheless, although some health authorities recommend avoiding foods containing non-essential additives (such as artificial colors and flavorings) wherever possible, little evidence exists at present to indicate that the health of Americans is suffering due to the chemical food additives currently in use.

Foodborne Disease

Ironically, while questions dealing with the safety of chemical additives generate most of the public's concern regarding food quality these days, most cases of illness or death due to food involve a number of old-fashioned foodborne diseases commonly referred to as "food poisoning".

Food poisoning can result from a variety of causes, including the following.

Natural toxins in food

The widely prevalent notion that all "natural" foods are safe and nutritious is a dangerous misconception. The faddish trend toward "living off the land" by collecting and eating various types of wild plants has led to a surge in food poisoning cases, according to some local public health officials. The fact is that there are many common plants, both wild and cultivated, which are poisonous, capable of causing ailments ranging from mild stomach disorders to a quick and painful death if consumed by the unwary. In addition, certain marine fish and shellfish species may contain toxins which induce severe illness or death. Some examples of plants or animals capable of causing a toxic reaction if eaten include:

> *Mushrooms*—mushrooms constitute a gourmet's delight, provided, of course, that the item in question is a non-poisonous variety. The problem is that there is no simple rule of thumb for distinguishing between those wild forms which are safe and those which are not. Although only a relatively few of the thousands of species found in North America are poisonous, they may look very much like non-poisonous species and frequently even grow together. One of the most poisonous types, the amanitas (one species of which is called the "Death Angel"), grow commonly in "fairy rings" in woods and on lawns. Just one or two bites of these alkaloid-containing amanitas can be fatal to an adult and, in fact, the vast majority of deaths due to mushroom poisoning are caused by these.

> *Castor Bean (Ricinus communis)*—this attractive shrub-like plant is commonly grown as an ornamental foundation planting as well as commercially for its oil. The leaves of the plant are only slightly toxic, but the colorful mottled seeds can be deadly, containing the toxin **ricin**. Children who chew on the seeds experience intense irritation of the mouth and throat, gastroenteritis, extreme thirst, dullness of vision, convulsions, uremia, and death. Only 1-3 seeds can kill a child; 4-8 are generally required to cause fatality in adults.

> *Jimsonweed (Datura stramonium)*—this common weed contains toxic alkaloids in all parts of the plant. The seeds and leaves are especially

dangerous; children have been poisoned by sucking nectar from the flowers, eating the seeds, or drinking liquid in which the leaves have been soaked. A very small amount can be fatal to a child.

Ergot (Claviceps purpurea)—this fungus which frequently infects cereal grains, especially rye, produces a toxic alkaloid, **ergotamine**, responsible for the serious type of food poisoning known as **ergotism** or "St. Anthony's Fire". When the fungal sclerotia growing on the rye grain are ground up with flour and subsequently consumed in bread, violent muscle contractions, excruciating pain, vomiting, deafness, blindness, and hallucinations can follow. One type of ergotism is characterized by severe constriction of the blood vessels, development of gangrene, and a painful death. Outbreaks of ergotism resulting in thousands of deaths were common until the 20th century when the decrease in home milling and institution of quality control in commercial mills reduced the level of flour contamination. Even so, small outbreaks of ergotism are still reported from time to time. Interestingly, federal controls do not apply to rye grown for the organic foods market.[13]

Aflatoxin—another mycotoxin (fungal poison) already discussed in Chapter 6, aflatoxins are produced by the mold *Aspergillus flavus* which grows on a wide variety of nuts, grains, and peanuts. When consumed, they can cause serious liver damage and are some of the most potent carcinogens known.

Certain Fish and Shellfish—several different types of food poisoning are associated with eating various marine organisms. **Ciguatoxin**, a poison associated with certain mostly bottom-dwelling fish living near reefs or rocky bottoms (e.g. red snapper, barracuda, grouper, sea bass, eel), has accounted for many food poisoning outbreaks in Florida and Hawaii. Ciguatoxin is not broken down by cooking; symptoms, including cramps, vomiting and diarrhea, followed by tingling and numbness in the tongue, lips, and mouth, as well as other signs of nervous system disorder, usually appear within 1-6 hours after eating. **Scombroid Poisoning**, generally associated with deep-sea fish such as tuna and mackerel, is caused by ingestion of a toxin produced by certain bacteria acting on the flesh of fish which aren't handled properly after catching. Onset of symptoms such as a flushing of the skin, headache, dizziness, a burning sensation in the mouth, hives, and the usual gastrointestinal discomfort, generally occurs very quickly, averaging ½ hour after eating. **Paralytic Shellfish Poisoning** (PSP) results from eating shellfish such as oysters, clams, or scallops contaminated with **saxitoxin**, a nerve poison produced by microscopic dinoflagellates (algae). *PSP* is characterized by numbness in the mouth and extremities, gastroenteritis, and in severe cases, difficulty in speaking and walking; such symptoms occur within 30 minutes to 3 hours after eating. In a small percentage of cases death may result. Protection of the public against *PSP* depends on effective shellfish sanitation and inspection programs in the states where harvesting occurs.

In addition to these natural poisons in seafood, the U.S. lately has witnessed a small but increasing number of foodborne parasitic diseases traced to the growing popularity of raw or undercooked fish preparations such as sushi and ceviche. Tapeworm infections are the most commonly reported problems, occurring predominantly along the West Coast where most victims admit to having eaten raw fish, mainly salmon. Symptoms of tapeworm infections, as well as time of onset, vary greatly from one person to another: some victims report experiencing severe cramps, nausea, and diarrhea almost immediately after eating; others may not develop symptoms for weeks or months. However, the majority of victims have no symptoms at all and only discover their infection when they pass the tapeworm, or segments of it, in their stool. Tapeworm infections can be eradicated with drugs, but roundworm infections (anisakiasis) are much more serious since there is no effective medication available. Such infections are very painful and may require surgery to remove the parasite. Consumers can easily avoid such problems simply by thoroughly cooking fish until it is flaky (internal temperature should be at 145°F for 5 minutes) or by freezing it at -4°F for 3-5 days before eating in order to kill the worms.

Microbial contamination

While some important pathogenic foodborne diseases (e.g. trichinosis) are caused by parasitic worms and others (e.g. hepatitis A, Norwalk virus) by viruses, by far the greatest number of foodborne disease outbreaks can be traced to ingestion of food containing certain pathogenic bacteria or to bacterial toxins pre-formed in the food before it was consumed. Although bacterial food poisoning can, and occasionally does, occur with foods prepared and eaten at home, public health officials are most concerned with the potential for large-scale poisoning inherent in the current trend towards more frequent eating outside the home and with the rapid growth and sheer size of the food service industry in the U.S. today. As the number of meals eaten away from home increases, the task of preventing foodborne disease grows more challenging.

It should be noted in passing that food *spoilage* is not the same thing as food poisoning. Spoilage involves the decomposition of foods due to the action of natural enzymes within food, to chemical reactions between food and containers, or to the activities of certain types of bacteria, fungi, or insects, resulting in unpleasant odors, taste, or appearance of the food. However, spoilage organisms do not produce toxins which would cause human illness if they were consumed, nor does eating food containing such live organisms induce sickness. The same cannot be said of food poisoning bacteria, whose presence is not betrayed by the appearance, smell, or taste of the food. The old term "ptomaine poisoning" often used in reference to food poisoning is a misnomer—there is no such thing. Ptomaines are foul-smelling chemical compounds produced by bacterial decomposition of proteins. Eating food containing ptomaines will not produce any illness.

Bacterial foodborne diseases are classified either as *Infections* or *Intoxications,* depending on whether illness is caused by consumption of large numbers of live organisms or by ingestion of pre-formed bacterial toxin, respectively. The more common types of bacterial food poisoning have rather similar symptoms—symptoms which almost everyone has experienced at one time or another: diarrhea, abdominal pain, vomiting, dehydration, prostration, and often fever and chills in the case of bacterial infections (not, however, with intoxications). Onset of such symptoms usually occurs within 1-24 hours after eating the contaminated food, depending on the type of bacteria involved and the amount of food ingested. The most common foodborne bacterial infection is:

Salmonellosis—often referred to by more descriptive appellations such as "Delhi Belly" or "The Tropical Trots", salmonellosis is the most common bacterial foodborne disease in the U.S., estimated in recent years to afflict about 4 million Americans annually. Thanks in part to changes in lifestyle and to the way in which livestock is raised and processed, the incidence of this foodborne illness is steadily increasing. Caused by a number of species of the genus *Salmonella*. the disease is typically associated with eating poultry, meat, or eggs harboring large numbers of the rod-shaped bacterium. Nevertheless, numerous outbreaks have been traced to foods not generally associated with the disease: the largest salmonellosis outbreak in U.S. history, affecting an estimated 200,000 persons (16,000 laboratory-confirmed cases; many more unreported) in Illinois and several other Midwestern states in the spring of 1985, was traced to milk (although potentially an excellent medium for the growth of *Salmonella* and other foodborne pathogens, milk today is considered one of our safest foods due to pasteurization and high standards of sanitation in the dairy industry; less than 1% of all foodborne disease outbreaks in recent years have been traced to contaminated milk). Other unusual sources have included cocoa beans and marijuana (both were contaminated with animal feces harboring the pathogen). .

Inside the small intestine, colonies of *Salmonella* continue to grow and invade the host tissue, irritating the mucosal lining. Sudden onset of disease symptoms most commonly occurs within 12-24 hours after eating the contaminated food, with 18 hours being the most common time interval; discomfort may persist for several days and some victims may remain carriers for months after all outward symptoms have disappeared, shedding bacteria in their feces and remaining capable of infecting others. Severity of the disease ranges from very mild to very severe, with young children, the elderly, and travelers often the most adversely affected. Among otherwise healthy adults, fatalities due to salmonellosis are rare (victims only *wish* they were dead!) but do occur occasionally—the Illinois outbreak claimed at least 2 lives, possibly several more. In addition to the obvious short-term effects of the ailment, salmonellosis sufferers may also develop serious chronic disorders as a result of their infection. About 2-3% of victims later contract chronic arthritis, while a much smaller percentage develop painful septic arthritis when the *Salmonella* bacteria invade the joints. Outbreaks of salmonellosis are of particular concern in hospitals or nursing homes where victims are already in a weakened state and where the consequences of an infection are most severe.

Exhibiting characteristics of both an infection and an intoxication is:

Clostridium perfringens—because outbreaks of this foodborne ailment are usually associated with quantity food preparation in restaurants or institutions, *Clostridium perfringens* is often referred to as the "cafeteria germ". This illness is sometimes categorized as a foodborne infection because live bacteria multiply within the host; alternatively, it may be classified as an intoxication because the disease symptoms are caused by a toxin which is either produced by live bacteria inside the body or already present in the food at the time of consumption. In either case, very large numbers of bacteria or large amounts of toxin must be ingested to produce *C. perfringens* food poisoning. Cooked meat and poultry that have been left unrefrigerated for several hours have frequently been traced as the source of an outbreak, as have meat pies, stew, and gravies. Disease symptoms generally become evident 8-22 hours after eating; fortunately, *C. perfringens* poisonings are relatively mild and of brief duration, discomfort generally lasting only a day or two. This type of food poisoning is becoming increasingly common as more and more meals are eaten outside the home.

Among bacterial foodborne intoxications the most important are:

Staphylococcus aureus—sometimes known as "Roto-Rooter Disease" because of its violent onset, *Staphylococcus* intoxication is estimated to account for between 20-40% of all food poisoning cases. The causative bacteria are present in pimples, boils, hang-nails, wound infections, sputum, and sneeze droplets. People thus constitute the prime source of these organisms which flourish in such proteinaceous foods as cooked ham, sauces and gravies, chicken salad, egg salad, cream pies and pastries, etc. Growth of the bacteria within the food medium results in production of an enterotoxin (poison of the intestinal tract) which is not destroyed when the food is cooked. When consumed, the toxin causes irritation and inflammation of the stomach and intestine, resulting in vomiting and diarrhea. Since illness is produced by a poison already in the food at the time of eating rather than by bacterial growth within the victim's intestine, the effects of bacterial intoxication appear more rapidly than do those of an infection. People consuming *Staphylococcus* toxin may experience the sudden onset of vomiting and diarrhea within as little as 30 minutes after eating, although a period of 2-4 hours is more common. As is the case with most foodborne illness, individual differences in susceptibility will result in some people becoming quite ill after eating the tainted food, while others may not be affected whatsoever.[14] Due to the nature of the symptoms and to the fact that duration of the illness is relatively brief, seldom persisting for more than a day or two, sufferers of staph intoxication frequently blame their miseries on "the 24-hour flu" rather than on the true culprit—contaminated food. Deaths from this foodborne disease are extremely rare and most victims recover quickly without any complications developing.

Botulism—the most serious of all bacterial foodborne diseases, botulism is caused by the spore-forming soil bacterium *Clostridium botulinum* which, growing under anaerobic conditions, produces a deadly neurotoxin, the most poisonous substance known. Outbreaks of botulism have been most frequently associated with home-canned, low-acid foods such as beans, corn, beets, spinach, mushrooms, etc. This is because many home canners fail to realize that a long processing time (or a shorter time at high pressure in a pressure cooker) is necessary in order to kill the heat-resistant bacterial spores. If the spores survive, they can germinate and, in the absence of oxygen, multiply within the food medium, producing the deadly poison. If food contaminated with the botulism toxin is boiled for 15-20 minutes, the poison will be destroyed, but all too frequently such food is eaten uncooked or only briefly warmed, with disastrous results. In recent years a number of botulism outbreaks have been traced to commercially processed foods as well, mostly smoked fish or vacuum-packed items. Some recent botulism outbreaks have been traced to highly atypical sources, indicating a need for caution in situations where the causative bacteria encounter a warm, oxygen-free environment. In the fall of 1983, one of the worst botulism outbreaks in U.S. history resulted in the hospitalization of 28 victims (one of whom subsequently died) who had eaten "patty melt" sandwiches at a restaurant in Peoria, IL. Surprised investigators ultimately identified sauteed onions as the cause of the problem. Contaminated with *C. botulinum* spores from the soil in which they grew, the onions were fried in margarine which provided a protective air-free shield for germinating bacteria which proceeded to multiply in the incubating temperatures provided by the warming tray in the restaurant kitchen. By the time the onions were consumed many hours later, enough of the deadly botulinum toxin had been formed to cause the disease outbreak. In an unrelated incident in Baton Rouge, LA, the following year, a restaurant patron was stricken with botulism after eating a foil-wrapped baked potato, warmed up from the previous day. The foil wrapping had provided the anaerobic conditions which permitted growth of bacterial spores on the potato skin, while remaining at room temperature overnight allowed multiplication of the organism and production of the toxin.[15] Botulism is first evidenced by the usual gastrointestinal distress which generally appears within 12-36 hours, followed by the onset of neurological symptoms—double vision, difficulty in swallowing and breathing, stammering, and respiratory paralysis leading to death. Prior to the 1950s, the fatality rate among botulism victims stood at about 60%; more recently, thanks to prompt administration of antitoxin and to improvements in respiratory therapy, death rates have dropped to 15% or less—still high in comparison with other bacterial foodborne diseases.[16]

Box 9–5
Prevention of Foodborne Disease: Time-Temperature Control

When environmental conditions are favorable, the pattern of growth and multiplication of populations of pathogenic bacteria in food corresponds to the sigmoid curve described in Chapter 2. An initial lag period of about one hour is characterized by negligible

---

multiplication as the organisms adjust to their new conditions. This lag phase is followed by extremely rapid multiplication in the numbers of organisms until the supply of essential nutrients diminishes and toxic by-products accumulate. At this stage, growth levels off and the number of organisms remains relatively constant until eventually a progressive die-off of cells occurs. However, for this sequence of events to occur, certain environmental preconditions such as proper pH, moisture, essential nutrients, and temperature must be met. Of these, perhaps the most crucial in determining the rate of bacterial multiplication is *temperature*. The bacteria responsible for most foodborne disease outbreaks multiply most rapidly within a temperature range referred to as the "**Danger Zone**"—between **45° - 140°F**. Temperatures above 140°F will kill most actively growing bacteria, though bacterial spores and a few thermophilic species may survive. At temperatures below 45°F, growth of the bacterial populations associated with common foodborne illnesses either ceases entirely or is extremely slow; however, the organisms are not killed by cold temperatures and can remain viable for long periods of time, resuming multiplication when temperatures rise. Therefore, the most effective way to prevent buildup of bacterial numbers to levels high enough to cause food poisoning is to keep foods refrigerated, especially those proteinaceous foods which most frequently harbor pathogenic bacteria. Heating such foods thoroughly will kill bacteria which may be present in the food; the higher the temperature above 140°, the shorter the time the bacterial population will be able to survive (normal cooking times and temperatures are not sufficient, however, to break down *Staphylococcus* toxins).

To ensure complete heat penetration throughout the item being cooked, it is advised that internal temperatures reach the following minimum levels to guarantee that any pathogens present within the food are killed:

Poultry and stuffed meats	165°F
Pork	150°F
Other potentially hazardous foods	140°F

It should be noted that the internal temperature of the item being cooked, rather than the temperature of the oven or burner, is the crucial factor. In many instances, large roasts of beef, ham, or turkey still harbor viable pathogens after cooking because they weren't in the oven long enough for temperatures at the center of the roast to reach the recommended 140° level. In the same way, large pieces of cooked meat held in the refrigerator for cooling frequently have internal temperatures well within the growth range, even though the refrigerator thermostat registered at or below 45°F as advised. To promote rapid cooling, cooked meat should be sliced into thin layers and placed in shallow pans before being refrigerated.

The most effective methods that food handlers can follow to prevent foodborne disease, be it in the home, in restaurants, or at large public gatherings, is to complete the processing of food within an hour or two while the bacteria remain in the lag phase of growth and to cool foods rapidly if they are not to be consumed immediately. Bearing these principles in mind, it should come as no surprise that an analysis of food poisoning outbreaks revealed that 5 out of 6 factors which most frequently contribute to such illness are related to time-temperature control. The six factors most often implicated in bacterial food poisoning outbreaks are, in order of importance:

1. failure to refrigerate foods properly
2. preparing and cooking foods a day or more before they are to be served
3. failure to cook foods thoroughly
4. infected persons who practice poor personal hygiene handling food
5. improper hot holding (keeping foods in heating trays at temperatures under 140°F)
6. inadequate re-heating of cooked foods

Factors leading to food poisoning outbreaks:

Bacterial contamination of foods can occur at any time from the production of food in field or feedlot right up to preparation and serving of the meal. Thus strict adherence to principles of food sanitation are essential at every step from production to processing, transportation, storage, preparation, and service if food poisoning outbreaks are to be avoided. Bacteria which caused foodborne disease are common inhabitants of the intestinal tracts of humans and domestic animals, present in healthy and sick individuals alike; some are naturally present in soils as well. When discharged in fecal material, these organisms can survive for long periods in litter, feces, trough water, and soil. Livestock feed is often contaminated with *Salmonella* organisms introduced when infected animal by-products are rendered and added to the feed mixture. Animals can become infected from any of these sources and thus bring such pathogens into slaughterhouses and poultry processing plants. Just one infected organ or carcass or animal feces can contaminate cutting equipment or workers' hands and thereby can transfer the bacteria to other carcasses or foods, a process referred to as **Cross-Contamination**. Once in a processing plant or food establishment, pathogenic bacteria can survive on the surface of equipment for long periods and thus constitute sources of food contamination over an extended time period. For this reason, cleaning and sanitizing of grinders, choppers, slicers, etc., after each use and frequent washing of workers' hands are important measures in preventing cross-contamination.

Foods, particularly those of animal origin, often contain pathogens such as *Salmonella* and *Clostridium perfringens* when they enter the kitchen. Fifteen to 30% of commercial egg products and of raw dressed poultry contain *Salmonella* (it has recently been reported that even whole, uncracked eggs may harbor *Salmonella* organisms transmitted from infected hens via their ovaries into the developing egg. For this reason, much to the dismay of Caesar salad and eggnog lovers, health agencies are now strongly recommending against the consumption of raw or undercooked eggs). Half the red meat in supermarkets harbors *Clostridium perfringens*. Once in the kitchen, additional opportunity for contamination of food is presented by the food handlers themselves. The primary reservoir of the *Staphylococcus* organism is the human nose; if kitchen workers cough or sneeze near foods, the bacteria are readily transferred to an appropriate growth medium. If food handlers have infected cuts on their hands, boils, bad cases of acne or other skin eruptions, *Staphylococcus* bacteria likewise can be transferred to food. Similarly, since approximately 40% of all healthy people carry *Salmonella* organisms in their gastrointestinal tract and regularly shed the live bacteria when they defecate, failure of kitchen workers to wash their hands thoroughly after using the bathroom can result in contamination of foods with this pathogen.

Since so many foods contain at least some disease-causing bacteria, it is fortunate that bacterial counts or toxin levels within the ingested food have to be relatively high in order to induce symptoms of food poisoning. By maintaining conditions which inhibit the multiplication of bacteria within the food medium, (i.e. by keeping foods at temperatures below 45°F or above 140°F), most food poisoning outbreaks can be avoided. Unfortunately, though such preventive measures are relatively simple, relating primarily to personal hygiene and time-temperature control (see Box 9-5), they are all-too-frequently neglected by householders and commercial food establishments alike. Thus bacterial food poisoning, which fundamentally is a result of improper food sanitation and should not even exist in affluent modern societies, will undoubtedly remain our most prevalent food-related health problem.

Box 9–6
Is Irradiated Food Safe?

Controversy has raged for years over the pros and cons of utilizing ionizing radiation to kill pests and parasites in food products and to extend the shelf life of fruits, vegetables, meat, and fish. Already employed on a small scale in 27 other countries, food irradiation has been vigorously opposed by some U.S. consumer groups fearful of possible health and environmental implications of "zapping" sizeable portions of the American food supply. Nevertheless, the Food and Drug Administration, after 40 years of research and extensive deliberation on the issue, is convinced of the safety of using radiation as a food preservative and is gradually expanding its legal applications.

Employed since the mid-1960s to control insects in wheat and flour, as well as to prevent sprout development in potatoes, irradiation now can be used to kill trichina worms in fresh pork, control insects and slow ripening in fruits and vegetables, and to kill pests in dry herbs, spices, and tea. In permitting such uses, the FDA has specified maximum radiation levels for treating foods and requires that such products on the retail market bear the easily recognizable international logo, indicating to the consumer that the food in question has been irradiated. Food irradiation facilities must adhere to strict safety regulations promulgated by the Nuclear Regulatory Commission and the Occupational Safety and Health Administration (OSHA), and manufacturers must follow prescribed record-keeping requirements.

Some of the objections to food irradiation raised by concerned consumers are based on misinformation about what the process actually entails. The most common irradiation methods employ gamma rays, X-rays, or electron beams which, unlike pesticides, accomplish the task for which they were intended without leaving any residue and without rendering the food itself radioactive. Consumers handling or eating irradiated food are exposed to no radiation whatsoever. Some critics of the process worry that radiation results in certain chemical changes in the food, producing new radiolytic products which may be toxic. FDA concedes that small amounts of radiolytic chemicals are indeed produced, but insists that 90% of these are natural components of food and the remaining 10% are chemically analogous to naturally-occurring substances in food. FDA disputes any toxic hazard to the public posed by such chemicals, stating that the amounts are far too small to pose any risk. Charges that irradiation can alter the texture, flavor, or nutritional value of foods are countered by observations that cooking, canning, or freezing produce equivalent changes.

In a world where pests and spoilage continue to claim a sizeable share of each year's harvest, and with increasing concerns regarding toxic chemical residues on food, the desirability of expanding the use of irradiation for food preservation deserves careful and dispassionate consideration by the American consumer.[17]

REFERENCES

[1] Janssen, Wallace F., "America's First Food and Drug Laws", *FDA Consumer,* June 1975.

[2] Tannahill, Reay, *Food in History,* Stein and Day, 1973.

[3] Wirth, David A., "FDA Flip-Flops on Antibiotic Hazard", *Environment,* vol. 25, no. 5, June 1983.

[4] Norwood, Christopher, *At Highest Risk,* Penguin Books, 1980.

[5] Weir, David, "The Boomerang Crime", *Mother Jones,* Nov. 1979.

[6] Hornblower, Margot, "U.S. Firms Export Products Banned Here As Health Risks", *The Washington Post,* Feb. 25, 1980.

[7] "Better Regulation of Pesticide Exports and Pesticide Residues in Imported Food is Essential", *U.S. General Accounting Office,* Washington, DC, June 22, 1979.

[8] *"Regulating Pesticides in Food: The Delaney Paradox"*, National Research Council, National Academy Press, Washington, DC, 1987.

[9] Mott, Lawrie, and Karen Snyder, *"Pesticide Alert: A Guide to Pesticides in Fruits and Vegetables"*, Natural Resources Defense Council and Sierra Club Books, 1987.

[10] Weir, David, and Mark Schapiro, "The Circle of Poison", *The Nation,* Nov. 15, 1980.

[11] Lecos, Chris W., "Sulfites: FDA Limits Uses, Broadens Labeling", *FDA Consumer,* October 1986.

[12] Tannenbaum, Steven R., "The Ins and Outs of Nitrites", *The Sciences,* New York Academy of Sciences, January 1980.

[13] Klein, Richard M., *The Green World: An Introduction to Plants and People,* Harper & Row, Publishers, 1979.

[14] Koren, Herman, *Handbook of Environmental Health and Safety,* vol. 1, Pergamon Press, Inc., 1980.

[15] Miller, Roger W., "How Onions and a Baked Potato Became Sources of Botulism Poisoning", *FDA Consumer,* October 1984.

[16] Gunn, Robert A., ed., *Botulism in the United States, 1899–1977,* U.S. Department of Health, Education, and Welfare, Public Health Service, Centers for Disease Control, May 1979.

[17] Lecos, Chris W., "The Growing Use of Irradiation to Preserve Food", *FDA Consumer,* July/August 1986.

10

Radiation

"What man's mind can create, man's character can control."
—Thomas Alva Edison

"The release of atom power has changed everything except our way of thinking."
—Albert Einstein

Late in the autumn of 1895, a German physics professor, Wilhelm Roentgen, was busily pursuing a line of research which would soon revolutionize medical science and transform mankind's understanding of the nature of matter and energy. Roentgen was experimenting with a cathode-ray tube, a device perfected by the English scientist Crookes two decades earlier which consisted of a glass vacuum tube through which flowed a high voltage electric current. By chance, Roentgen noticed that emissions from the tube caused a nearby sheet of paper coated with a fluorescent chemical to glow, and he observed that these emanations could be blocked to varying degrees by materials of different densities. Calling his wife to place her hand on a photographic plate, Roentgen turned on the cathode ray tube; when the plate was subsequently developed, Roentgen amazed the world with a picture of his wife's bones inside her hand. Realizing that he had stumbled upon a form of radiation whose existence was hitherto completely unsuspected, Roentgen appropriated the Greek symbol for the unknown and called his discovery "X-rays". Within a few days after publication of his findings, the medical profession put the fluoroscope and "roentgenogram" to use—the shortest time gap between announcement of a major medical discovery and its practical application yet recorded.

The implications of Roentgen's announcement far transcended the field of medicine, however. Upon hearing of Roentgen's findings, the noted French scientist Henri Becquerel became intrigued by the relationship between X-rays and fluorescence and thereupon directed his attention to naturally phosphorescent minerals. In February of 1896, just two months after publication of Roentgen's report, Becquerel placed some crystals of a uranium compound on a photographic plate wrapped in black paper and demonstrated that the

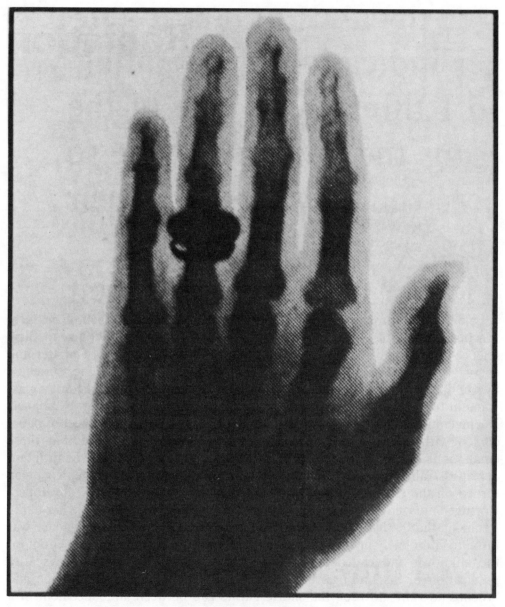

World's first X-ray: this is the "roentgenogram" which Wilhelm Roentgen took of his wife's hand, thereby demonstrating the existence of the mysterious emanations which he named "X-rays".

emanations from the uranium exhibited the same characteristics as Roentgen's X-rays. Becquerel's work was quickly picked up by Marie and Pierre Curie who termed the mysterious phenomenon "radioactivity" and who soon succeeded in isolating two new radioactive substances, polonium and radium, from uranium ore.[1] Thus the independent discovery of both man-made and natural radioactivity within a 3-month time span quickly led to the birth of a whole new field of scientific inquiry with far-reaching implications in physics, biology, medicine, and, unfortunately, warfare.

Ionizing Radiation

Early investigations of radioactivity quickly revealed that the observed emissions were of several different kinds. Some consisted of subatomic particles—protons, neutrons, or electrons—released when atoms spontaneously decay; these came to be known as *Particulate Radiation,* a group which includes *Alpha* and *Beta particles*. Other emission, such as Roentgen's *X-Rays* and naturally-occurring *Gamma Rays,* were shown to consist of highly energetic short wavelengths of *Electromagnetic Radiation*, a form of energy which also includes ultraviolet light, visible light, infrared waves, and microwaves. Alpha and beta particles, as well as X-rays and gamma rays, are today referred to as *Ionizing Radiation* because the particles or rays involved are sufficiently energetic to dislodge electrons from the atoms or molecules they encounter, leaving behind ions, i.e. electrically-charged particles. While certain forms of non-ionizing radiation such as ultraviolet light and microwaves can have an adverse effect on living organisms and will be discussed later in this chapter, ionizing radiation's ability to destroy chemical bonds gives it special significance in relation to both human health and environmental pollution. It is recognized today that when certain particularly vulnerable cells (e.g. fetal cells, sex cells) are exposed to ionizing radiation, birth defects or mutations can result; in any cell, radiation-induced alteration of DNA can lead to cancer. Although discovery of ionizing radiation was immediately hailed as a momentous medical and scientific event, subsequent investigations regarding what is frequently called our "most studied and best understood pollutant" have revealed the importance of extreme caution in dealing with radioactive materials.

Radiation Exposure

Exposure to ionizing radiation is an inescapable circumstance of life on this planet. Every individual, to a greater or lesser extent, comes into contact with ionizing radiation from three general types of sources: naturally-occurring, naturally-occurring but enhanced by human actions, and man-made.

Natural Sources—Although the fact was not realized until Becquerel's discovery in 1896, earth, air, water, and food all contain traces of radioactive materials which constitute a ubiquitous source of naturally-occurring, or "background", radiation. Some of the more significant sources of background radiation include:

> *cosmic radiation*—high energy particles composed primarily of protons and electrons continually stream toward the earth both from outer space and from the sun following episodes of solar flares. An appreciable amount of such cosmic radiation is blocked by the layer of atmosphere surrounding the globe, so that exposure to cosmic radiation is considerably less at sea level than at high altitudes (annual exposure to cosmic radiation approximately doubles with each 2,000 meter increase in altitude above sea level). For this reason, residents of Denver receive about twice as much cosmic radiation as do inhabitants of Los Angeles or Miami. While the natural tendency is to assume that something which has always been with us must be harmless, some biologists assert that perhaps 25% of all spontaneous mutations are caused by cosmic radiation.

Box 10-1
Types of Ionizing Radiation

Although any exposure to ionizing radiation is potentially dangerous, the degree and nature of harm varies depending on the type of radiation involved. Early studies of radioactivity revealed that ionizing radiation comprises several different types of emissions, the most biologically significant of which include:

Alpha particles, basically helium nuclei consisting of 2 protons and 2 neutrons, are relatively massive particles which, although the most energetic type of radiation, are the least penetrating. Such flimsy barriers as a sheet of paper, clothing, or even human skin can stop them. The greatest threat to health involving alpha radiation occurs when alpha-emitting particles (e.g. plutonium, radium, radon) are inhaled, ingested with food or water, or taken into the body through a cut or wound. Once in contact with delicate internal tissues, alpha radiation can cause intense damage within a localized area. Theoretical projections of large numbers of lung cancer deaths following a nuclear power plant melt-down are based on assumptions of pulmonary damage caused by inhalation of alpha-emitting plutonium dust.

Beta particles, consisting of single electrons, are more penetrating than alphas, capable of passing through the skin to a depth of about a half-inch. Like alphas, however, they are most dangerous when ingested. Since several beta-emitters (e.g. strontium-90, iodine-131) are chemically similar to naturally-occurring bodily constituents, they may substitute for those elements and concentrate in living tissues (e.g. bones, thyroid), where they continue to emit radiation for an extended period of time, increasing the risk of cancer or mutations. Most fission products in spent fuel rods or in reprocessed nuclear wastes are beta-emitters.

Gamma rays are the most penetrating form of ionizing radiation and generally accompany beta radiation. Shielding with a dense material such as lead is necessary to prevent gamma radiation from penetrating the body and harming vital organs. Short-lived beta emitters such as krypton-85 generally exhibit the highest levels of gamma radiation.

X-rays, though slightly less penetrating, have basically the same characteristics as gamma rays.

radioactive minerals in the earth's crust—radioactive compounds of uranium, thorium, potassium, and radium are found in soils and rocks in many parts of the world. People living in areas such as the Rocky Mountain region of the U.S. are exposed to background levels of radiation several times higher than are inhabitants of areas such as the Midwest or East Coast where radioactive minerals are much less abundant. Such an advantage may be lost, however, if easterners or midwesterners choose to live in homes or work in buildings constructed of granite, which gives off a considerable amount of radiation. Brick, too, is a source of radiation exposure due to its radioactive mineral content—a person living in a brick house experiences double the level of background radiation as does a person in a home built of wood.[2] Because of the extensive use of stone for streets and buildings, cities in Europe generally have significantly higher levels of background radiation than do their counterparts in the eastern United States.

Coal deposits frequently contain a number of radioactive elements which are released into the atmosphere when the coal is burned. At a time when many large coal users are contemplating switching to low-sulfur western coal as a means of reducing sulfur emissions, it is interesting to note that western coal contains about 10 times more radionuclides than do eastern or midwestern deposits.[3]

Fig. 10-1

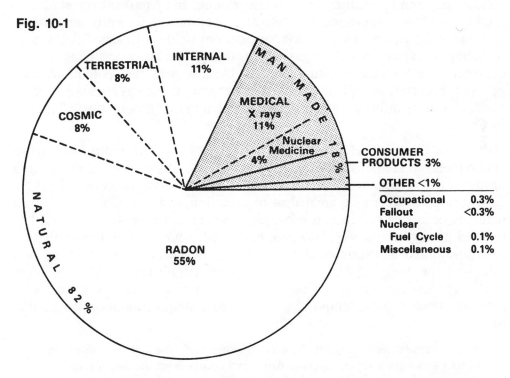

The percentage contribution of various radiation sources to the total average effective dose equivalent in the U.S. population.

Source: National Council on Radiation Protection and Measurements Report No. 93.

radionuclides in the body—a number of radioactive substances enter the body by ingestion of food, milk, water, or by inhalation and are incorporated into body tissues where their concentration may be maintained at a steady state or gradually increase with age. Plants growing in soil containing radioactive minerals readily take up such isotopes as radium and potassium-40 and in areas where people live on radioactive soils, consuming locally-grown foods further increases radiation exposure. In regions where groundwater is in contact with radioactive rock strata, well water used for domestic drinking supplies may constitute a significant source of indoor exposure to the radioactive gas radon. Another unavoidable source of radiation exposure is carbon-14, a naturally-occurring isotope of carbon, which is inhaled with the air we breathe and is incorporated into the tissues of all living organisms (a fact which has useful implications for scientists who employ C-14 dating techniques to ascertain the age of ancient plant and animal remains).

Enhanced Natural Sources—This category of sources, while not fundamentally different from the group discussed above, is considered separately because of the impact human activities have on levels of exposure which would, under other conditions, be much lower. Examples of enhanced natural sources include uranium mill tailings, phosphate mining, and jet airline travel (due to increased exposure to cosmic radiation at high altitudes). Recently, national attention has focused on what experts consider our single most significant source of radiation exposure—radon gas which, though naturally-occurring, can be considered an "enhanced natural source" because it reaches potentially dangerous concentrations only in enclosed environments such as houses and mine shafts (for more information on radon, see section on "Indoor Air Pollutants" in Ch. 12).[4]

Man-Made Sources—Human beings have evolved and multiplied in an environment where constant exposure to low levels of ionizing radiation was a universal experience. With the exception of indoor radon concerns which are currently the subject of a great deal of attention and remedial action, most naturally-occurring radiation is relatively constant and cannot be controlled or reduced in any feasible way. However, man-made sources of ionizing radiation have multiplied at exponential rates during the years since Roentgen first exhibited the X-ray of his wife's hand to an astonished world. It is these man-made sources, which *can* be controlled, which constitute the focus of a growing concern today about the impact of ionizing radiation on human health.

medical applications—by far the greatest source of exposure to man-made ionizing radiation for the average American comes from the use of medical X-rays and radiopharmaceuticals for both diagnostic and therapeutic purposes. Today approximately 75% of all Americans receive one or more medical or dental X-rays annually. Radioactive isotopes of phosphorus, technicium, iodine, iron, chromium, cobalt, selenium, and others are widely employed in hospitals for therapy and diagnosis, with as many as one-fourth of all patients in some hospitals receiving applications of some form of nuclear medicine. In addition to X-ray machines and radionuclides, the health professions utilize other such radiation-producing devices as teleradioisotope units and accelerators (e.g. cyclotrons, linear accelerators) to generate subatomic particles for radiotherapy. While radiation has provided medical science with an extremely valuable tool, its occasional misuse has been accompanied by some serious health problems; thus a thoughtful weighing of risks vs. benefits should precede any decision regarding the application of ionizing radiation for medical purposes.

nuclear weapons fall-out—since the explosion of the first atomic bomb in 1945 until the signing of the Limited Test-Ban Treaty in 1963, atmospheric testing of nuclear weapons by several of the major powers, primarily the U.S. and the U.S.S.R., resulted in significant amounts of radioactive fall-out worldwide. Such fall-out consists of a number of atomic fission products, including strontium-90, iodine-131, cesium-137, and radioactive krypton. Weapons fall-out is not always evenly distributed, however. Local fall-out close to the test site can be quite intense for about a day following the explosion, a fact which became obvious after the March 1, 1954, detonation of a multimegaton U.S. bomb over Bikini Atoll in the Pacific. Heavy fall-out of large radioactive particles and dust contaminated several inhabited islands nearby, as well as a Japanese fishing boat sailing in the vicinity. Many of the Marshall Islanders and the fishermen developed burns, skin lesions, and loss of hair as a result of radiation exposure and one of the islands, Rongelap, had to be evacuated and remained unoccupied for a number of years following the incident. In some cases air currents or rainstorms can cause radioactive particles and gases to precipitate unevenly. The greatest concern about weapons fall-out is focused on those isotopes which enter the human system in food and are incorporated into body tissues. Strontium-90 and iodine-131 enter the food chain when contaminated plant material is consumed by cows and passed on to humans in milk. Strontium tends to displace calcium, being incorporated into bones, while iodine localizes in the thyroid gland; both thereby constitute internal sources of exposure, continuing to emit radioactive particles inside the body over a period of weeks or months in close proximity to vital organs. Radioactive cesium also is ingested in both meat and milk and remains in the body for several months before being metabolized.[5] During the peak period of weapons testing, an average individual's radiation exposure due to bomb fall-out was 13 millirems annually, a figure which has been steadily falling since 1963.[6] According to a recent report by the National Council on Radiation Protection and Measurements, annual fall-out exposure currently averages less than 0.01 mSv (1 mrem) and, barring a resumption of atmospheric testing of nuclear weapons, will continue to decline. Having reached such negligible levels, nuclear weapons fallout need no longer be taken into account in calculating total human radiation exposure.

nuclear power plant emissions—public opposition to construction of nuclear power plants often centers around fears concerning radioactive emissions both to the air and in wastewater released from such plants.

Radioisotopes such as tritium (H^3), iodine-131, cesium-137, strontium-90, krypton, and others are indeed released to the environment during routine operation of a nuclear power generator, but the quantities involved are extremely minute, the average dose to individuals living within a 10-mile radius of the plant being 0.8 mSv (8 mrem), an amount considerably lower than that received from background radiation.[7]

consumer products—in addition to the sources mentioned above, very small amounts of exposure are received from luminous instrument dials (radium, tritium), home smoke detectors (Americium), static eliminators (polonium), airport security checks (X-rays), TV receivers (low energy X-rays), gas lantern mantles (thorium), and tobacco products (polonium). Of these sources, the most significant is tobacco; the radioactive polonium particles in cigarette smoke lodge primarily in the bronchial epithelium of the upper airways—the site of most lung cancers—thereby further contributing to the health risk posed by other carcinogenic and toxic substances in tobacco smoke.[8]

Until recently it was estimated that the average American receives approximately half of his/her annual radiation exposure from naturally-occurring background radiation and half from man-made sources, primarily medical applications. However, a growing realization of the extent to which citizens everywhere are exposed to radon in their homes has prompted a drastic revision in calculations of the contributions of various radiation sources to total average exposures. Due to estimates that as much as 55% of our annual radiation burden results from radon exposure alone, it is now believed that fully 82% of the average American's exposure originates from background (including enhanced) radiation, only 18% from man-made sources.[9] For any one individual, of course, the ratio can vary widely. A person living in an area of unusually high natural radioactivity (e.g. Salt Lake City, Denver) or sleeping in a basement bedroom where radon levels are exceptionally high might receive an even larger portion of his total exposure from background sources, while a person undergoing radiation therapy or working inside a nuclear power plant would receive a disproportionate share of his exposure from man-made sources.

Health Impacts of Ionizing Radiation

The advent of X-ray technology for diagnosing and treating human maladies, so eagerly and immediately seized upon by the medical profession, was soon shown to be a two-edged sword so far as its impact on human health was concerned. The first reported case of X-ray induced illness involved an American physician, Grubbé, who also manufactured cathode-ray tubes and who had been using them to study chemical fluorescence. When Grubbé heard of Roentgen's discovery he promptly began self-experimenting with X-rays and within a few weeks reported acute irritation of the skin on his hand. Subsequently the skin began peeling off, cancer developed, and eventually his hand had to be amputated. Grubbé's case was not an isolated one. By 1897, scarcely a year after the new technology came into use, 69 cases of X-ray induced injuries had been documented from various clinics and laboratories in different parts of the world.[10] Reports of health damage due to radiation from natural sources were not long in following. Becquerel himself reported a reddening of the skin on his chest as a result of carrying a vial of radium in his vest pocket. He and the Curies subsequently used a radium extract to produce a skin burn on the forearm of a male volunteer, thereby demonstrating that X-rays and natural radioactivity have essentially identical biological effects.[11]

In spite of an increasing awareness of the hazards, as well as the usefulness, of ionizing radiation, the first few decades of the 20th century witnessed numerous cases of radiation-induced illness or death resulting from carelessness, faulty equipment, or simple ignorance. Perhaps the most infamous example involved the approximately 40 women who developed bone cancer and leukemia some years after working in factories where they were employed to paint watch dials with radium so the numbers would glow in the dark. Using their lips to maintain a fine point on the brush, the women thereby accidentally swallowed small amounts of radium with each lick, radium which was absorbed into the bloodstream and eventually localized in their bones. Even more surprising in retrospect was the medical practice, widespread during the 1920s, of prescribing intravenous injections of radium for such ailments as arthritis, syphilis, tuberculosis, and mental disease; rather than curing such ills, the treatment resulted in more cases of bone cancer. Starting in about 1925, doctors began irradiating children's scalps to treat ringworm, their heads and throats for enlarged tonsils and adenoids, their faces to banish acne. Even as late as the 1960s some physicians used low-voltage X-rays to shrink the thymus gland (located in the neck) of infants in the erroneous belief that such treatments would cure colds. Unfortunately, such X-rays could not be precisely focused. As they spread out they irradiated not only the target tissue but the thyroid gland as well. The thyroid is one of the most radiation-sensitive organs in the body, and about 10 or more years following exposure (19 years seemed to be the peak period) significant numbers of these now-teenagers or young adults developed thyroid cancer as a result of this ill-advised application of radiation therapy.[12]

One segment of the population at special risk during the early years of work with radioactivity was the medical community itself, particularly radiologists whose enthusiastic use of their new machines exposed not only their patients but also themselves to large amounts of radiation on a daily basis. By the mid-1940s, physicians were succumbing to leukemia at double the rate seen in the general population, an incidence researchers attributed to the extent of their exposure to X-rays; an even more revealing statistic was the fact that among physicians, radiologists who regularly worked with X-ray machines exhibited a leukemia mortality rate ten times that of their medical colleagues.[13]

Box 10-2

Half-Life

Not all radioisotopes are dangerous for the same length of time. Each radioactive element is characterized by its own unique half-life ($t\frac{1}{2}$)—a period of time during which half of the amount originally present, undergoing radioactive decay, is transformed into something else. The concept of half-life, in essence, is the reverse of exponential growth. Assume, for example, that one has a gram of cesium-137 whose half-life is 30 years. After 30 years, only ½ gram would remain; in 60 years, ¼ gram; in 90 years ⅛ gram, and so forth. Obviously the term half-life is not synonymous with safety—½ gram of cesium-137 still presents a hazard. Indeed, highly radioactive substances may have to go through 10 or more half-lives (i.e. 300 years in the case of cesium) before their level of radioactivity is low enough to pose no significant health threat. However, the half-life concept has considerable relevance in assessing relative hazards and in devising waste management strategies.

Isotopes with very short half-lives are intensely radioactive initially; that is, they are experiencing a very high number of transformations at any one point in time. However, within a few days or weeks they go through so many half-lives that they no longer present a significant risk. The best management strategy for such wastes is simply to isolate them from human contact during the brief period when they are dangerous. Isotopes with extremely long half-lives will be radioactive virtually forever, but the level of emissions at any one point in time is relatively low; one can briefly handle a piece of long-lived uranium or thorium ore with little concern for radiation injury. The most difficult management problems involve those isotopes with intermediate-length half-lives, elements such as plutonium which, with a half-life of 24,000 years, remains hazardous for hundreds of thousands of years. Human contact with such radioisotopes must be accompanied by stringent safety precautions and ultimate disposal of such material must be carried out in such a way that it remains isolated from the general environment for extremely long periods of time.

Some representative half-lives

Element	Half-life	Element	Half-life
Radon-222	3.8 days	Cesium-137	30 years
Iodine-131	8.1 days	Radium-226	1600 years
Phosphorus-32	14 days	Carbon-14	5800 years
Krypton-85	11 years	Plutonium-239	24,000 years
Tritium	12 years	Uranium-235	710,000,000 years
Strontium-90	29 years	Thorium-232	14,000,000,000 years

Observations of radiation-induced health problems such as those just described led to extensive research into safer methods of utilizing this valuable but dangerous tool. Since the early 1940s, improvements in equipment design and increasingly stringent standards relating to allowable exposure have significantly reduced the incidence of overt cases of radiation damage. Nevertheless, concerns regarding unnecessary use of X-rays for diagnostic purposes and new understanding regarding long-term effects of low-level exposure require that individuals must be alert to the dangers implicit in any degree of radiation exposure and take an active role in deciding whether such exposure is justified.

Dosage

Since ionizing radiation can neither be seen nor felt, human exposure is measured in terms of the amount of tissue damage it causes. Under the International System of Units, the term **gray (Gy)** is the unit of absorbed dose, used to quantify the amount of energy from ionizing radiation absorbed per unit mass of material (the gray is replacing the term "rad" which is still in temporary use; a gray is equivalent to 100 rads). The most common unit for measuring radiation damage in humans, however, is the **sievert (Sv)**, a figure obtained by multiplying the absorbed dose in grays by a factor called the **relative biological effectiveness (RBE)**. This measurement reflects the fact that the health impact of radiation depends not only on the amount of energy absorbed, but also on the form of that energy. For example, X-rays and gamma rays which pass through tissue striking only occasional molecules along their path have an RBE of 1; beta particles have RBEs ranging from 1 to 5, depending on their energy level, while the relatively massive alpha particles have an RBE of 10, indicating their greater potential to damage living tissue. For practical purposes, human radiation exposure standards are set in terms of **millisieverts (mSv)**, an amount one-thousandth of a sievert, since these represent levels of exposure most commonly encountered by the average individual. Just as the gray is a relatively new term for what formerly was called the rad, sieverts and millisieverts are gradually replacing units, still used in many references, called "rems" and "millirems" (mrem). Under the new system a sievert is equivalent to 100 rems. The average amount of whole-body radiation exposure for a person in the U.S. from all sources is estimated to be approximately 3.6 mSv (360 mrem) a year or 0.01 mSv (1 mrem) per day.

There is little evidence that present average levels of exposure to ionizing radiation are having a serious adverse effect on the health of the general public. It is well known, however, that higher doses can be extremely injurious to living tissues. Types of radiation-induced biological damage include mutations, birth defects, impairment of fertility, leukemia and other forms of cancer, infections, hemorrhage, cataracts, and reduced lifespan. Humans, and mammals in general, are far more sensitive to ionizing radiation than are lower forms of life. The same degree of damage which a dose of 0.5 Sv (50 rems) can cause in a mammalian cell requires 1000 Sv (100,000 rems) exposure in an amoeba or 3000 Sv (300,000 rems) in a paramecium. The frequent reference in horror films to cockroaches inheriting the earth in the aftermath of all-out nuclear war is reflective of the fact that insects also have a very high level of tolerance to ionizing radiation.[14]

Dose *rate*, the time span during which a given amount of radiation is delivered, is extremely important in determining the extent of tissue damage incurred, perhaps more important than total dose. Radiation absorbed over an extended time period is demonstrably less harmful than the same amount received during a brief time span, indicating the existence of bodily repair mechanisms.

Health effects of ionizing radiation can be subdivided into those types of damage caused by high-level and low-level exposure, respectively. **High-level radiation exposure** is defined as a whole-body dose of 1 Sv (100 rems) or more, delivered within a relatively short period of time—minutes or hours. Such exposure will produce obvious symptoms of radiation sickness within a period ranging from a few hours to several weeks, symptoms ranging in severity from temporary nausea to death, depending on the dosage. Human effects of high-level exposure have been determined from studies of victims of the Hiroshima-Nagasaki atom bomb explosions, from experience with radiation therapy, and from observations of the results of nuclear accident victims. The 135,000 unfortunate Soviet citizens exposed to large amounts of radioactive debris resulting from the 1986 disaster at Chernobyl constitute a particularly valuable study group for radiation biologists because the radiation doses they received were measured at the time of the accident, unlike the wartime situation in Japan where exposures were estimated after the event. As one British radiation specialist remarked, "The human experiment has now been done. At last we can test our hypotheses."[15] Study results indicate the following consequences of varying levels of acute whole-body radiation exposure:

1-2 Sv (*100-200 rems*)—at this level of exposure, symptoms are generally so mild as to be unnoticeable in ordinary clinical examinations; heartbeat may be more rapid than usual and some nausea and vomiting may be experienced. At levels close to 2 Sv, miscarriages of early pregnancies or temporary sterility of males may occur.

2-4 Sv (*200-400 rems*)—onset of nausea and vomiting beginning a few hours after exposure and lasting about one day; mild weakness and fatigue persist for a few days to 3 weeks, followed by 3-4 weeks of such symptoms as sore throat, fever, general weakness, and in some cases development of purplish blotches on the skin as the white blood cell count drops. About 3 weeks after radiation exposure, loss of hair occurs. Recovery generally begins around the 5th week and is complete within 3-6 months.

4-6 Sv (*400-600 rems*)—the same sequence of events occurs as in the 2-4 Sv range, except that the onset of specific symptoms is more rapid and the decrease in white blood cell count more severe. Most persons receiving this dosage will die from infections and internal bleeding, though in some individuals bone marrow transplants may save the patient.

6-10 Sv (*600-1000 rems*)—within a few hours after exposure severe vomiting, stomach cramps, and diarrhea commence, indicative of damage to the gastro-intestinal tract. After the first day or two, the exposed person may begin to feel better, but within about one week nausea and vomiting return, progressing to bloody diarrhea, shock, and death within 10-14 days after exposure, due to destruction of the gastrointestinal lining.

10 Sv (*1000 rems*) *and above*—doses of this magnitude have their primary impact on the central nervous system. A burning sensation occurs minutes after exposure, quickly followed by severe nausea and vomiting and occasionally by loss of consciousness. Within the hour the victim

experiences loss of muscular coordination, mental confusion, and prostration; a period of seeming improvement may occur for several hours, but
5-6 hours after exposure watery diarrhea commences, together with a bluish
discoloration of the skin, resulting from inadequate oxygen in the blood.
Shock sets in a few hours later and death occurs approximately 20-38 hours
following the acute radiation exposure.[16]

Levels of ionizing radiation capable of inducing the above-mentioned effects
would most likely occur only in the extreme situations represented by a nuclear

---

Box 10-3

Fatal Attraction

The pretty, luminous blue powder which Brazilian scrap dealer Devair Ferreira carried
home from his junkyard to display to fascinated family members and friends constituted a
tragic case of fatal attraction. Now regarded as the world's second-worst radiation
accident, surpassed only by Chernobyl, the bizarre chain of events which unfolded in the
central Brazilian city of Goiania in September of 1987 resulted in the radioactive
contamination of 244 victims, 4 of whom died soon after exposure and dozens of others
who suffered varying degrees of radiation sickness.

When two scavengers entered an abandoned clinic where a radiotherapy machine for
treating cancer patients had been left unattended, their only intent was to earn a few
cruzeiros by selling the stainless steel canister it contained for its scrap metal value. Little
did they realize that the harmless-looking item contained 1400 curies of cesium-137.
Several days later, a junkyard worker opened the canister and discovered a glowing blue
salt-like substance inside. With no inkling of the hazard it presented, Ferreira took the
intriguing substance home, keeping it in his living room for a while and subsequently
distributing it to friends. His little 6-year-old niece Liede was particularly entranced with
the glittering powder, rubbing it all over her body to play "Carnival". With cesium-dusted
hands, she then proceeded to eat a sandwich and was later estimated to have received at
least 5X the lethal radiation dose for an adult. Ferreira's wife also received massive
exposure as a result of sleeping in cesium-contaminated clothing. During the next few days
many of Ferreira's friends who handled the material were afflicted with vomiting and
blistering of their skin. Finally Ferreira himself went to a clinic for treatment of his
mysterious malady and an alert health care worker, correctly identifying the problem as
radiation sickness, notified authorities of what was to prove a public health calamity. An
international team of radiation health experts was rushed to Goiania to deal with the
situation. Upon arrival, they found that the 20 patients who were most seriously ill had
received radiation dosages ranging from 1-8 grays (100-800 rads); 19 of the 20 had
radiation burns and all were internally contaminated with cesium they had ingested or
inhaled. While doctors focused their attention on the human victims, government workers
concentrated on locating radioactive "hotspots" in the general environment. Contaminated houses were washed down and cesium-soaked soil scooped up into
concrete-lined drums—which then presented the government with a disposal dilemma,
since Brazil has no permanent nuclear waste disposal site.

Aside from the human tragedy this episode represents, the Goiania accident raises
disturbing questions about the adequacy of radiation safety standards, emergency
preparedness, and regulatory responsibility in developing nations where use of both
nuclear energy and nuclear medicine have been growing rapidly in recent years.[17]

---

bomb explosion, a nuclear power plant melt-down, or in severe industrial accidents involving mishandling of radioactive materials. Such effects are largely reflective of cell death which, if extensive, can be fatal to the entire organism.

At levels of radiation exposure below 1 Sv (100 rems), well within the range experienced by many individuals today, few, if any, harmful effects are readily apparent. Nevertheless, low-level doses of ionizing radiation are the focus of great concern because of their potential to cause cell damage rather than cell death—damage which can eventually lead to genetic defects, congenital abnormalities, or cancer.

Radiation-induced mutations

Exposure even to very low levels of ionizing radiation can result in gene mutations; indeed, experiments to date indicate that there is no threshold level below which no mutations would be expected (however, at very low levels of exposure the mutation rate will correspondingly be quite low). There is, rather, a direct linear relationship between increasing radiation dosage and an increased number of mutations, either at the gene or chromosomal level. Both diagnostic X-rays and radioactive isotopes used for treating various ailments have been shown to damage chromosomes. Nuclear power plant workers and medical personnel, particularly radiotherapy nurses, who receive small doses of radiation on a daily basis have been shown to exhibit a marked increase in the frequency of mutations in their chromosomes (these can be observed as breaks or changes in chromosome number when chromosome smears are made from a sampling of white blood cells). The number of such abnormalities is generally highest among individuals who have been occupationally exposed to radiation for a number of years, indicating that the effects of exposure are cumulative.

Of greatest concern from a genetic standpoint, of course, are the mutations which accumulate in the gonadal cells which are the precursors of eggs and sperm. The number of new mutations which an individual passes on to his children depends on the amount of radiation his sex organs have absorbed from the time of conception up to the moment each of his children is conceived. Most radiation-induced mutations are recessive; hence even though most are of a harmful nature, they are likely to persist in the human gene pool, increasing in frequency over several generations before carriers of the recessive gene mate, producing offspring who exhibit the mutant characteristic.

In addition to inducing mutations in sex cells, X-ray exposure has also been shown capable of causing chromosomal damage in developing fetuses. Because the majority of such instances involved diagnostic X-rays of women in the very early stages of pregnancy who were not yet aware of their condition, it is now recommended that irradiation of reproductive-age women be limited to the first ten days after the onset of their last menstrual cycle to prevent exposure of an unsuspected embryo. Males and females alike should insist on being provided with a gonadal shield (e.g. lead apron) to reduce the risk of sex-cell mutations whenever X-rays are administered.

Radiation and birth defects

A number of congenital abnormalities, as distinguished from defects caused by mutant parental genes, are known to result from X-ray exposure *in utero.* Sensitivity to radiation is many times greater during fetal development than at any subsequent period of a person's life, since rapid development and differentiation of tissues is occurring during this time (the more actively cells are dividing, the more vulnerable they are to radiation). The most pronounced impact of fetal irradiation is on the central nervous system, where the developing neurons are extremely radiosensitive. Once injured or killed by ionizing radiation, embryonic nerve cells cannot be regenerated—the damage is permanent. Thus it should not be surprising that some of the most commonly observed birth defects resulting from fetal irradiation are microcephaly (abnormally small head) and mental retardation. In addition to decreased head size, a general stunting of growth frequently results from radiation exposure in the womb and skeletal malformations, genital abnormalities, and eye problems may occur.

The nature and extent of fetal injury caused by radiation varies widely depending not only on dose but also on the precise stage of development. Because the fetal tissues are constantly growing and differentiating, the developmental response to radiation exposure on any given day may be quite different from what it would have been the day before or the day after. In general, as with other teratogenic agents, ionizing radiation is most harmful to the human fetus from the second week through the sixth week of pregnancy, with peak sensitivity occurring between days 32-37 (from the time of conception through the 10th-12th day, radiation exposure can cause fetal death; if not, the pregnancy will proceed normally, with no teratogenic effect). Overall, the early stage of fetal development is about ten times more radiosensitive than is the period shortly before birth.[18] In addition, there are individual genetically-controlled differences in sensitivity to radiation which make it unlikely that any two fetuses would respond in precisely the same manner to radiation exposure, even when the doses are identical.

Controversy persists among researchers concerning whether or not a "safe level" of radiation exposure exists in relation to the induction of birth defects (as opposed to mutations for which it is presumed there is no threshold). While acknowledging that some difficult-to-detect damage may occur at exposure levels even below 0.01 Sv (1 rem), most authorities agree that if exposures of 0.15 Sv (15 rem) or above occur during the first six weeks of pregnancy, chances of severe congenital abnormalities are so great that therapeutic abortion is advisable.

Radiation-induced cancer

The potential for health damage as a result of radiation exposure was first recognized in connection with the development of skin cancers among early radiologists, of whom nearly 100 fell victim to this disease within 15 years following the discovery of X-rays. Since then other forms of cancer, most notably leukemia, bone cancer, lung cancer, and thyroid cancer, have also been linked to radiation exposure.

Box 10-4

Just Say No

Each year in the U.S. approximately 600 million medical and dental X-rays are given, about one-third of which federal officials estimate are unnecessary. Since the effects of radiation exposure are cumulative, consumers have both the right and the responsibility to question the overuse of a technology which presents a hazard to their well-being. Fortunately, the degree of risk is small. While the ability of large doses of radiation to kill or injure living cells is well established, the levels absorbed in most diagnostic procedures today are far lower than those which in past decades resulted in radiation-induced cancers and leukemias among patients receiving radiation treatment for problems ranging from ringworm to enlarged thymus glands. In those situations, doses exceeding 1 Sv (100 rems) generally were employed—considerably more than today's average bone marrow dose of 0.1 Sv (100 mrem) from diagnostic use of medical X-rays (dose to the red bone marrow is the most critical radiation-safety consideration because of its relationship to leukemia induction). Even at high dose levels, the incidence of radiation-induced cancer and leukemia is low and is an acceptable risk in situations where the health benefit of X-ray examination to a patient is clear and where the health risk of *not* having the X-ray is much greater.

Nevertheless, since all radiation exposure is cumulative and since such exposure does present *some* risk, however small, of causing subsequent cancer or birth defects, the estimate that a significant number of all X-rays administered each year are unnecessary is a situation which merits serious scrutiny on the part of a concerned public. Why are so many Americans receiving excess exposure to X-rays? The finger of blame can be pointed in several directions:

1. **physicians' fear of malpractice lawsuits;** to avoid charges by a patient that he didn't do everything possible to detect the cause of a particular problem, a doctor may order X-rays which he knows will reveal nothing of diagnostic value but which can provide future documentation in court of his thoroughness.

2. **equipment malfunction;** not all X-ray machines are in peak operating condition. Older models particularly may not tightly focus beams on the area being irradiated. Studies of radiation equipment across the nation have revealed a variation in radiation exposure of more than 200-fold for the same type of examination. Equipment failure can also result in film being over- or underexposed, necessitating retakes.

3. **technician or physician error;** in three-fourths of the states, no special training is required to administer X-rays and any doctor or dentist can purchase X-ray equipment. Few practicing medical personnel have time to keep abreast of the latest advances in radiology and many received only minimal training during their medical school days. Mistakes by the technician in operating the equipment or in positioning the patient necessitate millions of retakes, resulting in additional radiation exposure to patients, and doctors' initially ordering wrong views account for millions more. Suboptimal use of protective shielding for patients remains a problem in the rush to complete examinations quickly.

With these facts in mind, patients whose physician or dentist orders X-ray examinations have every right to question whether such exposure is really essential and to ask how the information gained thereby will affect treatment; to request protective shielding if the area being X-rayed is near the thyroid gland, breasts, eyes, or reproductive organs; to ask for an additional copy for one's own records, especially when the problem relates to a chronic condition which may require consultation with other doctors; and to refuse to allow routine dental X-rays (especially for children, for whom a cavity in a baby tooth that will soon be lost anyway is less menacing than a dose of radiation) without first having the teeth visually examined and a dental history taken.

Ninety years of experience have amply demonstrated that use of medical X-rays is a 2-edged sword: a valuable diagnostic and therapeutic weapon, yet one whose use, in a small percentage of cases, can lead to radiation-induced malignancies or teratogenic effects. Where it is clear that benefits substantially outweigh risks, there should be no hesitation in utilizing such a tool. However, it's time for the American public to begin saying "no" to those 200 million X-rays taken each year which confer no benefit to the recipient whatsoever, while increasing his overall radiation burden.

Leukemia is perhaps the classic example of X-ray-induced malignancy. As early as 1911 a report of eleven cases of leukemia among radiation workers suggested a connection between the disease and their occupational exposure. Subsequently, epidemiological studies among radiologists, Japanese survivors of Hiroshima and Nagasaki, patients treated with X-ray therapy, and children who were irradiated in the womb when their mothers received diagnostic X-rays all confirm the association between exposure to ionizing radiation and the induction of leukemia. Leukemia, like other forms of cancer, is characterized by a latency period following the initial exposure, with development of disease symptoms in this case occurring, on the average, after 5-7 years (some as early as just 2 years after irradiation). Although the greatest number of cases have been traced to exposure dosages in the 0.5-10 Sv (50-1000 rem) range (there appears to be a linear relationship between dose and leukemia incidence rates), the fact that even very low doses may be carcinogenic is suggested by evidence that prenatal X-ray exposure to just 0.01-0.05 Sv (1-5 rems) can result in increased risk of childhood leukemia and other cancers. Interestingly, however, studies of Japanese children prenatally exposed to radiation from the 1945 blasts revealed no excess leukemias among that group.[19]

The precise mechanism by which ionizing radiation initiates cancerous growth remains imperfectly understood, though it is presumed that induced mutations in somatic (non-sex) cells represent the first step in a series of events leading to onset of the disease. Evidence on the amount of radiation required to induce a malignancy is scarce, particularly at doses less than 0.5 Sv (50 rems). Many authorities believe that proportionately fewer cancers are initiated at low doses of radiation exposure than at higher doses, owing to the ability of cells to repair some radiation damage, while other researchers present experimental evidence showing that the risk of radiation-induced leukemias, skin cancer, and thyroid cancer is greater after exposure to low doses of medical irradiation than following high-dose applications. These investigators hypothesize that high doses severely inhibit the irradiated cells' ability to divide and proliferate, whereas lower doses, especially when administered over a time period of several years, do not similarly impede the capability of malignant cells to multiply.[20] Nevertheless, for purposes of regulation, federal agencies subscribe to the linear dose-response curve which assumes a directly proportional increase in number of cancer cases with increasing radiation dosage and no threshold level below which cancer incidence would be zero. In the absence of definitive evidence, this approach is considered to provide the most prudent way of safeguarding public health. Currently, federal standards set 1.7 mSv/year (170 mR/year), excluding medical exposure, as the maximum permissible radiation dose for members of the general population as a whole, no more than 0.25 mSv (25mR) of which should come from a nuclear power facility. Individuals may receive up to 5 mSv/year (500 mR/year), while workers in radiation-related occupations are allowed average yearly exposures of 50 mSv (5 rems). Persons under the age of 18 are permitted no occupational exposure whatsoever. Such standards have been set for the intended purpose of protecting human health against the long-term radiation effects of cancer and genetic defects. These standards do not reflect levels of absolute safety but rather attempt to strike a balance between possible adverse effects of low-level exposure and the known benefits of nuclear power and other uses of radioactive materials. Recently the safety of current exposure limits has been called into question by new interpretation of data on exposure received by Japanese survivors at Hiroshima and Nagasaki. Post-war estimates of likely radiation levels at varying distances from ground zero, correlated with observed health effects, have formed the basis for radiation standards since the end of World War II. Results from new studies carried out over the past several years indicate that the original data considerably overestimated the radiation dosage received by persons in the affected area. It is now believed that the observable health damage experienced by survivors was caused by approximately one-half the amount of radiation exposure calculated previously. These findings, if correct, suggest that current radiation protection standards should be at least twice as stringent as they are in order to protect public health.[21]

It should be noted in passing that the above-mentioned consequences of low-level radiation exposure may also be manifested at higher rates among survivors of high-level radiation doses. Mutations, birth defects among offspring, a significantly heightened risk of leukemia and other cancers, as well as cataracts and a general shortening of life span due to premature aging, are realistic possibilities confronting individuals who have recovered from overt symptoms of radiation sickness.

Radiation and nuclear power generation

While medical uses of X-rays and radioisotopes constitute by far the largest amount of non-background radiation exposure, it is not these sources but rather the perceived health threat from nuclear power plants that has received the lion's share of public attention in recent years. Since 1957 when the first commercial nuclear power plant came on line in Shippingsport, PA, the percentage of electricity generated by nuclear energy in the U.S. grew rapidly until the mid-1970s, much more slowly after that time. At present approximately 110 nuclear power plants account for about 18% of all electrical energy produced in this country. Even before the serious accident in 1979 at the Three Mile Island power plant near Harrisburg, PA, and the catastrophe at Chernobyl in the U.S.S.R. in 1986, concerns about the safety of nuclear power had given rise to an active and vocal anti-nuclear movement. Chants of "Hell, no, we won't glow!" have been countered by dire warnings from pro-nuclear power forces that Americans are doomed to "freeze to death in the dark" if we don't proceed full steam ahead to develop the nuclear power option. In all likelihood, with construction costs soaring and demand for electricity declining, economic considerations will be the major factor determining the outcome of this national debate. Nevertheless, the impact of citizen protests and political considerations in shaping nuclear power policy was made evident in the announcement by N.Y. Gov. Mario Cuomo in May, 1988, that the recently-completed Shoreham nuclear power plant on Long Island would be dismantled before it ever generated a single kilowatt of electricity. This action, taken in response to local concerns about the feasibility of federally-required emergency evacuation plans in that densely-populated area, represents the first time a U.S. nuclear plant was abandoned before it was ever opened. Given the extent of emotionalism involved, it is important that citizens clearly understand the extent to which nuclear power generation contributes to the overall radiation burden experienced by the general public. Although most attention is focused on the power plants themselves, nuclear power production involves a number of steps, referred to as the *Nuclear Fuel Cycle,* several of which have greater relevance to the public safety issue than others.

Mining—the uranium which constitutes the fissionable fuel in all U.S. reactors is mined in 4 western states—New Mexico, Wyoming, Colorado, and Utah. The most significant radiation hazard involved in mining uranium is the increased risk of lung cancer from inhaling alpha-emitting radon gas and radon daughters (radioactive polonium and lead) attached to tiny particles of mine dust. Such exposure in the underground mines from which half of all U.S. uranium ore is extracted (the other half being from open-pit mines) has contributed to a lung cancer mortality among uranium miners which is 4-5 times higher than that prevailing among the general population. Closing off unused sections of mines, better mine ventilation, and encouraging miners to wear respirators can reduce, but not entirely eliminate, this hazard.[22]

Milling—the crushing and processing of uranium ore to produce the form of uranium oxide known as "yellowcake" leaves behind enormous quantities of sand-like mill tailings. At present more than 140 million tons of radioactive tailings exist at mill sites scattered across a number of western states, releasing radon into the air and leaching radium into the subsoil.[23] At many unprotected sites, wind has blown the loose material close to buildings and onto grazing land. In Grand Junction, CO, mine tailings were incorporated into cement which was used for foundations of homes, churches, and schools. For nearly 20 years until the problem was recognized, approximately 30,000 people living in these dwellings were exposed to levels of radon up to 7 times the maximum allowable level for uranium miners. On a smaller scale, a number of other western communities, including Denver and Salt Lake City, also have used radioactive tailings in constructing roads and the foundations of buildings. Among highly exposed individuals, annual radiation dosage from mill tailings is estimated at about 2.6 mSv (260 mrem).[24] Many authorities regard uranium mill tailings as the most neglected of all radioactive wastes and the source of greatest public exposure to ionizing radiation related to nuclear power production.

Conversion of yellowcake to gaseous uranium hexafluoride produces some solid or sludge-like wastes containing radium, some uranium and thorium, but presents a negligible health threat.

Enrichment of uranium to increase the concentration of the U-235 isotope from its original 0.7% (the bulk of uranium ore is U-238) to about 2-4%, the level necessary to sustain a fission reaction, results in the venting of small quantities of radioactive gases into the atmosphere and some discharge of diluted liquid wastes, but here again the environmental health impact is minimal.

Fuel fabrication—conversion of enriched uranium hexafluoride gas into solid uranium dioxide pellets which are then loaded into fuel rods entails virtually no release of radioactive material into the environment; exposure of fabrication plant workers to radioactive emissions likewise is low.

Power production—under normal operating conditions, radiation exposure to the general public emanating from nuclear power plants comes primarily from the deliberate release of controlled amounts of radioactive gases to the atmosphere. Gaseous fission products such as tritium and krypton build up in the fuel rods, leak through the cladding into the reactor building, and must be periodically vented. In addition, small amounts of radioactive materials may be discharged with wastewaters. Public exposure to such emissions has been calculated as ranging from a maximum individual dose of less than 1 mSv (100 mrem) to an average of 0.8 mSv (8 mrem) for those living within a 10-mile radius of the plant. Routes of such exposure include inhalation or skin contact with airborne radionuclides and ingestion of radioactive contaminants in food (especially fish from cooling lakes) and water.[25] Quite clearly, the radiation hazard to people living in the vicinity of a normally-operating nuclear reactor is minimal, considerably less than that from natural background sources.

The main fear among those opposed to further reliance on nuclear power, of course, is the potential, however remote, of catastrophic release of radioactive materials should a major accident occur. Although most people today realize that it is physically impossible for a nuclear power plant to explode like a bomb (for this to occur the U-235 fuel would have to be enriched to a concentration far above the level necessary to sustain a fission reaction for power production purposes), a *Core Melt-Down* which represents a worst-type accident scenario would be nearly as devastating. Overheating of the reactor core, such as might occur if water should cease to circulate among the fuel rods (a "loss-of-coolant" accident), could result in melting of the fuel rods and breaching of the containment vessel. The massive release of highly radioactive isotopes into the atmosphere, such as occurred at Chernobyl (see Box 10-5), or into groundwater supplies could cause widespread human exposure to lethal doses of radiation, contamination of the general environment with radioactive fall-out, and would initiate numerous leukemias and other cancers which would be manifested years later. Although physical destruction of buildings and property would not occur, the biological impact of a core melt-down would be nearly as serious as a bomb blast in terms of human health and environmental degradation. The "defense in depth" concept employed in the construction of nuclear plants, characterized by repeated layers of thick shielding materials and multiple safeguards designed to ensure safety even in the event of partial failure, are intended to prevent this situation from ever becoming a reality.

In spite of such precautions, thousands of mishaps have occurred both here and abroad since the advent of commercial nuclear power. Prior to the Three Mile Island incident, two of the most serious U.S. accidents occurred at the Enrico-Fermi experimental fast breeder reactor near Detroit where part of the fuel in the core melted in early October, 1966, and at Browns Ferry, Alabama, where in March, 1975, a fire ignited by an electrician's

---

Box 10-5
"China Syndrome" in the Ukraine

When Pennsylvania Gov. Richard Thornburgh visited the Soviet Union in 1979 to tour nuclear facilities in that country soon after the near-disaster at Three Mile Island, he was smugly informed that an accident such as the one which had devastated the nuclear power plant near Harrisburg could never happen in the U.S.S.R. "Safety is a solved problem in the Soviet Union," Thornburgh was told by one official who suggested that before long it would be possible to operate a reactor without risk in the middle of Red Square. On April 26, 1986, this optimism suddenly evaporated when reactor #4 near the Ukrainian town of Chernobyl experienced a "worst-case" accident which resulted in a breaching of the containment vessel and massive radioactive contamination of the environment with the equivalent of fallout from several dozen Hiroshima-type bombs (by contrast, the near-meltdown at Three Mile Island resulted in negligible amounts of radiation escaping from the containment structure).

The unlikely chain of events leading to this tragedy have been blamed largely on human error rather than on facility design, since the Chernobyl power station was among the newest facilities in the Soviet Union and one which boasted the best operating record of any nuclear power plant in the country. On the fateful day, operators at the plant were engaged in a special test to determine how long the station's turbines could continue generating power after the steam supply had been shut off. The technicians shut down one safety system after another, including turning off the emergency core cooling system and pulling out all the control rods (a Soviet investigating team subsequently reported that fully 6 serious rules violations had been committed). When the operators realized that the reactor was suddenly beginning to run out of control, it was too late to prevent disaster. Power levels soared to 120X normal levels, rupturing fuel rods within the core and causing the cooling water to vaporize. The resulting steam explosion blasted apart the 1000-ton concrete slab above the reactor and sent radioactive fuel particles hurtling into the sky. These flaming fragments kindled 30 separate fires around the power station complex and the graphite core of reactor #4 began to burn uncontrollably. Soviet firefighters who rushed to the scene performed heroically, neglecting their own safety as they fought desperately to get the fire under control and prevent its spread to nearby reactors. Most of the human fatalities occurring soon after the accident were among these men who knowingly braved fatal doses of radiation, standing their ground even as their boots stuck to the melting tar on the reactor roof. Efforts to extinguish the fire and stem the release of radioactive particles included the use of military helicopters which dropped thousands of tons of sand, clay, limestone, and lead into the burning reactor core. Although the fires were extinguished fairly quickly, it was not until 11 days after the accident, when liquid nitrogen was pumped under the reactor, that the core cooled sufficiently to reduce radiation levels sharply.

By this time the radioactive plume rising from the stricken reactor had spread over much of Europe. Detected first over Sweden, nuclear fallout was carried by shifting winds over most countries of eastern and central Europe, with some radioactive contamination reported from as far away as Scotland. In all, at least 20 countries reported levels of fallout high enough to constitute a potential public health threat (while traces of fallout were detected by monitors in the U.S., levels were so low as to constitute a negligible threat to the health of Americans).

Most directly affected by radiation exposure, of course, were those living in the vicinity of Chernobyl. Thanks to an efficient, if somewhat delayed, evacuation of towns in the region, about 135,000 people within a 19-mile radius of the plant were bussed to resettlement areas. It is doubtful that these people will ever be allowed to return to their homes, since dangerously high radiation levels are expected to persist for years. The area is now being used as a living laboratory by scientists studying the long-term ecological effects of radioactive contamination on biotic communities. Fortunately for the Ukrainians, favorable weather patterns at the time of the accident kept fallout levels considerably lower than they might otherwise have been. During the periods of most intense radioactivity, winds were blowing away from major population centers. Dry conditions meant that inhabitants were spared exposure to the radioactive pollutants which would have rained down on them if showers had occurred during that time. In addition, the intense fire which raged for more than a week created a "chimney effect" which carried radioactivity high into the atmosphere, ensuring its spread over neighboring countries but lessening the amount of local fallout. However, the absence of radiation sickness among these evacuees does not mean they have escaped health damage due to the accident. Those living within 19 miles of the plant are estimated to have received about 0.16 Sv dosage and Soviet authorities anticipate a significant increase in cancers and birth defects within the affected population over the next 50 years.

While the nuclear accident at Chernobyl was less devastating in terms of immediate health impact than might have been expected, its toll unquestionably represents the most disastrous release of radiation into the human environment since the advent of commercial nuclear power. A tally of costs shortly after the event included 31 deaths (2 additional fatalities have been reported since that time), 1000 immediate injuries, at least $3 billion in financial losses to the U.S.S.R. alone—not to mention the disrupted lives and fears of future radiation-induced illness among the almost 400 million exposed Europeans whose perceptions of electricity generated by "the friendly atom" will never be quite the same again.[26]

candle raged for 7 hours, destroying all the emergency cooling systems in one of the reactors at the complex. In both cases, a core meltdown was only narrowly averted. Each major accident has led to tightening of safety regulations; nevertheless, problems are still commonplace. In 1985 alone, U.S. power plants experienced 764 emergency shutdowns, of which 18 were caused by conditions serious enough to have caused damage to the reactor core. Overseas the operating record is no better, with emergency shutdowns in the developed nations as a whole averaging 1000 per year. France, the world's acknowledged leader in nuclear technology, also holds the world's record for the highest rate of forced shutdowns.[27]

Reprocessing—after a fuel assembly has been in operation for about a year, waste fission products accumulate in the rods to such an extent that the fission reaction can no longer be sustained, necessitating replacement of these "spent" rods with fresh ones. Spent fuel rods, highly radioactive, are initially placed in swimming pool-like cooling tanks where the isotopes with very short half-lives decay within a relatively brief time. The rods are still highly radioactive (and physically hot as well) due to longer-lived fission products still present and also contain appreciable amounts of unused fuel in the form of U-235 and plutonium which formed during the fission process within the fuel rods. To separate these two useful products from the other isotopes which constitute high level radioactive wastes, reprocessing material in the spent rods was envisioned as a vital part of the nuclear fuel cycle. In this process the fuel would be removed from the rods and dissolved in acid, the solution then being treated chemically to separate it into uranium, plutonium, and waste components. This operation represents a potential public hazard since volatile radioisotopes, particularly krypton, are released into the atmosphere and other radioisotopes are discharged with liquid wastes. Workers inside the reprocessing plant are also exposed to higher levels of radioactivity than are nuclear power plant workers, though conceivably safeguards could be taken to reduce this risk. Although reprocessing was considered a key part of the nuclear fuel cycle, reducing the amount of what would otherwise be considered waste and extending the fuel supply, a moratorium on commercial reprocessing was imposed by Pres. Ford in 1976 and continued by Pres. Carter due to the concern that such plants would be tempting targets for attack by terrorists attempting to obtain weapons-grade plutonium. Although Pres. Reagan subsequently lifted the ban, financial considerations have deterred private interests from re-entering the reprocessing business and at present no commercial reprocessing facilities exist in this country, despite cries from the nuclear power industry that they will soon have no place to store the spent fuel rods that continue to accumulate on-site.

Waste disposal—nuclear power production results in the generation of large quantities of both high- and low-level wastes, the former primarily in the form of spent fuel from reactors, the latter consisting of contaminated clothing, clean-up solutions, wiping rags, hand tools, etc. High-level wastes are extremely radioactive, highly penetrating, and generate a great deal of heat, hence must be handled without direct human contact. Currently, most high-level commercial wastes are being stored in cooling tanks at the power plants where they were produced (a relatively small percentage is in storage at facilities in Morris, IL, and West Valley, NY, once intended as reprocessing plants).

Responding to criticism that the lack of any clear-cut policy for permanent disposal of high-level radioactive waste could prove the Achilles' heel of the nuclear power industry, Congress in 1982 enacted the Nuclear Waste Policy Act. This legislation delegated responsibility for high-level radwaste management to the federal government and designated the U.S. Dept. of Energy as the lead agency to coordinate the effort to site, construct, and operate the nation's first permanent repository for such wastes. The politically-sensitive search for a location for this facility is now focused on Yucca Mountain, Nevada, where extensive characterization studies are underway to determine the site's geologic suitability for deep burial of solidified wastes. Although the Nuclear Waste Policy Act specifies that the facility be ready to begin accepting wastes by 1998, experts doubt that the repository will be completed before the first decade of the 21st century, if then. In the meantime, spent fuel rods continue to accumulate on site and some utilities warn that they may have to close down within the next several years for lack of a waste disposal alternative.

Low-level wastes, produced not only by nuclear power plants but also by hospitals, research labs, universities, etc., exhibit low but sometimes potentially hazardous concentrations of radioisotopes. They differ from high-level wastes in having significantly lower levels of radioactive emissions; they are not physically hot, generally require no shielding, and decay to harmless levels within 100-300 years (many high-level wastes remain dangerous for tens of thousands of years). Such wastes are disposed of primarily by burial in shallow landfills specifically licensed for this purpose. At present only 3 such facilities exist in the U.S.—in Beatty, NV, Hanford, WA, and Barnwell, SC. Three other sites were closed due to migration of radioactive materials beyond the landfill boundaries, in some cases contaminating soil and nearby waterways. Because the 3 existing sites don't have the capacity to accommodate the nation's output of low-level waste into the indefinite future, states are now in the process of negotiating regional "compacts" to provide for the establishment and operation of low-level radioactive waste facilities within their regions. Federal legislation, which places the responsibility for low-level radwaste management on state governments (as opposed to federal jurisdiction over high-level wastes) has given these regional compacts until 1993 to put their disposal facilities into operation. The success or failure of this effort will have a major impact on the sustained viability of the nuclear power industry, as well as on operations at thousands of hospitals, research laboratories, and industries which utilize radioactive materials.

Box 10-6

Radwaste Management Abroad

Engaged in an intense domestic debate over what to do with radioactive wastes, Americans have paid little attention to radwaste management policies being pursued elsewhere in the world. Since there are nearly 300 nuclear power plants currently operating in 25 other nations, disposal dilemmas pose challenges for policy-makers in many countries. Everywhere high-level wastes are proving the thorniest problem. While the United States is finally making at least halting progress toward developing a permanent high-level waste repository, no other countries have anything more than temporary storage facilities for these intensely hazardous by-products of nuclear power. Most national energy planners continue to assume that spent nuclear fuel will be reprocessed and that the remaining wastes will be solidified into a glass-like material and buried in deep geologic strata—very similar in concept to the disposal program underway in the U.S. However, such plans have not progressed beyond the research stage in most countries due to political opposition to siting such facilities in those densely populated nations. France currently has 2 reprocessing plants, handling spent fuel from its own 44 nuclear plants as well as from plants in a number of neighboring countries. The high-level wastes generated by this process are converted into solid glass blocks which the French intend to store in an engineered facility for 50-60 years, after which they plan to bury them in a currently non-existent repository deep underground (this repository will be used solely for French wastes, however; reprocessed, vitrified wastes from other countries will not be eligible for disposal in the French facility).

Other countries have made somewhat less progress than France in managing their high-level wastes. The United Kingdom recently opened a large reprocessing facility at Sellafield (formerly called Windscale) on the northwest coast. The U.K. intends to store the resulting vitrified wastes indefinitely in an engineered facility and has no plans at present for any permanent repository. In West Germany, where anti-nuclear sentiment is running high in the aftermath of Chernobyl, plans for a reprocessing plant in Bavaria have been cancelled; a permanent disposal facility deep in a salt dome in Lower Saxony will be developed if studies indicate the site is geologically suitable. Construction of an away-from-reactor facility for temporary storage of high-level radwastes is also planned.

Canada, like the U.S., continues to store spent fuel rods at reactor sites pending development of a permanent waste facility sometime in the 21st century.

Sweden, which has decided to forego further development of nuclear power and to phase out its 12 existing plants by 2010, will contract with other countries to handle its limited reprocessing needs and will eventually dispose of the high-level wastes by burial in a granite repository.

Densely populated, earthquake-prone Japan has the most ambitious nuclear power program in Asia but faces difficult radwaste disposal problems. Considerable antagonism toward Japan surfaced in the United Kingdom recently when the Japanese tried to hire British facilities to dispose of their wastes. Japan is currently searching for a suitable repository site and hopes to begin trial disposal of high-level waste canisters in about 25 years.

India, running a distant second to Japan in Asia for its reliance on nuclear energy, would like to construct small reprocessing facilities at each of its 6 power plants (8 more planned or under construction) and will utilize temporary storage on-site until development of a permanent deep burial facility at some unspecified future date.

Low-level radioactive waste disposal practices overseas are scarcely more advanced than those in the U.S. France currently boasts a state-of-the-art engineered structure designed to accept cement-encased low-level wastes and to prevent any possibility of leachates migrating away from the facility. Elsewhere, disposal methods include shallow land burial, placement in abandoned mine shafts, and ocean dumping.[28]

Ultraviolet Radiation

Wavelengths of the electromagnetic spectrum ranging between 40-400 nanometers in length are categorized as ultraviolet (UV) light. Although ultraviolet radiation is not of sufficiently high energy to ionize atoms and molecules, certain portions within this range are strongly absorbed by living tissues, particularly by cellular DNA which constitutes the major target of UV damage. Injury to the hereditary material of cells is the reason for the lethal or mutational effect which excess UV exposure can provoke in living organisms. Research has shown that the most detrimental effects to biological systems occur when UV radiation is in the 230-320 nanometer range (referred to as UVB as opposed to longer-wavelength UVA), peak absorption by DNA occurring at 260 nm. Much of the ultraviolet light naturally present in incoming solar radiation is filtered out by the layer of atmospheric ozone located about 20 miles above the earth's surface (see Ch. 11). Living organisms have developed various defense mechanisms to protect themselves against the amounts that do penetrate—shielding devices such as fur, feathers, shells, or darkly-pigmented skin, as well as light-avoidance behavior patterns among a variety of species. Of equal importance has been the evolution of enzymatic mechanisms for repairing UV-induced damage to DNA when levels of injury are not excessive. Without this cellular repair ability it is doubtful whether many organisms could survive existing levels of UV exposure. The importance of such mechanisms can be seen in the example of individuals suffering from the genetic disease xeroderma pigmentosum. Lacking the enzyme needed for repair of radiation-damaged DNA, victims of this ailment have to remain indoors throughout daylight hours or risk the development of multiple fatal skin cancers. There appears to be a tenuous balance between continual UV assault on the hereditary material and its biochemical repair. If the cell's capacity to deal with such damage is overwhelmed, the cell will die.

Since ultraviolet light cannot penetrate very deeply into living tissues, the major concern in reference to UV injury to humans involves the induction of skin cancers, particularly in lighter-skinned individuals who lack protective melanin granules in their epidermal skin layers.

After World War II, when the tyranny of fashion decreed that pale skin was "out" and the bronzed look "in", the apparently irresistible urge among fair-complexioned citizens to spend hours broiling themselves under the sun or at rapidly-proliferating tanning parlors, while at the same time wearing increasingly skimpy clothes outdoors, has resulted in an alarming increase in the incidence of skin cancer in Western countries. Whereas a child born in the U.S. in 1930 had about a 1 in 1500 risk of developing skin cancer within his/her lifetime, for a white child born today that risk has soared to 1 in 100 (for blacks the danger is much lower—less than 1 in 1000). The main villain behind these grim statistics is increased exposure to UVB radiation, a known carcinogen and mutagen. Three major types of skin cancer account for the approximately 500,000 new cases of the disease diagnosed in the U.S. each year. **Basal cell carcinoma** (400,000 new cases/year) and **squamous cell carcinoma** (80,000-

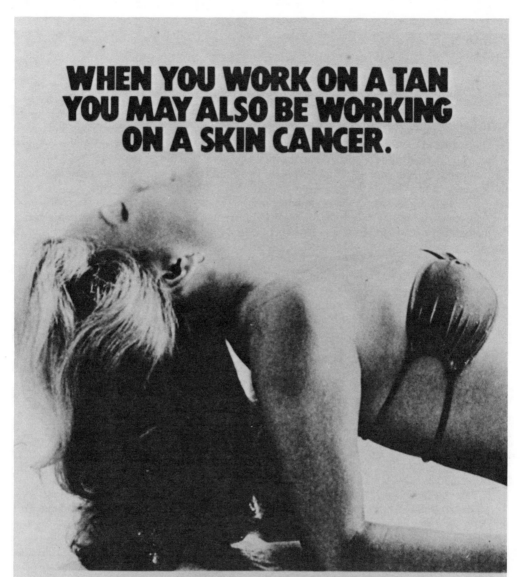

WHEN YOU WORK ON A TAN YOU MAY ALSO BE WORKING ON A SKIN CANCER.

You can get a golden tan in a matter of hours.

Skin cancer takes a little longer.

But if you stick to it—summer after summer in the sun—your day, unfortunately, might come.

1 out of every 7 Americans will develop some form of this disease. And the sun's radiation is the leading cause.

It can be disfiguring. Sometimes fatal. But—and here's the good news—it can almost always be cured. Provided it is detected and treated in time.

But why take chances? If you must be in the sun, avoid long exposures. Wear protective clothing. And use an effective sunscreen.

For more information on prevention and early detection, send a stamped, self-addressed (business-size) envelope to The Skin Cancer Foundation, Box 561, New York, New York 10156.

THE SKIN CANCER FOUNDATION
Know the signs of skin cancer.

Health education efforts such as this poster from The Skin Cancer Foundation are hampered by the dictates of fashion which promote the "bronzed look" as the ideal of beauty—regardless of the permanent skin damage and possible cancer which are its ultimate result. [Copyright, © *The Skin Cancer Foundation*]

Why Johnny Should Wear Sunscreen

For generations, plenty of fresh air and sunshine has been the standard prescription for raising healthy children. Recently, however, the sunshine portion of that formula has been disputed by dermatologists witnessing a dramatic rise in the incidence of skin cancer among young and middle-aged patients. Growing awareness that children are particularly vulnerable to UVB-induced skin damage and the fact that youngsters generally spend much more time outdoors than do adults (it is estimated that the average child receives 3X the annual UVB dose of an average adult) have prompted warnings that parents should do more to protect their little ones from the hazards of UV exposure.

Efforts are underway to educate not only mothers and fathers but also teachers, coaches, recreation counselors, and children themselves of sun-protection strategies. Admonitions include not allowing infants or children to become badly sunburned, keeping children indoors between 11 a.m.-3 p.m. (daylight saving time) when the summer sun is most intense, and covering them with long-sleeved shirts, slacks, and hats while playing outdoors. From a health protection standpoint, these are undoubtedly sound suggestions, but inconvenience of implementation makes it unlikely that they will attract many adherents. An alternative recommendation which could have a major impact on reducing a child's risk of developing skin cancer later in life could be adopted with minimal effort, however—insisting that children regularly use sunscreen with an SPF (sun protection factor) of 15 or higher. It is well recognized that sunscreens are very effective in preventing sunburn (in addition to the discomfort it produces, sunburn is suspected as being the triggering event in the development of malignant melanoma); animal research results indicate that sunscreens are also instrumental in reducing the risk of basal and squamous cell carcinomas. It has been calculated that regular use of sunscreen with SPF 15 (sunscreens with lower SPF values are regarded by skin specialists as providing insufficient protection for users of any age, regardless of skin type) from infancy through age 18 would reduce an individual's lifetime risk of basal and squamous cell carcinomas by fully 78%. Additional benefits would include fewer sunburns, slower aging of the skin, and possibly a lower risk of melanoma.

The fact that few children currently use high SPF sunscreens indicates that extensive public education efforts are needed to spread the word that the irreparable skin damage that can be caused both by chronic and acute sun exposure can be prevented by applying a dose of common sense—and sunscreen.[29]

100,000/year) represent the vast majority of skin cancers, accounting for fully one-third of all cancers occurring in the U.S. today. Chronic exposure to sunlight (actually the UVB component of sunlight) is recognized as the cause of over 90% of these two cancers. They appear, predictably, on portions of the body receiving the greatest sun exposure—face, neck, ears; back of the hands—and until recently were unusual in people under the age of 50. Now, however, numerous cases have been diagnosed among people in their 20s and 30s and occasionally even in teenagers. Not surprisingly, they are also being found on the legs, chest, and back of victims as the sunbathing mania takes its toll.[30] Fortunately, the majority of such cancers can be treated if detected early, but each year several thousand cases prove fatal when their neglect leads to invasion of underlying tissues. **Malignant melanoma** is much less common than basal cell or squamous cell carcinomas, but far more deadly. Each year recently about 23,000 Americans have been diagnosed as having malignant melanoma and in 1986 the disease killed 5600 victims (mortality rate of about 25%). Among Caucasians the incidence of the disease has been increasing by about 5% per year for the past 3-4 decades.[31] Unlike the non-melanoma skin cancers, malignant melanoma appears to develop as a result of occasional severe sunburn, rather than by prolonged, low-dose exposure to sunlight. A blistering sunburn experienced during childhood or adolescence seems to double or triple the risk of subsequently developing malignant melanoma. Interestingly, while basal cell and squamous cell carcinomas develop only on sun-exposed portions of the body, malignant melanomas frequently occur on areas normally covered. They also tend to occur at a younger age than do the other two forms of skin cancer, the highest percentage of malignant melanomas occurring in victims under age 50. Because of the suspected link between childhood sunburn and melanoma, groups such as The Skin Cancer Foundation are urging parents to be particularly careful in protecting youngsters from excessive sun exposure.

Ill effects of UV-light exposure are not limited to cancer and sunburn. Premature wrinkling, drying, and mottling of the skin are among the less desirable consequences of UV exposure. In recent years the growing popularity of tanning parlors has been accompanied by claims from the owners of such establishments that they provide a safe alternative to sunbathing because they utilize UVA radiation rather than UVB and hence cannot result in burning. Nevertheless, tanning parlor patrons are exposing themselves to several other serious risks. While the link between UVA and skin cancer is still somewhat controversial, the ability of UVA to cause premature aging of skin and to induce cataracts is indisputable. UVA weakens the immune system and enhances the effect of sunlight: individuals who sunbathe outdoors shortly after a stint in a tanning parlor frequently suffer extremely severe sunburns. Photosensitive reactions to either tanning parlors or outdoor sunbathing can occur when unwary sun-worshippers expose themselves to UV light while

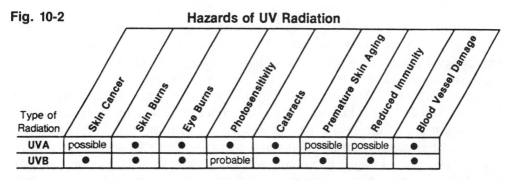

Fig. 10-2   **Hazards of UV Radiation**

Type of Radiation	Skin Cancer	Skin Burns	Eye Burns	Photosensitivity	Cataracts	Premature Skin Aging	Reduced Immunity	Blood Vessel Damage
UVA	possible	●	●	●	●	possible	possible	●
UVB	●	●	●	probable	●	●	●	●

Source: Food & Drug Administration, U.S. Dept. of Health and Human Services/Public Health Service

taking antibiotics, antihistamines, birth control pills, even certain cosmetics. Such a toxic reaction is generally manifested as an unusually severe sunburn immediately following exposure to UV light. Weighing serious long-term health risks against short-term fashion benefits, dermatologists are unanimous in their recommendation that all UV exposure, whether on the beach or at a tanning salon, be avoided to the greatest extent possible.

Ultraviolet light has some beneficial as well as harmful effects. A certain amount of skin exposure is necessary to promote the bodily synthesis of vitamin D, a deficiency of which can result in the development of rickets, a bone deformity. The germicidal properties of UV light have recommended its use in operating rooms to reduce danger of bacterial or viral infections. Ultraviolet light applications have also been successfully employed to treat such bacterial skin diseases as acne and boils.[32]

Microwaves

Electromagnetic radiation comprising wavelengths ranging from approximately one millimeter to one meter (intermediate between infrared and short-wave radio wavelengths) is termed microwave radiation. Since microwave energies are so low, such radiations are typically characterized by their frequencies which, in the case of microwaves of biological interest, generally fall between 100 and 30,000 megahertz (MHZ).

Humans today are continuously bombarded with microwaves from such diverse sources as military radar installations, radio and television transmitters, communications and surveillance satellites, radar and radio-frequency transmitters at airports and on planes and ships, microwave ovens, telephone and TV-signal relay towers, walkie-talkies, video display terminals, automatic garage door openers, etc. Whether or not microwave radiation, particularly at lower levels of exposure, presents a public health threat remains a matter of controversy among researchers. Unlike X-rays, microwaves are non-ionizing; instead, when absorbed they cause an increased rate of vibration in the molecules of the absorbing material, resulting in the production of heat. Depending on frequency, microwaves are differentially absorbed by bodily tissues. Those of very low energy (below 150 MHZ) simply pass through the body without being absorbed; those of intermediate frequency (150-1200 MHZ) are absorbed by the deeper tissues without any noticeable heating of the skin. This poses a danger of serious bodily harm, since internal organs can receive highly damaging doses of microwave radiation without the victim realizing that anything is wrong. As microwave frequency increases, tissue penetration decreases and at 3500 MHZ warming of the skin can be felt; above 10,000 MHZ only the surface of the skin is heated and no penetration of the body occurs.

Differential absorption of microwave energy by bodily tissues is to a large degree a function of their water content. Moist tissues such as skin, muscle, and the intestines absorb more microwaves than do bones and fatty tissues. Sensitivity of specific organs to microwaves depends not only on how readily such radiation is absorbed, but also on how effectively blood circulating through the organ can dissipate the excess heat. Experiments have shown that body parts with poor· circulation—the eyes, gastrointestinal tract, testes, urinary bladder, and gall bladder—are the areas most susceptible to injury from microwaves.[33]

Excessive heating of internal organs is the best understood type of microwave-induced injury. One extreme case involved a 42-year-old radar repairman who stood in the beam of a radar transmitter while working within 10 feet of the antenna. He felt a sensation of heat in his abdomen which became intolerably painful in less than a minute. He quickly moved aside, but within 30 minutes he began to experience acute abdominal pains and vomiting and soon lapsed into shock. Despite prompt hospitalization and subsequent surgery, he died 11 days later from tissue destruction caused by absorption of microwave energy, his doctor reporting that his small intestine appeared to be "cooked".[34]

That high levels of microwave absorption can cause serious biological damage is not disputed. Much more controversial is the question of microwave radiation damage from prolonged low levels of exposure. The federal government has set 10 milliwatts/cm^2 of body area as the maximum permissible level for continuous exposure to microwaves, but a number of researchers claim to have evidence showing that much lower levels of exposure can cause a wide variety of ill effects, including cataracts, cancer, chromosomal abnormalities, birth defects, heart attacks, and a tendency among irradiated men to father only girl babies. Unfortunately there has been little support in this country for research into the long-term health effects of microwave exposure. It is interesting, however, that the Soviets and East Europeans who have been studying the biological effects of microwaves for many years have set a level of permissible exposure 1000 times lower than current U.S. regulations permit.

REFERENCES

[1]Cooper, George, Jr., "The Development of Radiation Science", *Medical Radiation Science,* Dalrymple, Glenn V., Me. E. Gaulden, G. M. Kollmorgen, and H. H. Vogel, Jr., eds., W. B. Saunders Co., 1973.

[2]Spiers, F. W., "Radioactivity in man and his environment", *Nature of Radioactive Fallout and Its Effects on Man,* U.S. Atomic Energy Commission, U.S. Government Printing Office, 1957.

[3]Carter, L. J., "More burning of coal offsets gains in air pollution control", *Science,* 198, 1977.

[4]*"Ionizing Radiation Exposure of the Population of the United States,* National Council on Radiation Protection and Measurements, Report No. 93, September 1, 1987.

[5]Hall, E. J., *Radiation and Life,* Pergamon Press, 1976.

[6]Eisenbud, M., *Environmental Radioactivity,* Academic Press, 1973.

[7]National Council on Radiation Protection and Measurements Report No. 93, op. cit.

[8]Ibid.

[9]Ibid.

[10]Eisenbud, op. cit.

[11]Cooper, op. cit.

[12]Norwood, Christopher, *At Highest Risk,* Penguin Books, 1980.

[13]Environmental Defense Fund and Robert H. Boyle, *Malignant Neglect,* Vintage Books, 1979.

[14]Giese, A. C., *Cell Physiology,* W. B. Saunders, 1962.

[15]Hawkes, Nigel, Geoffrey Lean, David Leigh, Robin McVie, Peter Pringle, and Andrew Wilson, *Chernobyl: The End of the Nuclear Dream,* Vintage Books, 1987.

[16]Maxfield, W. S., G. E. Hanks, D. J. Pizzarello, and L. H. Blackwell, "Acute Radiation Syndrome", *Medical Radiation Biology,* Dalrymple et al. eds., W. B. Saunders Co., 1973.

[17]Roberts, Leslie, "Radiation Accident Grips Goiania", *Science,* vol. 238, Nov. 20, 1988.

[18]Sternglass, E. J., *Low Level Radiation,* Ballantine, 1972.

[19]Upton, Arthur C., "Radiation Carcinogenesis", *Medical Radiation Biology,* Dalrymple et al. eds., W. B. Saunders Co., 1973.

[20]Basso-Ricci, S., "Cancer following medical irradiation: The validity of Gray's hypothesis", *Panminerva Medica,* vol. 27, 1985.

[21]Hawkes et al., op. cit.

[22]*Health Implications of Nuclear Power Production,* World Health Organization, 1977.

[23]Carter, L. J., "Uranium mill tailings: Congress addresses a long-neglected problem", *Science,* 202, 191, 1978.

[24]National Council on Radiation Protection and Measurements Report No. 93, op. cit.

[25]Ibid.

[26]Flavin, op. cit.; Hawkes et al., op. cit.; Hohenemser, Christoph, and Ortwin Renn, "Chernobyl's Other Legacy", *Environment,* vol. 30, no. 3, April 1988.

[27]Flavin, Christopher, "Reassessing Nuclear Power: the Fallout from Chernobyl" *Worldwatch Paper 75,* Worldwatch Institute, March 1987.

[28]*The Nuclear Waste Primer,* League of Women Voters Education Fund, Nick Lyons Books, 1985.

[29]Stern, Robert S., M.D., Milton C. Weinstein, Ph.D., and Stuart G. Baker. ScD., "Risk Reduction for Nonmelanoma Skin Cancer with Childhood Sunscreen Use", *Archives of Dermatology,* vol. 122, May 1986.

[30]Schreiber, Michael M., "Exposure to Sunlight: Effects on the Skin", *Comprehensive Therapy,* vol. 12, no. 5, 1986.

[31]"Sunburn and Melanoma", *The Lancet,* May 23, 1987.

[32]*Biological Impacts of Increased Intensities of Solar Ultraviolet Radiation,* National Academy of Sciences and National Academy of Engineering, 1973.

[33]Dalrymple, Glenn V., "Microwaves", *Medical Radiation Biology,* Dalrymple et al., eds., W. B. Saunders Co., 1973.

[34]Brodeur, Paul, *The Zapping of America,* W. W. Norton & Co., 1977.

PART III

PART III

ENVIRONMENTAL DEGRADATION
How we foul our own nest

"The fouling of the nest which has been typical of
man's activity in the past on a local scale now seems to
be extending to the whole system."
—Kenneth Boulding

Air pollution, water pollution, excessive levels of noise, and the accumulation
of disease-breeding refuse are not phenomena unique to the latter half of the
20th century. Wherever humans have congregated in appreciable numbers, the
burning of fuel, the thoughtless disposal of excreta and material wastes, and the
din arising from a multitude of human activities have created conditions which
adversely affected the health and well-being of the very people responsible for
those conditions. For most of mankind's history, environmental degradation
was primarily local in scope, concentrated in the relatively few places where
humans established urban centers. The extent of pollution in these cities,
however, often far exceeded the levels of filth plaguing our environmentally-
conscious society of today. Streets and gutters clogged with human body wastes,
animal excrement, and garbage were a result of both overcrowding and a
transferrence to the city of more casual rural practices. By the time of the
Industrial Revolution in the late 18th and early 19th centuries, belching
smokestacks from thousands of factories and the noise of machinery and
transport vehicles further degraded the quality of urban life. Indeed, back in the
"good old days" health and sanitary conditions due to air and water pollution
and to inadequate (or nonexistent) refuse collection and disposal were far worse
than anything with which we are familiar in the 1990's. When repeated epidemic
outbreaks of waterborne disease killed thousands of citizens or when smog-
laden air caused millions to wheeze, cough, and occasionally die, society's more
enlightened civic leaders began to question mankind's shortsightedness in
fouling his own nest. Many of the most important reforms in civic life which
occurred late in the last century involved implementation of public health
measures to deal with water pollution, refuse collection, and smoke abatement.
However, throughout this period when urban pollution levels were rising, the

countryside remained relatively uncontaminated, except for those areas where a local industry—perhaps a metal smelter or pulp mill—created noxious conditions within its own sphere of influence.

The changes which transformed local pollution problems into national ones have occurred largely in the years since the end of the Second World War. Reverse migration from urban centers into sprawling suburbia was made possible by a quantum increase in the number of automobiles ("infernal combustion engines") whose exhaust fumes guaranteed that air pollution would no longer be restricted to areas of smoke-generating heavy industry. The escalating energy demands of a growing, affluent population were accompanied by construction of massive new power plants, most of them coal-burning and many located in regions of the country previously noted for pristinely clean air. Perhaps most significant was the vast outpouring of new, synthetic chemical products, many of them toxic compounds, which do not break down readily and can be transported immense distances by air currents, water, or in the tissues of living organisms to wreak their havoc far from their place of origin. In spite of the warnings of a few farsighted individuals, several decades of experience were required before society as a whole became aware of the insidious nature and now-massive scope of environmental degradation.

During the decade of the 1970s, a national awakening regarding issues of ecology and environmental health produced a flood of federal and state legislation aimed at pollution abatement. The battle has been joined and some successes have already been achieved, but it has become increasingly evident that the problem of environmental pollution is far more complex than originally perceived. Issues not even considered until fairly recently—issues such as acid precipitation, carbon dioxide accumulation, ozone layer depletion, contamination of groundwater with toxic organic chemicals, and the fearsome dilemma of what to do about abandoned chemical waste dumps—present policy-makers, scientists, and citizens with thorny technical and political problems. Solutions to older questions pertaining to community waste disposal practices, air pollution abatement measures, or stormwater runoff control are well understood but often fail to be implemented due to fiscal constraints.

The concluding chapters of this book attempt to delineate the nature of the pollution problems confronting American society in this final decade of the 20th century and to describe the legislative tools with which we are now attempting to combat the contamination of our nation's air and water resources in order to prevent future generations from perpetuating the "fouling of the nest" which so endangers the health and well-being of mankind.

11

The Atmosphere

"When I look at thy heavens, the work of thy fingers, the moon and the stars which thou hast established; what is man that thou art mindful of him. . .?"
—Psalms 8:3-4

The airy canopy above the earth which so inspires poets and painters is a physical characteristic of our planet unique in the solar system. Its existence makes possible the rich diversity of life forms found on Earth, making this globe a veritable Oasis in Space.

Questions regarding the origin of Earth's atmosphere have intrigued scientists for decades. It is generally assumed that the earth formed almost 5 billion years ago when particles in a gigantic whirling cloud of dust and gases were pulled together into an aggregate body by enormous gravitational forces. This infant planet had an atmosphere consisting primarily of light gases such as hydrogen and helium, very similar to the present-day atmosphere on the larger planets of Jupiter and Saturn. However, due to Earth's smaller size, gravitational forces were insufficient to retain these elements and they subsequently dissipated into space. This original atmosphere was gradually replaced by a secondary atmosphere produced through the outgassing of volatile materials from the interior of the earth as the once-molten orb began to cool. Modern phenomena such as volcanic eruptions provide vivid evidence that such outgassing continues right up to the present day.

While there is widespread agreement among scientists that the primitive earth's atmosphere was significantly different in chemical composition from that of the present, opinions vary as to precisely which compounds were the major constituents of the early atmosphere. For many years it was widely accepted that a mixture of hydrogen, methane, ammonia, and water vapor would have provided the most congenial environment for the origin of life; these must have been the predominant gases in pre-biotic times. Recently, however, this assumption has been challenged by observations that gases ejected by volcanoes consist largely of carbon dioxide and water vapor, leading to the conclusion that, unless volcanoes operated very differently in the past than they do today, the main component of Earth's early atmosphere was carbon dioxide, just as it is today on our neighboring planets of Mars and Venus. This concept of a carbon dioxide-rich primitive atmosphere, with mere traces of ammonia and notably devoid of free oxygen, constitutes the prevailing view at present. The origin of our modern oxygen-rich atmosphere is traced to the evolution of green plants, about 2 billion years ago, whose photosynthetic activities resulted in the uptake of considerable quantities of atmospheric carbon dioxide and the subsequent release of free oxygen—a necessary precursor for the evolution of higher forms of life.[1]

Although the chemical constituents of the atmosphere have existed in roughly their present proportions for at least several hundred million years, these constituents are in a constant state of flux, reacting with the continents and oceans to form our weather patterns, constantly being removed and recycled (see Ch. 1 on "Geochemical Cycles") as a part of great natural processes. The intimate interrelationships between the atmosphere and land, water, and living things make it relevant to refer to such interactions as the *Earth-Atmosphere System.* This system is essentially a closed one—every material which goes into the air, though it may circulate and change in form, nevertheless remains within the earth-atmosphere system. This fact has disquieting implications for humans who have always viewed the skies as a convenient garbage dump for their volatile wastes—unfortunately the concept of a pollutant, or any other substance "vanishing into thin air" is an impossibility.

Composition of the Atmosphere

The modern atmosphere consists of a mixture of gases so perfectly and consistently diffused among each other that pure dry air exhibits as distinct a set of physical properties as is possessed by any single gas. By volume, the composition of dry air can be broken down as follows:

78% Nitrogen (N_2)
21% Oxygen (O_2)
0.9% Argon (Ar)
0.03% Carbon Dioxide (CO_2)
trace amounts—neon, helium, krypton, xenon, hydrogen, methane, and nitrous oxide

Of the four major atmospheric components, only two, oxygen and carbon dioxide, directly enter into biological processes. Oxygen is required by most living organisms for the production of energy in the process known as aerobic respiration; carbon dioxide constitutes the carbon source for photosynthesis—a series of photochemical reactions whereby the energy of sunlight absorbed by chlorophyll molecules in green plants is harnessed in the synthesis of a simple sugar from carbon dioxide and water. Atmospheric nitrogen, on the other hand, can be utilized only by a few species of nitrogen-fixing bacteria and blue-green algae, while argon is chemically and biologically inert and thus plays no significant role in the biosphere.

Regions of the Atmosphere

Although the composition of its component gases is uniform throughout the atmosphere from sea level to an altitude approximately 50 miles (80 km) above the earth's surface, scientists subdivide this extent into 3 distinct regions based on temperature zones.

Troposphere—extending from sea level to an altitude about 8-9 miles above the earth (slightly less above the poles, more above the equator) is the region known as the ***Troposphere***. Virtually all life activities occur within this region and most weather and climatic phenomena occur here. In addition to the usual gases, the troposphere also contains varying amounts of water vapor and dust particles. Within the troposphere temperature steadily falls with increasing altitude, a decrease of 5.4°F per 1000 feet (10°C/km). The upper limit of the troposphere is known as the ***Tropopause***.

Stratosphere—above the troposphere lies the ***Stratosphere***, a region distinguished by a temperature gradient reversal. Here the temperature slowly rises with increasing altitude until it reaches 32°F (0°C) at a height of about 30 miles (50 km), the upper boundary of the stratosphere known as the ***Stratopause***. Unlike the troposphere, the stratosphere contains almost no water vapor or dust. It is the site, however, of the ***Ozone Layer***, a region characterized by higher-than-usual concentrations of the rare gas ozone (O_3), an isotope of oxygen (O_2). The ozone layer extends from about 10-30 miles above the earth's surface, being most concentrated between 11-15 miles. Amounts of ozone vary depending on location and season of the year. Ozone concentrations are lowest above the equator, increasing toward the poles; they also increase markedly between autumn and spring.

Mesosphere—above the stratopause is the region known as the ***Mesosphere***, where temperature once again begins to fall with increasing altitude.

Since the air becomes progressively more diffuse as the altitude above the earth increases, it is difficult to say precisely where the atmosphere ends. In terms of mass, 99% of our atmosphere lies within 18 miles of the earth's surface—an astonishingly thin blanket nurturing beneath it all the life known to exist in the universe.[2]

Radiation Balance

In addition to providing the major source of certain chemical elements

Fig. 11-1

Regions of the Atmosphere

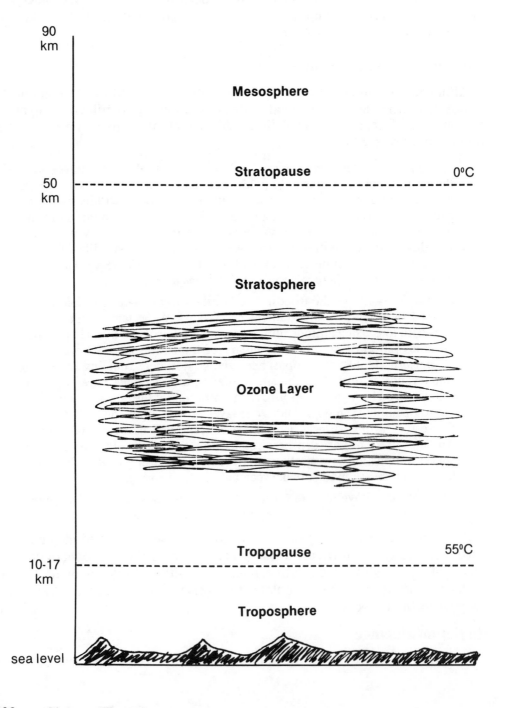

necessary for life, the atmosphere performs a vital role in controlling the earth's surface environment by regulating both the quality and quantity of solar radiation which enters and leaves the biosphere.

The source of all energy on earth, of course, is the sun, but solar energy can be subdivided into several categories, depending on wavelength of the various forms of radiation involved:

TYPE OF RADIATION	% OF TOTAL ENERGY	WAVELENGTH (in micrometers)
Ultraviolet rays	9	0.1 - 0.4
Visible light rays	41	0.4 - 0.7
Infrared rays (heat)	50	0.7 - 3000

These forms of electromagnetic radiation travel outward from the sun at a rate of 186,000 miles (300,000 km) per second, taking slightly over 9 minutes to reach the earth. Although none of the sun's energy is lost as it travels through space, once it begins to penetrate earth's atmosphere, both a depletion and diversion of solar radiation begin to occur.

Most of the ultraviolet radiation present in sunlight is absorbed by the ozone layer as it passes through the stratosphere, though some of the UV wavelengths longer than 0.3 micrometers (the so-called UV-B region) manage to penetrate to the earth's surface where they can produce sunburn and skin cancers. The ozone layer itself is actually created by ultraviolet light, since UV radiant energy causes ordinary oxygen molecules to break apart, releasing single atoms of oxygen which then react with intact oxygen molecules to form ozone.

Since, as was explained in Ch. 10, ultraviolet radiation can have serious adverse effects on living organisms, the existence of the ozone layer is of great biological significance.[3]

Visible light rays and infrared radiation penetrate through the upper stratosphere unaffected by the ozone layer. However, as the atmospheric gas molecules increase in density closer to the earth, these molecules cause a random scattering of the incoming visible light waves (infrared waves are not so affected and for the most part continue to stream directly toward the earth). Entering the troposphere, additional scattering and diffuse reflection of visible light waves occur due to contact with dust particles and clouds (a clear sky appears blue because the shorter blue wavelengths are scattered to a greater extent than are the longer red wavelengths and thus reach our eyes from all parts of the sky). Additional amounts of incoming solar radiation are lost by reflection from the upper surfaces of clouds, oceans, or from the land (particularly when covered with snow or ice). Energy losses also occur by absorption of infrared radiation (heat waves) by carbon dioxide and water vapor as sunlight enters the lower atmosphere. This heat absorption results in an increase in air temperature. Although the carbon dioxide content of the air is constant everywhere, the amount of water vapor varies considerably and is the main factor accounting for differences in the amount of infrared absorption in various climatic regions (e.g. arid regions experience greater temperature extremes during a 24-hour period than do more humid areas at the same latitude because the low water vapor content of desert air minimizes the absorption of the infrared waves). Altogether, scattering, reflection, and absorption of sunlight can result in the loss of as little as 20% of incoming solar radiation when skies are clear to nearly 100% under conditions of heavy cloud cover. On a global yearly average it is estimated that the earth-atmosphere system absorbs about 68% of the total incoming solar radiation, 32% being lost due to the factors mentioned above.

In order to maintain a global radiation balance, energy absorbed by the earth from incoming sunlight must be equalled by outward radiation of energy from the earth's surface. This so-called "ground radiation" occurs in the form of infrared waves longer than 3 or 4 micrometers (referred to as "longwave radiation") which are continually being radiated back into the atmosphere, even at night when no solar radiation is being received. Some of the infrared waves leaving the earth (those in the 5-8 and 12-20 micrometer range) are absorbed by water vapor and carbon dioxide in the atmosphere, a portion of which are re-radiated back to the earth's surface, thereby keeping the earth's climate warmer than it would otherwise be. This phenomenon, known as the **Greenhouse Effect**, has extremely important climatic implications which will be discussed in more detail later in this chapter.

While incoming and outgoing units of radiation are often not in balance at any one particular time and place (indeed, such imbalances provide the forces behind our constantly-changing weather patterns), an equilibrium of such units for the world as a whole during any given year exists, resulting in the maintenance of annual average global temperatures which fluctuate very little from year to year.[4] One of the most pressing concerns among atmospheric scientists today is that human activities may be altering the global radiation balance in ways which may have far-reaching climatic consequences.

Human Impact on the Earth-Atmosphere System

Geologic records give ample indication of drastic climatic changes at various times in Earth's long history, the most recent being four successive periods of widespread glaciation (the "Ice Ages"), the last of which ended only 10,000 years ago. Obviously mankind had nothing to do with past fluctuations in the global heat balance, but our impact today may no longer be so negligible. Temperature measurements compiled over many decades clearly indicate that possibly significant changes in climate are already underway; the extent to which human activities are provoking or enhancing such trends is presently the topic of heated academic debate.

The major causes of human-induced atmospheric change are:

1. changes in the concentrations of natural atmospheric components

Fig. 11-2

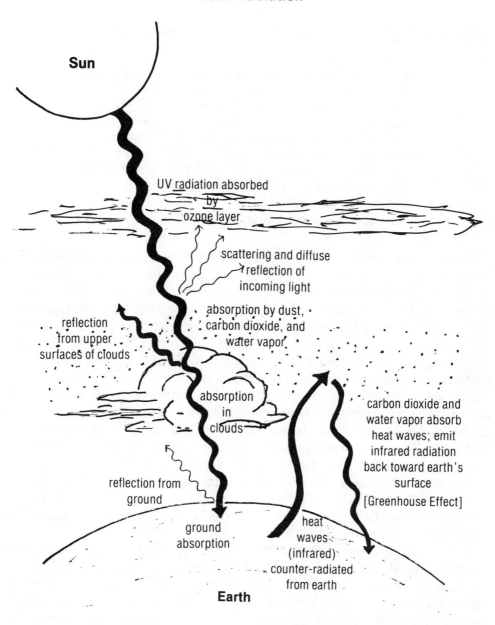

**Reflection and Absorption
of
Solar Radiation**

2. introduction into the atmosphere of pollutant gases and particles not usually found there in significant amounts.

The following examples illustrate two of the most difficult issues modern man confronts as the impact of human activities on the earth-atmosphere system inexorably intensifies.

Rising Levels of Atmospheric CO_2—Moving Toward a Warmer World?

> "The inhabitants of planet earth are quietly conducting a gigantic environmental experiment. So vast and so sweeping will be the impacts of this experiment that, were it brought before any responsible council for approval, it would be firmly rejected as having potentially dangerous consequences. Yet, the experiment goes on with no significant interference from any jurisdiction or nation. The experiment in question is the release of carbon dioxide and other so-called greenhouse gases to the atmosphere."[5]
> —Wallace S. Broecker
> geochemist, Columbia University

As mentioned earlier in this chapter, the relative concentrations of the four major atmospheric gases—nitrogen, oxygen, argon, and carbon dioxide—have remained constant for at least several hundred million years. Within recent decades, however, concern has been expressed that a decrease in oxygen levels and an increase in the amount of atmospheric carbon dioxide might be occurring due to the sharp rise in combustion of fossil fuels (a process which consumes O_2 and releases CO_2), to the world-wide destruction of forest cover, and to the poisoning of oceanic photoplankton by pollution of the seas (plants are the source of atmospheric oxygen and also capture and store huge amounts of CO_2, thereby removing it from the atmosphere). Fortunately, recent studies of the oxygen balance have shown that no oxygen depletion has yet occurred and forces operating at the present time are deemed far too insignificant to constitute a real threat so far as oxygen supply is concerned.[6] The fears regarding carbon dioxide increase, on the other hand, have proven to be well-founded and the prospect of a long-term global warming due to CO_2-induced enhancement of the Greenhouse Effect promises to be one of the biggest environmental issues of the late 20th century.

Levels of atmospheric CO_2 have been gradually rising ever since the dawn of the Industrial Revolution as a result of the ever-increasing use of coal, oil, and gas to power the world's factories and vehicles. When fossil fuels are burned, one of the primary combustion products is carbon dioxide; the combustion of one ton of coal, for example, releases 3 tons of CO_2. In past ages, excess carbon dioxide released through volcanic outgassing was gradually absorbed into the oceans and eventually incorporated into carbonate rock or was photosynthetically "fixed" by green plants. These natural processes, however, are now being overwhelmed by the sheer volume of excess carbon dioxide being released. While fossil fuel combustion has received most of the attention—and blame—in relation to rising CO_2 concentrations, another factor of almost equal importance has been the widescale destruction of natural vegetation, particularly tropical forests, as land is cleared for farming, mining, timber production, or urban development. Both forests and the organic matter in soil humus hold immense quantities of carbon which are oxidized and released as carbon dioxide when vegetation is destroyed. Recently space satellite monitors have revealed that the impact of forest destruction on CO_2 release may be even greater than previously realized. Data collected over the Amazon basin indicate that the thousands of fires deliberately set every year by settlers and ranchers clearing the Brazilian rain forest are generating such enormous quantities of gases and particles that they alone may account for at least one-tenth of the carbon dioxide released by human activities each year.[7] The equilibrium which has prevailed for millennia has been disrupted, with the result that atmospheric CO_2 levels are now sharply increasing. Now measured at 346 ppm, the concentration of atmospheric carbon dioxide has risen by 25% since the mid-19th century, a full 7% of this increase occurring in the years since 1958. Many scientists predict that a continuation of existing trends will result in a doubling of CO_2 from pre-industrial levels by the middle of the next century; even if coal use were to be curtailed, EPA officials assert that a doubling of carbon dioxide concentrations would only be postponed for a few decades.

The sense of alarm felt by those monitoring this situation relates not to any adverse effect which CO_2 might exert on human health—the gas is not a toxic pollutant but a natural and necessary constituent of the biosphere—but rather is due to the impact increasing levels of carbon dioxide will have on global climate. As mentioned earlier in this chapter, atmospheric CO_2 plays a vital role in moderating the earth's temperature, a phenomenon known as the Greenhouse Effect. Just as the glass in a greenhouse permits light to enter but prevents the escape of heat, thereby warming the air within, so the absorption of infrared ground radiation by carbon dioxide and its subsequent re-radiation back toward the earth helps to maintain an average global temperature of 58°F; without CO_2 in the atmosphere, the earth's average surface temperature would fall to about 0°F, making the existence of life as we know it impossible. However, as carbon dioxide levels increase, more infrared radiation will be absorbed and over time average global temperatures will correspondingly rise. Studies recently completed by the U.S. Environmental Protection Agency, the National Academy of Sciences, the National Aeronautics and Space Administration (NASA), and the National Center for Atmospheric Research have all independently concluded that the projected doubling of CO_2 will cause an average temperature increase of about 1.5-4.5°C (3-8°F) by about 2030 A.D.—an unprecedentedly short time for a climatic change of this magnitude.

To many people, the prospect of temperatures a few degrees higher than they are at present seems little cause for dismay—particularly when they happen to be contemplating such a scenario during a January blizzard. The major impact of a global warming trend, however, would not be felt in terms of human physical discomfort but rather in a possibly drastic alteration of world-wide rainfall and temperature patterns.

While climatologists are unable to make accurate detailed predictions regarding CO_2-induced climatic changes in specific areas of the globe, their computer modelling studies support widespread agreement that while temperatures everywhere are rising to some extent, the global warming trend is not evenly distributed. It is expected that the high latitude regions of the northern hemisphere will experience the greatest temperature increases (perhaps twice as high as the world average), particularly during the winter months. In the mid-latitude regions also (including the continental United States) greenhouse warming will exceed the global average, with winter temperatures increasing more than summer temperatures. Regional changes in rainfall patterns are even more difficult to predict, but computer models suggest that our grandchildren's generation may witness heavier precipitation in the already-wet equatorial regions, more winter precipitation in the polar regions, much drier summers in the midwestern U.S. (the drought of '88 may be a harbinger of worse to come!), and drier winters in California. Along with such widespread regional climatic alteration, more localized weather changes such as the frequency and intensity of storms will also be pronounced. From an economic standpoint, major climatic change could bring benefits to some regions, severe hardships to others. A northward shift of agricultural zones might enhance crop yields in Canada and the Soviet Union while turning the American "Breadbasket" into a dustbowl.

While some have suggested that rising concentrations of CO_2 might actually boost food production by increasing photosynthetic rates, the combination of excessive heat and drought could counteract this effect. It is believed that a mere 3.5° temperature rise in the tropics could cut rice yields by more than 10%. The extent to which greenhouse warming will affect agricultural production will depend in large measure on the rate at which these climatic changes occur. Most of the world's major food crops are already adapted to a wide range of environmental conditions and if climatic change is gradual, agricultural scientists will have time to develop new, even more tolerant varieties. However, if changes are rapid, the prospect for world harvests is far less comforting. Climate change will impose even greater stresses on natural ecosystems, since many non-agricultural plant and animal species are quite sensitive to temperature change and might disappear in the event of major warming. For others, reduced levels of precipitation could be the factor causing species loss. Extinction of natural predator species could cause problems for agriculture by favoring more resilient pest species. Since world agriculture is now so highly adapted to existing conditions, any change at all is bound to be disruptive, at least in the short term. At a time when world food reserves are marginal, any threat to sustained high crop yields is a cause for serious concern.

A second even more dramatic consequence of global warming will be a world-wide rise in sea level due both to the thermal expansion of water as temperatures in the ocean rise and to the melting of the Greenland and Antarctic Ice Sheets. Although this development could be a boon to navigation in the Arctic (the fabled "Northwest Passage" might become a practical alternative to the Panama Canal!), its impact on densely-populated coastal regions worldwide will be devastating. A sea level rise of just 6 feet (and most estimates predict significantly greater increases than this) would totally obliterate many low-lying coral islands. Entire populations in the Marshall Islands, Maldives, and parts of the Caribbean face the prospect of their homelands disappearing beneath the waves within the foreseeable future. Along the edges of continents, town and cities built on barrier islands, river deltas, or low-lying shorelines can anticipate a similar scenario unless they soon embark on multi-billion dollar coastal defense construction projects. In many desperately poor, densely populated regions of the world, such expenditures are obviously impossible. It is anticipated that Egypt may lose 15% of its arable land to encroaching seas by the mid-21st century; in Bangladesh even a 3-foot rise in sea level will inundate one-sixth of the country's land area. When one pauses to consider the number of major world cities now located at or near sea level, the impact of such a rise on human settlement patterns becomes clear. Although sea level will advance gradually (no one foresees the likelihood of Boston or Galveston or Miami being submerged overnight!), even a slight increase can have significant consequences. Some experts feel that a 6-inch rise during the present century has been responsible for much of the coastal erosion which has occurred. Hurricanes (which are predicted to become more frequent and more severe as ocean temperatures increase) will be much more damaging to beach communities as sea levels rise; studies suggest that ocean levels only a foot or two higher than at present could turn a moderately bad hurricane into a killer. Seaside resorts such as Atlantic City, NJ; Ocean City, MD; Myrtle Beach, SC; and Galveston, TX—built on low-lying barrier islands—will be at special risk from storms in the years ahead.

Since the early 1970s, climatologists have been raising increasingly strident warnings about the impending greenhouse warming, urging that policymakers take action to forestall this so-called "Doomsday Issue". While the general public until recently tended either to ignore such predictions or to regard them as plot material for a science fiction novel, there has been a steadily growing consensus among the experts that global climatic change has already begun. Testifying before a Senate subcommittee during the torrid summer of 1988, James Hansen of the NASA Goddard Institute for Space Studies told the assembled lawmakers that "The greenhouse effect has been detected and is changing our climate now". Hansen cited the fact that the four hottest years on record have all occurred in the 1980s. Such statements add a sense of urgency to demands that governments shake off their inertia and launch efforts to reduce the concentration of greenhouse gases which will otherwise produce significant climatic change within the next 50 years. As Howard Ferguson, a meteorologist with the Canadian Atmospheric Environmental Service remarked, "All the greenhouse scenarios are consistent. These numbers are real. We have to start behaving as if this is going to happen. Those who advocate a program consisting only of additional research are missing the boat." Calling for action is easier than implementing such changes, however. At the International Conference on the Changing Atmosphere, held in Toronto in June of 1988, representatives from 48 countries recommended an action agenda which called for:

1. stabilizing emissions of CO_2 (it is estimated that attaining this goal would require a greater than 50% reduction of existing emission levels) through the implementation of energy conservation measures and by a shift from fossil fuels to clean energy sources. As an interim goal, industrialized nations are urged to reduce their CO_2 emissions 20% by the year 2005.
2. greatly increasing funding for research and development of renewable energy technologies such as biomass conversion, solar, wind, and geothermal power, and safer forms of nuclear power generation.
3. working vigorously to halt deforestation, particularly in the tropics, and to increase substantially on-going efforts to plant new trees.
4. limiting emissions of greenhouse gases other than CO_2, particularly CFCs.
5. requiring that products be labeled to permit consumers to judge the impact their manufacture and use will have on atmospheric contamination.

Action to implement these long-term policies must begin immediately on a global scale if the changes already underway are to be minimized. The obstacles to success are great, since the basic problem stems from the energy use decisions of billions of individuals in every nation of the world. Some observers conclude that it is already too late; the degree of world-wide cooperation and coordination necessary to achieve any meaningful reduction in CO_2 releases would, in their view, be impossible to attain in a world "hooked" on fossil fuels. Instead of a crash fuel-switching effort, such voices call for accelerating research on CO_2 and its effects and for a policy to improve society's ability to adapt to changing circumstances, preparing the economy for the consequences of global warming. Perhaps the best summation of the differing assessments of what society's response to greenhouse warming ought to be was given by Harvard planetary scientist Michael McElroy who told his colleagues at the Toronto Conference:

"If we choose to take on this challenge, it appears we can slow the rate of change substantially, giving us time to develop mechanisms so that the cost to society and the damage to ecosystems can be minimized. We could alternatively close our eyes, hope for the best, and pay the cost when the bill comes due".[8]

Box 11-1

Trace Elements and the Greenhouse Effect

As if the climatologists don't have enough to worry about with the seemingly inexorable rise in carbon dioxide levels, researchers have recently reported that increasing atmospheric concentrations of several trace gases threaten to enhance the Greenhouse Effect to an extent almost as great as that of the far more abundant CO_2. Although present only in parts per billion, as opposed to carbon dioxide's 340 parts per million in the atmosphere, trace gases such as the chlorofluorocarbons, methane, and nitrous oxide are a cause for concern because they are far more efficient than CO_2 at absorbing infrared radiation. One type of CFC, for example, absorbs 8 times more strongly than does CO_2. The absorptive potential of these trace gases is directly proportional to their atmospheric concentration—a doubling in the amount of these substances will result in a doubling of their infrared absorption. There is now solid evidence to indicate that concentrations of these gases are indeed on the rise. Monitoring carried out by the National Oceanic and Atmospheric Administration indicates a 6% yearly increase for chlorofluorocarbons (CFC_s), a 1.5% annual rise in methane levels, and a 0.2% increase in nitrous oxides. Experts at the World Meteorological Organization estimate that an increase of chlorofluorocarbon concentrations to 1 part per billion, plus a doubling of methane and nitrous oxide levels, would warm the atmosphere by 0.9°C. Other researchers have estimated an even greater degree of warming as a result of trace gas concentrations. Such increases, whatever the precise figure, would of course be over and above the 1.5-4.5°C temperature rise caused by increased carbon dioxide levels. Because the sources of trace gas emissions are so varied—ranging from the evaporation of solvents, refrigerants, and spray-can propellants in the case of CFCs to microbial activity in the intestines of cattle and termites in the case of methane, as well as to the burning of fossil fuels—controlling their release will be difficult, if not impossible. Research on the role of trace gases in affecting climate change is still in its infancy, but preliminary indications are that their impact may be significant.[9]

Depletion of the Ozone Layer

Although ozone is one of the rarest of atmospheric gases, its presence in the stratosphere is of vital importance in protecting life on earth from the damaging effects of solar ultraviolet radiation. As mentioned earlier, the ozone layer is created when UV energy splits the oxygen molecule and the freed atoms rejoin other oxygen molecules to form ozone (O_3). At the same time, the highly reactive ozone is being broken down again to normal oxygen (O_2); thus the ozone layer is maintained in a state of dynamic equilibrium, daytime increases being balanced by night-time decreases.

Fig. 11-3

FORMATION OF OZONE IN THE STRATOSPHERE

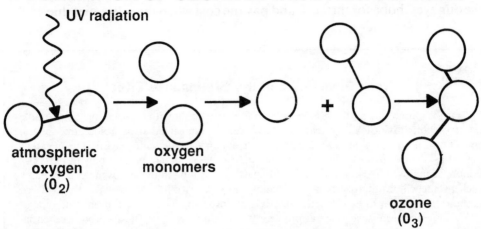

UV radiation

atmospheric oxygen (O_2)   oxygen monomers   +   ozone (O_3)

Since the early 1970s, fears have been growing that certain pollutant emissions into the atmosphere are beginning to disrupt this equilibrium, threatening the long-term integrity of the ozone layer. Although initially attention focused on the damage potential of nitrous oxides emitted with jet airplane exhausts (particularly from supersonic transports such as the Anglo-French Concorde) and the use of nitrogen fertilizers, it gradually became apparent that a far more serious threat to the ozone layer is posed by the widespread use of a group of synthetic chemicals called chlorofluorocarbons (CFCs), one of the best known of which is the refrigerant Freon. Used in a number of industrial processes, as solvents and refrigerants, in making plastic foams, and as spray can aerosol propellants until their use for this purpose was banned in 1978, CFCs are particularly troublesome because they are such stable chemicals; when released into the environment through vaporization or leakage from enclosed systems or by direct spraying into the air, as in the case of aerosol containers, CFCs do not break down but instead drift upward through the troposphere into the stratosphere where the molecules are finally broken down by solar radiation, releasing atoms of chlorine which react with and destroy ozone. The chlorine-ozone reaction is a catalytic one, meaning that the same chlorine atom can repeat the reaction with tens of thousands of ozone molecules. This, plus the fact that the chlorine atoms will remain in the atmosphere for 100 years or more, explains why CFCs' destructive impact on the ozone layer will be much greater than emission levels might suggest.

Depletion of the ozone layer is worrisome from a human health perspective because of stratospheric ozone's role in absorbing biologically damaging ultraviolet radiation. It is now well-established that for each 1% decrease in atmospheric ozone, penetration of UV radiation to the earth's surface will increase by 2%. Since over 90% of non-melanoma skin cancers are associated with exposure to UV radiation in sunlight, any increase in ultraviolet exposure is expected to result in a rising incidence of skin malignancies. A National Academy of Sciences report in 1982 estimated that for every 1% decrease in the concentration of atmospheric ozone, there will be a 2-5% increase in cases of basal cell carcinomas (currently about 400,000 new cases/year in the U.S.) and a 4-10% increase in squamous cell carcinomas (approximately 100,000 new cases annually). The impact of rising UV exposure on the incidence of more dangerous malignant melanomas is unclear.[10] A USEPA analysis released in 1988 suggested that from now through the year 2075, increasing levels of UV exposure due to ozone layer depletion could result in as many as 200 million additional cases of skin cancer, as well as damage to the body's immune system.

Revelations of a significant "hole" in the ozone layer over Antarctica (see Box 11-2), where declines in ozone concentration as great as 50% during early spring have been confirmed, have lent a sense of urgency to questions regarding the extent of ozone depletion worldwide. For the past 20 years, the U.S. government has been collecting data on atmospheric ozone from ground-based survey stations and the Nimbus-7 satellite. In March of 1988 NASA's Ozone Trends Panel released a disquieting report derived from a re-analysis of this data which revealed a much more significant decline in ozone levels than had previously been suspected. The panel reported that stratospheric ozone over the U.S., Europe, Japan, China, and parts of the USSR has decreased by as much as 3% since 1979. Australia and New Zealand are experiencing ozone level declines of 4%, while over the Scandinavian countries, atmospheric ozone during winter months has dropped 6%.[11]

After years of controversy among scientists, the chemical industry, and government policymakers as to the extent of ozone depletion, the identity of the main culprits, and the most effective approach for halting—or at least slowing down—the process, consensus is gradually emerging that ozone depletion is real, that it presents a major threat to life on this planet, and that global cooperation is required to combat a phenomenon which threatens us all. A major step forward to meet this challenge was taken in September, 1987, when diplomats from 31 nations, meeting in Montreal, Canada, signed an international accord aimed at controlling the chemicals most responsible for ozone layer depletion. The Montreal Protocol calls for the freezing of CFC consumption at 1986 levels by 1990, to be followed by a 50% reduction in the production of these chemicals by the end of the century. The treaty went into effect in January, 1989, after ratification by nations representing more than two-thirds of the world's CFC production. Although the U.S. Senate ratified the protocol in the spring of 1988, making the United States the first nation to do so, misgivings are already being expressed by some members of Congress and the scientific community that the CFC reductions called for in the treaty fall short of what is needed. They urge that the U.S. push for a complete halt in CFC production by 1999, rather than the 50% cut called for in the Protocol. Other critics worry about exemptions in the treaty's mandatory cuts which allow developing nations to *increase* their CFC production up to 10% a year through 1997 and would permit the USSR to complete construction of two CFC manufacturing plants. A reassessment of the terms of the protocol will be made in 1990 to determine whether new scientific findings justify more stringent regulations.

Box 11-2

A "Hole In The Sky"

When Chicken Little warned his barnyard friends that "the sky is falling!", he probably wasn't referring to ozone layer depletion. A modern version of this classic children's tale, however, might well substitute a penguin for the hero and shift the scene to the icy vistas of Antarctica where the most tangible—and alarming—evidence yet of damage to our protective ozone shield has been attracting the attention of atmospheric scientists worldwide.

The story begins in 1985 when members of the British Antarctic Survey announced the existence of a large hole in the ozone layer over the South Pole. Although the gap was temporary, opening in early September (Antarctic spring) and closing by mid-October as the southern atmosphere grew warmer, it had been increasing in size each year since the British researchers first noticed it in 1981 and by the time of their startling revelation represented a 40% decline in ozone concentrations. Shocked NASA scientists, whose extensive atmospheric sampling program had given no indication of massive ozone depletion, re-examined their satellite data and discovered their British colleagues were right—Nimbus 7 had picked up the same information but its computers had been programmed to disregard extremely low ozone measurements on the assumption that they represented sampling errors!

NASA confirmation that the ozone hole was real led to intensified research efforts to learn what was going wrong in the polar skies. U.S. scientific teams sent to McMurdo Bay in 1986 and 1987 confirmed that the ozone hole was enlarging—by 1987 the ozone level decline had reached 50%. Conflicting theories regarding the cause of this depletion—chemical pollution, cyclical solar flares, and natural atmospheric variation were the main contenders for chief villain—were vigorously debated by researchers. Recent discovery within the ozone hole of chlorine levels 400-500X greater than those on the outside tilt the weight of evidence toward the chemical pollution theory and may prove to be the "smoking gun" which establishes a direct cause-and-effect link between CFC emissions and ozone layer destruction.

While the Antarctic "hole in the sky" has provided a fascinating topic for scientific research and journalistic headlines, its societal implications are more than a little disturbing. For years policymakers have assumed that even if the chemical wastes we so carelessly dump into earth's air and waters should begin to overwhelm the assimilative capacity of Nature, any adverse effects will develop gradually and will prompt remedial measures before the damage is too great. The extreme rapidity and extent of ozone depletion over Antarctica, however, has led to troubled questions about the overall global equilibrium. Perhaps the insults humanity is currently heaping upon an already burdened environment will go unperceived until we add that proverbial "straw that broke the camel's back" and the balance is suddenly shifted in favor of swift and irreversible change. It is this possibility that haunts policymakers and adds a sense of urgency to efforts at limiting emissions of ozone-destroying pollutants.

Box 11-3

Ozone Enemy #1

The almost-perfect chemicals, chlorofluorocarbons (CFCs) are used in hundreds of products we encounter constantly in our daily lives. The freon in our refrigerators and freezers is a CFC; the blowing agents used to inject the bubbles which give buoyancy and lightness to styrofoam egg cartons, fast-food containers, disposable plates and cups, foam cushions and carpet pads are CFCs; solvents used to clean delicate microchips, for grain fumigation, electronics manufacturing and dry cleaning contain CFCs; CFCs are found in home and automobile air conditioners and, in most countries, comprise the propellants in aerosol cans dispensing everything from French perfume to insecticides to deodorants. So how has such a universally-acclaimed product of modern industry suddenly found itself at the top of environmentalists' "hit list" of pollutants posing a threat to the global eco-system? Why are CFCs the target of an international effort to phase out their production by the end of the century?

The answer lies in one of the properties of CFCs which makes them so useful to industry—their extreme chemical stability. When released, CFCs don't break down; instead they persist in the environment for as long as 150 years, eventually migrating into the upper atmosphere where, upon contact with solar UV radiation, they break apart, releasing highly active chlorine atoms which catalyze the breakdown of ozone. As if this weren't bad enough, they also act as "greenhouse gases", trapping outgoing heat waves and contributing to global warming (while CO_2 is the major contributor to the so-called Greenhouse Effect, CFCs are believed to be responsible for about 20% of the predicted rise in earth's temperature).

As evidence of large scale, pollutant-induced atmospheric changes continued to accumulate during the late 1970s and early 1980s, calls for banning CFC production and consumption became more vocal. In 1978 Congress responded by prohibiting the use of CFCs as propellants in aerosol spray cans; Canada and the Scandinavian countries followed the U.S. example, but elsewhere in the world use of the chemicals continued without restriction. Indeed, the large chemical companies manufacturing the product took the position that CFCs, like citizens in a free country, should be considered innocent until proven guilty, and they continued to insist that conclusive evidence linking CFC use with ozone layer depletion was lacking. They stressed the profound economic impact which a phaseout of CFC production would surely have. In the U.S. alone, the value of goods and services related in some way to CFC use totals about $28 billion annually; approximately 715,000 American workers are employed in jobs directly dependent on the availability of chlorofluorocarbons.[12]

Nevertheless, by 1988 the weight of evidence incriminating CFCs as the prime cause of ozone layer destruction could no longer be denied. E.I. du Pont de Nemours & Co., the corporate giant which invented CFCs and currently sells one-fourth of the world supply, announced its intention to try to eliminate production of CFC 11 and 12 (the most heavily used CFCs and the ones considered most damaging to ozone) by the year 2000. Two other U.S. producers, Pennwalt Corp. and Allied Signal, Inc., also indicated they, too, saw the handwriting on the wall and intended to get out of the CFC business at some unspecified time (taking a cue from the giants, McDonald's fast-food chain also declared its intention to phase out the use of CFC related packaging materials in its U.S. establishments). Accordingly, a scramble to find ozone-safe alternatives to CFCs is now underway, but the effort won't be easy or cheap. None of the chemicals now being researched as substitutes for CFC 11 and 12 are as efficient or durable as the current products. Some work but are unacceptable because of toxicity, flammability, or high cost. As the search for alternatives intensifies, the short-term demand for existing CFCs is strong, and prices—and profits to CFC producers—are expected to rise (du Pont promises to use most of its increased earnings for research into CFC substitutes). Replacements for CFCs, once they're found, will also be costly—and may not perform as well. Drastic steps to save the ozone layer are urgently needed—but they won't be painless.

Unfortunately, even full implementation of the treaty's requirements will not prevent further losses of ozone. Millions of pounds of CFCs already released are gradually drifting up toward the ozone layer and even with future cutbacks in CFC production, chlorine levels in the stratosphere are expected to increase four-fold within a century. Nevertheless, international efforts to protect the ozone layer are extremely significant in that they represent the first time in history that nations of the world have agreed to work together to prevent a disaster of global proportions before it's too late.

Box 11-4
Eco-Catastrophe—"Nuclear Winter"

The ultimate ecological catastrophe by any definition would be an all-out nuclear war among the superpowers which many authorities fear could ultimately result in the extinction of most higher forms of life on earth. For the most part, voices warning of massive death and destruction should the nuclear genie ever be unleashed focus on the short-term effects of blast, firestorm, radiation sickness, and social disruption. Horrible though these very real consequences of a thermonuclear exchange would be, it is probable that a sizeable portion of the world's population would survive the initial period of hostilities and would then be confronted with the harsh realities of a post-nuclear world. According to recent studies conducted by several prominent scientists using computer models, atmospheric contamination following a nuclear war would be extensive enough to produce world-wide climatic change so severe as to make survival of the human species doubtful.

Immediately following a large nuclear exchange, thousands of dust clouds would be produced by the initial blasts; such dust is generated when a nuclear explosion at or near the ground ejects and fragments soil particles and rock or when air currents created by the blast result in blowoff and sweep-up of surface dust. Nuclear surface explosions produce finer dusts than do volcanic eruptions and hence can be expected to produce even more significant atmospheric disturbance than the latter. In addition to blast-generated dust, a nuclear fireball emits light of such intensity that numerous fires are ignited both in urban areas and surrounding forests and grasslands. The combustion of large amounts of petroleum products and plastics within urban areas would be particularly significant, due to the black, sooty smoke they emit. The vast amount of smoke generated by raging fires would be added to the enormous quantities of fine dust entering the atmosphere during the days following a nuclear exchange. Such dust and smoke would spread over the mid-latitudes of the Northern Hemisphere at altitudes up to about 18 miles (30 km). Horizontal air currents, vertical wind shear, and continuing emissions from fires would cause a further spreading of nuclear dust and smoke throughout the troposphere and into the stratosphere, filling any gaps in the cloud cover within a week or two.

The result of this global pall of nuclear debris would be a sharp reduction in the average amount of solar radiation reaching the earth's surface, the precise amount of decrease depending on the total megatonnage of the nuclear exchange. The drop in light penetration would result in sharp declines in temperature occurring within 3-4 weeks following the initial explosions. Continental land areas would be most severely affected, with temperatures dropping by as much as 30°C or more. During the first month, widespread frosts and freezing events would occur, even during the summer (because of their great heat content and rapid misting of surface waters, the oceans would not experience a major cooling and would help to moderate the continental cold wave, particularly in coastal areas). Changes in precipitation patterns would also be dramatic. Decreases in rainfall could be as high as 80% over temperate zone and tropical regions, with failure of the summer monsoon in Asia considered likely. In addition to its impact on climate, reduced light intensity would adversely affect plant growth. If the nuclear explosion were in the 10,000 megaton range, light levels over much of the Northern Hemisphere would be below the minimum necessary for photosynthesis to occur for about 40 days. If such a scenario were to occur during the spring or summer growing season, the implications for food production, even in regions far removed from the explosion sites, would be disastrous. Over a period of months the nuclear dust and soot would gradually be removed from the atmosphere as dry deposition or would be washed out with precipitation.

This of course would expose populations to dangerously high levels of external radiation and would result also in human ingestion of biologically active radionuclides with food and water. It is expected that the period of cooling would last approximately one year, with a return to more normal climatic patterns after that time.

Atmospheric implications of a nuclear war include not only climatic effects, but also large-scale ozone layer depletion due to nitrogen oxides generated by blast-produced fireballs. Estimates on the amount of atmospheric ozone which might be destroyed in a large-scale nuclear exchange are on the order of 50%, suggesting a substantial increase in human exposure to damaging ultraviolet radiation. In addition, raging fires following nuclear detonations are expected to release a variety of toxic compounds such as cyanide, carbon monoxide, and dioxins when widely used synthetic organic chemicals burn and create a fog of poisonous pollutants.

Simultaneously confronted with piercing cold, near-darkness, food shortages, radiation poisoning, toxic air pollutants, and social disintegration, victims struggling to survive in the weeks and months following a thermonuclear war may well envy the dead.[13]

Box 11-5

Atmospheric Inversions

Shortly before Christmas of 1952, the city of London experienced a killer smog which even in that notoriously polluted metropolis was exceptionally severe. For a period of 5 days the cold, moist air hung over the city like a heavy wet blanket, with scarcely a trace of breeze to carry away the thickening cloud of smoke and fumes from millions of coal-burning fireplaces, factories, and motor vehicles. Even in the middle of the day, the pervading gloom was so thick that car-train collisions were common and a steam ferry ran into an anchored ship along the Thames River. When the fog finally lifted, health officials revealed the grim human toll of this episode—nearly 3000 excess deaths, most of them due to respiratory or heart disease, had occurred during the week of foul air.

The London situation was not solely a result of man-made pollutants being dumped into an overburdened atmosphere. The volume of emissions during the time period in question was not substantially different than at many other times during the year. Though London, like most other metropolitan areas, suffered regularly from unhealthy levels of contaminated air, pollution was seldom bad enough to cause acute respiratory distress as it did during this event. The chief villain in this situation, and in virtually every other air pollution "disaster" on record was an atmospheric anomaly known as an *inversion.*

Under normal conditions air is in a constant state of flux. As the air near the earth's surface is warmed it expands and rises, carrying with it pollutant particles and gases. Cooler, cleaner air moves in to replace it, setting up convection currents. These forces, combined with the earth's rotation, generate winds which further aid in dispersing pollutants.

The vertical extent to which warm air rises until it cools to the same temperature as the air above is referred to as the **mixing depth**—an expanse which corresponds with the upper boundary for pollution dispersal. The amount of mixing depth varies depending on the time of day and the season of the year, being greater during daytime and in summer than it is at night and during winter.

In contrast to this usual situation, a reversal of the normal pattern can occur in which the air closest to the surface of the ground is cooler than the layer above it. In such a situation the cool air, being heavier than warm air, is unable to rise and mix and remains atypically stable. This state of affairs is known as an **atmospheric inversion**—*a condition where a layer of cool surface air is trapped by an overlying layer of warmer air.* In such a case, the mixing depth will be minimal and pollutant emissions, if any, within the affected area can acumulate to levels which may threaten human health.

The two most important types of inversions are:

a) *radiation inversion*—this normal nocturnal situation often occurs on clear nights when absorbed daytime heat is radiated quickly out into space and the temperature of surface air drops below that of the air above it. Generally a radiation inversion presents little health threat because it breaks up as soon as the morning sun warms the earth, re-establishing normal convection currents. In most cases a radiation inversion simply doesn't persist long enough to permit build-up of dangerously high concentrations of pollutants.

b) *subsidence inversion*—more troublesome than radiation inversions are subsidence inversions, caused when a layer of air within a high-pressure mass settles down over a region, being compressed and thereby heated by the high pressure area above. At ground level the air temperature remains unchanged and hence is relatively cooler than the air layer directly above. Subsidence inversions are particularly worrisome because they may remain in place for days, the surface air becoming increasingly foul as time passes.

While inversions can occur at any time (southern California experiences inversions as often as 340 days of the year), they are more frequent and last longer during the fall and winter months. They are particularly common in valleys, since at night cool air flows down the hillsides and is trapped at the bottom. Not until the sun is directly overhead will the surface air be sufficiently warmed to break up the inversion layer, and in winter such an inversion may persist all day.

It should be pointed out that an atmospheric inversion per se is a perfectly natural occurrence and presents no threat to human health—*if* there are few sources of pollutant emissions within the affected region. Inversions become major problems only when they occur in industrialized or densely settled areas where noxious pollutants can steadily accumulate to dangerous concentrations.

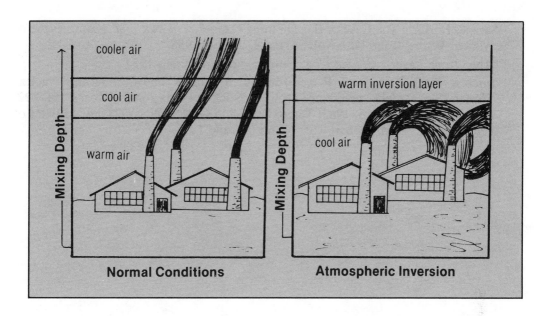

| Normal Conditions | Atmospheric Inversion |

REFERENCES:

[1]Budyko, M.I., *"The Evolution of the Biosphere",* D. Reidel Publishing Company, 1986; Gribbin, John, "Carbon Dioxide, ammonia—and life", *New Scientist,* 94 (1305), 413-416, May 13, 1982.

[2]Strahler, Arthur N., and Alan H. Strahler, *Environmental Geoscience,* Hamilton Publishing Company, 1973.

[3]Panofsky, Hans A., "Earth's Endangered Ozone", *Environment,* vol. 20, no. 3, April 1978.

[4]Strahler et al., op. cit.

[5]Mintzer, Irving M., *"A Matter of Degrees: the Potential for Controlling the Greenhouse Effect",* World Resources Institute, Research Report #5, April 1987.

[6]Broecker, Wallace S., "Man's Oxygen Reserves", *Science,* vol. 168, June 26, 1970.

[7]Woodwell, G. M., et al., "Global Deforestation: Contribution to Atmospheric Carbon Dioxide", *Science,* vol. 222, no. 4628, December 9, 1983; Simons, Marlise, "Man-Made Amazon Fires Tied to Global Warming", *The New York Times,* Aug. 8, 1988.

[8]Mintzer, op. cit.; Jager, Jill, "Anticipating Climatic Change: Priorities for Action", *Environment,* vol. 30, no. 7, September 1988; Revkin, Andrew C., "Endless Summer: Living with the Greenhouse Effect", *Discover,* vol. 9, no. 10, October 1988.

[9]Hoffman, John S., and Michael Barth, "Carbon Dioxide: Are We Ignoring a Vital Environmental Issue?", *The Amicus Journal,* Natural Resources Defense Council, Summer 1983.

[10]Maugh, Thomas H., "New Link Between Ozone and Cancer", *Science,* vol. 216, April 23, 1982.

[11]Savage, Harlin, "The Case of the Thinning Ozone", *The National Voter,* League of Women Voters of the U.S., vol. 38, no. 2, August 1988.

[12]"The Ozone Layer", *Chemecology,* vol. 16, no. 8, October 1987.

[13]Turco R. P., O. B. Toon, T. P. Ackerman, J. B. Pollack, and Carl Sagan, "Nuclear Winter: Global Consequences of Multiple Nuclear Explosions", *Science,* vol. 222, no. 4630, December 23, 1983; Turco, R. P., and G. S. Golitsyn, "Global Effects of Nuclear War", *Environment,* vol. 30, no. 5, June 1988.

12
Air
Pollution

"If you visit American city,
You will find it very pretty;
just two things of which you must beware:
don't drink the water and don't breathe the air!"
—Tom Lehrer, lyrics from "Pollution"

Humans have undoubtedly been coping with a certain amount of polluted air ever since primitive *Homo sapiens* sat crouched by the warmth of a smoky fire in his Paleolithic cave. An inevitable consequence of fuel combustion, air pollution mounted as a source of human discomfort as soon as man began to live in towns and cities. It has become an extremely serious problem on a world-wide basis during the past century for two primary reasons: 1) there has been an enormous increase in world population, particularly in urban areas, and 2) since the early 1800s the rapid growth of energy-intensive industries and rising levels of affluence in the developed countries has led to record levels of fossil fuel combustion.

Prior to the 20th century problems related to air pollution were primarily associated, in the public mind at least, with the city of London. As early as the 13th century small amounts of coal from Newcastle were being shipped into London for fuel. As the population and manufacturing enterprises grew, wood supplies diminished and coal burning increased, in spite of the protestations of a long series of both monarchs and private citizens who objected to the odor of coal smoke. One petitioner to King Charles II in 1661 complained that due to the greed of manufacturers, inhabitants of London were forced to "breathe nothing but an impure and thick Mist, accompanied by a fuliginous (sooty) and filthy vapour, which renders them obnoxious to a thousand inconveniences, corrupting the Lungs, and disordering the entire habit of their Bodies. . .".[1]

In spite of such railings, English coal consumption increased even faster than the rate of population growth and by the 19th century London's thick, "pea-soup" fogs had become a notorious trade-mark of the city. Numerous well-meaning attempts at smoke abatement were largely ignored during the hey-day of laissez-faire capitalism, epitomized by the industrialists' slogan, "Where there's muck, there's money."

The same conditions which had made London the air pollution capital of the world began to prevail in the United States as well during the 19th and early 20th centuries. St. Louis, plagued by smoky conditions, passed an ordinance as early as 1867 mandating that smokestacks be at least 20 feet higher than adjacent buildings. The Chicago City Council in 1881 passed the nation's first smoke ordinance. Pittsburgh, once one of the smokiest cities in the U.S., was the site of pioneer work at the Mellon Institute on the harmful impact of smoke both on property and human health. In spite of gradually increasing public awareness of the problem, levels of air pollution and the geographical extent of the areas affected continued to increase. Although by the late 1950s and 1960s large-scale fuel-switching from coal to natural gas and oil had significantly reduced smoky conditions in many American cities, other newer pollutants— products of the now-ubiquitous automobile—had assumed worrisome levels. Today foul air has become a problem of global proportions; no longer does one have to travel to London or Pittsburgh or Los Angeles to experience the respiratory irritation or the aesthetic distress which a hazy, contaminated atmosphere can provoke. In the 1990's virtually every metropolitan area in the world—New York, Rome, Athens, Bombay, Tokyo, Mexico City—capitalists and Communists, industrialized and developing nations alike are grappling with the problems of how to halt further deterioration of air quality without impeding industrial productivity and economic development.

Sources of Air Pollution

Where is all this dirty air coming from? Not surprisingly, the sources of air pollution are quite diverse and vary in importance from one region to another. Some air contaminants are of natural origin; volcanic eruptions, forest fires, and dust storms periodically contribute large quantities of pollutant gases and particles to the atmosphere. In May, 1980, an EPA official jokingly remarked that Mt. St. Helens in Washington State should be cited for violating air quality standards due to the immense quantities of smoke and ash the volcano was spewing into the atmosphere. Considerable amounts of methane gas are released into the air when organic matter decays in the absence of oxygen, and some plant species produce volatile hydrocarbons which are thought to be responsible for the blue haze observed in the Smoky Mountains and other forest regions. However, most of the pollutants befouling our air today come from the man-made emission sources which have proliferated with the development of industries and transportation networks.

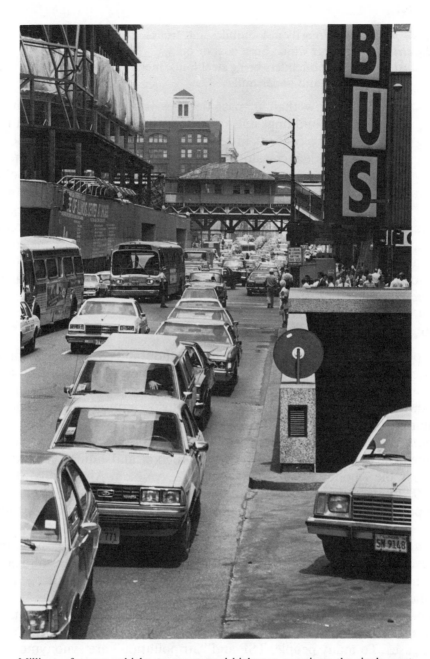

Millions of motor vehicles on streets and highways constitute the single most important source of air pollution in the U.S. Five of the 7 criteria air pollutants —carbon monoxide, nitrogen oxides, hydrocarbons, ozone, and lead—are associated primarily with auto emissions. [*Illinois Environmental Protection Agency*]

At present in the U.S. the largest sources of air pollution, in order of importance, are:

Transportation, primarily automobiles and trucks
Electric power plants which burn coal or oil
Industry, the major offenders being steel mills, metal smelters, oil refineries,
        pulp and paper mills

Of less importance now than in past decades is the contribution made by heating of homes and buildings and refuse burning. The general trend toward heating with oil, gas, or electricity instead of with coal greatly reduced pollution from space heating, while increasingly common municipal bans on home refuse burning, along with the utilization of sanitary landfills or non-polluting incinerators for community solid waste disposal, have accounted for a marked decline in emissions from trash combustion. Within any one region or community, of course, the relative importance of various emission sources may differ from the over-all national rankings noted above. In most metropolitan areas, automobiles contribute by far the largest amount of air pollutants; in small towns, by contrast, significant levels of contamination may be caused by just one polluting factory.

Major Air Pollutants

Air pollution, of course, is no single entity; thousands of gaseous, liquid, and solid compounds contribute to the atmospheric mess. The nature of some of these substances is well-known while others are only now being studied and their threat to human health assessed. The most common and widespread air pollutants include 7 which the federal government has designated *criteria pollutants*, requiring the Environmental Protection Agency to gather scientific and medical information on their environmental and human health effects. These are the 7 pollutants for which National Ambient Air Quality Standards (*NAAQS*) have been set, specifying the maximum levels of concentration of these pollutants allowable in the outdoor air. The seven criteria air pollutants appear below.

Total Suspended Particulates (TSP)—TSP, often referred to simply as "particulate matter", includes all pollutants which occur either in solid or liquid form, including dust, soot, pollen, and compounds containing nitrogen, sulfur, and metals. Particulates range in size from pieces of fly ash as large as a thumb-nail to tiny aerosols less than 1 micrometer in diameter—so small that they remain suspended in the air and are transported on wind currents as easily as are gases. To many people, TSP and "air pollution" are synonymous, since easily visible dark plumes of smoke and soot or clouds of dust are the only forms of air pollution of which they're aware. Marked reductions in TSP levels in a number of urban areas in recent years have led many citizens to conclude erroneously that air quality is no longer a problem, since most other air pollutants are invisible.

TSP is generated by a wide variety of activities—fuel combustion, road traffic, agricultural activities, certain industrial processes, and natural abrasion. The most visible damage caused by particulate matter is the layer of grime deposited on buildings, streets, clothing, etc. Prior to pollution-control efforts launched during the 1970s, it was estimated that in the most polluted areas of big cities as much as 50-100 tons of particulate matter per square mile fell each month.[2] TSP can obscure visibility and corrode metals; most important, though less obvious, is the fact that when inhaled, particulates irritate the respiratory tract. Most dangerous in this regard are the tiny aerosols ("fine particulates") which, because of their very small size, can evade the body's natural defense mechanisms and penetrate deeply into the lungs. In recognition of this fact, USEPA in 1987 replaced the original standard for total particulates with a revised standard which applies to those particles with a diameter of 10 micrometers or less (PM_{10}) which are small enough to penetrate to the highly sensitive alveolar region of the lungs.

Sulfur Dioxide (SO_2)—The major source of this colorless pollutant gas is fuel combustion, inasmuch as sulfur is present to a greater or lesser degree as an impurity in coal and fuel oil. When these sulfur-containing fuels are burned, the sulfur is oxidized to form SO_2. By itself sulfur dioxide is not particularly harmful, but it readily reacts with water vapor in the atmosphere to form other sulfur compounds such as sulfuric acid, sulfates, and sulfites which irritate the respiratory system, corrode metals and statuary, harm textiles, impair visibility, and kill or stunt the growth of plants. Sulfur dioxide is also one of the main precursors of acid precipitation, recognized now as an environmental threat of major proportions and a subject which will be dealt with in greater detail later in this chapter.

Carbon Monoxide (CO)—No other pollutant gas is found at such high concentrations in the urban atmosphere as is the extemely toxic, odorless and colorless carbon monoxide. Any type of incomplete combustion produces CO, but the most significant souce in terms of urban air pollution is automobile emissions (in indoor situations, cigarette smoking is a major source of carbon monoxide). When inhaled, CO binds to hemoglobin in the blood, displacing oxygen and thereby reducing the amount of oxygen carried in the bloodstream to the various body tissues. Depending on the concentration of CO in the air and the length of exposure, inhalation of carbon monoxide can result in adverse health effects ranging from mild headaches or dizziness at relatively low levels of exposure to death at high levels. Fortunately, the health effects of short-term carbon monoxide exposure are reversible, but people who work for many hours in areas of heavy traffic (e.g. policemen, toll collectors, parking garage attendants) are obviously receiving substantial doses. Some evidence indicates that blood absorption of CO slows down mental processes and reaction time, raising the suspicion that many rush-hour traffic accidents can be at least partially attributed to low-level carbon monoxide poisoning.

Nitrogen Dioxide (NO_2)—Formed when combustion occurs at very high temperatures, NO_2 enters the atmosphere in approximately equal amounts from auto emissions and power plants. Nitrogen dioxide is the only criteria pollutant gas which is colored. The yellow-brown "smoggy" appearance typical of southern California on bad days is due to the high concentrations of NO_2 in the air. At high levels of pollution, nitrogen dioxide has a pungent, sweetish odor. At commonly encountered ambient levels, NO_2 causes lung irritation and can increase susceptibility to acute respiratory ailments such as pneumonia and influenza. Nitrogen dioxide stunts plant growth and visibly damages leaves; it reduces visibility and, like sulfur dioxide, contributes to the formation of acid rain.

Ozone (O_3)—The main constituent of a group of chemical compounds known as **Photochemical Oxidants**, ozone and such fellow-travelers as peroxy-acetylnitrate (PAN) and various aldehydes are considered to be auto-associated pollutants even though they are not emitted directly from the tailpipe into the atmosphere. Instead, these substances form in a complex series of chemical reactions when nitrogen dioxide and hydrocarbons from auto exhausts react with oxygen and sunlight to produce a witch's brew of chemicals dubbed **Photochemical Smog.** First observed in the Los Angeles area in the 1940s (the bright sunlight, warm temperatures, frequent atmospheric inversions, and heavy traffic make southern California particularly well-suited for photochemical smog formation), photochemical smog is now often observed in other cities as well, especially on bright summer days ("Ozone season" is considered to extend from May 1 through September 30). Ozone, an early and continuing product of the photochemical smog reaction, is the chemical whose presence is used to measure the oxidant level of the atmosphere at any given time. Human exposure to this pungent, colorless gas causes irritation to the mucous membranes of the respiratory system, causing coughing, choking, and reduced lung capacity. Heart patients, asthmatics, and those suffering from bronchitis or emphysema are at special risk during periods of high O_3 levels. Ozone also cracks rubber, deteriorates fabrics, and causes paint to fade. The eye irritation and watering of the eyes frequently experienced during smog episodes is caused not by ozone but by PAN, another member of the photochemical oxidant family. Photochemical smog has caused extensive plant damage, killing or injuring plants directly or increasing their vulnerability to attack by insects. A classic example of photochemical oxidant damage to plants can be seen in the ailing ponderosa pine forests of the San Bernardino Mountains, about 70 miles downwind from Los Angeles. The profound impact of photochemical oxidants on agricultural yields was highlighted in a recent report issued by the World Resources Institute which documents crop damage due to air pollution, primarily ozone, as costing U.S. farmers up to $5 billion a year. Crops most seriously affected include soybeans, cotton, winter wheat, kidney beans, and peanuts.

Hydrocarbons (HC)—Over 1000 different compounds containing hydrogen and carbon atoms in various combinations, hydrocarbons include liquid, gaseous, and solid forms. Most present little health hazard at existing atmospheric concentrations, although a few such as benzene or benzo(a)pyrene

Fig. 12-1   **CRITERIA POLLUTANTS**

Pollutant	Form	Major Source	Effects
TOTAL SUSPENDED PARTICULATES (TSP)	solid or liquid	Combustion, industrial processes	1. acts synergistically with SO_2 as respiratory irritant 2. grime deposits 3. obscures visibility 4. corrodes metals
SULFUR DIOXIDE (SO_2)	gas	Coal-burning power plants, metal smelters, industrial boilers, oil refineries	1. respiratory irritant 2. corrodes metal & stone 3. damages textiles 4. toxic to plants 5. precursor of acid rain
CARBON MONOXIDE (CO)	gas	Motor vehicles	1. aggravates cardiovascular disease 2. impairs perception and mental processes 3. fatal at high conc.
NITROGEN DIOXIDE (NO_2)	gas	Motor vehicles Power plants	1. respiratory irritant 2. toxic to plants 3. reduces visibility 4. precursor of ozone 5. precursor of acid rain
OZONE (O_3)	gas	Motor vehicles (indirectly)	1. respiratory irritant 2. toxic to plants 3. corrodes rubber, paint
HYDROCAR-BONS (HC)	gas	Motor vehicles, evaporation from gas stations, etc.	1. precursor to O_3 2. some types are carcinogens
LEAD (Pb)	metal aerosol	Motor vehicles	1. damage to nervous system, blood, kidneys

are known to be potent carcinogens. Hydrocarbons are included among the criteria air pollutants chiefly because of their role as catalysts in the formation of photochemical smog. Strategies to control ozone pollution focus largely on reducing emissions of NO_2 and hydrocarbons, without which ozone could not be produced. In addition to auto emissions, major contributors to hydrocarbon pollution include vapors from gasoline stations, oil refineries, and painting and dry cleaning operations.

Lead (Pb)—The harmful health effects of this toxic metal (see Ch. 7) caused it to be added to the list of criteria pollutants several years after establishment of standards for the other six. Since most airborne lead can be traced to automobile emissions, the major control strategy for this pollutant is to phase out the use of leaded gasoline.

Hazardous Air Pollutants

In addition to the criteria air pollutants, a large number of less common, but much more hazardous, chemicals are released into the atmosphere from a wide range of industries and manufacturing processes. Although the sources of these emissions are more localized than are those of the criteria pollutants, the fact that many of them are either toxic or carcinogenic suggests that they deserve more attention than they have received thus far. In 1970 Congress directed the EPA to develop a list of industrial air pollutants which can cause serious health damage even at relatively low concentrations and to establish protective emission standards for those so listed. No deadline date for listing substances as hazardous was mandated, however, and implementation of the Congressional directive has been exceedingly slow. By 1989 only 8 pollutants had been listed, with emission standards set for just 7 of these: *Asbestos, Mercury, Beryllium, Benzene, Vinyl chloride, Arsenic* and *Radionuclides* (coke oven emissions have also been listed, but no standards have yet been promulgated). Approximately 20 other toxic pollutants are currently under review. Environmental health advocates have long been urging EPA to speed up this evaluation process, listing and setting standards for additional toxic air pollutants which pose a special hazard to public health.

Impact of Air Pollution on Human Health

If dirty skyscrapers or sick ponderosa pines were the only consequence of polluted air, concern about the phenomenon would undoubtedly be considerably less than it is today. The unfortunate fact is, however, that over the years there has been a steadily growing mass of evidence indicating that the quality of the air we breathe has a measureable impact on human health.

Some of the ill effects of air pollution have, of course, been known for a long time: Los Angelenos knowingly curse the smog as they wipe tears from their burning eyes; motorists hopefully roll up their car windows in heavy traffic, trying to avert a carbon monoxide-induced headache; and asthmatics resignedly brace for an attack when the weatherman proclaims an ozone alert. For many years discomforts such as these were shrugged off as necessary consequences of economic growth, since smoke-belching factories were acknowledged symbols of prosperity and progress. Only after several air pollution "disasters" made world headlines did the general public begin to realize the extent of the threat to human health posed by dirty air. The great London smog of 1952 (see Box 11-4 in the previous chapter) involved the largest number of casualties, but it wasn't the first such episode. Eighteen years earlier a very similar scenario unfolded in the heavily industrialized Meuse River Valley of Belgium. During a 3-day inversion, 60 persons died of the foul air, while thousands of others became seriously ill, coughing and gasping for breath. In the fall of 1948, the small (pop. 14,000) Pennsylvania town of Donora, near Pittsburgh, fell victim to a 5-day inversion. Situated in a heavily industrialized valley, Donora was enveloped in a cold, damp blanket of smoggy air, permeated with the smell of sulfur. During this time, fully 42% of the town's population suffered eye, nose, and throat irritation, chest pains, coughing, difficulty in breathing, headaches, nausea, and vomiting. When the inversion finally lifted, it was found that 20 people had died during the period.[3]

The Air Pollution-Health Connection: Research Difficulties

In episodes such as those just described, it has proven impossible to pinpoint a single pollutant—or a precise level of pollution—as responsible for a specific health response. All of the fatalities during these air pollution disasters were persons who were already suffering from heart or respiratory diseases (though in the case of Donora, at least, many otherwise healthy people became ill during peak pollution levels). It has been difficult to determine whether air pollution can cause permanent damage to healthy people or whether at normally-encountered levels, air pollution presents any significant health threat. The problem in determining precise cause-and-effect relationships regarding air pollution and human health is due in part to scientific ethics: it simply isn't possible to expose the most vulnerable members of our society—children, the elderly, asthmatics, etc.—to high levels of air pollution and watch to see what happens to them. In addition, because urban air contains so many different pollutants, it is very difficult to determine with certainty which pollutant at what level is causing a perceived health effect. The likelihood that synergistic effects play a role in determining the nature of a health response to polluted air is a further complicating factor, as is the overwhelming importance of cigarette smoking—i.e. how much of an individual's respiratory distress is due to the pollutants in city air and how much is due to self-imposed tobacco pollutants? In spite of these difficulties, a substantial body of evidence regarding the health effects of air pollutants has been assembled from 3 basic sources.

Animal studies—using experimental animals to test the pathological effects of varying doses of a single air pollutant is common procedure for determining dose-response curves. Such studies provide a valid method of assessing cause-and-effect relationships and provide a way of determining precisely how a given pollutant affects the structure and function of the respiratory system—something which would be much more difficult to do with human subjects since in most cases it involves sacrificing the experimental animal and performing an autopsy. The major weakness of animal testing, of course, lies in extrapolating the quantitative results of such tests to human exposure levels, since animals may be either more or less sensitive to a given pollutant than are humans.

Studies on human volunteers—when conducted under controlled laboratory conditions, exposure studies on volunteers can be used to determine at precisely what concentration a given pollutant can induce an acute (short-term) health effect. Since such studies are almost always performed on healthy adults and are limited to short-term, reversible effects they are of limited value in predicting how more sensitive individuals might respond or how long-term exposure might affect public health. Such tests with isolated pollutants also ignore the synergistic effects to be expected when numerous intermingled air pollutants are inhaled. Nevertheless, such tests do help to quantify human responses to individual pollutants.

Epidemiologic studies—by investigating the distribution of suspected air pollution-related ailments within a relatively large population, researchers can study the effects of real-life exposures in various subgroups. Such studies are more realistic than controlled laboratory experiments in terms of actual exposure experienced by the general public, but they are frequently difficult to interpret because of the impossibility of controlling variables. In epidemiologic studies it is seldom possible to attribute an observed health effect to any one specific pollutant, and differences among members of the community in such terms as age, health status, socio-economic level, and smoking habits compound the difficulties faced by epidemiologic investigators.

In spite of the inherent shortcomings of each method, results of all three lines of research today are converging to provide evidence which strongly supports the need for government regulation of air pollution in order to protect human health.

Air Pollutants of Major Health Importance

Not surprisingly, air pollution's major impact on health is the result of irritants acting on the respiratory tract. Not all air pollutants are equally harmful, however. Research indicates that the most serious health effects associated with polluted air can be attributed to one of the following.

Sulfur oxide/fine particulate complex—various oxides of sulfur (SO_2, sulfuric acid mist, sulfate aerosols) acting in synergistic association with tiny particulate aerosols consisting of metallic oxides, nitrates, sulfates, etc., have been incriminated in more air pollution-related deaths and diseases than any other group of contaminants in the ambient air; the fatalities which occurred during the air pollution disasters described earlier have been attributed to this complex of pollutants. Although sulfur dioxide by itself readily dissolves in the mucous membranes of the nose and throat, acting as a minor irritant of the upper respiratory tract, in association with fine particulates the gas is carried deep into the lungs where, in combination with water vapor, it forms sulfuric acid and is highly irritating to the sensitive pulmonary tissues. Other toxic materials may also be transported into the lungs on the surface of fine particles, being deposited within the lungs or dissolved and carried by the lymph or blood to other organs of the body.

Photochemical oxidants—pollutants such as ozone and nitric oxides, related primarily to auto emissions, are not highly soluble and thus can travel deeply into the lower respiratory tract, producing acute irritation of lung tissue and, in the case of the most abundant oxidant, ozone, inducing a thickening of the walls of the alveoli (terminal air sacs in the lungs) where the diffusion of oxygen into the bloodstream occurs.

When polluted air is inhaled, both the structure and the functioning of the respiratory tract can be altered. Some of the ways in which air pollutants can induce illness include the following.

Inhibit or inactivate natural body defenses—the human respiratory system is well constructed to restrict entry of foreign particles and to rid the body of such intruders if they succeed in penetrating the first lines of defense. As a result, the approximately 10,000-20,000 liters of germ- and particle-laden air inhaled by a person each day are effectively cleansed by the time they reach the lungs. Particles are removed both by deposition and by clearance, the precise site at which this occurs depending on particle size. Large particles (those over 1 micrometer in diameter) may be trapped by nasal hairs or are deposited on the walls of the nose or throat, while smaller particulates generally escape these defenses and travel deeper into the respiratory tract where the slower air movement causes all but the smallest to settle out on the surface of the trachea or bronchii (the conducting airways). Upon settling, the invading particles are trapped by mucus produced by cells lining the airways. They are then swept upward by the constant beating movement of millions of tiny **Cilia,** hair-like projections of epithelial cells lining the respiratory tract. This mucociliary action transports dirt and pathogens to the upper respiratory passages from whence they are expelled by nose-blowing, coughing, sneezing, or swallowing. The tiniest aerosol particulates which evade removal in this manner and are deposited on the lining of the **Alveoli** (terminal air sacs) may be attacked and devoured by specialized scavenger cells called **Macrophages,** thus removing them from the lungs. Although not always successful, these defense mechanisms are extremely important in shielding the respiratory system from assault. Research has shown that exposure to certain air pollutants can induce health problems due to the effect of these contaminants on the body's natural defenses. When pollutant gases, especially ozone, NO_2, or SO_2 are inhaled, the action of the cilia lining the airways may be slowed down or halted altogether. At high pollutant concentrations, patches of ciliated cells may be killed and slough off; function of the macrophage cells in the alveoli also may be inhibited. Any of these effects greatly reduces the body's ability to withstand invasion from pathogenic organisms such as bacteria or viruses. Thus a common health consequence of breathing polluted air is increased susceptibility to infectious airborne diseases such as pneumonia or acute bronchitis.

Cause constriction of the airways ("chronic airway resistance")—exposure to gases such as SO_2 may result in a swelling of the membrane lining the airways, thereby reducing the diameter of the opening and resulting in more labored breathing.

Induce fibrosis and thickening of alveolar walls—ozone is particularly effective in altering the wall structure of the delicate terminal air sacs. When ozone comes into contact with sensitive alveolar cells, tiny lesions are formed. The breaks subsequently heal, but in the process scar tissue is formed. Lung tissue becomes thicker and stiffer, making it more difficult for air to penetrate and thereby reducing functional lung capacity.

Breathing polluted air has long been associated with the development of a variety of health problems—an association which even today is but imperfectly understood. As with any type of illness, individual susceptibility to air

Fig. 12-2

Human Respiratory System

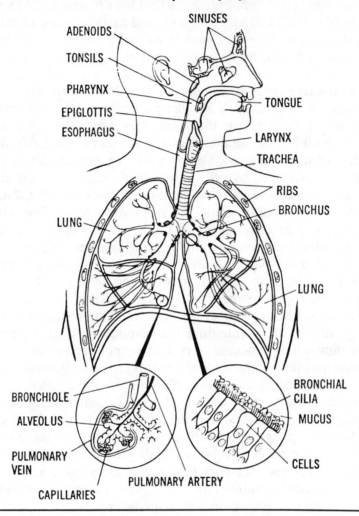

SINUSES

ADENOIDS

TONSILS

PHARYNX

EPIGLOTTIS

ESOPHAGUS

TONGUE

LARYNX

TRACHEA

RIBS

BRONCHUS

LUNG

LUNG

BRONCHIOLE

ALVEOLUS

BRONCHIAL CILIA

MUCUS

PULMONARY VEIN

CELLS

CAPILLARIES

PULMONARY ARTERY

Chronic Airway Resistance

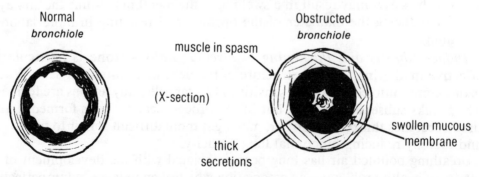

Normal
bronchiole

Obstructed
bronchiole

muscle in spasm

(X-section)

swollen mucous membrane

thick secretions

Source: American Lung Association, *Air Pollution Primer,* 1969.

pollution-induced disease varies widely depending on age, general health status, activity level, and genetic factors. In general, those segments of the population most vulnerable to the adverse effects of polluted air include the very young, the elderly, asthmatics and persons suffering from other respiratory or cardiovascular disease, smokers, and persons engaged in physical exercise demanding high levels of oxygen in the blood. Recent findings on the health consequences of air pollution include:

Death—the dramatic increase in death rates which occurred during such air pollution disasters as the episodes in the Meuse River Valley, Donora, and London provide the best evidence for a direct association between high levels of air pollution and an increase in human death rates. In each of these cases the sulfur dioxide/particulate complex appears to have been the prime factor accounting for the excess mortality. Investigations indicated that concentrations of SO_2 and TSP greater than 1000 $\mu g/m^3$ (3-5 times higher than current standards permit) are required to produce such death rates. Interestingly, follow-up studies conducted 9 years after the Donora episode revealed higher subsequent rates of both illness and death among Donora residents who had become sick during the 1948 event than among Donora citizens who did not experience ill effects at that time. Such findings indicate either that high levels of air pollution can shorten life expectancy or that people who are susceptible to pollution-induced disease may also be more vulnerable to serious illness.

Researchers have not been able to determine a well-defined threshold level of air pollution above which an increase in death rates is likely; however, they have observed that the number of deaths among cardiovascular patients tends to increase on days when pollutants of the SO_2/TSP complex reach high levels. A similar association, surprisingly, was not found with the photochemical oxidants, possibly because of the sizeable day-night fluctuation in oxidant levels.

It is more difficult to establish a connection between long-term lower-level exposure to polluted air with decreased life expectancy because of such confounding variables as residence time, smoking habits, pre-existing disease, and the like. Nevertheless, a number of studies conducted in various parts of the world over the past several decades point to an association between residence in areas affected by high levels of air pollution and higher-than-average mortality, particularly in regard to bronchitis deaths and sulfur oxide/particulate pollution.

Chronic Respiratory Disease—the development of long-term degenerative diseases such as chronic bronchitis and emphysema is a response to a cumulative complex of environmental insults, including childhood respiratory infections, exposure to occupational dusts, cigarette smoking, and the sulfur oxide/particulate group of air pollutants. Epidemiological studies pinpoint cigarette smoking as the major culprit but found that air pollution acts synergistically with tobacco smoke to increase the risk of chronic respiratory disease disproportionately among smokers living in polluted areas.

In addition to the connection between the development of chronic lung disease and air pollution, evidence is very clear-cut showing a direct association between high sulfur oxide/particulate levels and the aggravation of symptoms among patients already suffering from bronchitis and emphysema, victims feeling worse on days when pollution levels are high, better on days when contamination is low.

Acute Respiratory Disease—sulfur dioxide/TSP appears to induce not only chronic ailments but also short-term infections of the lower respiratory tract such as pneumonia and acute bronchitis in both adults and children. As in the case of chronic disease, the severity of attacks increased when pollution levels rose and eased as levels declined. It is assumed that the acute disease-air pollution association is a result of pollutant inhibition of the respiratory system's natural defenses against pathogenic invasion. Researchers theorize that the reason epidemiologic studies implicate only the SO_2/TSP complex and not the photochemical oxidants is because acute respiratory diseases are most common during cold weather when coal-burning pollutants are more prevalent than photochemical oxidants, contaminants generally associated with bright, warm weather. Laboratory experiments with animals show that high levels of ozone and NO_2 exposure can also predispose the respiratory system to pathogenic infections.

Cancer—although it is well-known that inhaled pollutants such as cigarette smoke, asbestos fibers, arsenic, nickel, etc., can cause lung cancer, it has proven much harder to assess the contribution of ordinary urban air pollution to cancer incidence rates. Here, as in the case of chronic respiratory disease, the overwhelming impact of smoking habits makes it difficult to distinguish the relative contribution of air pollution by itself to the development of a malignancy. While studies have indicated a higher incidence of lung cancer among urban as opposed to rural residents (the "urban factor") and while it is known that certain carcinogenic by-products of fossil fuel combustion such as benzo(a)pyrene and cyclopentapyrene (CPP) are commonly present in urban air, it has not yet been possible either to prove or disprove the suspicion that polluted air can cause cancer.

Lung Function—by causing chronic airway resistance, both SO_2/TSP, ozone, and, to a lesser extent, NO_2 can result in temporarily decreased lung function (O_3 and SO_2 in combination are particularly harmful in this respect). Reductions in ventilatory functioning are most pronounced when exposure occurs during periods of heavy exercise because a larger volume of air is inhaled at such times. Fortunately this type of damage is reversible and a return to near-normal lung function has been observed among affected persons when pollutant levels were lowered.

Heart Disease—due to its ability to bind to hemoglobin, thereby displacing oxygen and reducing the amount of this vital gas reaching the heart and other body tissues, carbon monoxide is the air pollutant which provokes the most severe reactions among heart patients. Studies have shown that more deaths

Box 12-1

Is the Air Safe to Breathe Today? Check the PSI!

In 1977 an amendment to the Clean Air Act required EPA to establish a national air monitoring network using a uniform air quality index. The Agency felt it was important to devise a method of conveying air quality data to the public in a way which would give people a clear understanding of how daily levels of air pollution might be affecting their health. Obviously, reporting levels in terms of micrograms per cubic meter for each criteria pollutant would be meaningless to the average citizen. Hence an interagency task force spearheaded by the Environmental Protection Agency and the Council on Environmental Quality devised a reporting tool known as the *Pollutant Standards Index (PSI)*.

POLLUTANT STANDARDS INDEX

INDEX VALUE	HEALTH EFFECT DESCRIPTOR	GENERAL HEALTH EFFECTS	CAUTIONARY STATEMENTS
401-500	HAZARDOUS	PREMATURE DEATH OF ILL AND ELDERLY. HEALTHY PEOPLE WILL EXPERIENCE ADVERSE SYMPTOMS THAT AFFECT THEIR NORMAL ACTIVITY.	ALL PERSONS SHOULD REMAIN INDOORS, KEEPING WINDOWS AND DOORS CLOSED. ALL PERSONS SHOULD MINIMIZE PHYSICAL EXERTION AND AVOID TRAFFIC.
301-400	HAZARDOUS	PREMATURE ONSET OF CERTAIN DISEASES IN ADDITION TO SIGNIFICANT AGGRAVATION OF SYMPTOMS AND DECREASED EXERCISE TOLERANCE IN HEALTHY PERSONS.	ELDERLY AND PERSONS WITH EXISTING DISEASES SHOULD STAY INDOORS AND AVOID PHYSICAL EXERTION. GENERAL POPULATION SHOULD AVOID OUTDOOR ACTIVITY.
201-300	VERY UNHEALTH-FUL	SIGNIFICANT AGGRAVATION OF SYMPTOMS AND DECREASED EXERCISE TOLERANCE IN PERSONS WITH HEART OR LUNG DISEASE, WITH WIDE-SPREAD SYMPTOMS IN THE HEALTHY POPULATION.	ELDERLY AND PERSONS WITH EXISTING HEART OR LUNG DISEASE SHOULD STAY INDOORS AND AVOID PHYSICAL EXERTION AND OUTDOOR ACTIVITY.
101-200	UNHEALTH-FUL	MILD AGGRAVATION OF SYMPTOMS IN SUSCEPTIBLE PERSONS, WITH IRRITATION SYMPTOMS IN THE HEALTHY POPULATION.	PERSONS WITH EXISTING HEART OR RESPIRATORY AILMENTS SHOULD REDUCE PHYSICAL EXERTION AND OUTDOOR ACTIVITY.
101-200	UNHEALTH-FUL	MILD AGGRAVATION OF SYMPTOMS IN SUSCEPTIBLE PERSONS, WITH IRRITATION SYMPTOMS IN THE HEALTHY POPULATION.	PERSONS WITH EXISTING HEART OR RESPIRATORY AILMENTS SHOULD REDUCE PHYSICAL EXERTION AND OUTDOOR ACTIVITY.

51-100	MODERATE		
0-50	GOOD		

The PSI system provides a simple, uniform method for local and state pollution control agencies to report daily levels of air pollution within a given metropolitan area and to relate these levels to general health effects which might be associated with such concentrations. The PSI converts the actual measured concentration of a particular pollutant to a simple number on a scale of 0 to 500. Intervals on this scale are related to the possible human health effects of the 5 major criteria air pollutants—TSP, SO_2, CO, NO_2, and O_3—as well as to a parameter known as Coefficient of Haze (COH). It also may show values for SO_2—TSP and COH-SO_2 combinations. On the PSI scale the 100 index value represents the short-term (24 hours or less) National Ambient Air Quality Standard for each pollutant. Thus any PSI value above 100 indicates that a violation of air quality standards has occured. The PSI intervals and their health effects have been established as shown on the chart on page 387.

The PSI index value reported is computed by converting the measured concentration of each air pollutant to a "subindex" value. The highest subindex is then reported as the PSI for that particular day. For example, if subindices of 95, 52 and 130 were obtained in Peoria, Illinois, for TSP, SO_2 and CO, respectively, the PSI for Peoria on that day would be 130 and the city's air quality would be reported as "unhealthful," with carbon monoxide being identified as the pollutant responsible, even though concentrations of the other pollutants were within air quality standard limits. If two or more pollutant subindices exceed the 100 value, then each of the pollutants in violation must be named. In large metropolitan areas where there are a number of monitoring sites, the highest single reading will be reported as the PSI for the entire area, an action based on the assumption that non-monitored areas of the community are also experiencing high concentrations (this conservative approach raises the possibility that one isolated pollution "hot spot" in a city could skew the reported PSI, indicating worse conditions than actually exist in the area as a whole; on the other hand, of course, an unmonitored area could have an undetected violation, in which case the reported PSI would be too low).

Public officials are expected to use the PSI as a tool in decision-making during health-threatening air pollution episodes. As PSI values rise, control actions such as restrictions on auto traffic, reducing or halting operations of coal-burning industries, and closing schools might be considered if weather forecasts indicate that prevailing conditions are likely to persist or worsen. Weather reports and media public service announcements are used to advise individuals with heart or respiratory ailments to limit physical activities and to remain indoors. Although the PSI is based strictly on human health considerations, local agencies might include reference to crop, livestock, or property damage at prevailing pollution levels when reporting PSI values.

Introduction of the Pollutant Standards Index system has made it much easier for the average citizen to obtain easily understandable and personally useful information on the quality of the air he or she breathes and has made it possible for regulatory agencies to obtain uniform, consistent, and comparable urban air quality data on a nationwide basis (e.g. a PSI of 110 in Chicago means the same as a 110 in Boston).

among heart attack victims occur during periods of high CO concentrations than at other times. Patients suffering from angina pectoris, a coronary disease in which there is an insufficient supply of oxygen to the heart during exercise, experience a much more rapid onset of pain during periods of increased carbon monoxide pollution. Preliminary investigations also suggest that ozone exposure can damage the fibers of the heart muscle.[4]

Fortunately, public recognition of the serious health hazards posed by air pollution have led to the establishment of air quality controls which have significantly reduced the high levels of contamination commonly encountered in urban air in former years. Although our air pollution problems are by no means solved, today in most parts of the United States and Western Europe it is very unlikely that another air pollution disaster such as that of Donora in 1948 or London in 1952 could occur again. For this we can thank the persistent efforts of a dedicated coalition of citizens and scientists who wouldn't allow the public to ignore the air pollution-health connection and the legislators, both state and federal, who had the political courage to impose mandatory controls on protesting polluters.

Pollution Control Efforts—The Clean Air Act

As air quality in the United States steadily deteriorated during the 1950s and 1960s, it became increasingly evident that a broad-based, concerted effort was needed to deal with what was increasingly perceived as a problem of national scope. Until 1955 any attempts to regulate pollutant emissions were based solely at the local or state level; in that year the first federal law dealing exclusively with air pollution offered research and technical support to states and municipalities, thereby initiating a policy of federal-state-local partnership in the pollution control effort. By 1963, worsening levels of air pollution generated pressure for more effective action and led to passage of the first Clean Air Act, which gave the federal government a modest degree of authority to attack *interstate* air pollution problems and which further increased the flow of federal dollars to state and local pollution control agencies. By 1965 recognition of the automobile's contribution to air quality problems precipitated the first setting of emission standards for automobiles and in 1967 the comprehensive Air Quality Act established a regional approach for establishing and enforcing air quality standards, though the main responsibility for control of emission sources (except for automobiles) remained at the state and local levels of government. This gradual transition from total reliance on state and local authorities to deal with air contaminants to an increasing federal involvement grew out of general recognition that the problems of air pollution were so immense, diverse, and complex that environmental improvement could be achieved only through intergovernmental cooperation at all levels.

Although such laws were well-intentioned, they relied on voluntary compliance by states, many of which were reluctant to adopt strict controls for fear of driving away industry, thereby forfeiting jobs and tax revenues. As a result, pollutant levels continued to rise and public outcry mounted. By 1970, spurred by a grass-roots demand that *something* be done about the environmental crisis facing the nation (a public outcry which culminated in the national observance of "Earth Day" on April 22, 1970), an historic turning-point was reached with Congressional passage of the Clean Air Act Amendments of 1970 (henceforth referred to here simply as the Clean Air Act). This landmark piece of environmental legislation provided the first comprehensive program for attacking air pollution on an effective nationwide basis. The Clean Air Act established a number of legal precedents which form the basis of the air quality control regulations in effect today. Among the most significant provisions of the Clean Air Act are:

- a requirement that the then-newly created U.S. Environmental Protection Agency (USEPA) set **national ambient air quality standards (NAAQS)** for the major air pollutants, since designated as particulate matter, sulfur dioxide, carbon monoxide, nitrogen dioxide, ozone, hydrocarbons, and lead. In setting standards, the EPA was instructed to review existing medical and scientific literature and to establish *primary standards* at levels which would safeguard human health, allowing a margin of safety to protect more sensitive segments of the population such as asthmatics, young children, and the elderly. These primary standards were to be set without regard for pollution control costs and were originally mandated to be attained by 1975; however, this deadline date for compliance was subsequently extended several times and finally was set at 1982 for most regions of the country, with extensions until 1987 possible for certain metropolitan areas having special problems controlling auto-related pollutants. In addition to the primary standards, EPA was told to set more stringent *secondary standards* which would promote human welfare by protecting agricultural crops, livestock, property, and the environment in general. No timetable for compliance with secondary standards has been set.

Fig. 12-3

National Ambient Air Quality Standards

Pollutant	Averaging time	Primary standard levels	Secondary standard levels
Particulate matter (PM$_{10}$)	Annual (geometric mean)	50 µg/m^3	50 µg/m^3
	24 hrs^b	150 µg/m^3	150 µg/m^3
Sulfur oxides	Annual (arithmetic mean)	80 µg/m^3 (0.03 ppm)	—
	24 hrs^b	365 µg/m^3 (0.14 ppm)	—
	3 hrs^b	—	1300 µg/m^3 (0.5 ppm)
Carbon monoxides	8 hrs^b	10 mg/m^3 (9 ppm)	10 mg/m^3 (9 ppm)
	1 hr^b	40 mg/m^3 (35 ppm)	40 mg/m^3 * (35 ppm)
Nitrogen dioxide	Annual (arithmetic mean)	100 µg/m^3 (0.05 ppm)	100 µg/m^3 (0.05 ppm)
Ozone	1 hr^b	240 µg/m^3 (0.12 ppm)	240 µg/m^3 (0.12 ppm)
Hydrocarbons (nonmethane)	3 hrs (6 to 9 a.m.)	160 µg/m^3 (0.24 ppm)	160 µg/m^3 (0.24 ppm)
Lead	3 mos	1.5 µg/m^3	1.5 µg/m^3

- EPA has proposed a reduction of the standard to 25 ppm (29 mg/m^3).
- A nonhealth-related standard used as a guide for ozone control.
- Not to be exceeded more than once a year.

Source: Information provided by the U.S. Environmental Protection Agency.

It is difficult to over-emphasize the importance of *national,* as opposed to state or local air quality standards. As experience prior to 1970 amply demonstrated, drifting air pollutants pay little heed to political boundaries, a fact which largely nullified feeble state attempts at improving air quality within their own borders. States or cities which *did* try to impose emission controls on polluters within their jurisdictions found that air quality gains were minimal due to airborne pollutants arriving from less concerned—or less courageous—states upwind. Threats by polluting industries to leave a particular state and relocate in a more lenient regulatory environment should controls be mandated made many state legislatures extremely reluctant to get tough with polluters. Establishment of uniform nation-wide standards has been a key element in improving air quality since 1970.

• *emission limitations for new stationary sources* of pollution (e.g. factories, power plants, etc.) were to be set by EPA. The intent in establishing **new source performance standards (NSPS)** is to reduce pollutants at their point of origin by ensuring that pollution controls are built in when factories and plants are newly constructed or substantially modified. Note that this requirement is not retroactive; that is, polluting power plants or factories already in operation at the time the Clean Air Act was passed are not affected by the NSPS guidelines. The new source performance standards are set on an industry-by-industry basis, taking into account such factors as economic costs, energy requirements, and total environmental impacts, such as waste generation and water quality considerations.

• tougher *emission standards for automobiles* and other mobile sources form an integral part of Clean Air Act requirements, inasmuch as 5 of the 7 criteria air pollutants originate chiefly from motor vehicle exhausts. Detroit eventually settled upon modified engine design plus installation of catalytic converters as the chief means by which American car manufacturers would reduce emissions (see Box 12-2). Claiming financial difficulties and the impossibility of meeting

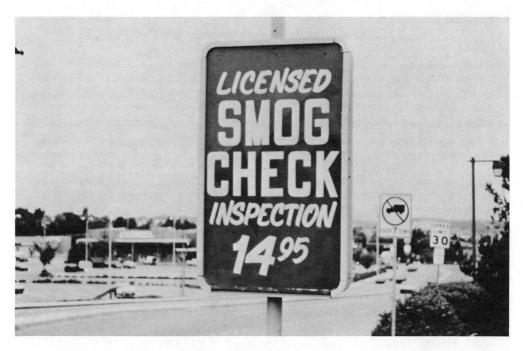

Auto emissions testing is now required in 64 urban areas in an effort to ensure that the pollution control equipment of in-use vehicles is functioning properly. [*Becky Anderson*]

the deadline imposed by Congress, the auto industry won several deadline extensions and a relaxed standard for NO_2 emissions. In spite of much foot-dragging on the part of industry, most new model automobiles can now meet federal standards and average emission levels are dropping. Attention focused on controlling auto emissions during the 1970s and early 1980s left unresolved the question of what to do about the sooty, odorous emissions from diesel-powered trucks and buses. Such emissions are of concern not only due to their unsightliness, but also because they include fine particulate pollutants which are possible human carcinogens. Recently USEPA promulgated strict standards for particulates emitted by heavy-duty diesel engines, beginning with 1988 models, and will require additional improvements for 1991 and 1994 model year engines.

Thanks to the Clean Air Act mandate, auto emission standards in the U.S. today are among the most stringent in the world. Canada, Japan, South Korea, and Australia have set permissible emission levels equivalent to those in this country and Brazil plans to match U.S. standards by 1997. Elsewhere in the world, regulation of auto emissions ranges from lenient in Europe to non-existent in many Third World countries. Even in the U.S., in spite of strict emission controls, further progress in abating pollution from motor vehicles will be difficult to achieve simply because of the enormous, and still growing, volume of traffic on American roads.

Box 12–2
Car Tampering Leads to Demand for I/M Programs

Much of the documented improvement in urban air quality since passage of the 1970 Clean Air Act has been achieved through strict pollution controls on motor vehicles—the prime source of carbon monoxide, nitrogen oxides, ozone, hydrocarbons, and lead. The device chosen by auto manufacturers to limit such emissions was the *catalytic converter*, installed in all non-diesel American cars since 1975. Within the catalytic converter carbon monoxide, hydrocarbons, and nitrogen oxides are burned at temperatures between 2000°-3000° F and thereby converted to non-polluting water vapor and carbon dioxide. Improvements in catalytic converters over the years since they were first introduced have made these devices highly efficient; according to the Motor Vehicle Manufacturers Association, the emission control systems on late model cars have decreased CO and HC emissions by 96% and NO_x by 76% below the levels emitted by vehicles without emission controls.

Unfortunately, the air quality gains achieved through use of the catalytic converter are now in jeopardy due to poor maintenance and illegal tampering with these devices by car owners who have removed their catalytic converters or replaced them with a so-called "test pipe" (dubbed a "cheater pipe" by state and federal officials). So widespread has the problem become that the EPA now estimates that 32% of cars on the road have been tampered with. In addition to instances of deliberate removal, many car owners are destroying the effectiveness of their catalytic converters through the use of leaded gasoline which poisons the palladium-platinum catalyst and pollutes the air with toxic lead particles.

That ordinarily law-abiding citizens by the millions are willfully engaging in practices which not only are illegal but also endanger public health is due to two serious misconceptions:

1. *catalytic converters reduce gas mileage and engine efficiency*—although some of the methods used by auto manufacturers to reduce pollutant emissions prior to 1975 did adversely affect performance and mileage, introduction of the catalytic converter solved this problem and newer model cars show great improvement in fuel economy. Late model cars feature engines that are computer controlled, with engine performance and emission control closely integrated. Thus replacement of the catalytic converter with a test pipe can damage the car's engine and in some cases even reduces gas mileage.

2. *replacing a catalytic converter with a test pipe and switching to leaded gas saves money*—although test pipes cost as little at $25 (compared to almost $500 for a catalytic converter) and leaded gasoline is a few cents per gallon cheaper than unleaded, over the lifetime of a car the owner actually saves money by using a well-maintained catalytic converter and unleaded gas. This is so because in this situation replacement time for spark plugs is nearly doubled, at least one less muffler and exhaust system is necessary, less frequent repair of other parts is needed, oil change intervals are increased, and less is spent for servicing the ignition and exhaust systems. Problems with leaded gasoline are likely to fade rapidly in the years ahead as USEPA's efforts to reduce the lead content of gasoline take effect. The current standard of 0.1 grams per leaded gallon (gplg) represents a 95% decrease from the 2.0 grams of lead/gallon in 1973 (unleaded gasoline, by definition, contains 0.05 gplg).

Because of poor car maintenance, use of leaded gasoline in catalyst-equipped vehicles, and car tampering, pollutant emissions from autos are substantially higher today than they theoretically should be given the percentage of cars on the road which were manufactured since installation of catalytic converters became mandatory. Studies have shown that removing the catalytic converter or rendering it ineffective through the use of leaded gasoline can boost HC emissions by about 500% and CO emissions by 400% per vehicle. These emissions have made it impossible for a number of metropolitan areas to attain the national ambient air quality standards for carbon monoxide and ozone, resulting in the threat of federal sanctions against such "non-attainment" areas. Penalties could include actions such as the withholding of federal funds for highway construction or bans on industrial development within the affected area. Recognizing that further reductions in auto-related pollutants in congested urban areas can be achieved only through strict transportation controls, regulatory agencies have promoted the adoption of auto *inspection* and *maintenance (I/M)* programs, whereby motorists are required to bring their cars to an approved testing station where a computer-linked probe inserted into the exhaust pipe measures pollutant emissions. Many I/M programs also include a tamper inspection and require that any missing or tampered pollution control devices be replaced before a car is certified as passing the test. Since the first statewide I/M program was instituted in New Jersey in 1974, 64 urban areas in 34 states and the District of Columbia have adopted this approach to reducing levels of automotive pollutants by ensuring that cars on the road have properly functioning pollution control devices. Today drivers in regions of the country still plagued by poor air quality accept the fact that they must periodically have their vehicles' emissions tested and, if these are found to be excessive, make any adjustments needed to reduce pollutant emissions to allowable levels. Now that the deadline for attainment of CO and O_3 air quality standards has passed, the number, size, and requirements of I/M programs may be altered as USEPA considers the potential for greater HC and CO reductions.

●a requirement for the development of *State Implementation Plans* (SIPs) gave state governments the primary responsibility for achieving and maintaining the national air quality standards. States must draft detailed strategies showing how they will reduce pollution levels to conform with standards in non-attainment (dirty air) areas and how they will maintain good air quality in those regions where pollution levels are already low. SIPs must list all the pollution sources within the state, estimating the quantities of each pollutant emitted annually, including both mobile and stationary sources. They must specify the emission limitations to be set for stationary sources, as well as timetables for compliance, and must include some kind of transportation control strategy for dealing with auto-related pollutants in areas of heavy traffic. States must have their SIPs approved by the federal EPA or be working with the Agency to improve a conditionally approved plan before they can issue a construction permit for any new polluting facility.

enforcement of the Clean Air Act is a prerogative of the federal government. Amendments added to the Clean Air Act in 1977 required the EPA to levy fines against facilities in violation of air quality requirements—penalties sufficiently stiff to cancel any economic benefits a firm might derive from delaying compliance. The Clean Air Act also gives citizens the right to file suit against polluters if the EPA fails to take action.[5]

Air Quality Trends

Deadline dates have come and gone, hot summers are still punctuated with ozone alerts, and a haze of smog still hovers over many of our cities. Nevertheless, nearly two decades after the Clean Air Act ushered in a "get tough" approach regarding air pollution control, overall trends are favorable. Although serious problems persist in many areas, American air quality is improving. A brief look at the situation regarding the 5 criteria pollutants measured by the Pollutants Standard Index highlights the present situation:

TSP
Installation of pollution control equipment such as electrostatic precipitators and "baghouses" or the enclosure of industrial processes such as stone crushing helped to reduce man-made particulate emissions by about 33% between 1975-1984. Ambient air concentrations of TSP dropped somewhat less, about 20%, during the same period, thanks to contributions from windblown dust, construction activities, and low-level fugitive emissions from factories. By the mid-1980s, the industrial Midwest and arid regions of the West were the areas recording the highest levels of TSP. In the nation as a whole, by 1985 only 145 counties were in violation of health-based primary standards for TSP.

SO_2
Sulfur dioxide levels had begun to fall even before passage of the Clean Air Act, thanks primarily to the transition from coal to oil and gas as primary fuels in this country. Between 1970-1980, SO_2 emissions dipped by an additional 15%, largely due to a shift from eastern to western coal, the latter

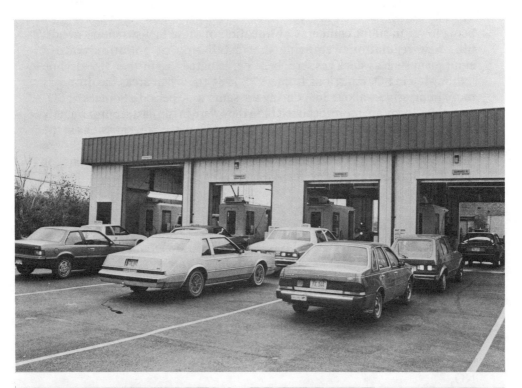

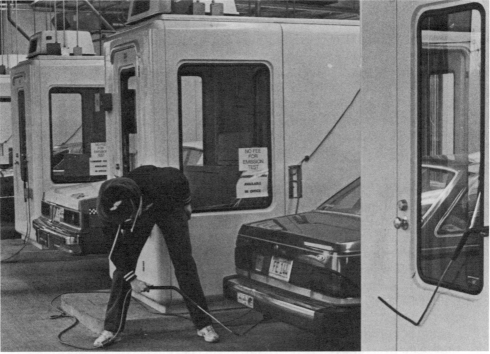

Inspection/Maintenance program: (a) vehicles await their turn for emissions testing in Chicago; (b) monitor inserted into tailpipe of automobile measures emissions of carbon monoxide and hydrocarbons. [*Illinois Environmental Protection Agency*]

being lower in sulfur content. Continuation of these fuel-switching trends, plus new regulations requiring the installation of pollution control equipment such as stack gas scrubbers, contributed to a further 16% decline nationwide in SO_2 emissions from 1975-1984 (in urban areas the drop was more impressive—about 36% during the same time period). Sources of SO_2 emissions today are more localized than they were in the past; approximately 200 large coal-burning power plants produce 57% of the SO_2 emissions in the entire country; in Western states, a relatively small number of smelters are the major SO_2 emitters. As these sources close, limit their operations, or install pollution control devices, violations of SO_2 standards will decline significantly.

CO

Imposition of auto emission controls, reducing CO emissions by over 90% from those of pre-1968 models, has resulted in a dramatic drop in the number of days each year when standards for CO are violated. Monitoring stations in heavily-trafficked urban areas recorded an 88% decline in the number of times the CO standard was exceeded at those sites from 1975-1984. Overall, ambient air levels of CO were down by about 34% during that time period. Nevertheless, 59 American cities still cannot meet the national standards for carbon monoxide, indicating the need for additional efforts to reduce levels of this troublesome pollutant even further.

NO_2

Trends for NO_2 emissions are more variable than are those for the other criteria pollutants. Nitrogen dioxide levels actually increased between 1975-1979, mainly because older model catalytic converters were not effective in reducing NO_2 emissions. Newer converters, modified engine design, and the use of lighter construction materials on motor vehicles, plus the installation of improved pollution control equipment on new coal-fired power plants, are helping to control NO_2 emissions. By the mid-1980s, ambient air levels of NO_2 were about 10% lower than they had been a decade earlier, and the Los Angeles region is the only part of the country that remains consistently in violation of federal standards for this pollutant.

OZONE

No criteria pollutant is proving more difficult to control than ozone. Although on a national basis ozone levels have been slowly declining, in 1987 68 urban areas had ozone levels higher than federal standards permit. Thanks in part to a record-breaking heat wave during the sultry summer of 1988, ozone readings in urban areas were at their highest levels in a decade. Unlike CO, which is a highly localized pollutant, ozone presents area-wide problems. Geographic regions most seriously affected at present are California, the Northeast, the Texas Gulf coast, and the Chicago-Milwaukee area. Several heavily populated regions, most notably southern California, have little hope of achieving compliance with federal ozone standards any time in the near future. Although its air quality has improved markedly since the 1950s, parts of the Los Angeles basin exceed the maximum permissible levels of ozone for 5 months out of every year (Los Angelenos are more fortunate than their neighbors South of the Border, however; in Mexico City, ozone levels exceed U.S. standards every day of the year).

The need for additional, more stringent efforts to devise transportation control strategies and to reduce evaporation from the industrial sources of volatile hydrocarbons which are the precursors of ozone formation is becoming increasingly obvious.

Fig. 12-4

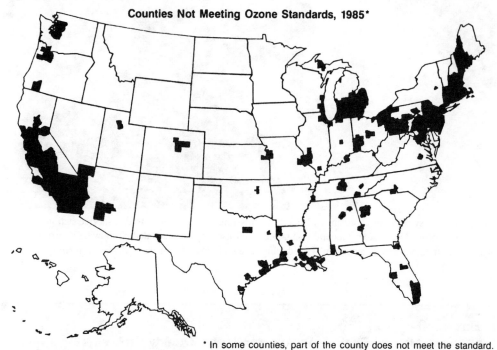

Counties Not Meeting Ozone Standards, 1985*

* In some counties, part of the county does not meet the standard.
Source: U.S. Environmental Protection Agency.

Overall, since passage of the 1970 Clean Air Act, air quality in most parts of the United States has improved significantly. In spite of population growth, increased traffic volume, and continued industrial development, pollutant emissions have declined and the number of days rated as "unhealthy" by the Pollutant Standard Index has dropped dramatically since the 1970s. Progress in cleaning up the nation's air has not been uniform—levels of some pollutants have dropped more than others and some regions of the country have experienced air quality trends better or worse than national averages would indicate. In some urban centers, air pollution levels are still high enough to constitute a public health threat. Nevertheless, the trends are encouraging; while declining levels of pollutant emissions are due in some measure to energy conservation, fuel-switching, and the demise of many smokestack industries, a large share of the credit must be given to the regulatory programs which have mandated significant investment in pollution control technologies. Although the battle to control air pollution is not yet over, progress to date proves that the Clean Air Act is working.[6]

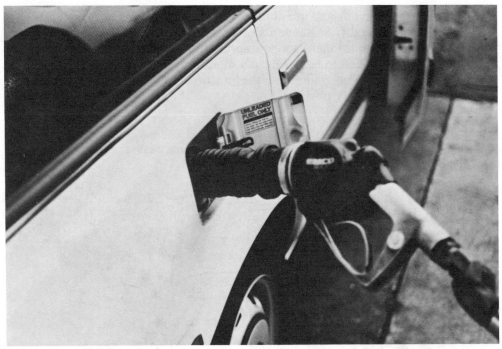

Vapor recovery systems for capturing hydrocarbon emissions are now being used at service stations in some cities where ozone levels exceed federal standards. Their use may be mandated nationwide if current ozone abatement strategies are unsuccessful in reducing levels of this irritant gas. [*Becky Anderson*]

Box 12–3
Alcohol Fuels—An Answer To Air Quality Problems?

The inability of many metropolitan areas to come into compliance with federal air quality standards using currently available emission control technologies is prompting a new look at the potential of alcohol fuels as a replacement for gasoline. Interest in such fuels first emerged in the 1970s when their use was promoted as a means of reducing America's reliance on foreign sources of petroleum while providing a boost to agricultural prices. With the phaseout of lead in gasoline, alcohol fuels appeared increasingly attractive as an alternative means of enhancing octane levels in gasoline. However, most of the discussion today about a shift toward alcohol-based fuels focuses on their ability to improve air quality, offering non-attainment areas a possible solution for avoiding likely federal sanctions for failure to reduce pollution levels sufficiently.

The two alcohol fuels most frequently mentioned as gasoline replacements, ethanol and methanol, though frequently discussed collectively, are actually quite different, both in terms of their characteristics and in their potential as alternative fuels.

Ethanol, sometimes referred to as "grain alcohol" because it is generally produced by distillation of corn, sugar cane, or sugar beets, is most commonly used in this country as "gasohol"—a 10% blend with gasoline (however, in Brazil, the world's largest ethanol producer, approximately one-third of all cars are powered by pure ethanol derived from sugar cane; the remainder of the Brazilian auto fleet runs on an 80/20 blend of gasoline and ethanol). While many advocates of gasohol use—particularly representatives from Corn

Belt states who view increased reliance on ethanol-based fuels as an economic bonanza for farmers—cite its advantages for improving air quality, impartial observers see no significant difference in pollutant emissions between gasoline and gasohol, which, after all, is only one-tenth ethanol. Although CO and HC emissions are somewhat less in cars fueled with gasohol, NO_2 may or may not be affected, and formaldehyde emissions may create a new emissions problem. Ethanol does offer a distinct advantage over gasoline as an octane booster; on the other hand, because it is water soluble, ethanol storage and transportation facilities must be assiduously maintained water-free in order to avoid contamination. From a supply perspective, there are definite limits on the extent to which ethanol could supply U.S. needs for transportation fuel. Currently ethanol comprises less than 1% of the energy powering motor vehicles in this country. It is estimated that the U.S. would have to devote 40% of its annual grain harvest to provide just 10% of the national demand for automotive fuel. Given our present resource base and worldwide food demand, it appears unlikely that we would decide to earmark such a major share of our total harvest to ethanol production. It has also been pointed out in numerous studies that the energy inputs required to produce ethanol (e.g. gasoline to run farm equipment, natural gas to produce fertilizers and pesticides, energy to ferment and distill the alcohol) are equal to or even exceed the energy output obtained from the final product. Overall, the prospects of ethanol replacing or supplementing the use of gasoline on the massive scale needed to improve national air quality are not particularly bright.

Methanol, by contrast, appears to be a far more promising option. Although commonly referred to as "wood alcohol" because formerly it was produced by the destructive distillation of wood, methanol today is derived primarily from the gasification of fossil fuels, primarily natural gas. Methanol has attracted considerable interest as an automotive fuel largely because its octane rating is even higher than that of ethanol—120 vs. 118 (compared to 87 for ordinary unleaded gasoline). Environmentally, cars burning pure methanol would have a very positive impact on air quality since they emit substantially less nitrogen oxides and hydrocarbons—the two major contributors to photochemical smog production—while their CO emissions are on a par with those of gasoline-powered engines. However, because methanol has only half the energy value of gasoline, its use outside polluted urban areas may be limited.

While most current methanol research is focused on the potential for totally replacing gasoline with pure methanol fuel (a change which would necessitate specially designed engines), methanol's main fuel use at present is as an ingredient in the production of the gasoline additive MTBE (methyl tertiary butyl ether), employed as an octane booster. Because it tends to separate when blended with gasoline and because it can damage conventional gasoline tanks due to corrosivity, methanol itself has not been approved for blending with gasoline.

From a health and safety standpoint, methanol presents some concerns which need attention before the fuel comes into widespread use. Corrosive, odorless, tasteless, and highly toxic, methanol poses problems of safe storage. Because methanol dissolves in water rather than floating on the surface like gasoline, the consequences of an accidental spill of methanol into a waterway would be very different from those associated with oil spills. Large-scale use of methanol hinges on the successful resolution of these concerns, as well as on development of the necessary infrastructure to produce, distribute, store, and market a new fuel. It also requires the production of autos designed to burn pure methanol and service stations to fuel such cars.

Nevertheless, if the admittedly significant technical problems can be overcome, methanol offers great potential to become a major transportation fuel in the years ahead. Produced from fossil fuels which are in abundant supply, methanol is already cost-competitive with gasoline and offers the promise of significant air quality improvements in areas grappling with ozone pollution problems.[7]

Acid Rain

While levels of the criteria pollutants in urban areas are gradually declining, another air quality problem which was virtually unrecognized and unmentioned at the time the Clean Air Act was passed is today widely acknowledged as one of our most serious and controversial environmental issues. The question of what to do about acid rain (more accurately referred to as "acid deposition", since the phenomenon includes not only rain but also snow, fog, dry SO_2 and NO_2 gas, and sulfate and nitrate aerosols) has become political dynamite, pitting region against region, nation against nation. To understand what the fuss is all about requires a brief look at the nature of acid rain, how it is formed, and the types of damage it causes.

What IS acid rain?

Rainfall by nature is slightly acidic due to its tendency to react chemically with atmospheric CO_2, thereby forming a weak solution of carbonic acid. Thus while distilled water has a pH value (See Box 12-4) of 7.0, a pH of 5.6 is considered normal for natural, unpolluted rain. Thus, by definition, any

Box 12-4

pH—Acid or Alkali?

The pH scale, ranging in number from 0 to 14, is used as a measure of the acidity or alkalinity of a solution. A value of 7.0 on the pH scale is neutral; increasing acidity is represented by falling pH values, while values above 7.0 are increasingly alkaline (basic). For example, a pH reading of 1 would indicate that the solution being tested is extremely acidic, while a solution with a pH of 13 is very alkaline. The pH scale is a logarithmic one; thus a solution with a pH of 4.0 is ten times more acid than one with a pH of 5.0 and 100 times more acid than one of pH 6. Since unpolluted rain is considered as having a pH value of 5.6, average readings of pH 4.1 in McLean County, IL, during the summer and fall of 1983 indicate levels of rainfall acidity approximately 50 times the normal value. The below-2.0 reading recorded in 1978 in Wheeling, West Virginia, represented a level almost 10,000 times more acid than unpolluted rainfall.

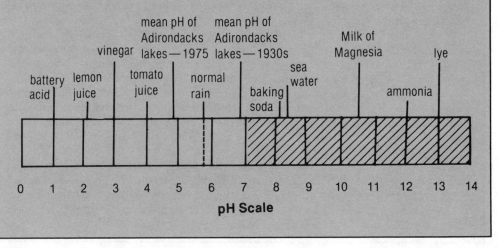

precipitation measuring *less than* 5.6 on the pH scale is considered acid rain. (some researchers who have been measuring pH levels in remote areas far from sources of industrial emissions suggest that the pH of unpolluted rain is closer to 5.0 than 5.6 and advocate a downward revision of what level of rainfall acidity should be considered "normal").

Extent of the Problem

Acid precipitation has been observed as a local phenomenon in the vicinity of coal-burning facilities for over a century. In fact, the term "acid rain" was first coined by an English chemist, Robert Angus Smith, to describe the corrosive brew falling on industrial Manchester more than 100 years ago. Only recently, however, has acid rain emerged as a regional problem, affecting areas far from the source of pollutant emissions. The alarm was first raised in 1972 by Swedish delegates attending the U.N. Conference on the Human Environment in Stockholm. After initial disbelief by many national governments, Swedish views about the extent and seriousness of this newly-recognized environmental threat have become widely accepted. On the basis of measurements taken during the past few decades, scientists believe that the pH of rainfall has been gradually dropping throughout large areas of both North America and Europe. Not only is rainfall becoming more acid in the affected areas, but the geographical extent of the problem is widening also. Early measurements of rainfall pH indicated that in the years 1955-56 only 12 northeastern states were experiencing acid precipitation. By 1972-73 the number of states experiencing average rainfall acidity below pH 5.6 extended over the entire eastern portion of North America, except for the southern tip of Florida and the far northern regions of Canada. In addition, acid rain was detected in several of the major urban areas of California and in the Rocky Mountain region of Colorado. Acid rain also affects most parts of Europe and has recently been identified as a serious concern in rapidly-industrializing areas of China. Indeed, although extensive monitoring has not been done outside North America and Europe, it is assumed that acid rain is a problem everywhere that coal and oil are intensively used.[8]

Today the average pH of rainfall ranges between 4.0-4.5 throughout the U.S. east of the Mississippi River; such values mark an approximately 50-fold increase in the acidity of precipitation within the past 30 years. Such average figures don't tell the entire story, however. Much lower readings have been obtained during some individual storm episodes, the lowest ever observed anywhere in the world being slightly under pH 2.0 (more acid than lemon juice) recorded during a 3-day drizzle in the fall of 1978 at Wheeling, West Virginia.[9]

Mystery of the Dying Lakes

During the 1960s and '70s fishermen, campers, and resort owners raised the first alarms concerning what was to become a major environmental tragedy. From the sparkling lakes of the remote Adirondacks, to the popular vacation-

Fig. 12-5

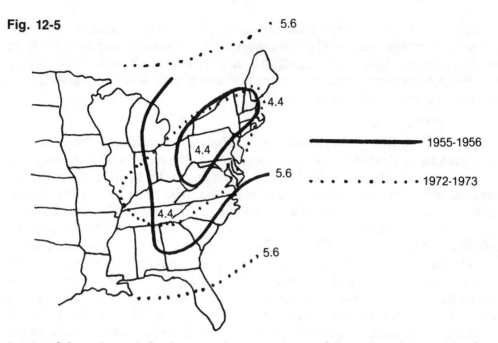

· 5.6

·4.4

4.4

5.6

4.4

5.6

—————— 1955-1956

· · · · · · · · · 1972-1973

lands of Ontario and Quebec, to the waterways of Scandinavia reports of the mysterious disappearance of once-abundant fish, amphibians, and aquatic insects began to generate public concern. The fact that such lakes and streams were far from any of the usual sources of water pollution which have traditionally been associated with fish kills only increased the bewilderment. To a casual observer the water remained blue and clear, uncontaminated by chemical spills or sewage overflows; beneath the surface, however, the affected lakes had become watery deserts, devoid of life. Today in the Adirondacks alone, 280 lakes once renowned for their trout fishing are devoid of fish; 2600 lakes in Minnesota's Boundary Waters Canoe Area are on the brink of suffering the same fate; in Canada 140 Ontario lakes are now fishless and the expectation is that within 20 years another 48,500 will be dead; 10,000 Scandinavian lakes no longer contain any fish and another 10,000 are threatened. Such lakes are acid dead, poisoned by pollutants falling from the sky in the form of sulfuric and nitric acid.

Formation of acid rain

Acid precipitation forms when its major precursors, sulfur dioxide and nitrogen dioxide, are chemically converted through a complex series of reactions involving certain reactive hydrocarbons and oxidizing agents such as ozone to become sulfuric or nitric acid. The reactions involved can take place either within clouds or rain droplets, in the gas phase, on the surface of fine particulates in the air, or on soil or water surfaces after deposition.[10]

Sulfur dioxide, one of the two pollutants primarily responsible for acid rain formation, is discharged into the atmosphere in amounts averaging 30 million tons annually in the U.S. Of this amount, approximately ⅔ originates from coal- and oil-burning power plants; the remainder is primarily from smelters and industrial boilers. A certain amount of SO_2 enters the atmosphere from natural sources such as volcanoes or mud flats, but such emissions contribute relatively little to the problem of acid rain; it is estimated that in the northeastern U.S. 90% of the sulfur in the air comes from man-made sources of pollution.

Nitrogen oxides, produced at the rate of about 25 million tons per year in the U.S., come predominantly from auto emissions, power plants, and industry. Unlike SO_2 emissions which have somewhat stabilized in recent years, NO_2 emissions continue to rise.[11]

So far as acid rain generation is concerned, sulfur dioxide emissions appear to pose the larger problem. It is estimated that about 65% of acid rain in the northeast is due to sulfuric acid as compared to only 30% from nitric acid (the remaining 5% is attributed to hydrochloric acid which may be emitted directly from coal-burning power plants and travels relatively short distances downwind).[12]

Long-distance transport

The aspect of acid rainfall which makes it such a politically-charged issue is the fact that the pollutant emissions which are the precursors of acid rain formation may be produced hundreds of miles from the regions suffering the effects of acid deposition. Because some pollutants can remain in the air for a relatively long period of time, they can be carried on the prevailing winds across geographical and political boundaries far from their place of origin—a phenomenon known as *long distance transport*. There are documented examples of acid rain-forming pollutants being carried more than 600 miles before being deposited on the earth's surface. Relations between Canada and the United States are currently under serious strain because much of the corrosive rainfall experienced by southeastern Canada (and by the northeastern U.S. as well) originates in the heavily industrialized Ohio River Valley and upper Midwest (fully one-fourth of all U.S. sulfur emissions come from Illinois, Indiana, and Ohio). Similarly, the acid rain currently wreaking havoc on lakes and forests in Norway and Sweden was produced primarily in central Europe and Great Britain. Such circumstances make the formulation of acid-rain control policies politically difficult because those bearing the cost of pollution-abatement strategies and those reaping the benefits are not one and the same. Illinois Congressmen, for example, are almost unanimous in their opposition to proposed federal legislation which would impose more stringent sulfur emission controls on coal-burning midwestern power plants. Citing the financial burden which would be passed along to Illinois electric consumers and the inherent threat controls pose to Illinois coal-mining interests, Illinois representatives are well aware that the environmental improvement achieved by such a measure would be enjoyed by citizens outside their own constituencies. Conversely, legislators from such states as New Hampshire and Maine, areas which have few large sources of emissions yet are suffering severe economic and ecological damage due to acid rain, have been among the most vocal in demanding regulatory action.

Ironically, pollution control technologies adopted early in the 1970s to reduce local levels of ambient air pollution had the unanticipated effect of increasing the long distance transport problem. The strategy adopted most often by utilities to reduce local SO_2 readings was to build extemely tall stacks which would discharge pollutant gases into the persistent air currents more than 500 feet above the ground. This approach was indeed effective in lowering local SO_2 levels, but it promoted long distance transport and thereby increased the scope and severity of acid rain in regions downwind. Although federal courts have declared use of these "superstacks" illegal, intense lobbying pressures from both utilities and the copper smelting industry has deterred EPA from doing anything about the 180 tall stacks now in use in the U.S.

Regional Vulnerability to Acid Rain

Although the entire eastern United States is now experiencing acid rainfall, not all areas are suffering adverse ecological effects, a factor which further contributes to the inter-regional animosity prevailing on this issue. An ecosystem's sensitivity to acid precipitation is determined primarily by the chemical composition of the soil and bedrock—an attribute referred to as the *buffering capacity* of that environment.

Buffering capacity refers to an ability to neutralize acids, the buffer acting to maintain the natural pH of an environment by tying up the excess hydrogen ions introduced by acid rain (buffering capacity is not inexhaustible, however; once the buffer is completely tied up, the pH will begin to fall). Regions such as New England, the Mid-Atlantic states, the Southeast, northern Minnesota and Wisconsin, the Rocky Mountain states, and parts of the Pacific Northwest are characterized by soils which are naturally already acidic or underlain by granitic bedrock; these areas are said to have a *low buffering capacity* and hence are very sensitive to the increased levels of acidity introduced by acid rain. By contrast, most parts of the Midwest, the Great Plains, and portions of the Southwest have predominantly alkaline soils and bedrock of limestone, giving them a *high buffering capacity.* This fact explains why states such as Illinois, which are currently experiencing rainfall almost as acid as that falling in New York or New England, are not suffering comparable ecological damage. It seems a cruel twist of fate that prevailing wind currents are transporting acid rain-forming pollutants to precisely those regions which are most sensitive to the harmful effects of increased acidification.

Environmental Effects of Acid Rain

Acid precipitation can cause a number of adverse environmental changes, the best-understood of which include the following:

> *Damage to Aquatic Ecosystems*—that acid rain can decimate the biotic communities inhabiting lakes, ponds, and streams in those regions where natural buffering capacity is low has been well documented in numerous studies. Most freshwater organisms do best in waters which are slightly alkaline—about pH 8. As lakes gradually become acidified due to steady

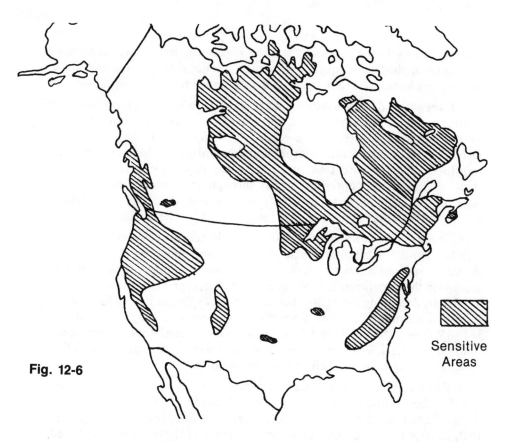

Fig. 12-6

Sensitive
Areas

inputs of acid rain, one aquatic species after another disappears. The first affected are the tiny invertebrates which constitute a vital link in aquatic food chains; at pH 6.0 the freshwater shrimp are eliminated; at pH 5.5 the bacterial decomposers at the lake bottom begin to die off, as do the phytoplankton, the producer organisms in aquatic ecosystems. Fish populations, the subject of most human attention, are somewhat more tolerant to increasing acidity; little change in their numbers is noticed until the pH drops below 5.5. Under pH 4.5 all fish species disappear, as do most frogs, salamanders, and aquatic insects.[13] Interestingly, falling pH levels seldom kill adult fish directly. The primary cause of fish de-population is acid-induced reproductive failure; pH values below 5.5 can prevent female fish from laying their eggs, and eggs which are laid frequently fail to hatch or result in the production of deformed fry (just as the early developmental stages of humans are the most vulnerable to the adverse influence of environmental contaminants, the same holds true for the larval stages of lower organisms). Interference with hatching is accentuated by the fact that the most critical developmental period usually coincides with the time of the annual snow melt when several months' accumulation of acid suddenly inundates the spawning areas in one massive dose, a situation known as *shock loading.* This large-scale reproductive failure leads to a situation in some lakes where the older fish grow larger and larger, thanks to decreased competition for food, and fishermen boast of their excellent catches until, with further increases in acidity, all the fish disappear. As a professor at the

University of Toronto succinctly states: "There is no muss, there is no fuss, there is no smell. The fish quietly go extinct . . . They simply fail to reproduce and become less and less abundant, and older and older, until they die out."[14]

Until recently it was assumed that acid rain's impact on aquatic environments was limited to freshwater ecosystems. In 1988, however, this assumption was shattered by a report published by the Environmental Defense Fund, a non-profit environmental organization, documenting acid rain-induced eutrophication of Chesapeake Bay. EDF cited evidence showing that nitrates entering the bay through acid precipitation were as important as farmland fertilizer runoff in stimulating the algal blooms which are degrading water quality in that important saltwater estuary.

Mobilization of Toxic Metals—contact with acidified water can cause tightly-bound toxic metals such as aluminum, manganese, lead, zinc, mercury, and cadmium to dissolve out of bottom sediments or soils and leach into the aquatic environment. Such metals, especially aluminum, can kill fish by damaging their gills, thereby causing asphyxiation. Acid-induced release of aluminum, even at concentrations as low as 0.2 mg/l, has resulted in fish kills at water pH levels which wouldn't have been lethal in the absence of the toxic metal. Toxic metals in the water also can bioaccumulate in fish tissues, making them dangerous for humans to eat.

Mobilization of poisonous metals also presents a direct threat to human health if the acidified lakes are a source of drinking water supplies. A resort owner from the Adirondacks testified before a Congressional committee that, in response to his children's complaints about the taste of water piped to their lodge, he had the water tested and found it contained 5 times the safe level for lead and 10 times that for copper. In other communities, acidified water which was originally free of toxic metals became contaminated upon passing through lead or copper plumbing systems—the low pH of the water caused corrosion of the pipes, resulting in leaching of toxic metals into the water. Homeowners who obtain their drinking water from roof catchments in areas affected by acid rain are also at special risk.[15]

Deterioration of Buildings, Statuary, and Metals—while it is extremely difficult to assign a precise monetary value to the impact of acid rain on materials, it is nevertheless acknowledged that the scope of the damage is large indeed. Most pronounced are the effects of acid deposition on stone and metal buildings and statues, on textiles, leather, and paint, and to some extent on paper and glass. Many monuments of great historic and cultural significance are today slowly disintegrating under the impact of airborne pollutants, of which various sulfur compounds are by far the most important. Corroding surfaces of the Statue of Liberty, the Washington Monument, the Capitol Building in Washington, D.C., Canada's Parliament buildings in Ottawa, and the Field Museum in Chicago all give evidence of the ravages produced by acid rain.[16]

Reduction of Crop Yields—the extent of acid rain damage to field crops is less clear-cut than with other types of acid-induced environmental damage, partly because few studies were conducted prior to 1979 and research on this topic is still considered to be in its infancy. Preliminary results indicate a wide range of responses, depending on the particular crop variety in question. Yields of some species appear to be diminished by acid rain, some are stimulated, while others show no change as pH levels of rainfall drop.[17] Since even slight reductions in yield can have a profound impact on farm economics, more research on acid rain and crop yields is urgently needed.

Damage to Forest Productivity—from the Adirondacks to the Green Mountains of Vermont to Scandinavia and West Germany's Black Forest, acid-laden rain and fog are contributing to death and reduced growth rates among an ever-increasing number of important tree species. Most affected are conifer forests at high elevations, frequently shrouded in acid fog or mist. At many sites above 850 meters in the White Mountains of New Hampshire or the Green Mountains of Vermont, over half the red spruce have died since the early 1960s. In Germany, the rate at which wide areas of forest have been similarly affected just within the past few years has been so dramatic that distraught German scientists have coined a word for the phenomenon—*Waldsterben* ("forest death"). Annual growth rings from trees in the affected areas show that the decline in forest vitality dates from the early 1960s. More recently, evidence of damage to deciduous trees at lower elevations, both hardwood and softwood species, has been documented.

The extent to which acid rain can be blamed for the decline of forests on two continents is currently a subject of intensive investigation by scientists in Europe and North America. While much remains to be learned, it appears that acid rain's role in the forest decline drama is an indirect one. Various theories have been advanced, including suggestions that acid rain may leach mineral nutrients out of the soil, ultimately leading to nutrient deficiencies in the tree which can increase its vulnerability to insect attack or other environmental stresses. Others theorize that pollutants in acid rain may kill the symbiotic fungi which live on tree roots, helping their host to ward off disease and assisting in water and nutrient uptake. Direct damage to leaves or needles by acidic droplets is a possibility, resulting in nutrients being lost from foliage faster than they can be replaced by root absorption. Some researchers suggest that ozone alone is the culprit, since it can damage chlorophyll and thus impede photosynthesis. Possibly the problem is due to the interaction of several of these mechanisms. Whatever the ultimate conclusions of the researchers may be, the extent and severity of forest damage now so readily apparent has increased environmentalists' conviction that we must act now to control acid rain before it's too late.

Acid Rain Controls

Since the early 1980s, a growing awareness of the extent and severity of the acid rain problem has led to increasingly vociferous public demands to "Stop Acid Rain!" through regulatory action. The primary focus of such mandates would be the coal-burning power plants which contribute the lion's share of sulfur dioxide emissions and about half of all nitrogen oxides (the remaining 50% come mainly from motor vehicles). Although the Clean Air Act imposes mandatory installation of pollution control equipment on new factories and power plants (i.e. "stationary sources"), nearly half the coal-burning plants in the U.S. were constructed before 1975 when regulations took effect and have no controls for either sulfur or nitrogen pollutants. Reports by the National Academy of Sciences and by the White House Office of Science and Technology Policy in the summer of 1983 concluded that a prompt tightening of emission controls is needed to avoid irreversible environmental damage and that reductions in SO_2 would result in directly proportional declines in acid rain (i.e. cutting sulfur dioxide emissions by half would result in a 50% acid rain reduction). Nevertheless, legislative efforts in Congress to require retrofitting of old polluting power plants with flue-gas desulfurization equipment (stack gas "scrubbers") which can remove up to 90% of the SO_2 were consistently resisted by the Reagan Administration, which insisted that more research into the causes and effects of acid rain was needed before imposing such a heavy financial burden on the utility industry. Aside from the political overtones inherent in the acid rain debate, evidence of the growing importance of nitrogen oxides as a major contributor to acid rain formation has added a new element to the debate. While scrubbers are very effective in reducing sulfur emissions, they have no effect whatsoever on nitrogen oxides. Several new "clean coal" technologies currently being demonstrated in full-size plants offer great promise in terms of reducing both SO_2 and NO_2 emissions simultaneously. Fluidized bed combustion, in which a turbulent bed of pulverized coal and limestone burns while suspended by an upward blast of air, and gasification/combined cycle, where coal is converted to a gas consisting primarily of hydrogen and carbon monoxide prior to combustion, both represent processes which would significantly reduce pollutant emissions and also improve power plant efficiency. As an added bonus, retrofitting old power plants with one of these clean coal technologies is cheaper and easier than retrofitting with scrubbers. It is estimated that repowering old plants with one of these newly-developed systems could cut NO_2 emissions by half and SO_2 by more than 80%. While general adoption of these technologies could provide society with an effective, economical means of solving the acid rain problem, government intervention in the form of mandated timetables will probably be needed to hasten the process.[18]

Indoor Air Pollution

While the attention of scientists, citizens, and government regulators has until recently been focused almost exclusively on problems of ambient air pollution, recent studies suggest that more serious air quality threats lurk much closer to home. It is now apparent that contaminants within private dwellings may pose a greater risk to human health than do outdoor air pollutants. In fact, levels of several health-threatening air contaminants are often significantly higher indoors than out. This is a particularly worrisome finding because the majority of people spend more of their time indoors than outside; thus their exposure to indoor air pollutants is nearly continuous. Such pollutants pose a special threat to the very young, the ill, and the elderly—the groups most susceptible to pollution's adverse health effects and also the ones most likely to spend long periods of time inside.

In recent years Americans' justifiable concerns about energy conservation may have worsened the indoor air pollution problem because thick insulation, triple-glazed windows, and magnetically sealed doors greatly reduce air exchange with the outside, effectively retaining and accumulating contaminants inside the home.

While most people tend to equate the risk of harm they might suffer from toxic pollutants to the total amount and toxicity of such substances, in fact the main determinant of danger is the dose actually received by the individual. Thus in reality large amounts of toxic pollutants such as benzene, formaldehyde, or carbon monoxide, for example, when emitted from a factory smokestack or the tailpipe of a car, pose minimal risk to the average citizen because they break down or are diluted in concentration before he/she is directly exposed to them. By contrast, much smaller amounts of the same chemicals, released in close proximity to individuals inside the confined environs of their homes or offices, have a quick, direct route into the body and hence pose a much greater overall risk of health damage. Studies carried out to date demonstrate that personal exposures and concentrations of indoor air pollutants exceed those occurring outdoors for all of the 15 most prevalent chemicals studied.[19] In addition, peak pollutant concentrations, as well as overall averages, are generally higher indoors than in the ambient air.

Some of the more common air pollutants known to be present in the home environment include:

> *Radon gas and its decay products*—when Stanley Watras started radiation-detection alarms ringing at the Limerick nuclear power plant near Philadelphia one December morning in 1984, he didn't realize that he was about to become a national celebrity, alerting Americans to a hitherto unsuspected menace within their own homes. The radioactive contamination that was detected on Watras when he arrived for work that fateful winter morning had obviously come from outside the nuclear facility, so Watras requested Philadelphia Electric, the utility company which owned the plant, to check his home in Colebrookdale Township. To everyone's amazement, tests revealed that the Watras home had levels of radon gas approximately 1000X higher than normal. Investigators estimated that Watras, his wife, and 2 young sons were receiving radiation exposure equivalent to 455,000 chest X-rays a year simply by living in their house. As officials of Pennsylvania's Division of Environmental Radiation hastened to determine the extent of the indoor radon threat, it quickly became apparent that the Watras family was not alone in its predicament. Throughout sections of eastern Pennsylvania, New Jersey, and New York, underlain by a uranium-rich geological formation known as the Reading Prong, thousands of homes exhibit elevated levels of radon. Nor is the problem limited to a few mid-Atlantic states—in the autumn of 1988 USEPA announced that their data indicate radon contamination problems span the country and urged that most homes be tested for the presence of

radon. While some scientists feel EPA figures overstate the number of homes affected, there is general agreement that indoor radon exposure represents a serious health hazard.

Box 12–5

A Hidden Menace in Your Home?

Radon detection businesses have been proliferating rapidly following EPA's announcement advising that homes nationwide be tested for the presence of this apparently ubiquitous indoor air pollutant. Concerned homeowners, deterred by the hefty fee charged by many entrepreneurs offering radon monitoring services, should be heartened to learn that they can purchase relatively inexpensive devices which will give a reasonably accurate indication of the extent of radon problems in the user's home.

The two most popular do-it-yourself home radon detectors are charcoal canisters—small containers of activated charcoal which should be opened and left in place for 3 to 7 days, then sealed and returned to the manufacturer for analysis—and alpha track detectors which are left in place for several weeks to as long as one year. Since radon levels can fluctuate considerably from day to day and season to season, alpha track detectors are good for determining yearly averages; charcoal canisters are useful for short-term screening tests, but since their results are indicative only of radon levels during the few days when the test was performed, they may over- or under-represent the actual extent of hazard over a more extended time period. Both devices, however, can be effectively used by non-professionals to give a rough approximation of radon pollution. If laboratory analysis reveals that radon levels are high, consultation with a radon abatement specialist would be advisable, but if the screening test indicates negligible amounts of the gas, the homeowner is saved the expense of contracting for a radon survey which might cost several hundred dollars.

Those interested in doing their own radon monitoring can improve the accuracy and relevance of the results by understanding a few basic concepts about radon. Because radon infiltrates into homes through the ground, basements are likely to exhibit the highest radon levels. For this reason, if residents want to know the peak concentrations to which they may be exposed, a monitoring device should be located in the basement (or lowest level of the dwelling), placed about 3-6 feet above the floor and away from walls, doors, or windows. However, if occupants spend little time in the basement and want a measurement more representative of the exposure they are receiving, monitors can be placed in living areas of the next highest floor. Another likely spot for monitor placement is near suspected sources of radon entry, such as sump holes or crawl spaces (however, don't use charcoal canisters in humid environments such as bathrooms and kitchens; the charcoal absorbs moisture and test results will not be accurate). Since monitoring devices are relatively cheap ($7-$12 each for charcoal canisters, depending on the vendor), it may be advisable to use 2 or 3 simultaneously in different areas of the house. Radon concentrations in most states tend to be highest in winter, so this is the best time for using short-term monitoring devices.

In many parts of the country, home radon detectors are available for purchase at hardware stores or supermarkets. Local health departments or state agencies also maintain lists of companies offering mail-order services for radon monitoring devices. Most states have no certification programs for radon abatement personnel; similarly, there are no mandatory standards which radon monitoring equipment or testing labs are required to meet; nevertheless, manufacturers may voluntarily submit their products or facilities for USEPA evaluation. Therefore, it's a good idea for those considering purchase of a radon detection device to check whether the company under consideration has passed the USEPA quality control tests.

Fig. 12-7

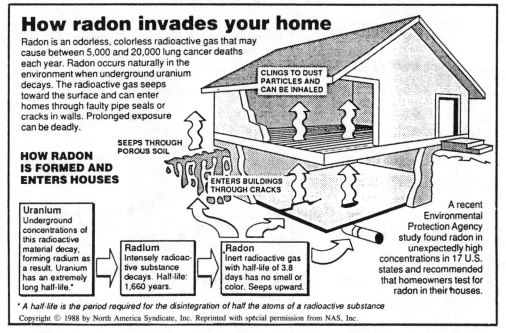

How radon invades your home

Radon is an odorless, colorless radioactive gas that may cause between 5,000 and 20,000 lung cancer deaths each year. Radon occurs naturally in the environment when underground uranium decays. The radioactive gas seeps toward the surface and can enter homes through faulty pipe seals or cracks in walls. Prolonged exposure can be deadly.

CLINGS TO DUST PARTICLES AND CAN BE INHALED

SEEPS THROUGH POROUS SOIL

HOW RADON IS FORMED AND ENTERS HOUSES

ENTERS BUILDINGS THROUGH CRACKS

Uranium
Underground concentrations of this radioactive material decay, forming radium as a result. Uranium has an extremely long half-life.*

Radium
Intensely radioactive substance decays. Half-life: 1,660 years.

Radon
Inert radioactive gas with half-life of 3.8 days has no smell or color. Seeps upward.

A recent Environmental Protection Agency study found radon in unexpectedly high concentrations in 17 U.S. states and recommended that homeowners test for radon in their houses.

A half-life is the period required for the disintegration of half the atoms of a radioactive substance

Radon originates from the natural radioactive decay of uranium. It is present in high concentrations in certain types of soil and rocks (e.g. granite, shale, phosphate, pitchblende), but most soils contain amounts high enough to pose a potential health hazard. Radon dilutes to harmless concentrations in the open air, but when it enters the confined space inside a structure it can accumulate to potentially hazardous levels. Since radon is a gas, it readily moves upward through the soil; small differences in air pressure between indoors and outdoors (very slight negative air pressure inside a heated building results from the "stack effect", created by air's tendency to rise whenever it is warmer than the surrounding atmosphere) cause the gas to seep into homes through dirt floors or crawl spaces, through cracks in cement floors and walls, through floor drains, sump holes, joints, or pores in cinder-block walls. Occasionally, radon gets into wellwater supplies and enters homes when water is used, particularly for showers or baths.

Radon is dangerous because it is radioactive, undergoing decay to produce a series of "radon daughters", the most troublesome of which are alpha-emitters, Polonium-218 and 214. These can be inhaled and deposited in the lungs where they constitute an internal source of alpha radiation exposure, increasing the risk of lung cancer. USEPA estimates that fully 10% of all lung cancer deaths in the U.S.—between 5,000 and 20,000 each year—are caused by indoor radon exposure. In some parts of the country where radon levels are unusually high, hundreds of thousands of Americans are receiving as much radiation exposure from radon in their homes as that received by the Soviet citizens who lived near Chernobyl at the time of the nuclear accident there in 1986. The extent of an individual's chances of developing radon-induced lung cancer depends on radon concentrations

Air Pollution   **359**

Fig. 12-8

Radon Risk Evaluation Chart

pCi/l	WL	Estimated number of lung cancer deaths due to radon exposure (out of 1000)	Comparable exposure levels		Comparable risk
200	1	440—770	1000 times average outdoor level		More than 60 times non-smoker risk
					4 pack-a-day smoker
100	0.5	270—630	100 times average indoor level		
					20,000 chest x-rays per year
40	0.2	120—380			
20	0.1	60—210	100 times average outdoor level		2 pack-a-day smoker
					1 pack-a-day smoker
10	0.05	30—120	10 times average indoor level		
					5 times non-smoker risk
4	0.02	13—50			
			10 times average outdoor level		200 chest x-rays per year
2	0.01	7—30			
					Non-smoker risk of dying from lung cancer
1	0.005	3—13	Average indoor level		
0.2	0.001	1—3	Average outdoor level		20 chest x-rays per year

Source: U.S. Environmental Protection Agency, *A Citizen's Guide To Radon*, August 1986.

inside the home and on the length of time one is exposed. It is thought that long-term exposure to slightly elevated levels of radon poses a greater cancer threat than does short-term exposure to much higher levels. Cigarette smoking has a synergistic effect in enhancing the radon/lung cancer risk by a factor of 10.

Historically, radon until recently was regarded as a health hazard only to uranium miners, so estimates of risk to residents of radon-contaminated homes have simply been extrapolated from standards set for occupational exposure in the mines. Indoor radon concentrations are measured as the number of picocuries of radiation per liter of air (pCi/1). Currently USEPA

Fig. 12-9

Points where radon can enter homes

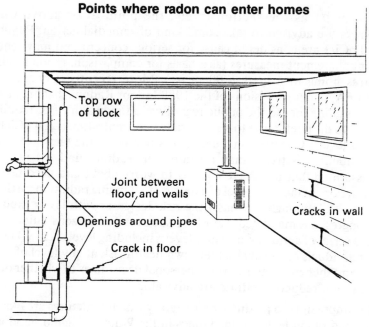

Top row
of block

Joint between
floor and walls

Openings around pipes

Crack in floor

Cracks in wall

Radon Reduction Methods

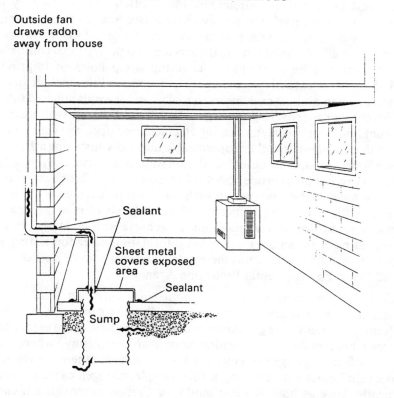

Outside fan
draws radon
away from house

Sealant

Sheet metal
covers exposed
area

Sealant

Sump

Source: U.S. Environmental Protection Agency, *Radon Reduction Methods*, August 1986.

regards 4 pCi/1 as the "action level", the point at or above which homeowners are advised to take some kind of remedial action. Readings above 20 pCi/1 are considered cause for serious concern and may require significant abatement measures (as a basis for comparison, radon levels in the Watras home measured 2700 pCi/1). More recently, Congress has directed EPA, under provisions of the 1988 Indoor Radon Abatement Act, to revise its guidelines to the public regarding radon health risks, requiring the Agency to drop reference to a single radon concentration (i.e. 4 pCi/1) as an "action level". Congressional concern is related to the fact that, under present guidelines, citizens may misinterpret readings under 4 pCi/1 as "safe", assuming that they have nothing to worry about and need take no remedial action. In fact, *any* level of exposure to ionizing radiation carries an associated risk, although obviously the risk decreases with lower exposure levels. Congress has mandated that EPA issue a revised citizens' guide which contains a series of action or guidance levels, including levels below 4 pCi/1, so that individuals can evaluate their own health risk at any level of radon exposure and then make an informed personal decision as to whether or not they feel radon reduction efforts are advisable.

Since it is impossible to predict with certainty which structures are likely to have elevated radon levels (some homes in the Watras neighborhood were essentially radon-free), the need for radon reduction measures can only be determined by actual measurements, which often can be done by the homeowner with relatively inexpensive devices (see Box 12–5). If test results indicate the need for some sort of radon remediation efforts, a variety of options are available. Most require the services of a professional contractor, though some can be as simple as covering sump holes or improving ventilation. More extensive—and expensive—possibilities include installing fans or air-to-air heat exchangers to replace radon-contaminated indoor air with outdoor air; covering any exposed earth inside homes with concrete, gas-proof liner, or sheet metal; sealing all cracks and openings with mortar, polyurethane sealants, or other impermeable materials; installing a drain tile suction system around the outer foundation walls of a house; or by installing a series of exhaust pipes inside hollow-block basement walls or baseboard to draw radon out of the voids within such walls before it can enter the living space. In structures with significantly elevated levels of radon, it may be necessary to utilize several methods to achieve sufficient reductions. Concerned citizens can obtain detailed information on radon testing and abatement matters by contacting their state radiation protection office or the United States Environmental Protection Agency.

Products of combustion: Carbon monoxide, nitrogen oxides, and particulates—these common outdoor air pollutants can reach very high levels inside homes where gas stoves or other gas appliances are used, where kerosene heaters or wood-burning stoves are operating, where auto emissions from a garage can enter the house, or where there are cigarette smokers. In homes with gas ranges, for example, nitrogen oxide levels are frequently twice as high as those outdoors. Carbon monoxide emissions from wood, coal, or gas stoves often exceed Clean Air Act standards for outside air. The growing popularity of woodburning stoves is a particular cause for concern, since wood is a much dirtier fuel than either oil or gas. Wood smoke contains approximately 100 different chemicals, at least 14 of which are the same carcinogens found in cigarette smoke. Cigarette smoking may constitute the most significant source of indoor air pollution in many homes; particulate levels may go as high as 700 micrograms/m³, far above the primary ambient air quality standard of 50, when there are smokers in a house. A study conducted by researchers at Harvard University found that household tobacco smoke is the main source of exposure to particulate pollutants for most children. It also demonstrated that whereas typical particulate levels in a home without smokers is 10-20 micrograms/m³, each smoker contributes an additional 25-30 micrograms/m³, more than doubling the base level amount.[20] Particulate matter and carbon monoxide are not the only indoor air pollutants generated by smokers—cigarette smoking represents the major source of human exposure to benzene, a known carcinogen and a listed toxic air pollutant. Nonsmokers living or working in the same room with a smoker are exposed to at least 5X the amount of benzene as those who work in the vicinity of coke ovens, the single largest industrial source.[21]

Formaldehyde—known to cause skin and respiratory irritation, formaldehyde is now suspected of being carcinogenic as well. A wide variety of household products contain formaldehyde, most notably urea formaldehyde foam insulation, particleboard, plywood, and some floor coverings and textiles. Levels of formaldehyde are particularly likely to be high in mobile homes where residents frequently complain of rashes, respiratory irritation, nausea, headaches, dizziness, lethargy, or aggravation of bronchial asthma. Within the same home, formaldehyde levels can fluctuate dramatically, depending on environmental conditions. A 15° F increase in temperature can result in a doubling of formaldehyde levels, while the lowest formaldehyde concentrations have been recorded on cold winter days; similarly, increases in relative humidity cause a corresponding rise in formaldehyde emissions. In terms of its effect as an irritant, there does not appear to be a threshold level for formaldehyde exposure.

The National Academy of Sciences estimates that as many as 10–20% of the population experiences some form of irritation due to formaldehyde exposure even at very low levels of concentration. The Consumer Product Safety Commission has advised consumers against using urea formaldehyde foam insulation, citing complaints from 5,700 persons who blame the product for causing various respiratory and health problems. A former Commission-imposed ban on such insulation was overturned in 1983.

Chemical fumes and particles released by numerous household products such as furniture polish, hair sprays, air fresheners, oven-cleaners, paints, pesticides, disinfectants, solvents, etc., can reach very high levels indoors. While relatively little research has been done on the health impact of inhaling these substances on a regular basis, it is known that several commonly-used household chemicals cause cancer in laboratory animals. Paradichlorobenzene, the active ingredient in moth crystals and many air

Fig. 12-10

Indoor and Outdoor Concentrations of Selected Toxic Organics

Bayonne and Elizabeth, New Jersey, Fall 1981

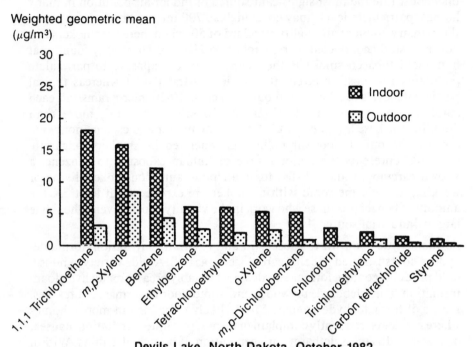

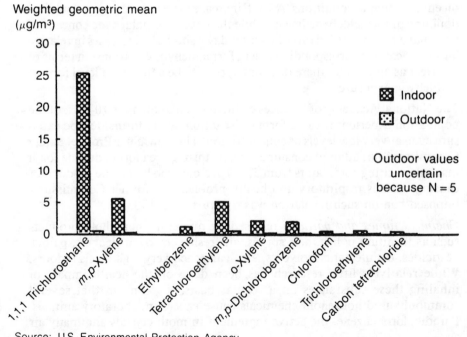

Source: U.S. Environmental Protection Agency.

fresheners and room deodorants, as well as limonene, another odorant, present perhaps the highest cancer risk among indoor organic chemicals. Tetrachloroethylene, a solvent used in dry cleaning, is another carcinogen to which household residents may receive significant exposure when wearing freshly dry-cleaned garments or by breathing emissions from closets in which such articles were stored.[22]

When used in accordance with instructions, most household chemicals are not known to provoke acute health effects. However, use of pesticides inside homes has occasionally resulted in a wide range of health complaints, including headaches, nausea, vertigo, skin rashes, and emotional disorders. Chlordane, which for almost 40 years was the most widely used insecticide for controlling termites, was recently taken off the market in response to hundreds of complaints about alleged chlordane-induced illnesses among residents following pesticidal applications in homes.

Biological pollutants—a diverse group of living organisms, most of them too small to be seen with the naked eye, can also pose serious air quality problems inside homes and public buildings. Bacteria and fungal spores can enter structures via air handling systems and occasionally cause disease outbreaks (the *Legionnaires' Disease* episode in Philadelphia in 1976 is the classic example of this sort of occurrence). Many allergies are associated with exposure to household dust which may contain fungal spores, bacteria,

Fig. 12-11 **A Day in the Life of . . . —One Person's Exposure to Respirable Particles, October 16, 1979**

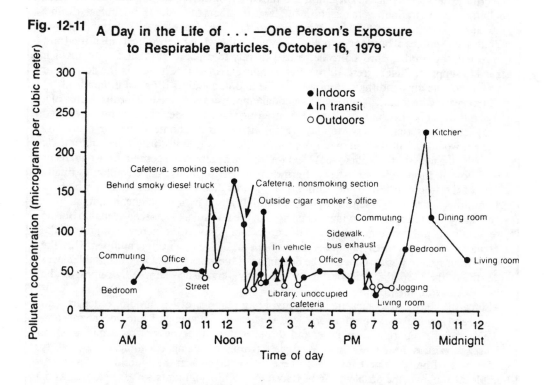

Source: U.S. Environmental Protection Agency.

animal dander, and feces of roaches or mites. Perhaps most significant in stimulating allergic reactions are live dust mites, tiny arthropods less than 1 millimeter in size which are found in enormous numbers on bedsheets and blankets where they feed on sloughed-off scales of skin. Humid conditions or the presence of stagnant water seem to favor buildup of large populations of these unwanted guests and their dissemination has sometimes been associated with the use of humidifiers or vaporizers which harbored fungal or bacterial growth.

Box 12–6

Sick Building Syndrome

"Faculty and students are working in an environment that could be detrimental or even fatal"—this allegation in a Hagerstown, MD, newspaper in December, 1984, frightened and angered parents of children attending Northern Middle School and prompted the PTA to demand that the 5-year old school be closed unless the situation was immediately corrected. The story which so inflamed public opinion originated with a report by a teacher who claimed that elevated levels of CO, CO_2, and SO_2 existed within the building, poisoning faculty and students. An investigation quickly launched by school authorities to determine the validity of the allegation and the extent of the problem found that although pollutant concentrations were insignificant, large numbers of students did, in fact, exhibit the classic symptoms of "sick building syndrome"—headaches, eye irritation, fatigue. While a few sources of outdoor air pollution entering the school were quickly identified and corrected, the problem proved to be related mainly to a poor ventilation system which failed to supply sufficient fresh air to several of the classrooms. Changes in the design and capacity of the air handling system were made and complaints dropped dramatically.[23]

In a separate incident, a group of white-collar employees working in a localized area of a large industrial facility had for years been suffering from a mysterious ailment they called the "Monday miseries". Every Monday evening after returning home from their jobs, many of them would fall ill with flu-like symptoms—high fever, chills, headache, and muscle pains. By the next morning they would feel well again, but the same complaints would recur the following Monday night. After suffering in silence for many years, employees finally brought the situation to the attention of plant authorities who identified the problem as "humidifier fever" (hypersensitivity pneumonitis) caused by microbial contamination of the humidification system serving that portion of the building. It was theorized that during weekends when the system was turned off, microbial populations increased rapidly in the stagnant water and were disseminated throughout the office area in large numbers when the ventilation system was activated at the beginning of the work week. Once the problem was identified, the "Monday miseries" were promptly vanquished simply by removing the humidifier from the premises.[24]

Since the mid-1970s, such incidents involving schools, office buildings, department stores, and hospitals have been reported with increasing frequency. Typical occupant complaints include reports of eye, nose, and throat irritation, dryness or reddening of skin, nausea, dizziness, headaches, mental fatigue, itching, wheezing, coughing, or respiratory infections. Although in perhaps 10% of these outbreaks, such as the "humidifier fever" example cited above, the problem can be traced to specific pollutants—e.g. microorganisms spread through ventilation systems, vehicle exhausts entering air intake vents, ozone emissions from photocopying machines, formaldehyde outgassing from wood panelling or furniture, carbon monoxide or particulates from cigarette smoking—these contaminants are seldom present in concentrations high enough to provoke the reported symptoms. Sick building syndrome, in the majority of instances, has been traced to inadequate ventilation and seems to be increasing in frequency thanks to modern building design aimed at energy conservation.

Unlike the situation in homes, most new non-residential structures are equipped with mechanical air handling systems and feature windows tightly sealed to restrict air infiltration from outside. Such ventilation systems recirculate air throughout the building, with a significant portion of the air being reused several times prior to being exhausted. The purpose of such reuse is to lessen energy costs for heating or cooling incoming fresh air. Building codes require that a specified minimum amount of outside air be provided in order to establish an acceptable balance between oxygen and CO_2 indoors, to dilute odors, and to remove contaminants generated within the structure. However, in some situations ventilation systems may be improperly installed, may have defective equipment, or may function poorly because of incorrect vent placement. When this happens, an insufficient amount of ventilation air will be supplied. In many cases, repairing or adjusting the air handling system to provide additional outside air will be sufficient to correct the problem; where this approach is unsuccessful, building design itself may be at fault. As investigations into the causes of "sick building syndrome" continue, information is begin gathered which will assist architects and engineers in designing structures which will be healthy workplaces.[25]

In general, the public has been slow to demand action on this problem because access to information about indoor air pollutants has been very limited and possibly because people don't want to believe that pollution problems have invaded the home. Nevertheless, an increasing awareness of the threat posed by indoor air pollutants has stimulated thinking on new ways of dealing with this recently-recognized problem. Monitoring and enforcing air quality standards inside 80 million American homes is obviously impossible. However, standards could be set to control pollutant emissions by modifying product design or manufacture. For example, the U.S. has set standards regulating emissions of formaldehyde from plywood and is considering regulating emissions from unvented fossil-fuel heating appliances; there have even been proposals to require catalytic converters on wood stoves! In the future, updated building codes which incorporate design features and materials which minimize release and retention of indoor air pollutants could ensure that most new structures have acceptable air quality. In the meantime, efforts must be made to educate homeowners and occupants on the impact personal behavior and consumer choices can have on the quality of the indoor environment. Decisions as to which products we buy, how we use certain appliances, our consideration for the health of others as reflected in personal smoking habits—all have a profound impact on indoor air quality and will ultimately determine the success or failure of any government effort to minimize indoor air pollution.[26]

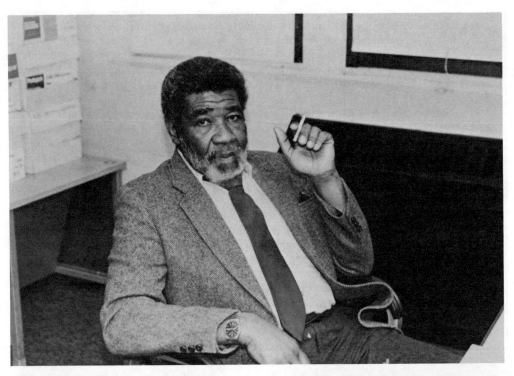

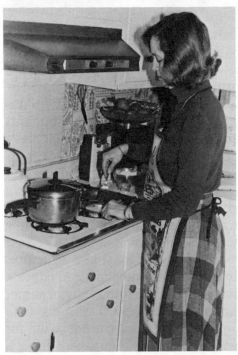
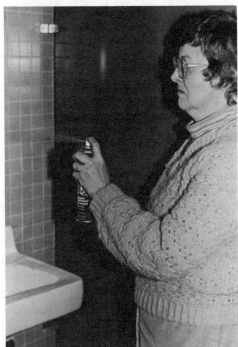

Sources of indoor air pollution: (a) cigarette smoking contaminates indoor air with levels of carbon monoxide and particulates far in excess of those found in outdoor air; (b) gas cooking ranges are an indoor source of both carbon monoxide and nitrogen oxides; (c) household chemicals, such as air fresheners and pesticide sprays, expose occupants to potential carcinogens and toxins. [*Author's Photos*]

Box 12–7

Preventing Future "Bhopals"

When 8000 unsuspecting citizens of Bhopal, India, died in agony and 300,000 others suffered debilitating injuries after a toxic cloud descended on their community, people in thousands of other cities wondered if they, too, might be living in close proximity to a chemical "time bomb". The accidental release of poisonous methyl isocyanate gas from Bhopal's Union Carbide pesticide-manufacturing plant on Dec. 3, 1984, represented history's worst-ever industrial accident. It would be comforting to assume that the disaster signified an isolated event in a Third World country where safety regulations are less stringently enforced than they are in the U.S., but the facts supply little such reassurance. If anything good can be said to have resulted from the tragedy at Bhopal, it is the recognition by policymakers and public alike of the potential for toxic accidents anywhere, anytime, and the need for contingency planning to deal with such emergencies should they occur. And toxic accidents *do* occur. Just 9 months after the Bhopal accident, a Union Carbide facility at Institute, West Virginia, experienced an accidental release of toxic fumes which caused 135 local residents to suffer nausea, dizziness, eye irritation, and breathing difficulties. In January of 1986, 2 people were killed and 18 injured in Ashtabula, Ohio, when a tank at Diamond-Shamrock's paint pigment plant exploded.

The U.S. Dept. of Transportation documents an average of nearly 11,500 transportation accidents involving hazardous materials every year and estimates that perhaps four times that many go unreported. Approximately a thousand of these accidents annually result in the release of toxic substances into the air—most commonly chemicals like chlorine gas, hydrochloric acid, or anhydrous ammonia—but sometimes including such extraordinarily hazardous substances as hydrogen cyanide, hydrogen fluoride, phosphorus trichloride, allyl chloride, hydrogen sulfide, bromine, or phosgene. In some cases these releases have presented a serious enough danger to necessitate large-scale evacuations. Between 1980-1986, approximately 60 incidents occurred in the U.S. that required the evacuation of 100 or more people.

Fortunately, loss of life due to accidental chemical releases in this country has been low thus far, but officials acknowledge that, until recently, contingency planning for technological hazards (as opposed to natural disasters such as floods or tornadoes) was entirely neglected. Admittedly, it is very difficult to prepare for airborne toxic releases—they can happen without warning, frequently involve substances which cause immediate death or illness, and can occur virtually anywhere, originating from fixed sites such as factories or from mobile sources such as trains or trucks. To a greater degree than would be the case with chemical spills into waterways or onto the ground, accidental releases into the air may require public evacuation, yet prior identification of the population at risk is difficult because the affected population is determined by the location of the release, time of day, weather conditions, direction of prevailing wind, and type of substance released. When Bhopal hit the headlines in 1984, it is doubtful that community leaders in the United States, faced with a similar disaster, would have responded any more effectively than did hard-pressed Indian officials. Thwarted by a paucity of basic information on exactly what toxic hazards existed in their midst, with virtually no prior experience in dealing with such incidents, and having scanty knowledge of how residents or those in positions of authority would be likely to react in an emergency situation, public officials could offer little reassurance to concerned citizens that they were prepared to deal with a "Bhopal" in their jurisdiction.

A major step toward overcoming these obstacles and improving communities' ability to deal more effectively with chemical accidents was taken with 1986 passage of **Title III: The Emergency Planning and Community Right-to-Know Act** (a portion of the Superfund

Amendments and Reauthorization Act). The provisions of this landmark piece of legislation should help local authorities improve contingency planning considerably by supplying badly-needed information on the nature and amounts of toxic materials manufactured, used, stored, or transported within their municipal boundaries. Provisions in Title III which should significantly enhance the ability of communities across America to deal more effectively with chemical accidents include:

1. Emergency Planning—state emergency planning commissions and local emergency planning committees with broad-based membership must be formed to develop and implement an emergency response plan; such plans were to be in place by 1988.
2. Emergency Notification—owners and operators of facilities where toxic chemicals are present must notify both the state commission and the local committees of any chemical release (above a certain level) into the environment.
3. Community Right-to-Know Reporting—facility owners and operators must provide information to the state and local committee and to the local fire department regarding the amounts, types, and general location of any toxic chemicals which they manufacture, use, or store at the site. They must supply material safety data sheets on every chemical in their inventory and must make this information available, upon request, to the general public.
4. Emissions and Release Reporting—owners/operators of large facilities must annually submit forms to USEPA, detailing any toxic chemical releases from that plant. EPA, in turn, is required to compile this information and make it available to the public through a computerized data base.

It is hoped that the information amassed through these new requirements will enhance the public's awareness and understanding of the chemical hazards present in their own communities and will provide local officials with the data they need for developing sound emergency preparedness plans to deal with potential airborne toxic releases.[27]

REFERENCES

[1]Evelyn, John, *Fumifugium,* (1661), London National Society for Clean Air, 1969.

[2]*Air Pollution Primer,* National Tuberculosis and Respiratory Disease Association, 1969.

[3]Waldbott, George L., *Health Effects of Environmental Pollutants,* C.V. Mosby Company, 1978.

[4]*Health Effects of Air Pollution,* American Thoracic Society, 1978.

[5]Sheiman, Deborah A., *Blueprint for Clean Air,* League of Women Voters Education Fund, Pub. No. 222, 1981.

[6]*"State of the Environment: A View Toward the Nineties",* The Conservation Foundation, 1987.

[7]Hornbeck, Ethel S., *"Alcohol Fuels: Environmental Impacts, Economics, and Policy Implications",* Petroleum Marketers Association of America, July 1987.

[8]*"Acid Rain: an unwelcome export",* UNESCO Courier, January 1985.

[9]Boyle, Robert, and R. Alexander Boyle, *Acid Rain,* Schocken Books/Nick Lyons Books, 1983.

[10]Rhodes, S.L., and P. Middleton, "The Complex Challenge of Controlling Acid Rain", *Environment,* vol. 25, no. 4, May 1983.

[11]Boyle et al., op. cit.

[12]Babich, Harvey, Debra Lee Davis, and Guenther Stotzky, "Acid Precipitation: Causes and Consequences", *Environment,* vol. 22, no. 4, May 1980.

[13]*Acid Rain: What It Is,* National Wildlife Federation, 1982.

[14]Weller, Phil, *Acid Rain: The Silent Crisis,* Between the Lines & the Waterloo Public Interest Research Group, 1980.

[15]Boyle et al., op. cit.

[16]Scholle, Stephen R., "Acid Deposition and the Materials Damage Question", *Environment,* vol. 25, no. 8, October 1983.

[17]Cohen, C.J., L.C. Grothaus, and S.C. Perrigan, "Effects of Simulated Sulfuric and Sulfuric-Nitric Acid Rain on Crop Plants: Results of 1980 Crop Survey", Special Report 670, Agricultural Experiment Station, Oregon State University, Corvallis, 1982.

[18]Mohnen, Volker A., "The Challenge of Acid Rain", *Scientific American,* vol. 259, no. 2, August 1988.

[19]Wallace, L.A., *Total Exposure Assessment Methodology (TEAM) Study: Summary and Analysis,* vol. 1, USEPA, 1987.

[20]Ware, J.H., et al., "Passive Smoking, Gas Cooking, and Respiratory Health of Children Living in Six Cities", *American Review of Respiratory Disease,* vol. 129, 1984, pp. 366–374.

[21]Smith, Kirk R., "Air Pollution: Assessing Total Exposure in the United States", *Environment,* vol. 30, no. 8, October 1988.

[22]Smith, op. cit.

[23]Helsing, Knud J., Charles E. Billings, and Jose Conde, "Cure of a Sick Building: A Case Study", *Indoor Air '87,* Proceedings of the 4th International Conference on Indoor Air Quality and Climate, Berlin (West), 17–21 August, 1987.

[24]Ganier, Mitchell, Phil Lieberman, Jordan Fink, and Dudley G. Lockwood, "Humidifier Lung: An Outbreak in Office Workers", *Chest,* 77:2, February 1980.

[25]Turiel, Isaac, *Indoor Air Quality and Human Health,* Stanford University Press, 1985.

[26]Nero, Anthony V., Jr., "Controlling Indoor Air Pollution", *Scientific American,* vol. 258, no. 5, May 1988.

[27]Kurzman, Dan, *"A Killing Wind: Inside Union Carbide and the Bhopal Catastrophe",* McGraw-Hill, 1987; Cutter, Susan L., "Airborne Toxic Releases: Are Communities Prepared?", *Environment,* vol. 29, no. 6, July/August 1987.

13
Noise Pollution

"An inability to stay quiet .... is one of the most conspicuous failings of mankind."
Bagehot, *Physics and Politics,* 1876

A few years ago a Gallup poll taken among urban residents revealed that most city dwellers view excessive noise as second only to water pollution among the environmental issues of greatest concern to them. In fact, these respondents ranked quiet surroundings on a par with low crime rate, friendly people, and good housing as qualities defining an ideal neighborhood. Quiet was considered more important than cleanliness, good schools, low traffic volume, and easily accessible shopping areas among those questioned;[1] another survey conducted annually for the U.S. Department of Housing and Urban Development found that central city residents more often name noise as an undesirable feature of their own neighborhoods than any other single characteristic. Noise, along with crime, was cited as one of the two major conditions which caused people to wish to move to another part of town.[2]

Sources of Noise

The noise which so bothers the city dwellers mentioned above is all-pervasive in modern life and is by no means restricted to urban centers, though noise levels in high-density metropolitan areas are consistently higher than in most suburbs or rural areas. The sources of noise are extremely varied and have been rapidly increasing in number during the past two decades as more cars, trucks, and motorcycles crowd our streets and highways, as more noise-generating

Fig. 13-1

Examples of Outdoor Day-Night Average Sound Levels in dB Measured at Various Locations

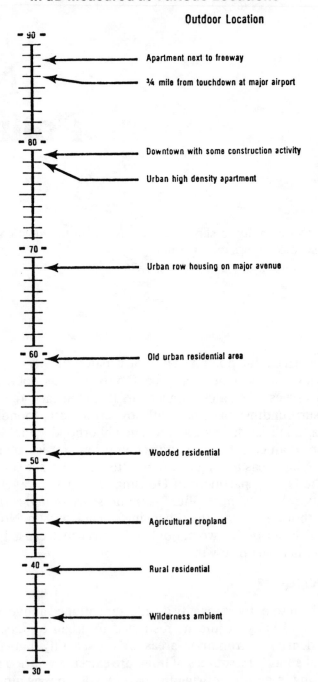

Outdoor Location

- 90 -
Apartment next to freeway
¾ mile from touchdown at major airport

- 80 -
Downtown with some construction activity
Urban high density apartment

- 70 -
Urban row housing on major avenue

- 60 -
Old urban residential area

Wooded residential
- 50 -

Agricultural cropland

- 40 -
Rural residential

Wilderness ambient

- 30 -

Source: U.S. Environmental Protection Agency, *Protective Noise Levels,* EPA 550/9-79-100, November 1978.

home appliances and motorized yard tools are purchased, and as sales of office and factory equipment boom. Although most people perceive community noise as a general din, originating from a multiplicity of sources, vehicular noise—particularly noise from motorcycles and large trucks—seems to be the source of noise most frequently perceived as annoying by community residents. Unfortunately, over-all noise levels are getting worse, in part because most machines are now more powerful than they were formerly and also because American lifestyles and transportation habits are changing in ways which inevitably result in more noise generation. We are also carrying noise with us to places which formerly were havens of peace and quiet. The advent of snowmobiles, trail bikes, and powerful motorboats have brought noise pollution to once-tranquil wilderness areas; amplified music now jars city parks when partying crowds forget that not everyone finds loud rock bands pleasureable; the increasing popularity of jet travel in preference to trains now subjects millions of people living near airports to ear-splitting levels of noise on a continual daily basis.

For the most part, levels of outdoor noise are directly related to population density—the larger the city, the noisier conditions are likely to be. Figure 13–1 gives an indication of average 24-hour noise levels at various urban, suburban, and rural locations. Predicted trends in noise levels to the year 2000 are not particularly encouraging. One of the two most important sources of excessive community noise, urban traffic, is expected to increase considerably during the next two decades. Projections prepared for the U.S. Department of Transportation estimates that the number of automobiles on the road will increase by 0.6-0.7% yearly through the end of the century and that average levels of automobile noise will also rise as diesel engines and 4-cylinder gasoline engines make up an ever-larger proportion of the motor fleet. Numbers of people affected by the other major community noise problem, aircraft noise, are expected to decline somewhat between now and the year 2000 if current noise emission regulations are implemented and special take-off procedures adopted; after 2000, the continued increase in air traffic is likely to witness a rise once again in the land area and population size exposed to aircraft noise.[3]

Noise as a Nuisance

Several years ago when an ABC television crew was filming a documentary entitled, "Death Be Not Loud", they interviewed a refined-looking New York businesswoman who related the following story:

> I got out at 40th Street and Madison after sitting 20 minutes in a traffic jam. And there was a car there from New Jersey blowing his horn. I walked over to him and said, 'Will you please stop that, it's impossible to go through, the traffic jam is from here as far as the eye can see.' He looked at me and blew his horn. I took off my shoe and hit his car. He did it again and I put another dent in his car. He turned to me and said, 'You're crazy, lady!' I said, 'I am, and you did it.' Whereupon he blew the horn again and I had the shoe on this time and I kicked his car. I really thought I was certifiable that day. But he

stopped blowing his horn.[4]

Noise obviously has strange effects on normally mild-mannered individuals, sometimes arousing them to violent, even murderous, acts. Some years ago a night clerical worker in New York was trying to sleep during the daytime but was kept awake by a group of boys playing noisily under his window. When they paid no attention to his shouts that they quiet down, the man fired a gun from his window, killing one of the youths. On another occasion, the owner of a lakeside summer cottage near Toledo, Ohio, became so enraged at a noisy motorboat making repeated passes near the shore that he fired a shotgun at the boat operator; luckily this time the results were not fatal. In a somewhat more humorous vein, a farmer in Idaho was once arrested for hurling potatoes at military planes as they swooped low over his field prior to landing![5]

Fig. 13–2
NOISE SOURCES CONSIDERED "HIGHLY ANNOYING"
(in areas away from the direct impact of freeway or aircraft noise)

pop. density under 3000/sq. mile		pop. density between 3000-20,000/sq. mile		pop. density over 20,000/sq. mile	
Source	%HA	Source	%HA	Source	%HA
1 Motorcycles	9.4	1 Motorcycles	13.2	1 Motorcycles	12.7
2 Helicopters	5.3	2 Large trucks	10.0	2 Autos	9.4
3 Autos	4.2	3 Autos	7.4	3 Large trucks	7.3
4 Construction	3.7	4 Construction	7.2	4 Construction	6.5
5 Airplanes	3.2	5 Sport cars	7.0	5 Sport cars	5.9
6 Sport cars	3.1	6 Constant traffic	5.5	6 Traffic noise	4.7
7 Large trucks	2.6	7 Small trucks	4.1	7 Buses	4.7
8 Power garden tools	1.8	8 Buses	3.5	8 Small trucks	4.1
9 Small trucks	1.5	9 Airplanes	3.4	9 Helicopters	3.9
10 Traffic noise	1.5	11 Helicopters	3.1	10 Airplanes	3.6
11 Buses	1.1	11 Power garden tools	2.1	11 Power garden tools	1.2
	55.9		62.2		66.0

%HA—percent of respondents highly annoyed by source
Source: U.S. Environmental Protection Agency, *The Urban Noise Survey* (Washington, D.C.: U.S. Government Printing Office, Aug. 1977), p. 38.

Just as beauty is in the eye of the beholder, the perception of a sound as "noise" (arbitrarily defined by some writers as "unwanted sounds") depends on the point of view of the individual listener. Unfortunately for those attempting to set up standards regulating noise exposure, the loudness of a noise and the annoyance it causes are not always directly correlated. As any college student partying near a residential neighborhood well knows, people *generating* loud sounds may frequently enjoy them, while those forced to listen against their will usually find the same noise profoundly objectionable. In general, a given individual most easily tolerates noise when:

1. he is causing it
2. he feels it is necessary or useful to him
3. he knows where it is coming from

To the extent that other persons exposed to the same sounds do not experience equivalent benefits from the noise, conflict between participating and non-participating groups is generated.[6]

While most people are well-acquainted with the feelings of annoyance and irritation which unwanted sounds can arouse, noise is frequently shrugged off as an inescapable part of modern life about which little can be done. It is becoming increasingly evident, however, that noise levels commonly encountered in thousands of cities, factories, places of recreation, and even inside homes represent far more than a simple nuisance. Noise today has become a public health hazard; more insidious than easily-recognized air and water pollution, noise is invisibly undermining the physical and psychological well-being of millions of people around the world. The remainder of this chapter will describe the ways in which noise affects human health, but first it is necessary to take a brief look at the physical nature of sound and at how noise levels are measured.

Nature of Sound

Sound is produced by the compression and expansion of air created when an object vibrates. The positive and negative pressure waves thus formed travel outward longitudinally from the vibrating source. Two basic characteristics of sound, *Frequency* (or *Pitch*) and *Amplitude*, are related to how loud and annoying a sound will be perceived.

Frequency describes the rate of vibration—how fast the object is moving back and forth. The more rapid the movement, the higher the frequency of the sound pressure waves created. The standard unit used today for measuring frequency is the *hertz* (Hz), equivalent to one wave per second passing a given point. Most people can hear sounds within a frequency range of 20-20,000 Hz, though there exists a great deal of individual variation in ability to perceive very low or very high frequency sounds.

Amplitude refers to the intensity of sound—how much energy is behind the sound wave. Sound waves of the same frequency can be heard as very loud or very soft, depending on the force with which they strike the ear. In technical terms, amplitude measures the maximum displacement of a sound wave from its resting, or equilibrium, position, but it is perceived psychologically as *Loudness*. The unit for measuring intensity, or amplitude, of sound is the *Decibel* (dB); the decibel scale ranges from 0, which is regarded as the threshold of hearing for normal, healthy ears, to 194, regarded as the theoretic maximum for pure tones. Because the decibel scale, like the pH scale, is logarithmic, 20 dB is 100 times louder than 0, 30 dB 1000 times louder, 40 dB 10,000 times louder, and so forth. Thus at high decibel levels, even a small reduction in decibel values can make a significant difference in noise intensity.

Loudness of a sound as perceived by the listener, however, does not depend entirely on its amplitude, being affected to some extent by its frequency as well. Although average hearing ability ranges from 10-20,000 Hz, not all of these frequencies sound equally loud to the human ear. Maximum sensitivity to sound occurs in the 1000-3000 Hz range, though human speech frequencies can vary from 300-4000 Hz. However, sounds at the very low or very high ends of the audible range seem much fainter to our ears than do those in the middle frequencies. Thus, for example, an extremely low-pitched sound must have an amplitude many times greater than a sound of medium pitch in order for both to be heard as equally loud. For this reason, decibel values are sometimes weighted to take into account the frequency response of the human ear. When this is done, the unit measurement designation may be written as dB(A). Figure 13-3 indicates approximate decibel values for a number of commonly-encountered sounds.

Fig. 13–3

Sound Levels and Human Response		
Common Sounds	Noise Level (dB)	Effect
Air raid siren	140	Painfully loud
Jet takeoff	130	
Discotheque	120	Maximum vocal effort
Pile driver	110	
Garbage truck	100	
City traffic	90	Very annoying, hearing damage
Alarm clock	80	Annoying
Freeway traffic	70	Phone use difficult
Air conditioning	60	Intrusive
Light auto traffic	50	Quiet
Livingroom	40	
Library	30	Very quiet
Broadcasting studio	20	
	10	Just audible
	0	Hearing begins

Source: U.S. Environmental Protection Agency

Noise and Hearing Loss

Almost everyone at one time or another has experienced irritation due to noise, but many people are unaware that the sounds which cause them so much annoyance may also be affecting their hearing. The EPA estimates that at least

20 million Americans are daily being exposed to levels of noise which are permanently damaging to their ability to hear. Most people are familiar with the temporary deafness and ringing in the ears which occurs after sudden exposure to a very loud noise such as a cap gun or firecracker exploding close to one's head. This type of partial hearing loss generally lasts a few hours at the most and is referred to as *Temporary Threshold Shift (TTS)*. However, it is not widely recognized that regular exposure to levels of noise commonly encountered in everyday life can, over a period of time, result in permanent hearing loss. Because damage to the ear is usually painless and seldom visible, few people recognize the injury they are incurring until it is too late. Research has shown that when daily noise levels average about 85 dB or more, permanent hearing loss can occur; for particularly sensitive individuals, average sound levels as low as 70 dB may be dangerous.[7] The noise of city traffic, jet planes, chainsaws, power lawnmowers, some household appliances, babies screaming, and even people shouting all exceed the decibel level considered as "safe".

Mechanism of Hearing Loss

Noise results in hearing loss through its destructive effect on the delicate hair cells in the Organ of Corti within the cochlea of the inner ear. These hair cells convert fluid vibrations in the inner ear into nerve impulses which are carried by the auditory nerve to the brain, resulting in the sensation of sound.

Fig. 13-4 **How We Hear**

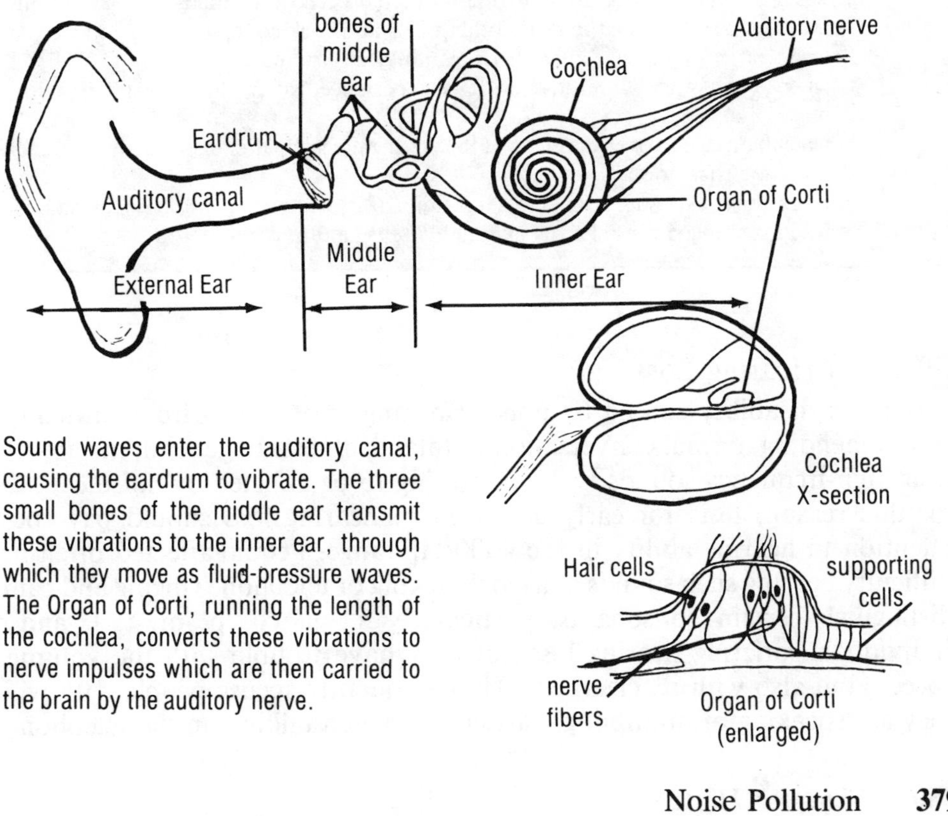

Sound waves enter the auditory canal, causing the eardrum to vibrate. The three small bones of the middle ear transmit these vibrations to the inner ear, through which they move as fluid-pressure waves. The Organ of Corti, running the length of the cochlea, converts these vibrations to nerve impulses which are then carried to the brain by the auditory nerve.

Progressive destruction of the hair cells and a correlated reduction in the number of associated nerve fibers can be caused either by aging (deterioration of hearing due to old age is referred to as **Presbycusis**) or by exposure to noise (noise-induced hearing loss is termed **Sociocusis**). Prolonged exposure to excessive noise levels results in damage to, or the complete collapse of, individual hair cells, thus affecting the transmission of nerve impulses. Although there are many thousands of hair cells in the Organ of Corti, when a large enough number are damaged hearing ability is inevitably affected. This type of hearing loss is irreversible and cannot be restored by the use of hearing aids. Since the ear, unlike the eye, has no automatic defense mechanism—no "earlid" to prevent unwanted sounds from penetrating—the only way to protect oneself against noise-induced hearing loss is to limit as much as possible one's exposure to a noisy environment.

Box 13–1

Warning Signs of Hearing Impairment

Perhaps the most difficult aspect of persuading people that the noise levels to which they are exposed present a real threat to their hearing is the fact that such a loss usually is gradual and because the inner ear has no mechanism for registering pain. Nevertheless, certain warning signs can indicate that noise levels are high enough to cause hearing impairment. If heeded, such warnings as the following can help to forestall serious damage:

1. when conversation is difficult or impossible because of high-level background noise (e.g. such as that in a discotheque or at a rock concert)
2. when ears ring or buzz after leaving a noisy environment
3. when Temporary Threshold Shift is experienced after exposure to very loud noise
4. when pain due to over-stressing of the eardrum occurs after exposure to extremely high-intensity noise
5. when noise exposure results in sensations of unsteadiness, dizziness, or nausea
6. when prolonged noise leaves one highly tense and irritable[8]

Effects of Hearing Loss

Hearing disability caused by noise can range in severity from difficulty in comprehending normal conversation to total deafness. In general, the ability to hear high-frequency sounds is the first thing to be affected by noise exposure; for this reason, tests for early detection of hearing loss should pay special attention to hearing ability in the 4000 Hz range. People affected often have difficulty hearing such sounds as a clock ticking or telephone ringing and cannot distinguish certain consonants, particularly s, sh, ch, p, m, t, f, and th. Individuals suffering hearing loss not only have trouble with the volume of speech, but also with its clearness. They frequently accuse people with whom they are speaking of mumbling, particularly when talking on the telephone or when background noises interfere with conversation; listening to the radio or television may become impossible. The psychological impact of such difficulties—the fear of being laughed at for misunderstanding questions or comments, the frustration of not being able to follow a conversation, the feeling of isolation or alienation experienced as friends unconsciously avoid trying to converse—are frequently as severe as the physical disability. Individuals experiencing hearing loss tend to become suspicious, irritable, and depressed; their careers suffer and social life becomes severely restricted, sometimes to the point of complete withdrawal.[9] In addition to these problems, a person with partial hearing loss may suffer sharp pain in the ears when exposed to very loud noise and may experience repeated bouts of *Tinnitus*—a ringing or buzzing sound in the head which can drive the victim to distraction, interfering with sleep, conversation, and normal daily activities.

Box 13-2

Mom Was Right About Rock Music!

In 1968 a study was launched in Knoxville, Tennessee to test the hearing ability of several different age groups of young people. The aim of the investigation was to determine the validity of suspicions that environmental noise might be having a detrimental impact on children's hearing. Because human hearing ability is generally optimum throughout the normal frequency range from the preteen years through the early 20s, it was assumed that measureable hearing loss for high frequency sound would be an indication that young people were being exposed to excessively high noise levels.

During the spring of that year, hearing tests were conducted within the public schools on 1000 children each from the 6th, 9th, and 12th grades. Among 6th grade students only 3.8% failed the high-frequency test—a figure which rose to 11% for the 9th and 12th graders. The same test was administered that fall to the incoming freshman class at the University of Tennessee in Knoxville, with the result that 32.9% failed! The test was repeated in the fall of 1969 to confirm the previous year's results; in spite of expectations that the 1968 freshmen results had been an anomaly and that 1969 readings would be lower, the failure rate nearly doubled in 1969 to 60.7%. Although the young people tested did not exhibit severe hearing disability—indeed, most who failed the test by a slight margin were totally unaware of any hearing loss—they nevertheless showed much higher levels of impairment than would have been expected for persons of their age (interestingly, the failure rate was much higher among males than females).

Although it was not possible to pinpoint the precise cause of reduced hearing ability, the researchers who conducted the investigation theorized that the popularity among teens and young adults of loud recreational activities such as listening to rock music, motorcycling, sport shooting, and car racing might be responsible for the observed trends.[10]

Stress and Related Health Effects

Hearing loss is the most obvious health threat posed by noise pollution, but it is by no means the only one. Exposure to unwanted noise involuntarily

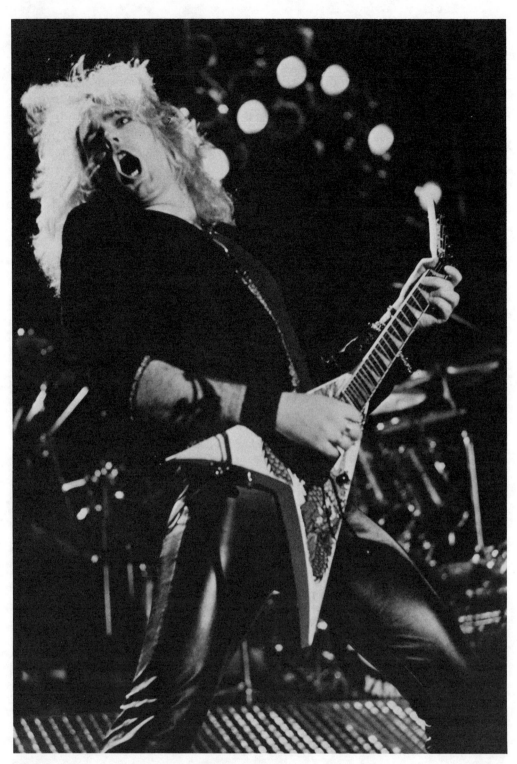

Routine exposure to noise levels as high as 140 decibels makes permanent hearing loss a common occupational hazard among rock musicians. [*Andrew Godzur*]

induces stress, and stress can lead to a variety of physical ailments including an increase in heart rate, high blood pressure, elevated levels of blood cholesterol, ulcers, headaches, and colitis.

Stressful reaction to loud or sudden noise undoubtedly represents an evolutionary adaptation to warnings signalling approaching danger. Bodily responses to the snarl of a predatory beast or the rumble of a boulder crashing down a mountainside cause a surge of adrenalin, an increase in heart and breathing rates, and the tensing of muscles—all physiological preparations for fight or flight which have important survival value. However, these same metabolic responses are today being triggered repeatedly by the innumerable man-made noises of modern society. As a result, our bodies are subjected to a constant state of stress which, far from being advantageous, is literally making millions of people sick—even though they may not attribute their problems to noise. While many individuals insist that they have "gotten used to noise" and are no longer bothered by it, the truth is that no one can prevent the automatic biological changes which noise provokes. Research into the association between noise exposure and stress-related disease has produced findings such as the following:

> workers exposed to high levels of occupational noise were found to exhibit up to 5 times as many cases of ulcers as would normally be expected among people in quieter surroundings.

> a 5-year study of factory workers revealed that employees assigned to noisy areas of the plant had a higher frequency of diagnosed medical problems, including respiratory ailments, than did workers in quieter sections of the same plant.

> exposure of a laboratory population of rhesus monkeys to noise levels typically experienced on a daily basis by factory workers resulted in a 30% elevation of the monkeys' blood pressure—a level which persisted for a long period after the experiment ended. Such findings indicate that adverse noise—induced health effects cannot be reversed quickly simply by removing the noise source.[11]

Teratogenic Effects of Noise

Contrary to earlier beliefs, it is now known that outside noise can penetrate the womb and provoke responses in the developing unborn child. A fetus responds to loud noise with an increase in heart rate and kicking. Pregnant women have reported that they felt considerably more fetal movement while listening to music in a concert hall, the kicking reaching a peak when the audience began to applaud![12] Although this type of direct fetal response to sound may not present any serious concern, indirect responses caused by noise-induced maternal stress are more worrisome. A study conducted in Japan suggests that expectant mothers living in noisy environments are more likely to give birth to underweight babies than are women from quieter areas. It is assumed that stress caused by high noise levels affected the production of certain maternal hormones responsible for fetal growth. Other studies have demonstrated that stress experienced by an expectant mother can cause blood vessels in the uterus to constrict, thereby reducing the supply of oxygen and nutrients to the developing child. A preliminary investigation among people living near a major airport indicate a higher-than-expected incidence of harelip, cleft palate, and spina bifida among children born in this area. Much more research is needed to define the extent of the relationship between noise and birth defects, as well as to establish how high noise levels must be to produce teratogenic effects.[13] Lacking definitive information, some doctors recommend that pregnant women try to avoid noise exposure to the greatest extent possible, one such expert offering the tongue-in-cheek advice that "any expectant mother should get out of New York".

Effects of Noise on Learning Ability and Work Performance

Noisy surroundings at home and school can adversely affect children's language development and their ability to read. High noise levels interfere with a youngster's capacity to distinguish certain sounds such as "b" and "v", for example, and can foster a tendency to drop the endings of words, thereby distorting speech. Research has shown that reading skills are seriously impaired when the student's surroundings are noisy. One study focused on children living in a noisy apartment complex found that the longer they had resided in that environment, the poorer was their reading development. The investigators conducting the study concluded that a noisy home environment has more of an impact on reading skills than do such factors as parents' educational level, number of children in the family, or the child's grade level. Another study which examined the effect of classroom exposure to noise revealed that in one school located adjacent to an elevated railway, students whose classrooms faced the track scored significantly lower on reading tests than did those whose rooms were on the opposite side of the school.

A comparable situation relating to decreased efficiency on the job faces millions of American workers. Several years ago the National Institute for Occupational Safety and Health conservatively estimated that over 2.5 million U.S. industrial workers were exposed to harmful levels of noise. Aside from the health aspects of this exposure, noise hinders the performance of tasks requiring high levels of accuracy (total *quantity* of work, as opposed to quality, does not appear to suffer appreciably). Very loud or sporadic noises seem to be the most disruptive, distorting time perception, increasing the variability in work performance, disturbing concentration, and making it more difficult to remain alert. The effects of working all day in a noisy environment frequently carry over into domestic life, making the worker more prone to aggravation and frustration when he or she comes home. Pent-up stress from daytime noise exposure may prevent relaxation in the evening, and if the home environment is noisy also, the worker may remain in a constant state of tension and irritability.[14]

Safety Aspects of Noise

Safety, as well as health, can be in jeopardy when noise levels are high. Several years ago a worker in an auto glass manufacturing plant caught his hand in a piece of equipment; he frantically screamed for help, but no one came to his aid because noise levels in the factory were so high that he couldn't be heard. As a result, he lost his hand. On another occasion, two people in Elizabeth, New Jersey, were struck and killed by a locomotive while watching Senator Robert Kennedy's funeral train pass through the city; they hadn't heard the warning whistle because of the noise from the Secret Service and news media helicopters. In an auto pressroom in Ohio, two workers were permanently disabled when noisy working conditions prevented their hearing warning shouts about

---

Box 13–3
Home No Longer a Haven?

While most of the public ire regarding noise sources has been directed at airport and traffic din, other health-threatening noisemakers can be found much closer to home. Household appliances and power tools such as chain saws, power mowers, dishwashers, hair dryers, vacuum cleaners, food processors, etc., generate decibel levels which can interrupt conversation, be disturbing to neighbors, or even result in permanent damage to the ears. Although most home appliances either are not loud enough or are used too briefly to impair hearing (permanent hearing loss is generally associated with noise levels in excess of 85 dB), prolonged use of certain power tools could contribute to hearing damage. The chart below indicates representative decibel levels for a number of common domestic noise sources.

Noise Around our Homes

Noise Source	Sound Level for Operator (in dBA)
Refrigerator	40
Floor Fan	38 to 70
Clothes Dryer	55
Washing Machine	47 to 78
Dishwasher	54 to 85
Hair Dryer	59 to 80
Vacuum Cleaner	62 to 85
Sewing Machine	64 to 74
Electric Shaver	75
Food Disposal (Grinder)	67 to 93
Electric Lawn Edger	81
Home Shop Tools	85
Gasoline Power Mower	87 to 92
Gasoline Riding Mower	90 to 95
Chain Saw	100
Stereo	Up to 120

approaching panel racks.[15] Many traffic accidents are thought to be caused by drivers' inability to hear emergency sirens. Both by interfering with shouts for help or by masking warning signals, high levels of background noise pose a very real threat to public safety.

Sleep Disruption

Sleep is a biological necessity for humans. We need sleep to repair the wearing out of bodily tissues and to rejuvenate them; deprivation or disruption of sleep can thus directly threaten both physical health and mental well-being.

Noise can prevent people from going to sleep, can waken them prematurely, or can cause shifts from deeper to lighter stages of sleep. While individual response to noise in relation to its impact on sleep varies widely, in general adults are wakened by noise more easily than are children; the elderly are more sensitive than the middle-aged; sick persons are more affected than healthy ones; and women are more easily disturbed than men.[16]

Noise Control Efforts

Historically, noise abatement efforts have consisted primarily of local ordinances directed at specific community nuisances. One of the earliest of such laws was a London ordinance which went into effect in 1829, allowing stagecoach horses to be confiscated if they disrupted church services![17] Over the years since then, cities have adopted a wide variety of local restrictions on noise sources. A brief sampling of such regulations include: requirements for mufflers on cars; prohibitions against construction activity, garbage collection, or lawnmowing during early morning or evening hours; bans on roosters or other noisy animals within city limits; bans on auto horn-blowing except for emergencies; prohibitions on truck traffic through residential neighborhoods; restrictions on amplified music outdoors; and many others with similar intent.

Municipal noise control codes are, of course, only useful if they are enforced. One of the best was that passed in 1971 by Chicago (the promotional advertising campaign which preceded the program's implementation concentrated on the theme, "SSSHHICAGO"). Under the new code strict decibel limits were set for cars and machinery; stiff fines and jail sentences were meted out to violators. The "Silent Service" team enforcing the law played no favorites—even churches were told to quiet down when citizens complained about the too-noisy chimes.[18]

The federal government entered the noise-control arena in 1972 with passage of the Noise Control Act—the first national law aimed at relieving over-stimulated American ears by regulating new commercial products which are considered to be major noise sources. These include medium and heavy-weight trucks, garbage trucks, buses, motorcycles, wheel and crawler tractors, truck refrigeration units, portable air compressors, power lawnmowers, jackhammers, and rock drills. Noise emission limits have been set or are under consideration for these products. In addition, noise labelling requirements for noisy products and for noise-reducing products were to be drafted by the EPA, which was also to carry out studies on the health impact of noise in order to provide an objective basis for the numerical noise standards which might be promulgated.

While representing a step in the right direction, the Noise Control Act unfortunately did little to help individual communities resolve their own unique noise problems. Recognizing that most actions taken to reduce noise levels are at the local level, Congress in 1978 passed a set of amendments called the Quiet Communities Act. This legislation authorized EPA to work in partnership with state and local governments, helping them to develop programs appropriate to their own special needs and abilities. Under the Act, federal money providing aid in the form of grants, seminars, and training programs is offered to lower levels of government. By encouraging self-help from local volunteers and through promoting the exchange of helpful information among cities, Congress hoped to tackle the noise problem by directly

Fig. 13-5

What You Can Do to Quiet Your Home and Yourself from Noise

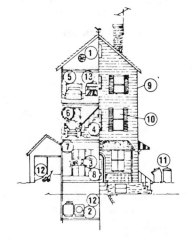

Inside

1. Install exhaust fan on rubber mounts
2. Use vibration mounts under electrical appliances like washer, dryer, and dishwasher
3. Put foam pads under blenders, mixers, and other small appliances (also your typewriter!)
4. Use wall to wall and stair carpeting with felt or rubber padding to dampen noise.
5. Use acoustical tile, spaced below ceiling
6. Install drapes to absorb sound
7. Buy quiet appliances
8. Install floor vinyl or thick linoleum to dampen sound

Outside

9. Eliminate noise leaks in walls by sealing holes or cracks
10. Caulk windows and install storm windows to cut down outside noise
11. Replace metal garbage cans with plastic ones

Protecting Your Ears

12. Wear ear protectors when you are using very noisy equipment or tools
13. Keep the stereo volume down

Source: Adapted from National Bureau of Standards Handbook 119, "Quieting— A Practical Guide to Noise Control, 1976."

involving citizens in an effort to improve the quality of life in their communities.[19]

Unfortunately, in spite of gradually increasing awareness that noise pollution is more than just a nuisance, noise control programs at both the federal and state level have been given a very low budgetary priority. Noise abatement departments are consistently understaffed and agency personnel have difficulty convincing both policy-makers and the public that noise pollution is really important. As one EPA official remarked, "Noise is something we grow up with, and it is very difficult to believe that such a common pollutant could be doing anything serious to our health or the environment." Until an aroused public insists that excessive noise is a community health hazard that must be controlled, it is unlikely that elected officials will give noise abatement efforts the attention they deserve.

REFERENCES

[1]"Urban Residents View Their Cities: A National Normative Study", Gallup Poll conducted for the Charles F. Kettering Foundation and the Charles Stewart Mott Foundation, Jan. 1978.

[2]U.S. Department of Commerce, Bureau of the Census, Annual Housing Surveys, 1973-76, *United States and Regions, Part B, Indicators of Housing and Neighborhood Quality,* prepared in cooperation with U.S. Department of Housing and Urban Development, Series H-150-73, Washington, D.C., U.S. Government Printing Office, August 1975.

[3]Council on Environmental Quality, *Environmental Quality: The Tenth Annual Report of the Council on Environmental Quality,* U.S. Government Printing Office, 1979.

[4]Lipscomb, David M., *Noise: The Unwanted Sounds,* Nelson-Hall Company, 1974.

[5]Ibid.

[6]Bugliarello, George, Ariel Alexandre, John Barnes, and Charles Wakstein, *The Impact of Noise Pollution,* Pergamon Press, 1976.

[7]U.S. Environmental Protection Agency, *Noise: A Health Problem,* Office of Noise Abatement and Control, August 1978.

[8]Lipscomb, op. cit.

[9]Perham, Chris, "The Sound of Silence", *EPA Journal,* U.S. Environmental Protection Agency, Office of Public Awareness (A-107), vol. 5, no. 9, October 1979.

[10]Ibid.

[11]Terry, Luther L., M.D., "Health and Noise", *EPA Journal,* U.S. Environmental Protection Agency, Office of Public Awareness (A-107), vol. 5, no. 9, October 1979.

[12]Kavaler, *Noise the New Menace,* The John Day Company, 1975.

[13]*USEPA,* op. cit.

[14]Ibid.

[15]Stansbury, Jeff, "Noise in the Workplace", *EPA Journal,* U.S. Environmental Protection Agency, Office of Public Awareness (A-107), vol. 5, no. 9, October 1979.

[16]Bugliarello et al., op. cit.

[17]Lipscomb, op. cit.

[18]Kavaler, op. cit.

[19]Culver, John C., "Opportunities in the Quiet Communities Act", *EPA Journal,* U.S. Environmental Protection Agency, Office of Public Awareness (A-107), vol. 5, no. 9, October 1979.

14
Water Resources

"All the rivers run into the sea, yet the sea is not full; to the place from whence the rivers come, thither they return again."
(Ecclesiastes 1:7)

Hydrologic Cycle

Although the ancient writer of Ecclesiastes expressed his scientific observations in poetic form, his statements relating to the cycling of water through the hydrosphere are basically correct, albeit overly simplified. Water moves in what is essentially a closed system, circulating from one part of the earth to another, changing in form from liquid to solid or gas and back to liquid again, yet remaining relatively constant in total amount. Water occurs as vapor in the atmosphere, as rain or snow falling on the earth or oceans, as ice locked in massive glaciers or ice caps, and as rivers, streams, lakes, seas, and subterranean groundwater. The manner by which water moves from place to place, changing from one form to another, is called the *Hydrologic Cycle.*

The hydrologic cycle, like virtually all other processes on earth, is powered by energy from the sun which causes water to evaporate from the surface of the oceans, rivers, lakes, and from the soil. The movement of this water vapor in the atmosphere is an important factor in the redistribution of heat around the earth. Because heat is absorbed when water evaporates, the atmosphere becomes a reservoir of heat energy. This heat energy then drives the hydrologic cycle which gives rise to the atmospheric forces involved in weather and climate.

Fig. 14-1   The Hydrologic Cycle

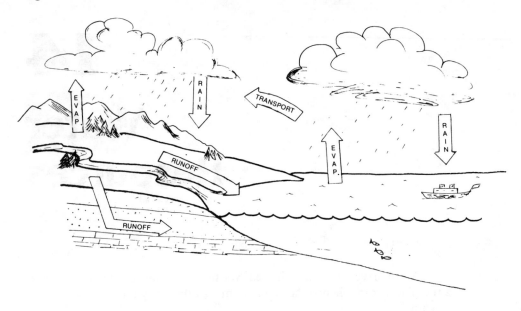

The principal processes involved in the hydrologic cycle are:

EVAPORATION of water from surface waters and from the soil.

TRANSPORTATION of water by plants; because both evaporation and transpiration produce the same result (i.e. the addition of water vapor to the atmosphere), the two processes are often collectively called EVAPO-TRANSPIRATION.

TRANSPORT of atmospheric water from one place to another either as water vapor or as liquid water droplets and ice crystals in clouds.

PRECIPITATION when atmospheric water vapor condenses and falls as rain, hail, sleet, or snow.

RUN-OFF, whereby water that has fallen on land finds its way back to the oceans, flowing either on or under the surface of the continents.

The amount of time required for the completion of the cycle can vary widely from place to place and from one part of the cycle to another. On the average, a water molecule spends 9 days in the atmosphere from the time it evaporates until it falls again as rain or snow.[1] However, if it happens to fall as a snowflake on the Antarctic ice sheet, it may remain there for thousands of years before it breaks off as part of an iceberg and melts into the ocean; conversely, if it falls during a desert thunderstorm, it might evaporate in an hour or two.

It has been calculated that all the waters of the planet are distributed roughly as follows:

97%—in the oceans
2%—in polar ice caps and glaciers
1%—in rivers, lakes, and groundwater, and water vapor
in the atmosphere

Note: The U.S. Geological Survey estimates the total amount of water on earth at 326,000,000 cubic miles, equal to 1,440,000,000,000,000,000 tons.

Obviously for humans it is the last figure in the column, less than 1% of the total, which is of greatest importance, since this is the source of the water we drink, bathe in, use for irrigation and for industrial processes. Of this small percentage of water on which human life depends, only a very small portion is found in the rivers, streams, and lakes of the world. Likewise, at any given moment only a minute amount of the world's water is found as atmospheric water vapor. The U.S. Geological Survey calculates that if all the water present in air were to fall at the same time, the earth would be submerged in water only 1 inch deep.[2] By far the greatest amount of all available freshwater, approximately 96.5% of the total, is found beneath the surface of the soil in the form of groundwater.

Water Quantity and Health

The human body's absolute dependence on regular intake of water is second only to its need for oxygen. While an individual can, if necessary, survive for a number of weeks without food, deprivation of water will result in death within a few days at the most. Water makes up approximately 65% of the adult human's body, a somewhat higher percentage in children. Blood consists of 83% water, while bones contain 25%. Water is essential for the body's digestion of food, transport of nutrients and hormones, and removal of wastes. Depending on a person's size, weight, degree of activity, and the prevailing level of temperature and humidity, an individual requires approximately 1-3 quarts of water daily just to maintain bodily functions. However, for a minimally-acceptable standard of living, 20-50 quarts of safe water are deemed essential for drinking, food preparation, cooking, dish-washing, and bathing. The use of sewer systems for safe removal of human wastes—wastes which present serious health hazards when mismanaged—also requires considerable amounts of water. In typical urban residential areas sewers will not function properly if per capita water use is less than 100 quarts a day. In industrialized countries and among the more affluent segments of the urban population in developing nations, water quantity is generally more than ample to meet these basic human needs; average daily water consumption in such situations ranges between 200-400 quarts a day per person. However, as many as 1.5 billion people in the Third World still lack access to adequate supplies of safe water. In many rural areas the problem is not that the water does not exist, but rather that the source of such water is far from the place where it will be used, requiring the expenditure of considerable time and energy to haul water from a river, well, or standpipe to the home. A study conducted by CARE in Kenya, East Africa, revealed that nearly a fifth of rural women spent more than 6 hours a day collecting water, leaving little time for more economically productive tasks such as farming or marketing. In a poor area of the central African nation of Cameroon, 50,000 persons had to share two standpipes; in many countries, rural women commonly walk 1-5 miles to fetch a pailful of water. In most urban areas of the Third World water supply systems are in place, but frequently they are in poor condition or are unreliable, functioning perhaps only a few hours each day; while walking distances for poor city dwellers is less than for their country cousins, such people nevertheless spend hours waiting in long lines for their turn at the standpipe.

In situations such as these, where safe water is in short supply or difficult or time-consuming to obtain, important aspects of personal hygiene and basic sanitation such as washing hands and eating utensils is frequently neglected. In addition, there is a strong temptation to utilize polluted sources of water if higher-quality supplies are not easily accessible. Some evidence suggests that households farthest from a water supply source tend to have the highest incidence of filth-related gastrointestinal disorders such as diarrhea.[3] Perhaps the most essential prerequisite to improving the health and living standards among the poor of the Third World is an increase in the quantity of readily-available safe water supplies.

Water Supply: Our Next Crisis?

During the past few years, numerous authorities on water issues have been warning that the coming water crisis which they forsee will make the so-called "energy crisis" seem pale by comparison. Recent water shortages, precipitated by drought, in such diverse areas as the Northeast (1980-81) and California (1976-77), are, these experts insist, but harbingers of more difficult times to come. At first glance, such gloomy predictions seem at variance with the facts pertaining to U.S. water supplies. On the average, the U.S. receives approximately 30 inches of rainfall annually, of which about 21 inches is returned to the atmosphere through evapotranspiration and 9 inches runs off into streams and other bodies of water. Water available for use—that found in rivers, lakes, and groundwater deposits—if equally divided would amount to more than 6000 gallons per day for each American.[4] Thus looking at the country as a whole, the United States today is not faced with a serious water supply problem. Available amounts of surface supplies and groundwater still far exceed the amount of water withdrawn for human use. Focusing on specific regions, however, a far different picture emerges. Water resources within the U.S. are not evenly distributed; whereas the Pacific Northwest receives about 80 inches of rainfall annually and the states east of the Mississippi River average about 40-45 inches, the Great Plains and Southwest are chronically water-short, the driest state, Nevada, receiving only 9 inches of precipitation in an average year.[5] Even within states where water supplies are generally adequate, periodic dry spells or increasing industrial and municipal demands may result in localized shortages.

Because water is characterized by high bulk and low cost, it cannot be easily or economically transported from water-surplus to water-deficit areas.

Basic elements of today's water woes

Compounding the problem of regional disparities in water supply is the fact that everywhere—both in water-short and water-abundant sections of the country—available supplies are being reduced both by pollution and by wastage. Pollution of water resources with chemical poisons or human wastes, a subject which will be dealt with extensively in the following chapter, does not, of course, reduce the amount of water present, but by making that water unfit for human use it diminishes the available quantity of the resource (see Box 14-1). A less dramatic but equally significant aspect of the growing water crisis is the wastage of water resources which has been encouraged in all parts of the country by historically low prices for water and a general belief that water supplies are inexhaustible. Some flagrant examples of water wastage include:

leaking water distribution systems—in many older cities the pipes, valves, and tunnels which carry water from a central treatment plant to thousands of homes, businesses, and institutions were installed during the 1800s or early 1900s and have for decades been in serious need of replacement. Unfortunately, the fiscal plight of most urban areas has resulted in continual postponement of these urgently needed renovations. Thus in Boston, for example, where the water distribution system was laid out beginning in the 1840s, lack of funds has made it impossible to replace more than 1% of its pipes each year. As a result, Boston loses an estimated 20% of the 150 million gallons of water entering its distribution system each day. Boston is not the only community with such problems, however. Other cities experiencing similar losses include Pittsburgh, 14%; Philadelphia, 12%; and Baltimore, 10%.[6] New York, which also has a crumbling pipe network, in addition loses millions of gallons of water every year when sidewalk hydrants are opened during hot weather by city residents who allow children to play in the cooling spray; such hydrants are seldom closed afterwards and may continue to gush high-quality water for weeks.[7]

inefficient irrigation systems—irrigated agriculture is the nation's single largest water consumer, particularly in the arid West. This region, where annual rainfall averages 20 inches or less, produces over 18% of the nation's total farm output,[8] but in so doing, according to the General Accounting Office (GAO), wastes about half the irrigation water used. Widely practiced methods involving the flooding of whole fields or the furrows between crop rows result in half or more of the water being lost through evaporation or seepage before it reaches crop roots. Sprinkler methods such as center-pivot irrigation are somewhat more efficient, with up to 70% of the water being taken up by the crop plant. The least wasteful method, drip irrigation, requires an expensive network of perforated pipes or plastic hoses which release water, drop by drop, at the base of each plant; up to 90% of the water reaches the root zone by this method, but the equipment expense (about $1000/acre investment) and the fact that it is suitable only for row crops or orchards has limited its acceptance by growers. Even with the least wasteful irrigation methods, however, questions are being raised as to whether it makes sense from a water policy standpoint to utilize vast amounts of a scarce regional resource to raise such crops as cotton and alfalfa which can be grown equally well on rain-watered lands to the east.

Reduction of useable water supplies through pollution and wastage guarantee that competition among major water exploiters—agriculture, industry, mining, energy development, municipalities—will result in rising prices for water and conflict over access to water, both among competing uses within a region (e.g. farmers vs. mining interests vs. urban developers) and between water-short and water-abundant regions (see Box 14-2).

Groundwater

Mention "water resources" and most people immediately think of rivers, lakes, and man-made reservoirs—surface water sources which are visible, accessible, and useful not only for direct consumption but for transportation and recreation as well. However, as pointed out earlier, over 96% of all available fresh water supplies occur in the form of groundwater, a resource whose immense importance is often overlooked and little understood by the general public. Approximately half of all Americans and more than 95% of farm

---

Box 14-2

Water Wars

Rights of access to water have been a source of conflict in arid lands from time immemorial; although today's water wars are being waged with legal briefs instead of swords or 6-shooters, the stakes are just as high and the emotions equally fierce.

To slake the thirst of rapidly-growing southern California and Arizona and to bail out thousands of farmers whose irrigated lands in Texas, Nebraska, and elsewhere are threatened by groundwater overdrafts, ambitious schemes have been proposed to construct massive networks of canals and reservoirs to transfer water from surplus to deficit areas. Examples of such proposals, all of which have generated intense controversy include:

- a scheme to divert vast quantities of water from Alaska and northwestern Canada to the southwestern U.S. and Mexico.
- the Texas Water Plan which seeks to water the High Plains of West Texas by pumping water out of the Mississippi, transporting it across Louisiana into a series of reservoirs and canals in eastern and central Texas, and then pump it uphill from northeast Texas to the High Plains where it would be used primarily for irrigation.
- a plan to divert water from the Northwest's Columbia River to the heavily over-utilized Colorado River Basin in the Southwest.

Any of these grandiose schemes would cost billions of dollars to execute and their mere suggestion has met fierce opposition from residents of the regions whose water would be diverted. Citizens of the Columbia River Basin have been particularly upset at the prospect of losing any of the water upon which their hydroelectric potential depends; in 1968 Congressional representatives from the region amended a Southwestern water project authorization bill, forbidding even a study of water transfers into the Colorado River system. Residents of the lower Mississippi Basin are likewise unwilling to sacrifice millions of acre-feet of their water for the sake of Texas corn production, and the prospect of Canadians relinquishing their waters to nourish California lawns and gardens is most unlikely.

Many taxpayers resent the idea that enormous sums of public money might be spent to subsidize over-development and profigate water use in an area of the country which 19th century explorer John Wesley Powell had warned was too dry to support a large population. The concept of massive interbasin water transfers at present remains unimplemented due to political obstacles, environmental considerations, and fiscal constraints. Nevertheless, boosters of Southwestern development still hold out hope that such plans will eventually be realized. As a University of Arizona hydrologist remarked, "It's the type of solution Americans like. It relieves them of individual responsibility to live within the limitations of their resources."

---

families depend on groundwater for their drinking water supplies (considering all uses, groundwater accounts for 25% of total U.S. water consumption).[9] This vast unseen reservoir flows very slowly toward the sea and is a major source of replenishment for most surface water supplies. Estimates indicate that most rivers receive as much of their flow from groundwater seepage as from surface run-off.

Groundwater supplies constitute an invaluable natural resource—one which has long been regarded as having certain inherent advantages over surface water supplies. Groundwater is usually cleaner and purer than most surface water sources. This is true because the soil through which it percolates filters out most of the bacteria, suspended materials, and other contaminants which find easy access to rivers and lakes. In addition, because evaporation is virtually nil and seasonal fluctuations in supply are small, groundwater supplies are dependable year-round. In terms of cost, groundwater has advantages also. The expense of digging a well is generally less than that of piping surface water to its place of use and because of its greater purity it is less expensive to treat prior to consumption.

Until recently, communities relying on groundwater for their municipal supplies tended to take this resource largely for granted, assuming that adequate quantities of high-quality water would always be available. Today, however, a sense of alarm is spreading with the realization that the twin evils of pollution and over-use are threatening the integrity of groundwater supplies. To understand how this situation has come about, it is necessary to take a brief look at the physical characteristics of our groundwater resource.

Nature of Groundwater

When rain falls upon the earth, that which is not taken up by plant roots or lost as surface run-off percolates downward through the soil until it reaches the water table. Contrary to what some people think, the water table is not a vast underground lake or river, but the upper limit of what hydrologists call the *Zone of Saturation*—an area where the spaces between rock particles are completely filled with water. Such moisture-laden strata are called *Aquifers* (Latin for "water carriers"). Above the zone of saturation lies the *Zone of Aeration*, where some soil moisture may be found as capillary water—useful for plants but incapable of being pumped out by man. The zone of saturation extends downward until it is limited by an impermeable layer of rock. Sometimes there are successive layers of groundwater separated by impermeable rock layers. Aquifers may range from a few feet to several hundreds of feet in thickness and they may underlie a couple of acres or many square miles. They may occur just below the soil surface or thousands of feet below the earth, though seldom deeper than two miles.

The amount of water that any given aquifer can hold depends on its porosity—the ratio of the spaces between the rock particles to the total volume of rock. Sand and gravel aquifers are examples of rocks with high porosity. Additionally, if water is going to move through an aquifer, its pores must be interconnected. To qualify as a good aquifer, a rock layer must contain many pores, cracks, or both. The rate of water movement through an aquifer varies, not surprisingly, with the type of rock: through gravel it may travel tens or hundreds of feet per day; in fine sand only a few inches or less per day. When hydrologists measure the flow of surface streams, they do so in terms of feet per second; when measuring groundwater flow, figures in feet *per year* are the rule.

Groundwater Pollution

During the past several years, instances of groundwater contamination due to such pollutants as toxic chemicals, fertilizers, road salt, and microbial pathogens have been discovered with increasing frequency in communities throughout the nation. Such findings have raised legitimate concerns among the public regarding both acute and chronic health effects and have resulted in the closure of hundreds of wells, affecting the water supplies of millions of Americans. In numerous cases involving synthetic organic chemicals, levels of contamination were many times higher than those found in the most heavily polluted surface supplies. Many researchers and government officials alike fear that these alarming discoveries may represent only the "tip of the iceberg". Their greatest concern is that because groundwater pollution is in a sense hidden, out of sight and difficult to detect without sophisticated chemical analyses, many contaminated wells undoubtedly are still serving as the water supply for citizens who remain unaware that the water drawn from their faucets contains tasteless, colorless, odorless, but nevertheless health-threatening poisons.

That the purity of groundwater supplies can be degraded by man-generated pollutants is largely due to unwise waste disposal practices or poor land management. Sources of groundwater contamination fall roughly into 3 categories:

> *Septic Tanks and Injection Wells*—here liquid wastes are discharged directly into the ground. If the location has been properly chosen, such discharges pose little hazard, but if located adjacent to or uphill from an aquifer or well, a potential for pollution exists. Contamination from septic tanks (of which there are about 19 million in use in the U.S.) can be both bacteriological and chemical, especially from detergents. A number of outbreaks of waterborne diseases such as typhoid, infectious hepatitis, and salmonellosis have been traced to well water contaminated by sewage from septic tanks.

> *Unintentional Contamination*—leaky sewage systems and holding tanks, urban street runoff, acid mine wastes, oil field brines, pesticides, and de-icing salts carry the potential for polluting groundwater as well as surface water. In Midwestern farming areas where large amounts of nitrogen fertilizers are used, well water should be periodically monitored for nitrate levels, since this substance has been linked to methemoglobinemia ("blue baby disease"). In some parts of the northeastern states where large amounts of road salts have been applied during the winter months, water supplies have become so contaminated with chloride ions that the towns using them had to seek other sources. Several states in New England have actually established annual budgets to allow for the replacement of affected wells.

Fig. 14-2   **Nature of Groundwater**

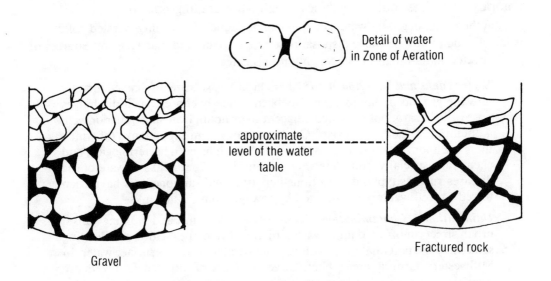

Zone of
Aeration

water table

Zone of
Saturation

(Aquifer)

groundwater flow

surface
water

Impermeable rock or clay

Detail of water
in Zone of Aeration

approximate
level of the water
table

Gravel

Fractured rock

How Water Occurs in the Rock

Source: U.S. Geological Survey, *A Primer on Ground Water*

Fig. 14-3 **Pollution of an Aquifer**

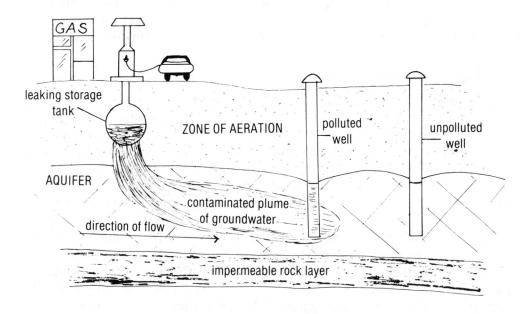

Leachates from Waste Disposal—seepage from landfills, waste ponds, or land application of sludges constitutes a severe groundwater pollution threat if such facilities are improperly sited. Industrial waste pits and lagoons pose particularly difficult problems because they are likely to contain extremely toxic materials such as arsenic, lead, cyanide, etc. In recent years the migration into aquifers of radioactive substances buried at supposedly secure sites has raised fears for which there exists no reassuring answer.

The most frightening aspect of groundwater pollution is the fact that by the time the problem is discovered, it is generally too late to do anything about it. Because of the very slow rate of flow, a contaminated aquifer will not be able to purify itself for many years, if ever, after the source of contamination is cut off (conversely, and for the same reason, contamination of one part of the aquifer does not necessarily affect the use of other parts of the aquifer). Once groundwater becomes polluted, it may be feasible to treat it to make it fit for consumption, but clean-up of the aquifer itself is generally impossible.

From the days of the late 1960s when environmental concerns began to escalate, until fairly recently, our justifiable concern about water pollution has focused almost exclusively on contamination of the nation's rivers, lakes, and oceans. Although the chemical and biological constituents of groundwater used for public drinking water supplies are monitored on a routine basis, scarcely any attention has been paid to monitoring the quality of our underground water resources as a whole. The need today is greater than ever before, because efforts to clean up the air and surface waters have resulted in greatly increased volumes of pollutants to be disposed of on land. Unless such disposal is wisely managed, we will simply be transferring the problem from one place to another. If groundwater becomes the ultimate repository for the toxic and pathological by-products of modern society, a healthful future for mankind is most unlikely.

Groundwater Depletion

As domestic water demand and per capita water consumption in the U.S. increased steadily over the past several decades, the water table has dropped alarmingly in many regions of the country. Across the nation as a whole, groundwater supply has remained relatively stable. The amount of recoverable groundwater in the U.S. is estimated at about 150 times the amount currently being tapped; not all of it is of good quality or in the areas of demand, however, and not all underground reservoirs are renewable resources. In certain parts of the country, particularly in the West, groundwater is being pumped out faster than it is being replenished, and water levels are steadily declining. Periodic fluctuations in the level of the water table are normal, with levels rising during wet periods and declining during dry spells (generally the water table is highest in late spring, sinks in summer, rises somewhat during the fall and reaches its lowest point just before the spring thaw). However, when the water table lowers persistently it means that more water is being taken out of the groundwater reservoir than is being returned to it through precipitation or stream flow. Such a situation is akin to mining an aquifer, and if continued over a period of time it can permanently deplete the groundwater supply.

Instances of groundwater "mining" have occurred even in such well-watered areas as the Chicago suburbs where rapid population growth and residential and commercial development have resulted in a sharp decline in groundwater reserves. Problems of groundwater depletion are most acute, however, in parts of the Great Plains and Southwest where the insatiable appetite of farmers for irrigation water and the water demands of householders and industries in the booming cities of the Sunbelt have resulted in serious groundwater overdrafts which are causing a rapid lowering of the water table throughout much of the

Box 14-3

Mining Fossil Water: The Ogallala Aquifer

The continued economic prosperity of 11 million acres of irrigated cropland extending from the High Plains of western Texas and eastern New Mexico northward into Oklahoma, Kansas, Nebraska, and eastern Colorado is today seriously in doubt. The groundwater supply which has converted the arid short-grass prairie into lush expanses of corn and cotton is being pumped at ever-increasing rates from what may be the world's largest reserve of underground water—the Ogallala Aquifer. This enormous sand-and-gravel formation was deposited millions of years ago as the eastern front of the Rocky Mountains eroded. The plentiful rains of Pleistocene times saturated the formation which later became sandwiched between an underlying layer of impermeable shale and a cap of erosion-resistant rock above, preventing escape of the entrapped water. Subsequently, the regional climate became drier and today little rain manages to percolate through the overlying strata to recharge the aquifer. The Ogallala, therefore, in a very real sense represents "fossil water"—a non-renewable resource, much like coal or oil which, once gone, is gone forever. The farmers who are pumping more water out of the Ogallala Aquifer each year than the entire flow of the Colorado River are mining groundwater, just as earlier exploiters of the West mined petroleum—and the ultimate outcome, i.e. exhaustion of reserves, will undoubtedly be the same. Given the current rates of extraction, the useful life of the Ogallala is estimated at approximately 40 more years, less in some areas. The water table has been dropping 6 inches to 3 feet a year and in many parts of the region irrigated acreage is already declining due to escalating costs of pumping water to the surface. Some experts predict that within a few years corn, the crop with the highest water demand, will vanish entirely from the High Plains. Although agriculturalists and public officials alike acknowledge that the Ogallala's reserves cannot last forever (farmers in the region qualify for a water-depletion allowance similar to the tax break given to oil-producers), the overuse of Ogallala water continues without any regulation. The prevailing attitude in the region seems to be one whereby each user, intent on immediate profit, tries to extract as much water as possible, assuming that when the well runs dry the federal government will be forced to rescue the regional economy with massive infusions of taxpayers' money.

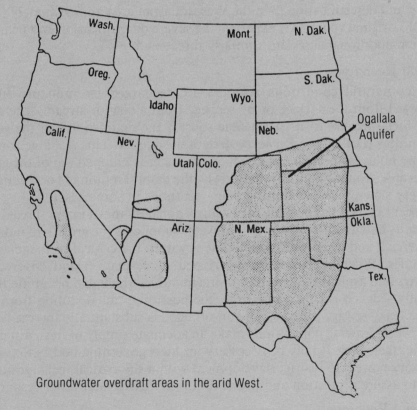

Groundwater overdraft areas in the arid West.

Source: U.S. Water Resources Council, *The Nation's Water Resources: 1975-2000,* Vol. 1: *Summary* (Washington, D.C.—U.S. Government Printing Office, 1978), p. 59.

region. The situation in the Southwest is particularly acute because the scarcity of major rivers makes groundwater an even greater necessity there than elsewhere in the U.S. While the nation as a whole depends on groundwater for 25% of its total consumption, reliance on this resource rises to 40% in California, 62% in Arizona, and 75% in West Texas. Tucson, Arizona, where annual rainfall averages 11 inches, is the largest city in the U.S. to rely entirely on groundwater for its municipal supply and is currently pumping its reserves out of the ground 5 times faster than they are being replenished. Groundwater overdrafts in the arid West are causing a number of serious environmental side-effects, the most visible of which is the drying up of many surface streams (recall that many rivers, particularly in dry climates, receive the bulk of their flow from underground sources with which they are in hydrologic contact). As groundwater reserves are depleted, land subsidence is occurring, accompanied by the formation of fissures and faults which disrupt irrigation canals and highways, as well as endangering buildings. Falling water tables are also resulting in the abandonment of hundreds of thousands of acres of irrigated land, as pumping costs become too great to make such farming economically feasible. These abandoned fields thereupon become subject to excessive rates of erosion and desertification.[10] In the West today an area approximately the size of the 13 original colonies is experiencing severe desertification and nearly half a million additional acres are similarly threatened.

Natural Recharge

Under natural conditions aquifers are recharged by moisture filtering downward from the surface or by seepage from a lake or stream. The area of land which, because of its permeable soils, is the main source of the ground-water inflow is called the *Recharge Area* of the aquifer. This recharge zone may be many miles from the point at which the water is pumped out of the ground; and because groundwater flows so slowly, the natural refilling of an aquifer may be a very slow process, requiring many centuries in some cases.

In recent years it has become increasingly apparent that a major threat to both the quality and quantity of our groundwater supplies is the growth of industrial, commercial, and residential development within the critical recharge areas of an aquifer. When such areas are stripped of vegetation and covered with buildings and asphalt the amount of precipitation which can penetrate the soil is greatly reduced. At the same time, the possibility for pollution from waste dumps, leaky sewage pipes, street run-off, etc., is substantially incresed—all at a time when growing populations make an adequate supply of fresh water more essential than ever. It may be necessary for local governing bodies to use their regulatory powers to restrict development within the critical recharge zones in order to assure protection and preservation of their groundwater resources.

Artificial Recharge

For many years, in various parts of the U.S., attempts have been made to recharge groundwater reservoirs artificially in order to increase or replenish the natural supply of groundwater. There are basically 2 ways of artificially recharging aquifers:

Water Spreading: The cheapest, most effective method involves releasing water over the ground's surface by means of flooding a large, relatively flat area or by releasing the water into basins, furrows, or ditches. This is done to increase the amount of water infiltrating the ground and percolating to the water table. Water spreading has been utilized to the greatest extent in California.

Pit, Shaft, and Well Recharge: In areas where hardpan, clay, or impermeable rock strata restrict water penetration, recharge by means of pits or shafts may be attempted. These are dug down through subsurface material into more permeable deposits below, from which water can filter directly into an aquifer. Recharging by means of a well, which pumps water from the surface to an aquifer below, may be practical where the water-bearing formations being depleted are deep and confined by impermeable layers or where lack of space, such as in urban areas, is a limiting factor. In the past, pit recharge was practiced in the Peoria, IL, area to replenish groundwater levels. Wells are being used to pump water used for cooling and air conditioning back into aquifers on Long Island where 3 million people rely totally on groundwater and where the supply is wholly dependent on precipitation falling directly on the island. In general, construction costs for implementing these methods are considerably higher than for water spreading and the amounts of water recharged are smaller, so they are justifiable only where the spreading method is not feasible. However, where land costs are high, pit recharge may be more economical than water spreading.[11]

It should be realized that the water used for artificial recharge purposes is always surplus water—water which has already been used for some other purpose or excess water from the high-flow period of a river. Thus, the practice of artificially recharging groundwater not only helps to raise the water table to normal levels, but also serves as a means for storing surplus water which otherwise would have run off into the sea.

Water Conservation

In recent years many ambitious, sometimes even visionary suggestions have been advanced for dealing with projected water shortages. Some of these ideas, such as proposed interbasin transfers of water, would be enormously expensive and would generate fierce political conflicts between donor and recipient regions. Others, such as the Rand Corporation's idea of towing plastic-covered Antarctic icebergs to southern California and to pipe the meltwater inland do not appear feasible in the near future. Technological advances in desalting seawater have resulted in a dramatic lowering of the cost for increasing water supplies by this method, but desalinated water is still far too expensive for use in irrigated agriculture. Efforts to enhance rainfall through cloud-seeding have received considerable government support for research and development, but concern about potential political and legal repercussions related to weather modification activities have kept the project in an experimental stage only. Agencies such as the National Research Council of the National Academy of Sciences doubt that weather modification technology could appreciably increase water supplies.[12]

In contrast to such high-technology, costly attempts to increase available water supplies, many authorities are convinced that the most sensible, economically feasible, and environmentally sound approach to prevent water shortages is to waste less of what we already have—in other words, to adopt a water conservation ethic. Contrary to popular belief, a call for water conservation is not a demand for citizens to change their lifestyle radically, nor does it necessarily imply deprivation. Rather, water conservation means making more efficient use of the resource available. Although demand curves for water have indeed been rising more rapidly than population curves during the past several decades, water *demand* and water *need* are not really the same thing. The amount of water required to support life, maintain public welfare, and produce food and consumer goods is much smaller than per capita water consumption charts would indicate. Statistics on water demand actually depict total water use without regard to how efficiently that water is being used, and future projections of water requirements assume that such demand will remain steady or increase. Recent trends indicate that such assumptions are not justifiable, because there are ways to decrease water use and still maintain a vigorous, productive society.

Because of historically low prices for water, there has been little incentive, except during short-term emergency situations, for implementation of water-saving policies. Nevertheless, many opportunities for water conservation exist. Regarding agriculture, the largest water consumer, new irrigation techniques could reduce the amount of water lost through evaporation by one-half to three-fourths. The second-largest consumer of water, industry, is beginning to look at ways of cleaning and reusing its wastewater or, in some cases, of changing production methods to less water-intensive processes. In some places

---

Box 14–4

Bathing with Friends and Related Activities
Water Conservation Begins at Home

Several years ago when a lengthy drought in the Northeast had seriously lowered the levels of reservoirs supplying water to New York City, officials of the Big Apple sponsored a contest for the best water conservation slogan. Among the hundreds submitted, one of the catchiest advocated, *"Save Water: Take a Bath with a Friend."* We can all smile at such tongue-in-cheek proposals, but the broader issues of water conservation are no laughing matter. The water demands of U.S. households, comprising about 8% of the nation's total water use, may seem insignificant compared to the amounts utilized by power plants, agriculture, and industry. However, considering that virtually all of the water consumed in the home is rendered unfit to use for other purposes (unlike power plant cooling water which is returned to a river or lake basically unchanged), the amount acquires increased importance.

Total water consumption in the home equals about 65 gallons per person per day (150 gallons/person if outdoor water consumption is included). Of this amount, only about 5% is used for drinking and cooking. The largest amount, 45%, is literally flushed down the toilet, 30% is consumed in bathing, and another 20% goes to wash dishes and clothes. Experts estimate that most people could reduce their water use by 15-20% without any drastic change in habits, simply by cutting down on waste. Some of the most effective ways to begin saving include:

1. *Eliminate leaks*—that dripping faucet, leaky pipe, or running toilet can waste hundreds or even thousands of gallons a month, yet in most cases is easy to repair. Toilet tanks can be checked for leaks by putting a few drops of food coloring in the tank; if color appears in the toilet bowl before it is flushed, this is evidence of a leak, probably caused by a plunger ball that needs to be cleaned or replaced. Washers on dripping faucets should be changed promptly. An over-all test for leaks consists of shutting off all water-consuming appliances in the house for 15 minutes, during which time someone should watch the lowest dial on the water meter. If the house is leak-free, the meter should not move at all; if it does and the problem cannot be located, a plumber should be called.

2. *Toilets*—since toilets account for almost half of daily household water use (5-7 gallons per flush), they should be used only to carry away body wastes, not as a wastebasket for kleenex and cigarette butts. The amount of water used with each flushing can be reduced by at least a gallon by placing inside the toilet tank a plastic container filled with water and a small stone or sand for weight. The container, of course, must be placed in such a way that it will not interfere with the mechanism. When installing a new toilet or replacing an old one, homeowners should be aware that there are newly-designed water-conserving toilets now on the market that use only 3-5 gallons of water per flush—a 30-40% reduction over the typical toilet.

3. *Bathing*—by taking showers instead of baths, keeping the duration of the shower less than 5 minutes, and by turning off the water while lathering, one can save 10-25 gallons of water per day.

4. *Bathroom sink*—most of the water used at the bathroom sink is wasted. Letting water run while brushing teeth, shaving, or washing hands and face can waste as much as 30 gallons per person per day. The best rule is simply to turn off the water when it is not being used.

5. *Dishwashing*—in general, electric dishwashers use less water than washing by hand; however, this advantage is offset if one rinses the dishes unnecessarily before loading the dishwasher. When washing by hand, soak first in a sinkful of soapy water and go sparingly on the rinse water.

6. *Garbage disposal*—this should be run only at the end of a meal or when full; do not use it for bones or peels that can just as easily be put in the trash. Better yet, compost fruit and vegetable waste in the garden.

7. *Laundry*—washing machines should be used only when there is a full load unless the washer has a variable load control. When washing clothes by hand, do not let the water run—fill a basin or tub and reuse the wash and rinse water whenever possible.

8. *Lawn care*—when watering is necessary, water in late evening or early morning when evaporation rates are lower; water slowly and thoroughly and let dry out between waterings. Allowing grass to grow slightly taller in the summer reduces water loss because the blades provide shade for the roots. Mulching in the garden is a big help in retaining soil moisture and reducing the need for frequent watering.

the steel industry has been able to cut its requirements by 90%. Renovation of disintegrating water distribution systems, as mentioned earlier, could save substantial amounts of water in many cities.

Perhaps equally important in reducing profligate water use among homeowners and businesses in many urban areas is the installation of water meters in each residence (several large cities do not meter water use, instead charging a flat rate to all users; under such a system individuals have no incentive to limit water use, since their water bill will be the same if they use 10 gallons of water or 10,000) and restructuring of water rates which in many areas are lower for large-volume users. In communities where water is already metered, an increase in water prices, though politically unpopular, may be the most effective method of reducing water demand. This policy has been pursued with some degree of success in Tucson, Arizona, where rate hikes convinced many householders that perhaps lush green lawns were a luxury desert dwellers could no longer afford and that cactus in the front yard could be equally attractive!

Experience in many parts of the country during drought emergencies—episodes marked, in many cases, by mandatory water-use restrictions—have shown that people *can* reduce water use significantly, with only minor inconvenience. During the mid-1970s drought in Marin County north of San Francisco, water conservation efforts, spurred by a 300% price increase, resulted in a drop in home water consumption from 122 gallons/day to 35 gallons/day over a 2-year period. Although efforts slackened somewhat after the drought ended, household water use several years later remained 25% lower than it had been prior to the drought.[13] The city of Elmhurst, IL, offers another good example of how a community beset with water supply problems launched a conservation program. A city of 50,000 in the Chicago suburbs, Elmhurst derives most of its water from deep wells. However, since the late 1950s, Elmhurst has been pumping water out of the ground faster than it is being naturally recharged. As a result, the water level in Elmhurst's wells has been steadily declining at an average rate of 14 feet per year. Because of the declining water table, Elmhurst sought permission to receive an allocation of Lake Michigan water. This was granted in 1977, on the condition that the city implement a number of water conservation measures. Elmhurst set a goal of reducing municipal water consumption by 10-15% and proceeded to achieve that objective through a combination of methods.

Perhaps most crucial to the success of the effort was a public education campaign which involved a newsletter mailed to all residents explaining the situation and offering conservation tips, a water bill mailing insert which explained the need for conservation, and extensive coverage by local media of the water supply problem and the need for conservation. Financial motivation for compliance was assured by the city's changing from a declining block rate charge to a uniform unit charge for water and sewage service. In addition, an excess facilities water rate was instituted after a study indicated that a small percentage of users were responsible for the high summer water demands.

Under this scheme, anyone whose water use during the summer exceeded base consumption rates by 30% would be charged at a higher rate. Recognizing that the two biggest users of water inside the home are toilets and bathing facilities, Elmhurst modified its plumbing code to require that all new plumbing installations and replacement fixtures meet certain water-conservation criteria. At the same time, a program was developed to retrofit existing toilets and shower heads with water-saving devices. Displacement dams for toilets, which can save approximately 1.6 gallons of water per flush, were distributed to every residence, as were a set of orifices for shower heads and dye tablets to check for toilet flush tank leakage. An ordinance was passed limiting use of water for outdoor purposes to 3 times weekly per home and then only between 8 p.m. and 8 a.m. Information was disseminated advising Elmhurst residents on proper methods of lawn maintenance and encouraging homeowners not to water their lawn unless it was newly seeded or sodded. By vigorously implementing reasonable conservation measures, Elmhurst saved both water and dollars and provided an example for other cities to emulate.

The people of Marin County and Elmhurst and of numerous other communities across the nation provide convincing evidence that water conservation practices can become an accepted way of life. Provided with the necessary "how-to" information and a cost incentive, citizens will validate the assertions of water managers who insist that the cheapest, quickest, and best way to secure more water is to conserve existing supplies.

REFERENCES

[1]Ehrlich, Paul, Anne Ehrlich, and John Holdren, *Ecoscience,* W. H. Freeman and Company, 1977.

[2]Powledge, Fred, *Water,* Farrar Straus Giroux, 1982.

[3]Jones, David, ed., *Water Supply and Waste Disposal,* Poverty and Basic Needs Series, Transportation, Water, and Telecommunications Department of the World Bank, September 1980.

[4]Powledge, op. cit.

[5]Pringle, Laurence, *Water: The Next Great Resource Battle,* Macmillan Publishing Co., Inc., 1982.

[6]Ibid.

[7]Powledge, op. cit.

[8]Sheridan, David, "the Underwatered West: Overdrawn at the Well", *Environment,* vol. 23, no. 2, March 1981.

[9]Council on Environmental Quality, *Contamination of Ground Water by Toxic Organic Chemicals,* January 1981.

[10]Sheridan, David, "The Desert Blooms—At a Price", *Environment,* vol. 23, no. 3, April 1981.

[11]Baldwin, Helen, and C. L. McGuiness, *A Primer on Ground Water,* U.S. Geological Survey, U.S. Government Printing Office, 1976.

[12]National Research Council, *Climate, Climatic Change, and Water Supply,* National Academy of Sciences, Washington, D.C., 1977.

[13]Pringle, op. cit.

15

Water
Pollution

"Praise be Thou my Lord for Sister Water
Who is very useful, precious and chaste"
—Canticle of Brother Sun 1225, St. Francis of Assisi

Back in the "good old days" when human settlements were relatively small
and far apart, the issue of water contamination seldom occupied much attention
on the part of the general public. Prevailing sentiment insisted that "the solution
to pollution is dilution", and popular wisdom held that "a stream purifies itself
every ten miles". While such statements have a certain amount of validity, they
lost their relevance as villages mushroomed into crowded cities and as the
expanse of countryside between towns steadily contracted under the impact of
urban sprawl. The rapid growth of human population and of industrial output
has resulted in a corresponding steady decline in water quality, as both
municipalities and industry regarded the nation's waterways as free, convenient
dumping grounds for the waste products of civilized society. During the present
century our careless waste management practices have turned most American
rivers into open sewers and many once-healthy lakes into algae-covered
cesspools. It is estimated that today fully 95% of all water drainage basins in the
country are polluted with such contaminants as toxic chemicals, human and
animal excrement, heavy metals, pesticides, silt, and fertilizers. The problems
posed by such pollutants involve far more than unpleasant sights and odors.
Waterborne disease outbreaks, massive fish kills, long-lasting changes in
aquatic ecosystems, and severe economic loss to sports- and recreation-based
industries—all are directly related to degradation of water quality by human
activities.

Water Pollution and Health

Although contamination of waterways with human and industrial wastes has a great many ramifications, none is of greater importance to policy-makers and citizens alike than the impact of water pollution on human health. While the nature of the problem differs somewhat in the developing nations vs. more industrialized societies, the extent to which polluted water adversely affects health and well-being is a world-wide source of concern.

Many health authorities now speculate that unless and until water quality is substantially upgraded, there will be no further improvement in public health and life expectancy such as that witnessed during the past 50 years or so. These experts estimate that perhaps as much as 80% of all illness in the world today could be prevented if everyone had access to safe water supplies and argue that it makes little sense to invest large amounts of money in building hospitals and training doctors if the people they intend to serve face renewed risk of disease every time they take a drink of water.[1]

In Third World countries, the most pressing health problems related to water quality involve contamination of waterways with the microbial pathogens found in human body wastes, a problem directly stemming from lack of adequate sewage disposal facilities. The gastrointestinal infections which occur when such pathogens are ingested are the leading cause of both death and sickness in most developing countries, contributing (along with malnutrition) to most infant fatalities and a large proportion of adult illnesses. Reducing the incidence of such disease requires not only water purification technologies, but also provision of sanitary waste disposal and education of the people regarding personal and household hygiene.[2]

In industrialized countries, disease caused by fecal pollution of waterways is no longer a major problem, though outbreaks of gastroenteritis traced to pathogenic contamination of drinking water do occur from time to time. Of greater concern today, however, is the potential long-term health threat posed by the multitude of organic and inorganic chemical substances, known to be present in most municipal water supplies today. Some of these chemicals are toxic, carcinogenic, or mutagenic; the biological effects of many remain unknown. Whether such chemicals pose a serious menace to public health at existing levels of concentration is a hotly debated issue—the fact that cancer rates seem to be higher in areas where water supplies are heavily polluted with synthetic industrial chemicals provides suggestive, but not conclusive, evidence.

An understanding of water pollution's impact on human health and well-being requires a look at the major sources and types of pollution and the problems posed by each. The remainder of this chapter will focus on such parameters and will attempt to delineate the challenges faced by regulatory agencies as they strive to protect public health through improving water quality.

Box 15–1
Schistosomiasis: Waterborne Scourge of the Third World

In 74 developing nations of Africa, Asia, and Latin America over 200 million people suffer recurrent fever, chills, and chronic weakness due to a waterborne ailment variously known as schistosomiasis, bilharzia, or snail fever. Next to malaria, schistosomiasis is today the world's most widespread serious infectious disease. Unfortunately, development projects in the Third World, particularly the construction of large dams and expanded irrigation networks, have greatly increased the number of people afflicted and have introduced the disease into areas formerly unaffected.

Schistosomiasis is caused by species of parasitic worms or "blood flukes," which pass different stages of their life cycle alternately inside snail and human hosts. First-stage larvae, hatching from eggs in the water, must find an appropriate species of snail which they then penetrate; within the snail the larva multiplies asexually, and within a one or two month period produces thousands of second-stage larvae which emerge from the snail into the water. These free-swimming, second-stage larvae have approximately 2 days in which to locate a human host, through whose skin they penetrate. Developing into small worms inside the human body, they travel through the circulatory system to the liver where they mature and mate. Subsequently they migrate to the bladder or the intestines, depending on the species, and there the female worms commence to lay 300-800 eggs daily for a period of 3 to 5 years. Some of these eggs are excreted in the urine or feces, while others are carried in the bloodstream to other parts of the body where they eventually die, causing inflammation and lesions. Since there is no multiplication of worms inside the human body, the seriousness of the infection depends on the number of second-stage larvae which penetrate the victim's skin. If the eggs which are excreted reach a body of slow-moving fresh water within a month, they hatch almost immediately and the cycle is repeated.

Although schistosomiasis is seldom fatal, its severely debilitating nature gravely impairs the productivity of infected individuals. Reducing the prevalence of schistosomiasis has been tackled via a broad-based effort to break the link in disease transmission—something which sounds simple enough in theory, but is very difficult in practice, given existing conditions of life in the developing world. Attempts to eradicate the snail hosts of the schistosome organisms have proven largely ineffective because even a few snails can produce enough schistosome larvae to infect a large number of humans. Therefore, snail-killing pesticides would have to be 100% effective in order to break the disease cycle—a near-impossible situation, since many snails could burrow into the mud to survive. Even in the unlikely event that the entire snail population in a given section of waterway is eradicated, there is nothing to prevent the influx of new snails from neighboring areas. In addition, the use of large quantities of pesticides incurs the risk of undesired environmental side-effects, while the cost of the chemicals is often beyond the means of financially-strapped Third World treasuries. Increasing the velocity of water flow in canals and irrigation ditches, fluctuating water levels, lining the edges of such waterways with concrete and removing water weeds along stream banks help to reduce snail numbers by altering their preferred habitat, but here again complete eradication is seldom possible.

An alternative approach to controlling schistosomiasis focuses on treating human victims of the disease with orally-administered drugs such as oxamiquine and praziquantel which produce high cure rates after a single dose. Although relatively expensive ($2-4 per dose), these drugs are effective against all species of schistosomes and kill many other parasitic worms as well; if used for projects sponsored by the World Health Organization (United Nations), they can be obtained at a considerable discount.

The most promising approach to control of schistosomiasis is generally thought to consist of an integrated program of chemotherapy, public health education, improved methods of sanitary waste disposal, provision of safe drinking water supplies, and modifying snail habitat, as described above. If human body contact with water could be avoided, larvae could not penetrate the victims' skin; if infected individuals could be persuaded to use latrines instead of urinating and defecating in or near the water, schistosome eggs would be unable to hatch. Unfortunately, avoiding contact with water is virtually impossible in Third World village society, where shallow waterways are used for bathing, swimming, doing laundry, planting rice, and washing cattle. Altering toilet customs appears a more feasible option, but centuries-old habits are hard to change, particularly among children and teen-age boys who are accustomed to urinating in the water while bathing and swimming. Efforts by civil authorities to reduce water contact by building bridges over canals, constructing public facilities for laundering, bathing, and recreation, and by providing safe drinking water offer some promise if the necessary funding can be obtained. National planners as well as international lending agencies must increase their efforts to break the cycle of disease which condemns a large portion of the developing world's population to life-long disability.[3]

Sources of Water Pollution

Pollutants can enter waterways by a number of different routes. Strategies for preventing water contamination must take into consideration the nature of the pollutant source and must devise appropriate methods of control for each source category. Congress has coined two terms—*Point Source* and *Non-Point Source*—to refer to the two general types of water pollution and pollution control regulations adopted within recent years have by necessity been tailored according to source.

Point Sources

Pollutants which enter a waterway from a specific point through a pipe, ditch, culvert, etc., are referred to as "point source pollutants". Typical point sources of water pollution include sewage treatment plants and factories. Point sources have been the most conspicuous violators of water quality standards, but because effluent from such sources is relatively easy to collect and treat, considerable progress has been made during the past decade in reducing this type of pollutant discharge. The two major categories of point source pollution— sewage treatment plants and industrial discharges—will be discussed in greater detail in a following section.

Non-Point Sources

Until recently non-point source pollutants—those which run off or seep into waterways from broad areas of land rather than entering the water through a discreet pipe or conduit—were largely overlooked as significant contributors to water contamination. However, when stringent effluent limitations on point sources failed to result in dramatic improvements in water quality, it became increasingly evident that in many waterways the largest pollutant contribution was coming from non-point sources. It is currently estimated that fully 99% of the sediment in our waterways, 98% of bacterial contaminants, 84% of phosphorus, 82% of nitrogen, and 73% of biochemical oxygen demand are contributed by non-point sources.[4] The majority of states have now identified pollutants from such sources as the main reason they have been unable to attain their water quality goals. Non-point source pollution (really just new terminology for old-fashioned runoff and sedimentation) results primarily from a variety of human land-use practices and includes the following:

Soil Erosion and Sedimentation—the single largest source of water pollution in the Midwest and in farming areas in general is soil erosion. While most people tend to think of erosion largely in terms of its adverse impact on agricultural productivity, soil entering streams or lakes can severely damage aquatic habitats as well. By increasing the turbidity of the water, sediment sharply reduces light penetration and thereby decreases photosynthetic rates of producer organisms; it buries bottom-dwelling animals, suffocating fish eggs and aquatic invertebrates. By serving as carriers of farm nutrients and pesticides, eroding soil particles introduce a wide variety of harmful chemicals into waterways, thus hastening eutrophication (see Box 15-2) and precipitating fish kills. Since at least half of all sediment comes from cultivated lands, the main approach to controlling this type of non-point source pollution is to promote soil-saving practices such as conservation tillage, terracing, and contour plowing which aim to keep soil on the land and out of the water.

Construction Activities—acre for acre, runoff from sites where homes, shopping centers, factories, or highways are under construction can contribute more sediment to waterways than any other activity. Over 200 tons of sediment per acre per year can wash off such sites into streams during the construction period, frequently carrying with them cement wash, asphalt, paint and cleaning solvents, oil and tar, and pesticides. Fortunately the actual construction time during which land surfaces are unprotected is relatively short and the amount of land exposed is small in comparison with farm acreage. Nevertheless, damage to water quality due to construction site runoff can be severe and long-lasting. Many municipalities are now mandating the use of readily available erosion control techniques on construction sites, the basic approach being to expose the smallest area of land possible for the shortest period of time and scheduling construction activities so that the minimum amount of land is disturbed during the peak runoff period in the spring. Using mulches and fast-growing cover vegetation, retaining as many existing trees and shrubs on the site as possible, roughening the soil surface or constructing berms to slow the velocity of runoff, and building retention basins to detain runoff water long enough to promote settling out of suspended sediment are all well-established management practices for reducing pollutant runoff from construction sites.

Animal Feedlot Runoff—when manure piles at animal feedlots are located near a stream or lake, heavy rains can wash large amounts of animal organic wastes into the water. Such feedlots can contribute 5 or 6 times as many nutrients to waterways as do point sources. Spreading of manure on fields

Approximately half of our water quality violations can be traced to stormwater runoff from broad land areas. Controlling pollution from these diverse sources is proving far more difficult than reducing pollutants from point sources. [*Illinois Environmental Protection Agency*]

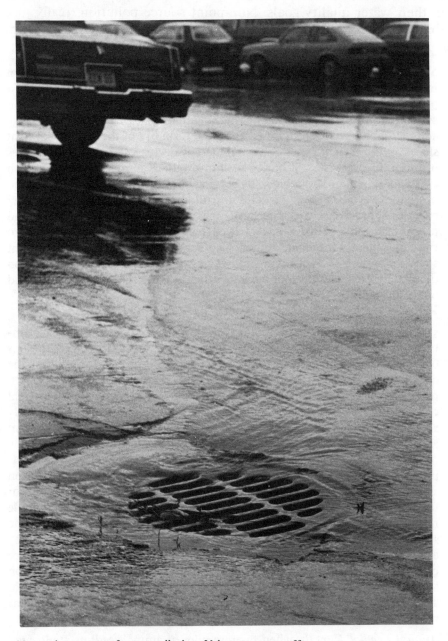

Non-point sources of water pollution: Urban street runoff

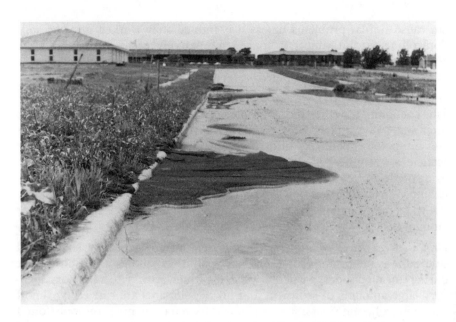

Non-point source of water pollution: Construction site runoff. [*Gary Fak*]

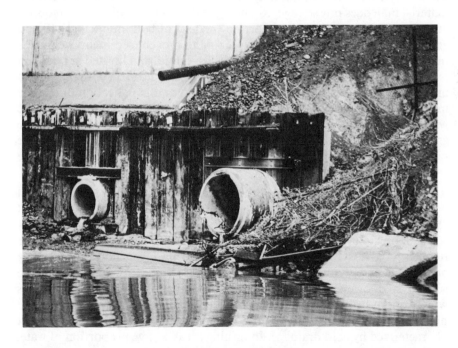

Point source of water pollution; effluents entering a waterway directly from a factory outfall, pipe, ditch, or sewage treatment plant outlet are the most visible source of water pollution. [*Illinois Environmental Protection Agency*]

can cause similar problems unless it is immediately worked into the soil. Controlling feedlot runoff is managed relatively easily by providing a diversion system which keeps clean water from running through the feedlot and redirects the flow of polluted water running off such areas.

Pesticide and Fertilizer Runoff—since these chemicals, which can poison fish, contaminate wells, and promote unwanted algal growth, most often enter waterways attached to soil particles, they can best be controlled by preventing soil erosion. Additional management strategies include: applying pesticides when there is little wind and the potential for heavy rain is low; using non-persistent, low-toxicity pesticides; disposing of containers properly; applying fertilizers only when they can be incorporated into the soil (i.e. not when the ground is frozen); and using any type of chemical in the proper amount and only when field checks indicate they are needed.

Urban Street Runoff—although people seldom consider city streets and sidewalks as important sources of water pollution, studies have shown that during storm episodes, particularly storms which terminate a long dry spell, very large amounts of sediment and other pollutants are carried by runoff water into adjacent rivers, streams, or lakes. Contaminants commonly found in urban runoff include sand, dirt, road salt, oil, grease, and heavy metal particles (lead, zinc, copper, chromium, etc.) from paved surfaces; pesticides and fertilizers from lawns; leaves, seeds, bark, and grass clippings; animal and bird droppings; and other substances too numerous to mention. In some situations, urban street runoff may carry a greater load of suspended organic material than does raw sewage. Reducing pollution from this source requires broad-based cooperation and effort on the part of both municipal officials and citizens: more frequent street-sweeping to prevent sediment accumulation on streets; proper disposal of pet wastes; careful and limited application of lawn and garden fertilizers and pesticides; litter control on both public and private property; judicious use of road salt and sand; application of organic mulches to reduce erosion on bare ground; incorporating more green space within the urban areas and along waterways to allow runoff to filter into the ground; use of surface ponds, holding tanks, rooftop catchments, subsurface tunnels, or similar structures to hold, retain, and gradually release stormwater.

Acid Mine Drainage—when the iron pyrite found in association with coal deposits is exposed to air and water during mining operations, a series of chemical reactions is initiated, culminating in the formation of a copper-colored precipitate (iron hydroxide) and sulfuric acid. The precipitate frequently covers the bottom of streams in mining regions, smothering bottom life and giving such streams a characteristic rusty appearance. The sulfuric acid lowers the pH of the water, eliminating many aquatic species which cannot survive or reproduce in the acidified water. Both operating and abandoned coal mines of either the underground or surface type are characterized by acid drainage. In mining areas a large proportion of water quality violations are due to this phenomenon.[5]

Fallout of Airborne Pollutants—the situation represented by acid rainfall (see Ch. 12) is but one example of pollution from the sky causing water quality problems. A great many of the particles released into the atmosphere by man eventually return to earth and enter rivers, lakes, or oceans either directly or in runoff. These airborne particles include many hazardous chemicals such as lead, asbestos, PCBs, beryllium, fluorides, and various pesticides. The contribution to water pollution by man-made chemical fallout is surprisingly large—the major portion of PCBs and other toxic chemicals in the Great Lakes and a substantial amount of the hydrocarbons found in the oceans entered these waters through airborne deposition.

As point source pollutants are increasingly on the decline due to improved pollution control technology and enforcement of effluent limitations, the non-point sources described above will present the greatest obstacle in attaining our nation's clean water goals. Controlling non-point source pollution unfortunately demands more than just a technological "fix"; it requires instead the cooperation of farmers, ranchers, and homeowners, municipal officials, developers, etc., in implementing better land management practices to prevent these diverse pollutants from running off the land and into the water.

Currently, the regulatory approach to controlling non-point source pollution emphasizes voluntary compliance. The federal government's role has been limited to providing state and local agencies with technical and financial assistance and to sponsoring research and development activities directed at combatting runoff-induced water degradation problems.

Box 15–2

Too Much of a Good Thing

Aquatic plants, like their terrestrial cousins, require certain mineral nutrients for healthy growth and metabolism. An excess of these essential elements, however, can result in a plant population explosion which leads to serious degradation of water quality and radical changes in the species composition of the overfed lake, pond, or stream. The process by which a body of water becomes over-enriched with nutrients and as a result produces an over-abundance of plant life is known as *eutrophication,* a classic and easily-recognized form of water pollution. Although eutrophication can occur in sluggish streams, bays, and estuaries, it is most common in lakes and ponds. This is so because lakes, unlike flowing bodies of water, flush very slowly; thus nutrient-laden wastewaters or runoff introduced into a lake tend to remain there for many years. For this reason, ⅔ of the nation's lakes today have serious pollution problems, most of them due to eutrophication.

The most characteristic sign that a lake is undergoing eutrophication is the formation of a green scum, consisting of millions of microscopic algal cells, on the surface of the water. This is only the most visible outward indication that something is amiss, however, for a closer look at what's going on shows that a number of drastic changes in lake ecology are taking place. An analysis of the eutrophication process reveals the following sequence of events:

1. *nutrient enrichment of the water* with dissolved nitrates and/or phosphates contributed by sewage treatment plant discharges, septic tank seepage, urban street runoff, or runoff from fertilized agricultural lands or animal feedlots.

---

2. *algal "blooms,"* stimulated by these nutrients, occur near the surface of the water, and over-populate the aquatic environment with enormous numbers of aquatic plants, particularly species of cyanobacteria (previously known as blue-green algae).

3. *death of large numbers of algae* which then settle to the bottom of the lake or pond.

4. *decomposer organisms, primarily bacteria, multiply rapidly* in response to the great increase in their food supply (dead algae); as they break down the algal tissues in a low-oxygen environment, they release methane and hydrogen sulfide gas, which accounts for the unpleasant odor of decomposition frequently associated with algae-choked ponds.

5. *levels of dissolved oxygen in the water are depleted* due to the very high rate of metabolic activity of the decomposer organisms; the drop in oxygen content is particularly rapid in summer because high temperatures promote more rapid metabolism and because warm water holds less dissolved oxygen than does colder water.

6. *fish and insect species requiring high levels of dissolved oxygen die and are replaced by species more tolerant of low oxygen conditions.* The kinds of fish and invertebrate species typical of a balanced aquatic ecosystem (e.g. bass, sunfish, trout) cannot live in waters where the dissolved oxygen concentration is below 5 or 6 ppm for any length of time; under low oxygen conditions, these species will give way to less desirable (from a human point of view) organisms such as sludgeworms, which can tolerate oxygen concentrations as low as 0.5 ppm and whose presence in bottom sediments is commonly used as a biological indicator of organic pollution.

7. *toxin secreted by cyanobacteria* imparts a foul taste to the water and may poison fish and livestock drinking from the lake if concentrations become sufficiently high.

Although eutrophication is a natural process of aquatic succession (see Ch. 1), its rate is greatly accelerated by the introduction of human-generated pollutants into aquatic ecosystems. Since people seem to prefer the cleaner water and more varied fish populations characteristic of the early developmental stages of a lake, it is in society's best interest to forestall the described course of events by preventing the nutrients which initiate the eutrophication process from entering the water in the first place.

Municipal Sewage Treatment

In 1854 the city of London was reeling under a severe epidemic of Asiatic cholera, a disease characterized by the sudden onset of profuse watery diarrhea and vomiting, resulting in rapid dehydration and death of approximately half of those afflicted. Not all parts of the city were equally affected, however. Within a district called St. James Parish, the cholera death rate hit 200 per 10,000 population, while in neighboring Charing Cross and Hanover Square districts fatalities were considerably lower. Dr. John Snow, a member of the commission of inquiry appointed to investigate the outbreak, noted that the vast majority of individuals who had died of cholera obtained their drinking water from a well on Broad Street; in other respects there seemed to be no fundamental difference between conditions in St. James Parish and nearby districts where cholera rates were low. Although the cholera bacillus and its method of transmission had not yet been discovered, Snow recommended that the handle of the Broad Street pump be removed to prevent further consumption of water from the well. Shortly thereafter, the cholera epidemic subsided. Subsequent investigations disclosed that prior to the outbreak, residents of one house on Broad Street had been ill with an unidentified disease. Their fecal wastes had been dumped in an open cesspool near the well—and the brick lining of the cesspool had deteriorated to the point that the liquid wastes could readily seep through the ground and contaminate the well water. The connection between poorly managed human wastes and serious human disease was clearly demonstrated.[6]

London's use of open cesspools as a method of sewage disposal was a well-established practice in many parts of the world until the late 19th and early 20th centuries. These pits in the ground simply collect wastes which are then stabilized by bacterial action. Seepage of liquids into the soil from such holes was common, and since no disinfection was used, contamination of wells and aquifers with human fecal pathogens frequently occurred. During the 19th century the growing popularity of flush toilets in urban areas resulted in greatly increased volumes of wastewater requiring disposal. This additional influx produced frequent overflowing of public cesspools and caused a further spread of filth and waterborne disease, particularly cholera and typhoid fever. Installation of sewer systems which carried wastes directly from homes into nearby rivers helped to alleviate problems of well contamination but caused severe degradation of surface water quality, resulting in the elimination of many forms of aquatic life and enhancing the risk of waterborne disease in communities downstream which used surface water supplies for drinking.

By the end of the 19th century rapid urban growth convinced city planners of the need for construction of sewage treatment facilities to alleviate the health and aesthetic problems created by the dumping of raw sewage into waterways. Today in the United States over ¾ of the population live in areas where domestic wastes pass through a sewage treatment plant before being discharged (the remainder, for the most part, rely on on-site septic tanks for sanitary waste disposal). Provision of adequate methods of sewage treatment, along with the chlorination of drinking water, has done far more to reduce the incidence of epidemic disease and to upgrade standards of public health than has the more widely acclaimed introduction of modern medicines and vaccines.

The aim of sewage treatment is to improve the quality of wastewater to a level at which it can be discharged into a waterway without seriously disrupting the aquatic environment or causing human health problems in the form of waterborne disease. Achieving these goals requires killing pathogenic organisms present in human wastes (within any human population there will always be some individuals suffering from various gastrointestinal diseases and releasing the causative bacteria, protozoans, etc., in their excreta; it is assumed, therefore, that domestic sewage entering the treatment facility is contaminated with pathogens capable of causing disease outbreaks) and, to the greatest possible extent, removing organic wastes or converting them to inorganic forms so that after discharge they will not deplete the oxygen content of the receiving waters as they decompose. To accomplish these ends, several levels of sewage treatment are necessary:

Primary Treatment

The used water supply of a community, averaging about 100 gallons/person/day in cities having separate storm and sanitary sewers, flows from homes and institutions into the municipal sewer system which carries the wastes to a treatment plant. At this point sewage consists not only of human feces and urine, but also of wastes from laundry, bathing, garbage grinding, and dishwashing, as well as all the miscellaneous articles which find their way into the sewer system—sand, gravel, rubber balls, leaves, sticks, dead rats, etc. Primary sewage treatment consists of several mechanical processes designed to remove the larger suspended solids through screening and sedimentation. Though there may be minor variations in the methods used by different treatment plants, in general the incoming flow first passes through one or more screens to remove large floating objects. Comminutors (grinders) may be used to reduce the solids to a uniform size so they cannot damage or clog equipment. After the waste-laden water has passed the screens, it enters a grit chamber where the reduced velocity of flow permits sand, gravel, and other inorganic material to settle out. Injection of air into the tank is sometimes provided to maintain aerobic conditions and to remove trapped gases. Following several hours in an additional sedimentation tank, the wastewater enters the secondary treatment system or, in those plants having only a primary level of treatment, is chlorinated and discharged into the receiving waters. The solid material (sludge) which settled out in the sedimentation tank is regularly removed, dried, and disposed of by one of several methods.

While primary treatment is unquestionably better than no treatment at all, it does not result in an effluent of sufficiently high quality to prevent degradation of the receiving waters. During primary treatment approximately 50-65% of suspended solids are removed and the BOD (see Box 15-3) is reduced by about 25-40%. Because the polluting potential of such wastewater is still quite high, the Environmental Protection Agency does not consider primary treatment by itself an adequate level of sewage treatment.

Secondary Treatment

Whereas primary treatment is based upon physical and mechanical methods of removing suspended solids from wastewater, secondary treatment depends on biological processes, similar to naturally-occurring decomposition but greatly accelerated, to digest organic wastes. Microorganisms, predominantly aerobic bacteria, are utilized in the presence of an abundant oxygen supply to break down organic materials into inorganic carbon dioxide, water, and minerals. This can be accomplished by means of *Trickling Filters*—beds of crushed stone whose surfaces are covered with a microbial slime consisting of bacteria, protozoans, nematodes, etc., which absorb the organic material as the wastewater is sprayed over the surface of the rocks—or by the more modern *Activated Sludge Process*. This involves "seeding" a tank of sewage with bacteria-laden sludge, pumping compressed air into the mixture and agitating it for 4-10 hours. During this time the microbes adsorb most of the colloidal and suspended solids onto the surfaces of the sludge particles and oxidize the organic material. After the process is complete, the sludge is separated from the remaining liquid by settling. Most of this sludge, consisting primarily of masses of bacteria, is removed, but some must be retained and fed back into the incoming sewage to perpetuate the process.

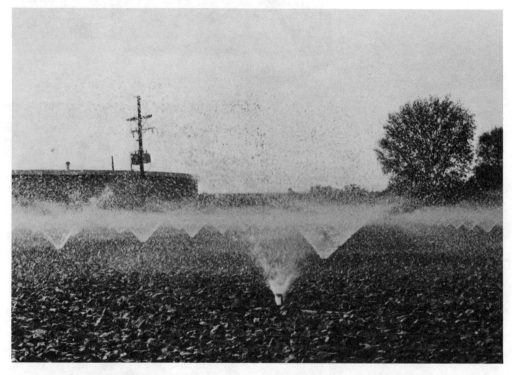

Trickling filter: a method of secondary sewage treatment in which wastewater effluent is distributed over a bed of rocks, the surfaces of which are covered by microorganisms that metabolize the organic nutrients in the wastewater, breaking them down into carbon dioxide and water. [*Author's Photo*]

After wastewater has passed through both primary and secondary treatment, the level of suspended solids and of BOD has been reduced by about 90% (however, cold weather can reduce the efficiency of pollutant reduction because it slows the metabolic rate of the microorganisms on which secondary treatment depends). Secondary treatment is not effective in removing viruses, heavy metals, dissolved minerals, and certain other chemicals.[7] A federally-imposed mandate requiring that all sewage treatment plants provide at least secondary wastewater treatment took effect in July, 1988.

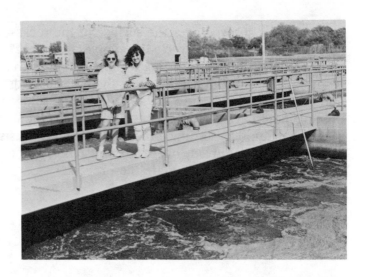

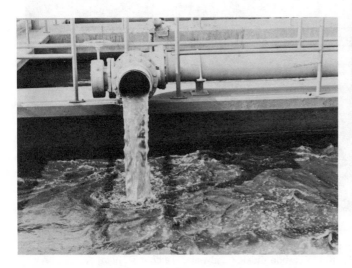

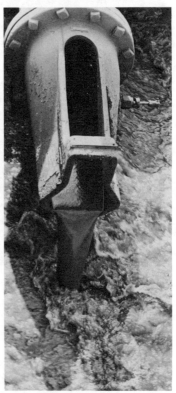

Activated sludge method: (a) a form of secondary sewage treatment in which wastewater effluent from primary treatment is mixed in aerated tanks with large numbers of bacteria ("activated sludge"). These bacteria feed on the organic nutrients, converting them to simpler inorganic substances. This process is energy-intensive, due to power requirements for running the pumps, but can achieve a very high degree of pollutant removal; (b) wastewater entering tank; (c) introduction of activated sludge. [*Author's Photos*]

Box 15-3

BOD

The most commonly used measurement of the amount of pollutant organic material in water is a parameter referred to as BOD—"biochemical oxygen demand". When bacteria act upon the organic matter in sewage or certain industrial wastes discharged into waterways, large amounts of dissolved oxygen are rapidly used up; this can result in fish kills and drastic alterations in the aquatic environment. Biochemical oxygen demand basically is an indication of how much putrescible organic material is present in the water or wastewater, with a low BOD indicating good water quality and a high BOD reflecting polluted conditions.

BOD is calculated by taking a sample of water, diluting it with fully-oxygenated water, and determining the amount of oxygen present at that time. The sample is then incubated in the dark at 20°C (68°F) for 5 days, after which the oxygen content is again measured. The difference between the initial and final readings, expressed in milligrams per liter (mg/l), is the BOD. Some representative BOD values are:

Pollutant	5-day BOD (in mg/l)
raw sewage	150-250
cannery wastes	5000-6000
discharges from pulp mills	10,000-15,000
wastewater from wool scouring	>20,000
treatment plant effluent	
(EPA standard—maximum average	30
for 30 consecutive days)	

Box 15-4

Border-Crossing Pollutants

Californians are currently grappling with a troublesome border-crossing issue which no immigration law can solve. Several miles of beautiful sandy beaches south of San Diego have been permanently quarantined since the early 1980s, while other stretches are closed intermittently, due to pollution by untreated sewage originating in Tijuana on the opposite side of the U.S.-Mexican border. Promoters of California tourism are concerned about the problem for economic reasons—the San Diego area plays host to 32 million visitors a year and officials fear that news of polluted seashore will drive these guests and their money elsewhere. From an ecological perspective the situation is worrisome also, since the wastewater threatens to degrade both San Diego Bay and U.S.-protected Tijuana Estuary—a unique saline ecosystem designated in 1982 as a National Estuarine Reserve and home to a number of endangered species.

The basic problem stems from the fact that the city of Tijuana, whose current population of 1.3 million is expected to double within 10 years, generates almost twice as much wastewater as its sewage treatment plant has capacity to handle. Consequently, the excess flow is simply discharged untreated into the Tijuana River and thence into the Pacific. To this amount is added raw sewage from smaller communities along the river and from broken pipelines leading to the treatment plant. Although the Mexican government had good intentions to expand Tijuana's sewage treatment capacity, financial constraints in that economically-troubled nation, as well as operational problems at the existing plant, have resulted in indefinite postponement of such plans.

Since Tijuana's problems adversely affect the environmental quality of its wealthier northern neighbor, numerous suggestions have been made that the U.S. help Mexico solve its wastewater treatment woes. A variety of proposals have been discussed, including U.S. funding of a new treatment plant in Tijuana, with effluent to be discharged through a jointly-used land and ocean outfall; construction on the U.S. side of the border of a treatment plant to be used solely by Tijuana; and construction of a joint facility on U.S. territory which could treat the wastewater from both Tijuana and the San Diego metro area (San Diego's own wastewater treatment performance is far from exemplary; its Point Loma wastewater treatment plant is at the top of EPA's Clean Water Act "hit list", accused of violating California's water quality standards for coliform bacteria and for discharging primary treated effluent into the ocean. San Diego is also charged with deficiencies in its pretreatment program and with poor sludge management and has been cited with more than 1800 spills of untreated wastewater from 1983-1988. According to a regional EPA official, "No other city in California has as far to go as San Diego to comply with the Clean Water Act"). No decision has yet been made on which, if any, of these long-range options to choose. Many Californians feel that solving Mexico's wastewater treatment deficiencies should not be the responsibility of U.S. taxpayers. Indeed, the most politically popular solution—and one which is currently being pursued—is the construction of what is referred to as the defensive pipeline or "U-turn pipe", a 2.3 mile "return to sender" conduit which will collect raw sewage flowing into the U.S. from Mexico and channel it back into Tijuana's wastewater system on the other side of the border. This strategy may alleviate some of the coastal pollution problems in southern California, but, in the absence of sewage treatment plant expansion in Mexico, would simply return the effluent to an already overloaded system. If utilized as an interim measure which would ultimately be integrated with one of the long-term options cited above, the U-turn pipe concept has merit; if viewed as the ultimate solution, as some San Diego politicians would like to do, the defensive pipeline falls short. Consensus of opinion among experts familiar with the situation favors construction of a facility to be used by both countries, insisting this would provide greater protection to the U.S. environment than the U-turn pipe alone is capable of doing. Such commentators see the defensive pipeline merely as the first step in what should be a joint cooperative effort to deal responsibly with the area's pollution problems. The ultimate response of policymakers to this troublesome issue could have far-reaching implications in other situations where pollution concerns straddle international boundaries.[8]

Advanced Wastewater Treatment ("Tertiary Treatment")

In situations where effluent from the secondary treatment process still contains substances which are causing water quality problems, when the sheer volume of effluent is large enough that the remaining 10% of suspended solids and BOD are sufficient to initiate eutrophication, or if the treated wastewater is to be used for purposes of drinking, irrigation, or recreation, then a third level of sewage treatment is required. Advanced wastewater treatment involves either one or a combination of several biological, chemical, or physical processes designed to remove such pollutants as phosphates, nitrates, ammonia, and organic chemicals. It also further reduces the concentration of remaining suspended solids and BOD to about 1% of that present in raw sewage. Some examples of tertiary treatment processes can be seen in Fig. 15-1.

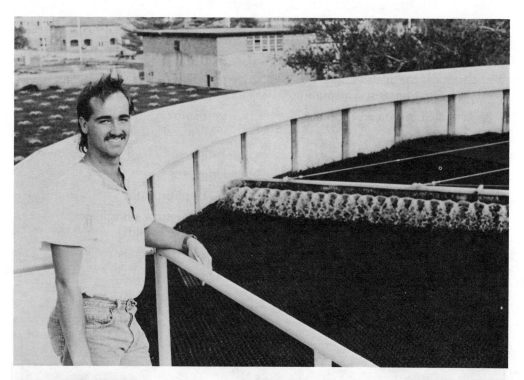

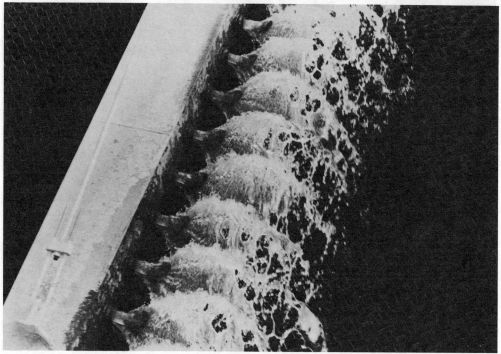

Nitrification tower: a method of advanced wastewater treatment for reducing the ammonia content of wastewater; (a) rotating bars distribute treated wastewater over the upper surface of a 40-50' high honeycomb-like plastic grid; as water trickles downward, aerobic nitrifying bacteria on the surfaces of the grid convert ammonia to nitrate; (b) close-up of nitrification tower grid surface. [*Author's Photos*]

Fig. 15-1

Tertiary Treatment Method	Pollutant Removed
Chemical coagulation, followed by filtration or sedimentation	phosphates, tertiary suspended solids, and BOD
Activated carbon adsorption	synthetic organic chemicals, tastes, odors
Ion exchange	ammonia
Air stripping	ammonia
Oxidation ponds and aerated lagoons	BOD, phosphates
Reverse osmosis	BOD, nitrates, phosphates, dissolved solids
Electrodialysis	dissolved minerals
Oxidation	organic material
Foam separation	organic chemicals
Land application	phosphates, nitrates, BOD, suspended solids

Box 15-5
Will Phosphate Detergent Bans Result in Sparkling Lakes?

For years controversy raged over which nutrient—nitrates or phosphates—was chiefly responsible for stimulating eutrophication. Both are necessary for plant growth, but the one present in the smallest amount is considered to be the limiting factor. In most situations involving aquatic environments, nitrates are far more abundant than phosphates; thus phosphates are generally regarded as constituting the limiting factor in determining whether rates of eutrophication are accelerated. When phosphate-laden effluents enter waterways, algal blooms are the usual result.

Phosphates can be contributed by various sources: they are present in fertilizer runoff, in human and animal body wastes, and in some industrial wastewaters; a small amount may be naturally present in groundwater, in marsh drainage, and in precipitation; urban runoff also contains not insignificant amounts of phosphorus compounds. In the early 1970s, when public concern about water pollution was at an all-time high, the largest portion of phosphates entering many waterways was traced to sewage treatment plant discharges, where 50-60% of the phosphorus loadings were contributed by laundry detergents used in millions of households. Since their introduction in 1945, detergents have largely replaced the use of soap for laundry purposes in the U.S. because of their superior cleaning ability in regions where hard water caused soap to form insoluble, greasy curds on clothes, leaving them grayish and dingy-looking after a number of washings. The major active ingredient in synthetic detergents which accounts for their resistance to hard water and their efficient cleaning power—their ability to leave clothing "whiter than white"—is the inorganic phosphate compound, sodium tripolyphosphate. By the early 1970s, detergents sold in the U.S. contained, on the average, about 12% phosphorus by weight, although some consisted of as much as 70% phosphate. Home washwaters entering the sewage system were thus heavily loaded with phosphates during those years and, in the majority of cases where municipal sewage treatment plants were not equipped to remove phosphates from the wastewater, these nutrients entered receiving waters along with the treated effluent and contributed to resulting algal blooms.

It was thus understandable that environmental activists of the period should focus considerable public attention on the phosphate detergent issue and demand that the industry do something to alleviate the problem. As a result, by the late 1970s the phosphate content of detergents had dropped by half and currently averages about 5%. Today the largest contributors of phosphorus to municipal wastewaters are human body wastes and food wastes, with detergents contributing only 20-30%.

Nevertheless, in areas where eutrophication of lakes was perceived as a critical problem, imposing legal limitations on the phosphorus content of laundry detergents was viewed by many as a quick, effective way of reducing phosphate loadings to overfed surface waters. Accordingly, as early as 1970 Canada enacted phosphate detergent limitations. Nine states in the U.S. followed the Canadian example, as Connecticut, Florida, Indiana, Maine, Michigan, Minnesota, New York, Vermont, and Wisconsin all attempted to ease their water pollution woes by mandating that detergents sold within their jurisdictions could not contain more than 8.7% phosphorus.

Since the 1970s, studies have been conducted on more than 400 lakes to evaluate the effectiveness of phosphate detergent bans in controlling or reversing eutrophication. The clear results of these investigations have proven quite disappointing to the advocates of such bans. The assumption of proponents that since phosphorus contributes to eutrophication, even small reductions in phosphate loadings should result in discernible improvements in water quality, can no longer be sustained. Because detergents are no longer the largest source of phosphates in domestic wastewater, the additional reductions in phosphorus loadings achieved by imposing limitations on their use simply are too small to have any impact on water quality. In areas where sewage treatment plant discharges are causing algal blooms, it is now considered more effective to implement relatively inexpensive advanced wastewater treatment processes which can remove 90% of the phosphorus in sewage, rather than imposing a phosphate detergent ban which could affect at most 20-30% of the phosphates present in wastewater. Beyond this, optimal control of phosphorus input to aquatic ecosystems demands much greater attention to sound land management practices in order to reduce the non-point source surface runoff and fertilizer applications which constitute the leading contributors of nutrients to waterways. Phosphate detergent bans, while superficially appealing as a "quick fix" to the problem of algae-choked lakes, have not proven to be the panacea we expected.[9]

Chlorination

Since the most common waterborn diseases are caused by pathogenic bacteria, viruses, or protozoans present in human excrement, one of the primary purposes of sewage treatment is to kill such organisms before they can infect new victims. Simple exposure to the hostile environment outside the human intestine is sufficient to reduce the number of bacteria appreciably as they pass through the treatment process. However, because a substantial number of live organisms still remain in the wastewater after primary and secondary treatment are complete, it has been standard procedure for many years to add chlorine to the treated effluent before discharge in order to eliminate any remaining disease-causing organisms. More recently, the policy of chlorinating all sewage treatment plant discharges has met with increasing

Fig. 15-2

Schematic Municipal Wastewater Treatment Process

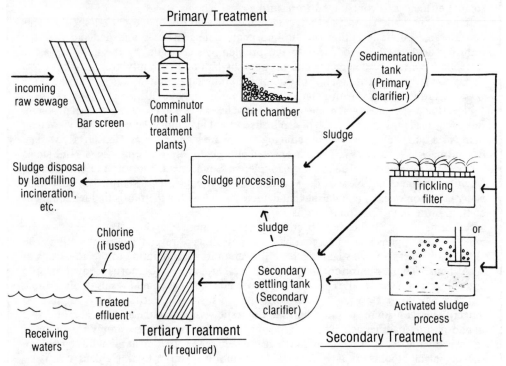

resistance and today over half of all states in the U.S. no longer require chlorination of wastewaters. The reasons for this change in accepted practice are several:

1. chlorine is effective in killing bacteria, but less so in relation to viruses, many of which survive this treatment.
2. chlorine is very destructive of fish and other forms of aquatic life, many of which are eliminated for a considerable distance downstream from sewage treatment plant discharge points due to the presence of this chemical in the water.
3. chlorine treatment is expensive and poses safety problems at the treatment plant in the eventuality of cylinder leaks or system disruption.
4. chlorine disinfects only a fraction of the wastes in streams because bacteria-laden runoff from farmland and urban areas enters waterways untreated.

Proponents of chlorinating sewage treatment plant discharges correctly point out, however, that this practice is effective in reducing outbreaks of disease which have been associated with swimming in sewage-polluted water or with the consumption of shellfish taken from waterways contaminated with bacteria-laden effluents from sewage treatment plants. Although disinfecting such effluent with chlorine does not sterilize the water, in the sense of killing every last microbe, it reduces their numbers significantly and thereby enhances the self-purifying capacity of natural waterways. As the controversy between wastewater chlorination opponents and proponents continues to rage, a compromise solution has been reached in some states where disinfection of discharge waters is required only during the summer bathing season, with the practice being discontinued during the winter when recreational contact with water is unlikely.[10]

Sludge Disposal

The more efficient sewage treatment processes are at cleaning pollutants out of wastewater, the greater is the amount of sludge requiring disposal. It is expected that by the year 2000 municipal sludge production will have reached 12 million dry metric tons as a result of continued population growth, increased efficiency of wastewater treatment systems, and more widespread compliance with Clean Water Act requirements. Because sludge itself can be a pollutant if improperly managed, its ultimate disposal and potential use must be handled in ways that will not endanger public health or the environment. Removed regularly at each step in the sewage treatment process, the watery sludge generally is first stabilized through aerobic or anaerobic digestion in order to reduce problems associated with odors and the presence of disease-causing organisms. To reduce its volume, the sludge is then thickened by either gravitational or mechanical processes. The concentrated liquid slurry must then be dewatered by one of several methods—drying on sand beds, vacuum filtration, pressure filtration, belt filtration, or centrifugation. At this point the sludge has the appearance of rich black dirt and is largely odor-free. This final product may be either landfilled, incinerated, co-composted with municipal yard wastes or woodchips, or applied directly to the land as a soil conditioner, provided it is not contaminated with heavy metals. Altogether, sludge treatment and disposal account for over 50% of the operating costs of a typical plant providing a secondary level of sewage treatment.

Since sewage treatment plants, particularly those in the larger metropolitan areas, generate enormous amounts of sludge during their normal course of operations, finding a place in which to dispose of this material poses major problems for many such facilities. Incineration of sludge can present problems of air pollution and in many communities open land for burying sludge is in short supply. Since the 1920s, a number of communities have utilized ocean dumping as a convenient and inexpensive method for disposing of their sludge, but in recent years this practice has been viewed with increasing public disfavor. At present 9 municipalities in New York and New Jersey, most notably New York City, collectively dump over 8 million tons of sewage sludge each year at a designated site located 106 miles off the New Jersey coast. Until 1987, the cities had used a dumpsite just 12 miles offshore; this area, known as the New York Bight, is generally regarded as one of the most degraded ocean

Fig. 15-3
Distribution of Municipal Sludge by Management Practice

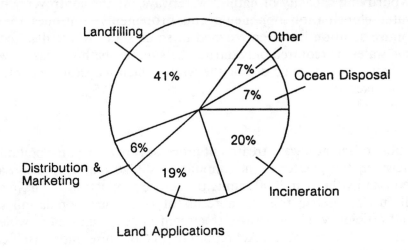

Source: U.S. Environment Protection Agency

bottoms in the world. Recent reports of diseased shellfish and high bacterial counts in seawater at the new site have prompted renewed concern about ocean dumping and widely publicized accounts of coastal pollution forcing closure of many popular East Coast beaches during the summer of 1988 generated intense election-year political pressure to end the practice once and for all.[11] Congress responded by passing the 1988 Ocean Dumping Ban Act, mandating that all dumping of sludge cease after Dec. 31, 1991. New York officials now face the daunting task of finding an alternative disposal method for the enormous quantities of sludge they generate daily and voice doubts that the Congressionally-imposed deadline can be met.

Elsewhere in the nation, a variety of innovative approaches to sludge disposal are being tried, most of them involving composting or land application. Over 200 municipal sewage treatment plants now have composting facilities either in operation or in some stage of development.[12] The end product of these operations resembles—and smells like—good, rich topsoil and is being sold or given away as a soil conditioner to home gardeners, farmers, and landscaping firms. Some cities, such as Milwaukee, Philadelphia, and Austin, TX, have employed imaginative marketing skills in promoting their product under such catchy tradenames as "Milorganite", "Philorganic", or "Dillo Dirt".

While sewage sludge contains sizeable amounts of phosphorus and nitrogen, both important plant nutrients, its usefulness to gardeners may be impaired by the presence of certain metals and toxic chemicals, especially if the sludge originated from a sewage treatment plant receiving industrial as well as domestic wastes. The contaminant of greatest concern is the toxic metal cadmium which is readily taken up from the soil by plants, particularly leafy vegetables, and can thereby pose a health risk to humans eatng crops grown on sludge-enriched soil. Mercury, zinc, lead, and copper can also be absorbed by plants and thus enter the food chain.[13] Unless an analysis of sludge content has shown it to be free of toxic contaminants, use of sewage sludge as a soil conditioner should be restricted to lawns, flower gardens, or other vegetation not intended for human consumption.

Innovative and Alternative Technologies (I/A)

Due to the high cost of advanced wastewater treatment and the obvious need to reduce the concentration of nutrients entering waterways from sewage treatment plants, Congress in 1977 passed an amendment to existing water pollution legislation, requiring communities asking for federal dollars to be used for sewage treatment plant construction to at least consider non-conventional disposal alternatives which would make use of the nutrients in sewage wastewaters. In other words, instead of returning nitrate- and phosphate-laden effluent to streams where it could cause eutrophication, sanitary districts are urged to look for innovative ways of reusing and recycling those nutrients in ways which are environmentally beneficial, energy efficient, and less expensive than standard methods of tertiary treatment.

By definition, "innovative" methods are those not yet proven to be successful but which offer promise of reducing costs, saving energy, or advancing the state of the art in waste treatment through new ways of containing pollutants, reclaiming and reusing effluents, making treatment more reliable or efficient, better managing toxic pollutants, finding more beneficial uses for sludge, and so forth. "Alternative" technologies, on the other hand, are different from the methods used in most conventional treatment plants but are approaches which are already being used successfully in various places. Alternative technologies include such practices as land treatment, water reclamation, artificial recharge of aquifers, use of wastewater in fish farms or tree plantations, etc.

Box 15–6
"DEEP TUNNEL": Chicago's Response to Combined Sewer Overflows

Deep under the streets of Chicago the 31-mile Mainstream Tunnel System constitutes a visionary—and highly successful—effort to solve a major water pollution problem facing many of our older cities: how to manage combined sewer overflows during periods of heavy rainfall. While most sewer systems installed in recent decades feature separate sanitary and stormwater conduits, the older sections of many urban areas still have combined sewers which carry not only sewage from households, but also stormwater runoff from city streets, rooftops, and lawns—all the water which isn't absorbed into the ground when it rains. Most sewage treatment plants are designed to accommodate the usual domestic wastewater flow (referred to as "dry weather flow"), usually with some built-in excess capacity. During storm episodes, however, water volume in combined sewers may be as much as 100 times greater than usual. Because the excess water would overwhelm the treatment capacity of the sewage plant, it is diverted past the facility and enters the

---

receiving stream untreated. Laden not only with human wastes but also with the wide variety of contaminants characteristic of urban runoff, combined sewer overflows seriously degrade the aquatic environment and are a common cause of water quality violations in older cities.

Beset by approximately 100 storm episodes per year which discharged raw sewage and stormwater into Chicagoland waterways and frequently caused flooding of streets and residential areas as well, the Windy City began looking for a long-term solution to its problem. Efforts to deal with this challenge in other communities suggested several alternative approaches: 1) separation of sewer systems in areas with combined sewers—a massive construction project presenting almost insurmountable difficulties in highly developed urban areas; 2) regular washing and sweeping of streets to reduce the pollutant concentrations in stormwater runoff; 3) construction of retention basins to hold stormwater runoff, gradually releasing it to the treatment plant in volumes which can be accommodated.

Chicago eventually settled upon one of the most ambitious and innovative public works projects ever undertaken. In the early 1970s, the city initiated its Tunnel and Reservoir Plan (TARP), the key segment of which is the Mainstream Tunnel, completed in 1985 and chosen by the American Society of Civil Engineers as the Outstanding Civil Engineering Achievement for 1986. The "Deep Tunnel", as it was promptly dubbed by the media, captures sewage-polluted stormwater from a 204-square mile urban area and stores it temporarily in 31 miles of tunnels at depths ranging from 240-300 feet below ground. After a storm has ended, this water is pumped back to the surface and sent at a controlled rate to sewage treatment plants prior to subsequent discharge into a waterway. Since the Mainstream Tunnel came on line, the frequency of combined sewer overflows and flooding throughout most of Chicago and 15 neighboring communities dropped dramatically—down 80% in its first year of operation. A second phase of TARP nearing completion will add to the Mainstream system about 18 miles of tunnels as well as several storage reservoirs, permitting capture of virtually all of the excess stormwater flow. No longer do engineers from around the world come to Chicago just to view its skyline—now they come to admire its sewer system as well![14]

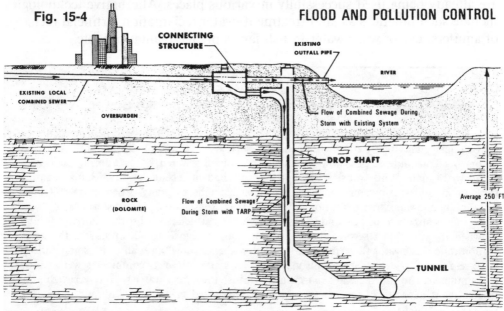

Fig. 15-4   **FLOOD AND POLLUTION CONTROL**

Schematic Representation of Chicago's Mainstream Tunnel (TARP)

Over 200 I/A projects have now been funded, the most popular method being land application of wastewater. This method involves spraying effluent which has received secondary treatment, as well as aeration and storage to kill remaining pathogens, onto forest, pasture, or crop lands. Land application not only helps to prevent system pollution by keeping nutrients out of the water, it utilizes those same nutrients as fertilizers for the plants on which it is applied. A further advantage of this method is that the wastewater is largely purified as it percolates through the soil to recharge the groundwater supply. The major concern about using such wastewaters for crop irrigation is the theoretical possibility that soil and vegetation might become contaminated with dissolved metals or other toxic compounds in the water. Experience with land application at Pennsylvania State University, Muskegon County, MI, Lubbock, TX, Bakersfield, CA, Lake George, NY, and in Germany, France, and Australia has not given evidence of any health problems related to this procedure.

Box 15–7

Designer Swamps

The coots and night herons delighting birdwatchers at the new freshwater marsh outside Arcata, CA, may not realize it, but they're part of a novel undertaking which promises to transform sewage treatment technology in small towns across the country. As their numbers grow and thrive in Arcata's carefully designed wetland, these waterfowl are living proof that the imperatives of restoring valuable ecosystems and providing for the nation's urgent wastewater management needs are mutually compatible.

Interest in the use of engineered wetland environments, or "designer swamps" as some like to call them, as an efficient, yet low-cost, alternative to conventional sewage treatment technologies has been growing rapidly in recent years. With the 1989 cutoff of federal dollars for the construction of municipal sewage treatment plants—a program which has channeled billions of dollars to local governments across the country since 1972—many of the 100 million Americans living in communities still served by inadequate sewage treatment facilities are considering planned wetlands as an affordable way of complying with stringent Clean Water Act standards.

Intended primarily to serve towns of 10,000 population or less, artificial wetlands can be built for less than half the cost of a conventional sewage treatment system, are far simpler and less expensive to operate, are as good or better at removing pollutants, and have the additional advantage of providing wildlife habitat. Adapting methods pioneered in Germany in the early 1970s, over 50 towns in the United States and Canada are now using artificial wetlands to treat sewage.

The process relies essentially on a marshland's ability to act as a natural filter. Following secondary treatment and disinfection at a conventional sewage plant, wastewater effluent (which still contains some suspended solids and inorganic nutrients) is allowed to move slowly through marsh vegetation—frequently bulrushes and cattails or, in warm climates, water hyacinth; as it flows, suspended solids settle out; microorganisms attached to the stems of aquatic plants metabolize dissolved organic wastes and plant roots take up inorganic nitrates and phosphates. Wetlands treatment also effectively breaks down pesticides, industrial solvents, and removes 90% of the heavy metals in wastewater.

The major limitation to such systems is the amount of land they require—about 20 acres for a town of 10,000 people. Unless a community already owns land on its outskirts, being able to afford, or even find, this much land may present serious difficulties. Perhaps the biggest obstacle to a rapid increase in the number of communities using artificial wetlands is sheer ignorance and inertia. Only recently have adequate design guidelines become available for engineers and regulators; municipal officials frequently are unaware of the advantages such systems offer; conventionally-trained engineers are frequently reluctant to embark on new, little-tried technologies and often lack the understanding of environmental conditions needed to factor these into their designs. Cynics might also wonder if engineers' general lack of enthusiasm might stem from the fact that cheaper artificial marshes translate into lower fees for engineering firms, since payment is typically calculated as a percentage of total project cost.

Nevertheless, with the evaporation of federal funds for sewage treatment plant construction and upgrading, and with stringent penalties for non-compliance with effluent requirements, it's likely that economically attractive, easy-to-operate "designer swamps" will become a fashion trend in the years ahead.[15]

Fig. 15-5   TYPES OF CONSTRUCTED WETLANDS

SURFACE FLOW SYSTEMS

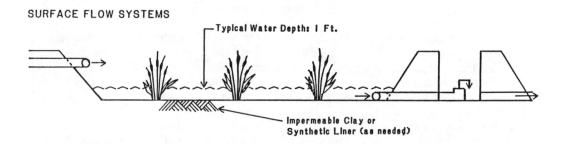

SUBSURFACE FLOW SYSTEMS

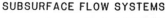
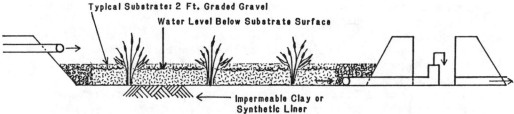

Source: Tennessee Valley Authority

Septic Systems

Approximately 25% of all Americans live in unsewered areas where they must utilize on-site septic systems for the disposal of wastewaters from bathrooms, kitchens, and laundries. A septic system consists of 2 basic parts: 1) a septic tank, buried in the ground at some distance from the house, to which it is connected by a pipe, and 2) a soil absorption field or buried sand filter.

The septic tank itself is a watertight container made of concrete or fiberglass with a minimum capacity of 750 gallons. Sewage entering the septic tank is partially decomposed by bacteria under anaerobic conditions. During this process, sludge settles to the bottom of the tank, while lighter solids and grease, as well as gases from the decomposing sludge, rise to the top to form a floating scum. The partially clarified liquid then passes through a pipe and the effluent is evenly dispersed among several perforated pipes in a carefully designed absorption field, which must be of adequate size and proper soil porosity to ensure that the effluent seeping out of the perforated pipe moves quickly enough to prevent ponding, but not so rapidly as to infiltrate aquifers, wells, or surface water supplies before contaminants in the effluent have been filtered out or oxidized.

Since more than half of the solids in the wastewater settle out during the retention period in the septic tank, the accumulation of sludge at the bottom, as well as the scum layer at the top, must be removed periodically. If this is not done, the sludge build-up reaches the point that solids are discharged into the absorption field, resulting in clogging and ponding. This accumulation of particulates and scum in the pores of the soil prevents proper drainage of the effluent and eventually results in failure of the system. In addition to improper maintenance of the septic tank, other reasons for septic failure are: use of a septic tank which is too small for the householders' needs, too great a usage of water in the house, insufficient size of the absorption field, and too impervious a soil.

Although a well-located, carefully constructed, and properly maintained septic system can be a perfectly adequate method of sanitary waste disposal (and is the only feasible option in most rural areas), malfunctioning septic systems frequently give rise to serious non-point source water pollution, as leachates containing pathogenic organisms and nutrients seep from absorption fields into water supplies. The rapid growth of rural subdivisions, many of which rely on septic systems installed on lots too small to provide adequate waste dispersal, ensures that pollution problems related to septic systems will continue to plague public health officials.

Industrial Discharges

Effluent discharges from almost 100,000 industrial sources nationwide affect 75% of all U.S. river basins (as high as 88% in the Great Lakes region) and constitute, along with municipal sewage treatment plants, the second major category of point source water pollution. Industrial discharges consist of a wide variety of pollutants which, for regulatory purposes, have been subdivided into

3 major categories:

> *Conventional Pollutants*—include organic wastes high in BOD, suspended solids, acids, oil and grease, etc. Such pollutants originate from food processing plants, pulp and paper mills, steel mills, oil tanker spills and cleaning operations, accidents involving offshore oil drilling, and so forth.

> *Toxic Pollutants*—a list of 129 specific toxic pollutants has been compiled by EPA; substances listed include heavy metals such as cadmium, mercury, and lead, PCBs, benzene, chloroform, cyanide, arsenic, 2,4-D, and a number of other pesticides. The electroplating and metal-processing industries, plastics manufacturers, and chemical companies are but a few of the industries discharging toxic effluents.

> *Non-Conventional Pollutants*—all the other pollutants not classified by EPA as either conventional or toxic are grouped into this third category—substances such as nitrogen and phosphorus, iron, tin, aluminum, chloride, and ammonia. As in the preceding categories, the sources of such pollutants can be traced to a wide variety of industrial processes.

Different levels of control are required for each general category of pollution and, for the most part, industry has a better record of compliance with existing water pollution regulations than do municipal dischargers (i.e. sewage treatment plants). At present the most serious water quality problems related to industrial discharges concern the toxic pollutant category. Due to EPA's slowness in promulgating the industry-specific effluent guidelines mandated by Congress, many industries continue to discharge toxic pollutants without violating standards; such industries technically are in compliance with the law because standards for the particular pollutants involved have not yet been finalized. Recent budget and personnel cut-backs at EPA have further hindered issuance of effluent guidelines and have hampered enforcement activities. A General Accounting Office investigation several years ago reported that non-compliance with discharge permit conditions is both frequent and widespread and recommended that stricter enforcement of existing laws is needed.[16] It should also be pointed out that the current permit system is not at all the same as a "zero discharge" policy. Permits specify the maximum allowable amounts of various pollutants which a given industry is allowed to discharge, the assumption being that below a certain concentration even toxic pollutants will be sufficiently diluted in the receiving waters to pose no acute threat to public health. Thus industries located along such waterways as the Niagara River in New York State may discharge as much as 7 tons of toxic chemicals into the river each day and still be in compliance with their permits.

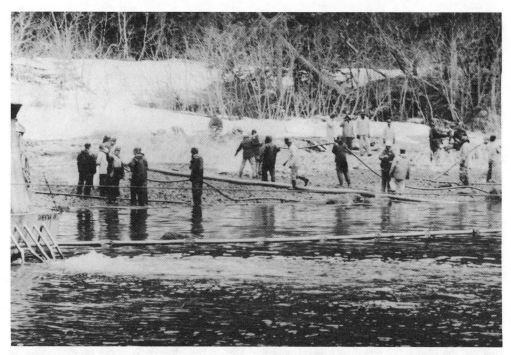

In April of 1989, crews were summoned to clean the beaches surrounding Alaska's Prince William Sound after what was the worst oil spill disaster in U.S. waters to date. [*USEPA*].

Box 15–8

Troubled Waters

Few environmental accidents capture media attention more dramatically than a massive spill of oil or chemicals into a major waterway. Frantic efforts to shut off water intake valves, dogged attempts to rescue bedraggled waterfowl, the weary task of cleaning befouled beaches—such scenes both anger and frighten a public concerned about local toxic hazards and raise questions regarding long-term ecological damage following such events. Two specific cases in point illustrate the fact that accidental industrial spills can happen virtually anywhere and can have far-reaching impacts.

The Rhine River flowing northward from Switzerland along the French border, through Germany and the Netherlands, and ultimately emptying into the North Sea, is one of the world's most polluted rivers. It became even more so on the night of Nov. 1, 1986. At about 7 o'clock that evening, alarms began ringing at a Sandoz chemical company warehouse near Basel, Switzerland. A raging fire had broken out in the building which contained 1000 metric tons of agricultural pesticides, as well as 300 tons of other chemicals. The blaze was spreading rapidly and efforts to control it with foam proved ineffective. Fearing the conflagration could spread to neighboring buildings, firefighters began pouring water on the flames. As chemical-contaminated runoff water streamed from the site, the capacity of surrounding catchment basins was overwhelmed and the polluted effluent poured into the adjacent Rhine. For days thereafter, horrified TV viewers around the world were given daily progress reports, as highly toxic mercury compounds, organophosphate insecticides, nitrocresol herbicides, and other dangerous chemicals drifted through Europe's industrial heartland, leaving massive fish kills in their wake. Fortunately no human deaths or illnesses resulted from the spill and subsequent reports state that no long-term effects on the health of the local population are expected. River-dwelling plants and animals were not so lucky; severe damage to aquatic organisms has been documented for a 155-mile stretch downstream from Basel. Although initial reports announcing the "death of the Rhine" were obviously exaggerated, observers warn it may be years before the water regains its pre-spill condition.

Just a year and 2 months after world attention was riveted on the Sandoz accident, the U.S. experienced one of the largest inland oil spills in its history. This time media cameras were trained on the Monongahela, 25 miles south of Pittsburgh, where just after dusk on Jan. 2, 1988, a 4-million gallon steel tank owned by Ashland Oil Company collapsed, releasing a massive flood of diesel fuel which surged over the containment dikes in all directions onto surrounding land. About 750,000 gallons of the oil entered storm sewers on adjacent property and from there flowed directly into the Monongahela River. As required by the Clean Water Act's National Contingency Plan, Ashland immediately notified federal authorities about the accident and within the hour contractors were on the scene. However, by the time equipment was brought to the river, the oil slick had passed the first lock and dam 12 miles downstream, generating strong fumes as it went. Being considerably lighter than crude oil, the diesel fuel emulsified rapidly in the water, complicating collection efforts (ultimately, only about 175,000 gallons of the spilled fuel were retrieved from the river). For the next several weeks, as the oil slug flowed from the Monongahela into the Ohio and toward the Mississippi, cities all along the Ohio River Valley scrambled to protect their water supplies. Sewage treatment plants were not affected, but water intakes as far west as Cincinnati were forced to close due to the spill. Cooperative water-sharing arrangements within the affected areas eased the burden on stricken communities. Pittsburgh sent water from its unimpacted Allegheny River plant to hard-hit nearby towns. In Wheeling, WV, whose water treatment plant was closed for 2 days, workers jerry-rigged a pipeline to bring water to the city from two Ohio towns. In communities with well fields located near the river, water quality was monitored round the clock; in towns where surface intakes were shut down, tank trucks or bottled water supplies were sent in and non-essential businesses such as laundromats and car washes temporarily closed. Brewing companies—Miller's, Anheuser-Busch, and Strohs'—made friends in several communities by sending in trailer-truckfuls of water in unlabelled beer cans! As in any disaster situation, the darker side of human nature found expression also. State environmental officials in both Pennsylvania and West Virginia reported several instances of "midnight dumpers" exploiting the spill by discharging hazardous wastes into the river, assuming such actions would pass unnoticed amidst the general chaos.[17]

Like the Rhine spill, the Monongahela incident took a heavy toll of waterbirds and fish along the Ohio, a river which in recent years has enjoyed a resurgence of aquatic life. However, if experience from ocean oil spills is any indication, the long-term ecological impact of the spill may be less serious than commonly feared. Studies of marine spills show that while petroleum is toxic to many organisms, there is no strong evidence that oil spills have done any permanent damage to the world's ocean resources. While such events can have a catastrophic short-term impact on biotic communities, recovery begins within a matter of months and, in most cases, such communities have returned to their pre-spill appearance within a year or two.[18] Nature's resiliency should not justify complacency in careless storage or transport of hazardous chemicals but does give reassurance to communities victimized by toxic spills that the impact of such disasters will not haunt them forever.

Direct vs. Indirect Discharges

Current water pollution laws distinguish two categories of industrial waste discharges: *Direct Discharges* which go directly into a receiving stream or lake and *Indirect Discharges* which are discharged into the sewer system where they first pass through the municipal sewage treatment plant (referred to in official jargon as a POTW—"publicly-owned treatment works") before entering a waterway along with sanitary wastewater effluent. When citizens think about industrial pollutant discharges, they generally envision the direct type—pipes from a factory leading straight to the water's edge, pouring a poisonous brew onto the back of some hapless fish. In point of fact, however, the majority of industrial dischargers, some 60,000 in the U.S., are of the indirect type, discharging at least 200 million pounds of hazardous wastes into sewer systems every year, according to USEPA estimates.[19] In cases where indirect industrial discharges consist primarily of biodegradable organic wastes, sending them to the sewage treatment plant is appropriate, since the same processes which decompose human excreta are effective on other organic materials as well. In situations involving toxic substances, however, indirect discharges via the sewer system can cause a number of very serious problems:

Structural Damage to Sewer System and Treatment Plant—Industrial discharges of strong acids or alkalis can corrode both sewer pipes and equipment at the POTW. Some chemicals react to produce toxic fumes which can present a serious health threat to workers at the treatment plant, and certain volatile substances can generate a build-up of gas in the sewers, occasionally resulting in explosions. An event of this type occurred in Louisville, KY, in February of 1981 when an industrial discharge of hexane exploded in the sewers, injuring 4 persons and causing over $10 million worth of damage.[20] A similar situation took place the same year in Cincinnati, OH, when wastewater containing both hydrochloric acid and volatile organic solvents was discharged into city sewers by a large paint factory. The acid corroded the concrete sewer pipe, causing it to collapse and leaving a hole in the street 24 feet in diameter. When workers entered the sewer 3 days later to try to repair the damage, several were overcome suddenly by nausea, dizziness, vomiting, and eye and nose irritation due to exposure to chemical vapors. All work had to be stopped until the discharges were halted and fumes had dissipated.[21]

Interference with Biological Treatment Processes—When toxic chemicals such as the synthetic organic pesticides pass through a sewage treatment plant, they have the same effect on the microbes responsible for the secondary treatment process as they do on the target pests—they kill them, and in so doing render the sewage treatment plant ineffective. In 1977, again at the ill-fated Louisville POTW, pesticide wastes illegally dumped into a city sewer caused a total breakdown in treatment at the huge plant. As a result, for nearly 2 years until the cleanup was completed, 100 million gallons of untreated sewage were discharged into the Ohio River every day and taxpayers were confronted with a repair bill amounting to millions of dollars.

Sludge Contamination—Certain toxics such as cadmium, mercury, lead, and arsenic may pass through the sewage treatment plant without damaging equipment or the microbes responsible for digesting organic wastes. Nevertheless, they pose major problems because they accumulate in the sludge, seriously complicating disposal options. Sludge contaminated with heavy metals must be given expensive treatment to ensure that these substances do not leach into the groundwater if the sludge is landfilled, become air pollutants if incinerated, or enter the food chain if such sludge is used as a soil conditioner for growing crops.[22]

Violation of POTW Effluent Limitations—Because sewage treatment plants, like industries, must comply with the terms of their discharge permit, specifying effluent limitations, toxic chemicals which pass through the treatment plant and pollute the receiving waters make it necessary for the POTW to install methods of advanced wastewater treatment to prevent such violations from occurring. This, of course, is a costly undertaking, the expense of which will be borne by the taxpaying public.

Need for Pretreatment of Indirect Discharges

Problems such as those just described led Congress to legislate a national **Pretreatment Program** which would require indirect dischargers of industrial wastes to detoxify their effluent before it entered the sewage system. EPA has been charged with setting discharge standards for various categories of industries (e.g. the electroplating industry, textile mills, plastics manufacturers, etc.) while local POTWs were assigned most of the work in developing, implementing, and enforcing the program. Although originally mandated in 1972, the pretreatment program was extremely slow in getting started, in part because EPA did not formulate basic rules for the program until 1980. Implementation of the program by local sanitary districts moved into high gear by the mid-1980s and today most industries discharging wastewaters to municipal sewers have some form of pretreatment program in place.

Industrial Accidents, Spills, and Runoff

In addition to direct and indirect effluent discharges, some industrial pollutants enter waterways due to transportation accidents, leaks in chemical containers, tanker spills or oil rig blow-outs, or chemical runoff from industrial wastes sites during storm episodes. Control over toxic and hazardous pollutants from these sources should be achieved through implementation of so-called "best management practices" specified in an industry's discharge permit.

Drinking Water Quality

If George Gallup or Lou Harris were to conduct a sidewalk poll on what major concerns the average man or woman on the street might have regarding water pollution, it's a safe bet that eutrophication of Lake Erie, fish kills in the Mississippi, or problems at the Louisville sewage treatment plant would rank far down on the list. Among the vast majority of respondents, the #1 water quality priority undoubtedly would be assurance that the water flowing from their kitchen or bathroom faucet was safe to drink.

Such public concerns stem from the recognition that human health is directly threatened by impure drinking water. There exists today a growing realization that the quality of drinking water is inextricably linked to the quality of our environment as a whole, inasmuch as air pollutants, leachates from landfills, sewage, toxic chemicals, etc., all can invade water supplies. The following examples indicate a few of the ways in which various contaminants in drinking water can affect human health:

- in Perham, Minnesota, eleven out of thirteen employees at a new office-warehouse complex became seriously ill with gastrointestinal problems soon after beginning work in the recently opened premises. Two of the victims had to be hospitalized and were diagnosed as suffering from arsenic poisoning. It was subsequently discovered that the new well which had been drilled to supply the building with drinking water was located just 20 feet from a long-forgotten village dump where, almost 40 years earlier, farmers had dumped approximately 50 pounds of arsenic-containing grasshopper bait. At one spot arsenic concentration in the soil was as high as 40%, while an analysis of well water samples showed arsenic concentrations of 21,000 parts per billion (safe drinking water standards for arsenic are set at 50 ppb).[23]

- severe diarrhea lasting 10 days or longer made life temporarily miserable for 240 citizens of Camas, Washington, in the spring of 1976. Stool analyses showed that the cause of their distress was a flagellated protozoan, *Giardia lamblia,* a parasitic species which inhabits the intestines of various vertebrate animals. Further investigation by health officials traced the source of infection to the city water supply which came from a remote mountain stream where *Giardia*—infected beavers were believed responsible for polluting the water with feces containing protozoan cysts. Inadequate pretreatment of raw water at Camas' water treatment plant was eventually pinpointed as the cause of the town's giardiasis outbreak.[24]

- the incidence of liver disorders among residents of rural Hardeman County, Tennessee, became suspiciously high after Velsicol Chemical Company began burying pesticide wastes in a nearby landfill. An increasing number of complaints by families in the area that their water tasted "funny" finally prompted an analysis of well water which constituted the sole source of drinking water for 40 rural households. The results confirmed residents' worst fears: the wells were highly contaminated with endrin, dieldrin, aldrin, and heptachlor—all carcinogenic organic pesticides which people in the area had been unwittingly drinking for several years.[25]

- in New Delhi, India, drinking water from a river contaminated with untreated sewage led to an epidemic of 28,000 cases of infectious hepatitis. Although the water had been filtered and chlorinated to kill bacterial pathogens, the hepatitis virus survived this treatment, resulting in the disease outbreak.[26]

Microbial Waterborne Disease

Prior to the late 19th century, outbreaks of epidemic waterborne disease in every part of the world claimed a heavy toll in human lives and suffering. As late as the 1880s, typhoid killed 75-100 people per 100,000 population in the United States each year. A major outbreak of the disease in Chicago in 1885 claimed 90,000 victims and persuaded city officials to divert the flow of Chicago's sewage from Lake Michigan, also the source of municipal drinking water supplies, into the Sanitary and Ship Canal (completed in 1900) and ultimately to the Illinois River and the Mississippi—a policy decision which had the unintended side effect of seriously degrading the quality and attractiveness of the Illinois River. Cholera also was a feared disease in 19th century America; a major outbreak in the Mississippi Valley during the 1870s claimed many lives and large numbers of westward-bound settlers died of cholera along the wagon trails.

Box 15-9

Blue Baby Disease

Fecal pathogens and organic chemicals are not the only drinking water contaminants capable of causing illness. A number of inorganic substances—arsenic, heavy metals, and road salts, to cite a few—are known to have caused illness among unknowing consumers. In 1945, a young pediatrician in Iowa City published a landmark article in the Journal of the American Medical Association in which he attributed the cause of a mysterious ailment called "blue baby disease" to contamination of drinking water supplies with nitrates. In the years following this discovery, numerous cases of blue baby disease were reported, primarily from rural areas of the Midwest. In 1950, Minnesota alone listed 144 cases with 14 deaths during one 30-month period.

Blue baby disease, more correctly termed **methemoglobinemia**, is induced when an infant is given powdered formula or other infant foods mixed with nitrate-contaminated water, generally water from shallow wells polluted by fertilizer or feedlot runoff or by seepage from septic systems. Nursing mothers who drink water with high nitrate levels could possibly pass this on to their babies in breast milk, but such an occurrence is very rare; in fact, where surveys have shown private wells to be polluted with nitrates, doctors urge new mothers to breast-feed their infants. It should also be noted that, unlike situations involving bacteria or other pathogens in drinking water, boiling nitrate-polluted water to rid it of contamination is not advised, inasmuch as this simply results in concentrating any nitrates present.

Where wells are polluted, all residents of a household consume the contaminated water, yet only infants under the age of 6 months are at risk of acquiring blue baby disease. This is because during the first few months of life babies typically possess low levels of the enzyme which reduces methemoglobin. Concentrations of the enzyme increase with age and reach adult levels about 6 months after birth.

Better understanding of the disease and regular monitoring of public drinking water supplies for nitrate content since 1945 have reduced the incidence of methemoglobinemia in recent years. Nevertheless, random surveys in the Plains states have revealed a high proportion of private farm wells containing nitrate levels in excess of the 10 ppm EPA standard. Methemoglobinemia thus remains a potentially dangerous problem for babies in rural America—a fact tragically underlined in June of 1986 when a 7-week-old baby girl in South Dakota died of the disease, making her the first such victim in the U.S. in over two decades. When her family's well water was subsequently tested, laboratory results showed 150 ppm nitrate.[27]

Typhoid and cholera are the most serious of several bacterial, protozoan, and viral diseases known to be transmitted to humans through water contaminated with human (and, in some cases, animal) fecal material. Other bacterial waterborne diseases include dysentery, paratyphoid, and salmonellosis—ailments which, like typhoid and cholera, can also be contracted by eating food harboring bacteria of fecal origin. Whereas typhoid and paratyphoid are characterized by headache, body pains, high fever, and constipation alternating with diarrhea (all symptoms being less severe in paratyphoid), cholera, dysentery, and salmonellosis are all typified by severe diarrhea and vomiting. Viral diseases spread by contaminated drinking water include infectious hepatitis and poliomyelitis, while amoebic dysentery and giardiasis are among the more prevalent waterborne diseases of protozoan origin.

Water Purification

Toward the end of the last century, a growing awareness of the link between waterborne pathogens and disease outbreaks prompted municipal officials in North America and Europe to institute various methods of drinking water treatment—primarily filtration and chlorination—which largely succeeded in eliminating the serious water-related epidemic diseases of the past. Nevertheless, the organisms which cause typhoid, cholera, dysentery, and other gastrointestinal ailments are still in our midst, ready to make their presence known whenever a breakdown in water treatment processes affords opportunity for such pathogens to penetrate our technological lines of defense.

Unlike sewage treatment, which is intended to reduce levels of wastewater contamination to the point where the effluent can be returned to a stream without provoking serious health or ecological damage, drinking water treatment theoretically should entirely remove all contaminants in the water, or at least reduce them to acceptable levels. All drinking water, regardless of its source, should be treated prior to consumption, since it can never be safely assumed that such water is totally free from contamination.

Although the precise details of drinking water treatment vary from plant to plant, depending largely on the quality of the local raw water supply (i.e. water from polluted surface sources will require more extensive treatment than does well water drawn from a high quality uncontaminated aquifer), the basic steps in the process can be described as follows:

> *Sedimentation*—incoming raw water is detained in a quiet pond or tank for at least 24 hours to allow heavy suspended material to settle out.

> *Coagulation*—alum (hydrated aluminum sulfate) is added to the water to cause smaller suspended solids to form flocs which then precipitate to the bottom of the tank.

> *Filtration*—through beds of sand, crushed anthracite coal, or diatomaceous earth further reduces the concentration of remaining suspended solids, including many bacterial cells and protozoans.

> *Disinfection*—most commonly with chlorine (ozone, bromine, iodine, or

ultraviolet light can also be used for disinfection), is the most important method utilized for killing pathogens in water. However, disinfection in the absence of the preceding steps is not highly effective because organic materials and suspended solids in the water interfere with the germicidal action of the chlorine. In addition, occasional outbreaks of hepatitis in cities where water has been disinfected indicate that chlorine is not as effective in killing viruses as it is against other disease organisms.

In many water treatment plants, particularly those utilizing well water, preliminary treatment also includes aerating the water to remove iron and dissolved gases such as hydrogen sulfide which impart objectionable tastes and odor to the water. In parts of the country where water contains excess amounts of dissolved calcium or magnesium (i.e. where the water is "hard"), lime and soda ash are added to precipitate these minerals out of solution, thereby "softening" the water. Ion exchange is an alternative method which can be used for this purpose. Finally, many treatment plants today add fluoride to the finished water to reduce the incidence of tooth decay.[28]

To ensure that the water treatment process is working efficiently, laboratory tests of finished water samples are carried out on a regular basis. Historically, the presence of appreciable numbers of coliform bacteria in a water sample has been used as an indication that the water is unsafe to drink. In fact, coliforms themselves rarely cause disease; however, because they are common inhabitants of the intestines of warm-blooded animals, present in greater numbers than the pathogenic bacteria, and because they can survive for longer periods of time in water than do the latter, coliforms serve as indicators that the water is contaminated with fecal material and hence potentially hazardous. In other words, the presence of fecal coliform bacteria in a water sample warns health officials that less abundant, but more harmful organisms such as the dysentery bacillus or hepatitis virus might also be present, since all of these organisms live in the intestinal tract and are expelled with fecal material. Recently, however, the validity of the coliform test in establishing the safety of a water supply has been called into question with the finding that pathogenic viruses may still be present in samples which the standard coliform test indicated were bacteriologically uncontaminated.

New Concerns About Drinking Water

Standard water treatment processes, designed primarily to remove bacteria, hardness, and odors from water supplies, have been outstandingly successful in reducing the incidence of acute waterborne disease in 20th century America. Not that gastrointestinal problems related to drinking water are unknown — each year several thousand cases of waterborne disease are reported to the Centers for Disease Control and in all probability many others occur but are not reported. Nevertheless, the major epidemics and high death rates so characteristic of centuries past are unlikely to recur, barring a calamitous breakdown in the social order.

However, in spite of the considerable improvement in drinking water quality from a bacteriological perspective, the American public today is justifiably

---

Box 15–10

The Safe Drinking Water Act

In 1969 a study of community water supplies conducted by the U.S. Public Health Service revealed that 56% of nearly a thousand public waterworks surveyed were not constructed or operating properly, 51% failed to disinfect their water, and 16% exceeded one or more of the federal drinking water standards. Most of the violations, it was pointed out, were found in small communities which lacked the funds to provide the trained employees and modern equipment necessary to improve their operations; as a result, 2.5 million people in the areas surveyed were provided with water of inferior quality, while 300,000 of these were drinking water that was potentially dangerous. Concerns raised by these findings were augmented by EPA revelations a few years later that public drinking water supplies in New Orleans, drawn from the heavily polluted Mississippi River, were contaminated with a number of toxic organic chemicals. A follow-up study by the Environmental Defense Fund reported that New Orleans residents drinking treated city water exhibited the second-highest rate of bladder and intestinal cancer in the country. While it cannot be proven that carcinogenic chemicals in drinking water are the direct cause of cancer incidence in Louisiana, the EDF report fueled public concerns about the potential health impact of toxics in water and helped spur passage of the **1974 Safe Drinking Water Act**—the only federal law which focuses on drinking water in a comprehensive manner.

Under the Act, USEPA must establish **Maximum Contaminant Levels (MCLs)** for specified pollutants found in the drinking water of any community water system (defined as one having at least 15 service connections used by year-round residents or regularly serving 25 or more people). The Safe Drinking Water Act sets uniform guidelines for drinking water treatment and requires that public water systems follow a prescribed schedule for monitoring and testing the quality of their treated water and report the results of such testing to the appropriate state agency.

By 1986, in spite of the recognition that over 700 organic, inorganic, biological, and radiological contaminants had been detected in water supplies around the United States, standards had been set for only 23 drinking water pollutants—and the majority of these had been established by the Public Health Service in the 1960s. Impatient with USEPA's tortoise pace, Congress amended the Safe Drinking Water Act, requiring that the Agency follow a strict timetable and set MCLs for an additional list of specified pollutants, bringing the number of regulated drinking water contaminants to 83 by June, 1989.

Setting MCLs is the first step toward ensuring a safe water supply—enforcing the law is another matter. A recent lawsuit filed against EPA by the National Wildlife Federation charges that the federal agency has failed in its responsibility to enforce SDWA provisions. Citing over 100,000 violations of drinking water standards or of testing and reporting requirements in community water systems serving 37 million people during 1987, National Wildlife complains that EPA has taken enforcement action in less than 3% of these cases. The Federation also faults EPA for insufficient oversight of individual state programs and inadequate progress reports to Congress. Whatever their validity, such charges highlight the necessity for citizens to remain vigilant regarding drinking water issues, to learn more about the quality and management of their own community's water supply, and to take action on water quality issues of local concern.[29]

Fig. 15-6

Contaminants To Be Regulated by EPA by June 1989*

Microbiological Contaminants

Turbidity*	Viruses
Total Coliforms*	Standard Plate Count
Giardia lamblia	*Legionella*

Volatile Organic Chemicals

Trichloroethylene*	Vinyl Chloride*	Trichlorobenzene(s)
Tetrachloroethylene	Methylene Chloride	1,1-Dichloroethylene*
Carbon Tetrachloride*	Benzene*	cis-1, 2-Dichloroethylene
1,1,1-Trichloroethane*	Chlorobenzene	trans-1, 2-Dichloroethylene
1,2-Dichloroethane*	Dichlorobenzene(s)*	

Synthetic Organic Chemicals

Endrin*	Carbofuran	Pentachlorophenol
Lindane*	1,1,2-Trichlorethane	Picloram
Methoxychlor*	Vydate	Dinoseb
Toxaphene*	Simazine	Alachlor
2,4,-D*	PAHs (Polynuclear Aromatic	EDB (Ethylene Dibromide)
2,4,5-TP (Silvex)*	Hydrocarbons)	Epichlorohydrin
Total Trihalomethanes*	PCBs (Polychlorinated	Dibromomethane
Aldicarb	Biphenyls)	Toluene
Chlordane	Atrazine	Xylene
Dalapon	Phthalates	Adipates
Diquat	Acrylamide	Hexachlorocyclopentadiene
Endothall	DBCP (Dibromochloropropane)	2,3,7,8-TCDD (Dioxin)
Glyphosate	1,2-Dichloropropane	

Inorganic Chemicals

Arsenic*	Silver*	Vanadium
Barium*	Fluoride*	Sodium
Cadmium*	Aluminum	Nickel
Chromium*	Antimony	Zinc
Lead*	Molybdenum	Thallium
Mercury*	Asbestos	Beryllium
Nitrate (as N)*	Sulfate	Cyanide
Selenium*	Copper	

Radiological Contaminants

Radium 226 and 228*	Beta Particle and Photon	Natural Uranium
Gross Alpha Particle Activity*	Radioactivity*	Radon

*asterisked substances are currently regulated; all except the VOCs may be revised.
Source: Environmental Protection Agency

alarmed about the safety of water supplies due to recent revelations of toxic chemicals in drinking water. With purification processes aimed at preventing the microbial diseases of the past, few water treatment plants are equipped to remove—or even to detect—the newer synthetic organic chemicals now acknowledged as present in drinking water supplies across the country. Although these substances may be present in concentrations measured in parts per million (ppm) or even parts per billion (ppb), the fact that many of them are known to be mutagenic or carcinogenic raises unanswered questions concerning the long-term health effects of ingesting small amounts of poison on a daily basis. A direct cause-and-effect relationship between toxic chemicals in drinking water and human health damage has not yet been conclusively demonstrated, but circumstantial evidence and the testimony of people who, unknowingly, consumed high levels of poisonous chemicals with their water for a number of years, indicate no reason to be complacent about the situation.

Trihalomethanes

The kinds of synthetic organic chemicals (SOCs, as they are now called) contaminating the Mississippi, and most other rivers as well, consist of various herbicides, insecticides, industrial solvents and cleaning fluids. Another major category of SOCs is the group of compounds known as *Trihalomethanes* (THMs). Including such substances as chloroform, bromoform, and dichloro-bromomethane, THMs, unlike other synthetic organic chemicals, are formed at the water treatment plant itself when chlorine, added to water for disinfectant purposes, reacts with natural organic compounds in the water (e.g. plant parts, humus). Any drinking water supply which has been chlorinated, particularly if the raw water was from a surface source containing substantial amounts of organic material, is likely to contain THMs. In fact, the presence of chloroform has been detected in almost every water system tested for this chemical—and chloroform, at least in high doses, is known to cause liver and kidney disorders, central nervous system problems, birth defects, and cancer. Concerns about possible health damage due to THMs have led some to suggest abandoning chlorination of drinking water altogether, but unless another form of disinfection is substituted, renewed outbreaks of bacteriological diseases would undoubtedly accompany such a change in practice. Chloramines, chlorine dioxide, and ozone are all non-THM-producing disinfectants which could be used in cities having problems with trihalomethanes; all, however, are more expensive than chlorination and may be less efficient.

Recent research indicates that THM concentrations in finished water can be substantially reduced by simply adjusting the chlorine dose, improving filtration practices to remove as much of the organic material in the water as possible, or by adding chlorine after filtration rather than before, in order to reduce contact time between the chlorine and any organic compounds in the water, thus preventing THM formation. In most areas measures such as these will be sufficient to keep THM levels within standards prescribed by the Safe Drinking Water Act. For a few cities with very severe THM problems, however, it will probably be necessary to adopt more advanced technologies such as GAC filtration or a biologically activated carbon (BAC) process which absorb THMs and other synthetic organic chemicals, as well as some natural organics, thereby removing them from the finished water. The high cost of such technology and continuing controversy over the extent of the health risk posed by THMs has delayed widespread adoption of these additional treatment processes.

Lead

That ingestion or inhalation of lead can cause human poisoning resulting in a wide range of health problems has been known for many years (see Ch. 7). Government initiatives to lower the lead content of housepaint and to phase out the use of leaded gasoline were prompted specifically by the desire to reduce human exposure to this toxic metal. However, recent scientific findings have identified a hitherto-unrecognized source of environmental lead—water from our own kitchen or bathroom sinks. Indeed, in many areas of the country, household drinking water is *the* major route of lead exposure. The USEPA estimates that more than 40 million Americans are drinking water containing more than the legally permissible level of lead (20 parts per billion).

This situation does not mean that municipal water treatment plants are doing a poor job, for in almost all cases lead enters drinking water *after* it leaves the purification plant or private well. The problem arises within the home plumbing system as a result of corrosion when water passes through lead pipes or through pipes soldered with lead. This type of reaction is particularly likely with "soft" water; corrosion is also increased by the common practice of using water pipes for the grounding of electrical equipment, since electrical current traveling through the ground wire hastens the corrosion of lead in the pipes.

The age of a home's plumbing system is a major determinant of whether or not a lead problem exists. In older structures—those built prior to the 1930s—lead was commonly used for interior piping as well as for the service connections that joined the house to a public water supply. Obviously if a home has lead plumbing, a potential problem exists. After 1930, copper piping largely replaced lead for residential plumbing, but such pipes were typically joined with lead solder; it is this solder which many authorities consider the main contributor to drinking water contamination with lead. Over time, the amount of lead leaching into water from plumbing decreases because mineral deposits gradually form a deposit on the inside of the pipes, preventing water from coming into direct contact with the solder. For this reason, homes with the greatest likelihood of having high lead levels are those less than 5 years old (unless the plumbing is made of plastic, in which case there's no problem).

Although tell-tale signs of corrosion (rust-colored water, stained dishwasher or laundry, frequent leaks) or recognition that the house falls into one of the high-risk age categories mentioned above can alert residents to a potential problem, the only way to make a definite determination of excess lead levels is to have the water tested at a certified laboratory (unfortunately, this is not a cheap procedure).

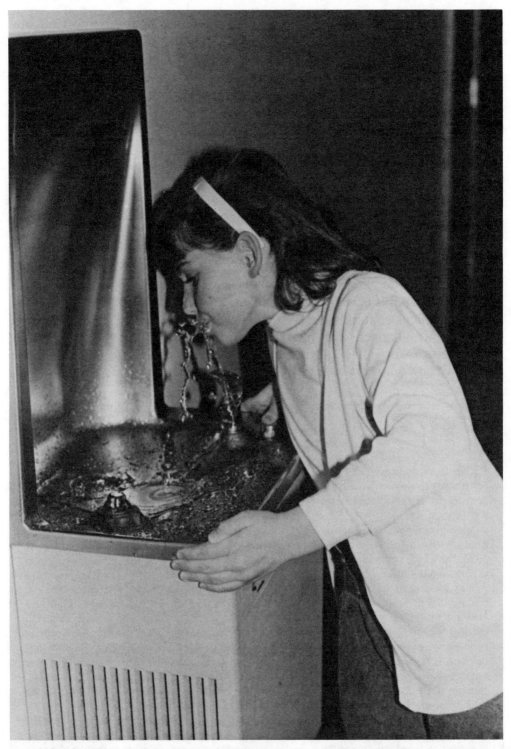

The EPA reports that lead-lined water coolers in some schools are exposing children to lead levels many times higher than federal drinking water standards. Congress has mandated that manufacturers of coolers with lead components must repair or replace such coolers by Nov. 1989. [*Author's Photo*]

If lab analysis confirms high lead levels, abatement options short of total replacement of the plumbing system are somewhat limited. Reverse osmosis devices and distillation units can be installed at the faucet but are quite expensive and of variable effectiveness (faucet filters containing carbon or sand, as well as cartridge filters, are totally useless for removing lead). Lead exposure can be minimized by 2 simple actions which should be taken by anyone who has, or suspects, a lead problem:

1. Don't drink water which has been in contact with pipes for more than 6 hours. The longer water has been standing, the greater the amount of lead likely to be present. Before using such water for drinking or cooking, flush out the pipes by allowing water to run for several minutes or until it is as cold as it will get (this water need not be wasted—it can be used for washing, watering plants, etc.).
2. Don't consume or cook with hot tap water, since lead dissolves more readily in hot water than in cold. If you need hot water, draw it cold from the tap and use the stove to heat it.

In response to this newly-recognized health hazard, Congress has prohibited the use of solder containing more than 0.2% lead (formerly, solder was 50% lead) and has banned any pipe containing more than 8% lead in new installations or for repair of public water systems. In addition, a number of states have now banned all use of lead materials in drinking water systems.[30]

Box 15–11

Pass the Perrier, Please!

Like Europeans who say they drink wine because the local water makes them sick, Americans in droves have been turning to bottled water because they don't like what's coming from their kitchen tap. A 1988 survey by the International Bottled Water Association revealed that 15% of households across the country use bottled water on a regular basis, choosing from over 600 brands. From 1986 to 1988 U.S. consumption of the product tripled and at current rates of increase, sales are expected to exceed $2 billion by 1990. Demand is greatest in the Southwest, with trendy California buying 3X the national average—one out of every 6 residents in the Golden State now drinks bottled water.

Why the rush to the supermarket for a product much more cheaply available from public water supplies? Primarily because many consumers perceive bottled water as safer and tastier than tapwater—and because skillful marketing, particularly of certain imported brands, has made consumption of bottled water fashionable. That health and aesthetic factors are important determinants of bottled water's appeal is obvious from the fact that demand is highest in those areas where taste and odor problems are prevalent or where reports of groundwater contamination have prompted health concerns among consumers. But can health-conscious buyers be sure that the bottled water they're purchasing is any safer than the tapwater they spurn?

Many public water commissioners vigorously argue that promotional claims of bottled water being more "wholesome" than tapwater are misleading, citing the fact that public water supplies are strictly regulated and monitored, hence are every bit as "healthy" as the commercial brands—and cost a fraction of the price. They also point out that certain

---

bottled "mineral waters" contain levels of dissolved minerals (e.g. barium) high enough to threaten the health of some consumers. Even from a taste standpoint, many municipal supplies are as good or better than the highly-touted bottled product. The public water supply in cities such as New York and Los Angeles, for example, consistently rank among the best-tasting waters in the nation, commercial brands included.

Bottled waters, like community water supplies, are heavily regulated by the federal government, in this case by the Food and Drug Administration, which classifies the product as a "food". While not requiring labels to state the source of the water, FDA regulations do require that water be taken from protected sources, be bottled in facilities following food plant regulations, be processed under federally-approved manufacturing processes, and be delivered to consumers in sanitized containers (**Note:** FDA regulations apply only to firms operating in more than one state). In addition to FDA-imposed requirements, domestic bottled water must meet EPA's drinking water standards and must comply with any state-imposed regulations. Like any food processing facility, all bottled water plants in the U.S. are visited by government inspectors at least once a year (imported brands, however, are not subject to Safe Drinking Water Act standards nor to FDA plant inspections).

While it is probably true that in most communities the public water supply is of high enough quality to make bottled water a non-essential status symbol, the industry fills an important role as a provider of an alternative source of safe drinking water when emergency situations render a public supply unsafe or when special health or dietary needs require low sodium or low nitrate water—or when consumers' demands that their water taste good and look clean are not met by their municipal source of supply.[31]

Controlling Water Pollution: The Clean Water Act

Although water pollution had been recognized as a major environmental problem in the United States for many decades, it was not until 1972 that a tough, comprehensive federal program to deal with this issue was enacted by Congress. Known originally as the Federal Water Pollution Control Act Amendments (Public Law 92-500), this landmark piece of legislation underwent some "mid-course corrections" in 1977, at which time its name was changed to the Clean Water Act. Prior to passage of this law, our nation's water pollution control strategy, such as it was, focused on attempts to clean up waterways to the point that they could be used for whatever purpose state governments had determined their function should be (e.g. drinking water, swimming, fishing, navigation, etc.). Thus each stream or portion of a stream might have a different water quality standard, and if that standard was not being met, it was up to the state water pollution control agency to determine which discharger was responsible for the violation and to seek enforcement action. This system was totally ineffective for a number of reasons: designations of desired stream use were frequently modified to retain or attract industrial development; insufficient information was available on how pollutant discharges were affecting water quality; blame for violation was difficult, if not impossible to assess when more than one source was discharging into a waterway; little attention was paid to the effects of pollution on the aquatic environment as a whole; and only contaminants entering a waterway through pipe discharges were given much attention. Undoubtedly the most serious drawback of the pre-1972 water pollution control strategy was the lack of enforcement power. State agencies had to negotiate with all the polluters along a given waterway, trying to persuade each individual source to reduce its discharges to the point at which water quality standards for the particular river or lake in question could be met. Not uncommonly, when industries disliked what they were being told, they would threaten to close down and move to a less-demanding state. Also, due to the nature of river basins, many states discovered that in order to improve their own water quality, they had to persuade states upstream to pollute less.

Passage of the Clean Water Act radically altered this approach to water pollution control and took a new philosophical stance toward the problem, reflected in the 1972 Senate Committee's statement that "no one has the right to pollute . . . and that pollution continues because of technological limits, not because of any inherent right to use the Nation's waterways for the purpose of disposing of wastes." Stressing the need to "restore and maintain the chemical, physical, and biological integrity of the Nation's waters", Congress declared as national goals the attainment, wherever possible, of water quality "that provides for recreation in and on the water" (popularly referred to as the "fishable-swimmable waters" goal) by July 1, 1983, and the elimination of all pollutant discharges into the nation's waterways by 1985 ("zero discharge" goal). These goals are not the same as legal requirements—they cannot be enforced and will certainly not be attained by the dates indicated; nevertheless, they are useful in providing objectives toward which to strive and against which progress in improving water quality can be measured. A number of regulations designed to meet these goals were subsequently formulated by EPA, the most important of which include:

Effluent Limitations for Industrial Dischargers—set by EPA for each specific type of industry and based on that industry's economic and technological capabilities.

National Pollutant Discharge Elimination System (NPDES) Permits—renewable every 5 years, required for all point sources of pollution. These permits specify the maximum allowable amounts of pollutant discharges, their content, a schedule for compliance with effluent limitations, and self-monitoring and reporting requirements.

Municipal Sewage Treatment Plant Discharge Limitations—aimed at upgrading the level of sewage treatment to at least secondary treatment; these requirements were made more palatable to local governments by enactment of a multi-billion dollar construction grants program whereby the federal government would give cities 75-85% of the cost of expanding or building new public sewage treatment facilities.

Comprehensive River Basin and Regional Water Quality Management Planning by states for both point and non-point sources of water pollution was required; state planning grants to fund such efforts were authorized.

Water Quality Standards—the Clean Water Act retains the pre-1972 concept of water quality standards and specifies an "anti-degradation" policy requiring that high-quality waters be protected from degradation; the Act also mandates states to review their water quality standards every 3 years, upgrading them in an effort to achieve the fishable-swimmable goal.[32]

Progress in moving toward the goals set forth by Congress is monitored by the Environmental Protection Agency's National Water Quality Surveillance System, consisting of approximately 1000 fixed stations nationwide, and by the U.S. Geological Survey's National Stream Quality Accounting Network, a system of about 500 stations. At each of these sites a wide range of variables (e.g. fecal coliform bacteria, dissolved oxygen, phosphorus, lead, mercury, cadmium) are measured on a regular basis. An analysis of the data collected by these stations since 1975 indicate that so far as river quality is concerned, there has been little over-all change. Some waterways, such as the Potomac River near Washington, DC, the Mississippi at St. Paul, MN, and the Delaware River at Philadelphia have shown marked improvement in levels of dissolved oxygen and less frequent algal blooms. In the Great Lakes, PCB concentrations in fish have been declining; phosphorus loadings to Lake Erie have dropped by 50%, largely due to improved sewage treatment. On the other hand, the quality of many other waterways has worsened over the past two decades. Nutrient and toxic chemical overloads in Chesapeake Bay threaten the continued productivity of that most valuable estuarine environment; the lower Mississippi remains grossly polluted; the degraded condition of Boston Harbor became a subject of national attention during the 1988 Presidential campaign. In contrast to phosphate concentrations which, on a nationwide basis, appear to be holding steady, nitrate levels have been rising. In some locations arsenic and cadmium levels have increased, while lead and mercury have declined.[33]

While progress in restoring the quality of our nation's waterways shows a mixed bag of results, the fact that overall surface water quality has not deteriorated during a period when both population and the GNP have continued to grow gives evidence that the billions of dollars spent on water cleanup efforts are having a positive impact. Nevertheless, although the Council on Environmental Quality reported in 1983 that a majority of U.S. surface waters are today "fishable and swimmable", the nation still has a long way to go before the goals of the Clean Water Act are fully met. While many of the conventional sources and types of water pollution are now being dealt with fairly adequately, newer problems such as toxic chemical pollutants and difficult-to-control runoff from farms, construction sites, and city streets have stymied pollution abatement efforts. A sustained—and costly—public commitment to water cleanup is essential if the lofty aims of the Clean Water Act are to be realized.

REFERENCES

[1]Quigg, Philip, W., *Water: The Essential Resource,* National Audubon Society, 1976.

[2]Jones, David H., ed., *Water Supply and Waste Disposal,* Poverty and Basic Needs Series, Transportation, Water, and Telecommunications Department of the World Bank, September 1980.

[3]Tucker, Jonathan B., "Schistosomiasis and Water Projects: Breaking the Link", *Environment,* vol. 25, no. 7, September 1983; Liese, B., "The Organization of Schistosomiasis Control Programmes", *Parasitology Today,* vol. 2, no. 12, 1986.

[4]Gianessi, L.P., et al., *"Non-Point Source Pollution: Are Cropland Controls the Answer?",* Resources for the Future, Washington, DC, 1986.

[5]McCaull, Julian, and Janice Crossland, *Water Pollution,* Harcourt, Brace, Jovanovitch, Inc., 1974.

[6]Cholera Inquiry Committee, *Report on the Cholera Outbreak in the Parish of St. James, Westminster, During the Autumn of 1854,* J. Churchill, London, 1855.

[7]Koren, Herman, *Handbook of Environmental Health and Safety: Principles and Practices,* Pergamon Press, 1980.

[8]Seamans, Pam, "Wastewater Creates a Border Problem", *Journal of the Water Pollution Control Federation,* vol. 60, no. 10, October 1988.

[9]Maki, Alan W., Donald B. Porcella, and Richard H. Wendt, "The Impact of Detergent Phosphorus Bans on Receiving Water Quality", *Water Research,* vol. 18, no. 7, 1984; Lee, G.F., and R.A. Jones, "Detergent phosphate bans and eutrophication", *Environmental Science and Technology,* vol. 20, no. 4, April 1986.

[10]Shertzer, Richard H., "Wastewater disinfection—Time for a change?", *Journal of the Water Pollution Control Federation,* vol. 58, no. 3, March 1986.

[11]Swanson, R.L., and M. Devine, "Ocean Dumping Policy", *Environment,* vol. 24, no. 5, June 1982; Johnston, Robin, "Concern grows over effects of ocean dumping", *The Christian Science Monitor,* July 25, 1988.

[12]Goldstein, Nora, "Steady Growth for Sludge Composting", *Biocycle,* vol. 29, no. 10, Nov./Dec. 1988.

[13]Koren, op. cit.

[14]Robison, Rita, "The Tunnel that Cleaned up Chicago", *Civil Engineering,* July 1986.

[15]Goldstein, Bruce E., "Sewage Treatment, Naturally", *World Watch,* vol. 1, no. 4, July/August 1988; Klockenbrink, Myra, "Small Towns Build Artificial Wetlands to Treat Sewage", *The New York Times,* Nov. 29, 1988.

[16]Sheiman, Deborah A., *Blueprint for Clean Water,* League of Women Voters Education Fund, Pub. No. 639, 1982.

[17]Fawcett, Howard H., "What We Learned from the Rhine", in *Hazardous and Toxic Materials: Safe Handling and Disposal,* 2nd ed., John Wiley & Sons, 1988; Nichols, Alan B., "Oil accident ignites response debate", *Journal of the Water Pollution Control Federation,* vol. 60, no. 4, April 1988.

[18]National Research Council, *"Oil in the Sea: Inputs, Fates, and Effects",* National Academy Press, 1985.

[19]*The National Pretreatment Program: An Important Link to Clean Water and a Cleaner Environment in Your Community,* League of Women Voters Education Fund, Pub. No. 644, 1983.

[20]Banks, James T., and Frances Dubrowski, "Pretreat or Retreat?", *The Amicus Journal*, Natural Resources Defense Council, Spring 1982.

[21]"Sewer Collapse and Toxic Illness in Sewer Repairmen—Ohio", *Morbidity and Mortality Weekly Report*, U.S. Department of Health and Human Services/Public Health Service, vol. 30, no. 8, March 6, 1981.

[22]Banks, op. cit.

[23]*Hazardous Waste Disposal Damage Reports*, USEPA, No. SW-151, June 1975.

[24]Centers for Disease Control, *Foodborne and Waterborne Disease Outbreaks, Annual Summary 1976*, U.S. Dépt. of Health, Education, and Welfare, Public Health Service, October 1977.

[25]Powledge, Fred, *Water*, Farrar, Straus, Giroux, 1982.

[26]McCaull, op. cit.

[27]Comley, Hunter H., MD, "Cyanosis in Infants Caused by Nitrates in Well Water", *Journal of the American Medical Association*, vol. 129, September 8, 1945; Johnson, Carl J., et al., "Fatal Outcome of Methemoglobinemia in an Infant", *Journal of the American Medical Association*, vol. 257, no. 20, May 22/29, 1987; Lukens, John N., MD, "The Legacy of Well-Water Methemoglobinemia", *Journal of the American Medical Association*, vol. 257, no. 20, May 22/29, 1987.

[28]Koren, op. cit.

[29]*"Safety on Tap: A Citizen's Drinking Water Handbook"*, League of Women Voters Education Fund, 1987.

[30]USEPA, *"Lead and Your Drinking Water"*, OPA-87-006, April 1987.

[31]Tonge, Peter, "Clean Enough to Drink", *The Christian Science Monitor*, January 3, 1989; *"Safety on Tap"*, League of Women Voters Education Fund, 1987.

[32]Sheiman, op. cit.

[33]Wolman, M. Gordon, "Changing National Water Quality Priorities", *Journal of the Water Pollution Control Federation*, vol. 60, no. 10, October 1988.

Solid and Hazardous Wastes

> "Nowhere in the world is there such a waste of material as in this country. In our eagerness to get the most results from our resources, and to get them quickly, we destroy perhaps as much as we use. Americans have not learned to save; and their wastefulness imperils their future. Our resources are fast giving out, and the next problem will be to make them last."
>
> —Austin Bierbower, "American Wastefulness",
> *Overland Monthly* 49, April 1907

The above quotation from a popular magazine in the early years of this century gives evidence that the "waste not, want not" attitude so highly valued in our nation's younger days has long since been replaced by the philosophy of a Throwaway Society. The inevitable result of Americans' proclivity to "use once and throw away" has been an ever-increasing volume of waste material which, for both sanitary and aesthetic reasons, must be regularly collected and disposed of in a manner which will not degrade the environment or threaten public health.

Waste Disposal Trends

Human generation of wastes is, of course, as old as humanity itself. Anthropologists and archaeologists have gleaned illuminating information about the everyday lives of our primitive ancestors by excavating the rubbish heaps outside early cave dwellings and other ancient settlements. Among rural or nomadic peoples, however, discarded wastes seldom accumulated to an extent great enough to threaten human well-being. The advent of the first cities after the Agricultural Revolution of approximately 10,000 years ago presented mankind with his first serious problems of refuse disposal. The poor sanitary conditions and frequent epidemics which characterized city life from ancient times until the late 19th century derived primarily from the perpetuation of country habits in a crowded urban environment. Human body wastes, garbage, and discarded material items alike were typically left on the floor of homes or thrown into the streets. A rudimentary awareness of the link between refuse and disease led to the establishment in Athens, Greece, of what was perhaps the first "city dump" in the Western world around 500 B.C.; this innovation was accompanied by what is believed to be the world's first ban against throwing garbage into the streets, as well as by a regulation requiring scavengers to dump wastes no closer than a mile from the city walls. The Athenian example regarding waste management was not widely emulated, however. Throughout the Roman period and the Middle Ages in Europe open dumping of wastes in streets or ditches remained the prevailing method of urban waste disposal. Attempts by municipal authorities to cope with mankind's slovenly habits were limited and sporadic. In 1388 the English Parliament prohibited dumping of wastes in public waterways; after the 13th century, Parisians were no longer permitted to throw garbage out their windows (they obviously pitched it elsewhere, however, for by 1400 A.D. the mounds of garbage outside the city gates of Paris were so high that they obstructed efforts by the military to defend the city). As medieval towns gradually developed into modern cities, and particularly after the onset of the Industrial Revolution in Europe at the end of the 18th century, the solid waste problem became even more acute. Urban areas became grossly over-crowded, polluted, noisy, and dirtier than ever. Rising levels of affluence among some segments of society, as well as sheer growth in population size, resulted in the generation of increasing amounts of waste. It gradually became apparent to civic leaders that the accumulation of filth and refuse in urban centers was directly related to disease outbreaks. Thus by the late 19th century, city-sponsored efforts at improving urban sanitation were launched both in Europe and North America. Refuse, previously regarded simply as a nuisance, was finally perceived as a major pollution problem which posed a serious human health threat—a problem so massive that it could be effectively tackled only by municipal governments, not simply by private individuals acting on their own initiative.[1]

Throughout the 20th century the "garbage problem" has continued to mount, in spite of steadily rising expenditures to manage such wastes in an acceptable manner. Unfortunately, victory in our war against waste is nowhere in sight. The rate of solid waste generation continues to increase several times more rapidly than the rate of population growth, suggesting that the major forces determining waste output today are an affluent lifestyle and changes in marketing techniques (e.g. multiple packaging) which result in more waste materials to be discarded. While tossing garbage into the streets is no longer considered socially acceptable, modern methods of waste disposal, for the most part, are not a great deal more advanced than they were a century ago. Today steadily increasing volumes of refuse, coupled with the realization that many of these wastes are of a toxic or hazardous nature, have lent renewed urgency to the need for finding safer, more effective methods of collecting, storing, transporting, and disposing of the unwanted by-products of modern society.

Sources of Solid Wastes

Solid wastes are generated in all sectors of the national economy. Major categories of waste generators include the following.

Agriculture

In terms of sheer volume, agricultural sources contribute the single largest group of solid wastes requiring disposal. Crop residues, manures, nut shells, fruit pits, corn cobs, vegetable and fruit peelings, tree trimmings, grain hulls, etc., are all wastes associated with farm production and food processing. For the most part, however, such wastes do not present major disposal problems; generally the stubble remaining in fields after harvesting is either plowed under or allowed to decompose on the surface (in no-till cultivation systems), thereby enriching the soil and retarding soil erosion. Some crop residues are utilized as animal fodder—there is a large market for potato, sugar beet, sugar cane, and citrus wastes for processed feeds. Tree prunings, sugar cane and soybean wastes, as well as many other types of crop stalks and stubble are frequently burned in the field to reduce their volume and to eliminate insect and fungal problems. Nut shells, fruit pits, rice hulls, wood chips, and even dried grounds from the processing of instant coffee are often burned as fuel, sometimes supplying an important energy source for the facilities where the primary product is processed. Some crop wastes such as peanut and pecan shells, cocoa bean husks, sawdust, and ground corncobs are utilized as mulches.[2] Certain types of agricultural wastes do present disposal hazards—pesticide containers can cause toxic contamination if not properly managed and animal feedlot wastes pose a serious water pollution threat—but by and large, waste generated by the agricultural sector of the economy does not constitute a serious waste disposal problem.

Mining

Over 2 billion tons of mineral wastes are produced annually by the mining of coal, phosphate rock, clay, iron, lead, and other minerals. On the average, about 60% of all the materials mined end up as waste rock or mine tailings—a figure which rises as high as 99% in the copper mining industry. In addition to the visual blight they present, mine wastes in the form of culm piles or slag heaps piled near homes or buildings constitute a serious safety hazard in the event of destructive slides. Loose mine tailings can also be blown about by the wind or wash into nearby waterways, thus causing pollution problems.[3] One of the mining industry's most baffling waste management problems pertains to shale oil mining. In order to extract the viscous hydrocarbon, the strip-mined shale rock must be crushed and heated to about 800°F, at which point the shale oil liquifies and flows out. In the heating process, however, the shale rock expands (a phenomenon aptly dubbed the "*Popcorn Effect*") to 1.2 times its former volume. Thus the option of simply returning the waste rock to the pit from which it was dug will not suffice—there is more rock after mining than there was originally! The dilemma of what to do with the enormous quantities of mine tailings which would be generated by large-scale exploitation of U.S. shale oil reserves has been perhaps the most vexing environmental problem confronting the shale oil industry.

Industry

Wastes from manufacturing operations are extremely varied and increasing at a rate of approximately 3% a year.[4] It is estimated that between 10-15% of industrial wastes are of a hazardous nature, requiring extra care in their storage and disposal. The special nature of industrial hazardous waste management will be discussed in greater detail in a following section.

Municipalities

> "All over the nation it's as plain
> as the eye can see or the nose can smell
> that we have to change our ways."
> —Robert P. Casey
> Governor of Pennsylvania, 1988

The tragi-comic voyage of the Islip (NY) "garbage barge" during the spring and summer of 1987 did more than any other single event to focus national attention on rapidly mounting problems of urban waste disposal. Loaded with over 3000 tons of commercial trash banned from a local landfill reserved for residential refuse, the "*Mobro*" cruised the Atlantic and Gulf coasts for 5 months, searching for a disposal facility which would accept the odorous cargo. Its odyssey well-chronicled by a bemused national media, the barge's load was angrily rejected in North Carolina, Florida, Alabama, Mississippi, Louisiana, Texas, Mexico, Belize, and the Bahamas. This modern-day version of the "*Flying Dutchman*" finally returned to New York where its overripe cargo was ultimately burned in a Brooklyn incinerator. The public interest generated by this spectacle raised hopes among beleaguered municipal administrators that perhaps at last citizens would begin to heed their warnings about an impending garbage crisis in our nation's cities.

Urban wastes, generated by millions of individual households, businesses, and institutions, constitute only about 5% of all solid wastes generated in the United States each year (agricultural and mining wastes together make up 91% of the total, while industrial wastes contribute about 4%), according to EPA statistics. Nevertheless, the amounts involved are staggering and steadily increasing. It is estimated that U.S. cities today collect and dispose of somewhere between 150-180 million tons of wastes annually, representing an average of *about* 4 pounds of refuse per person per day.

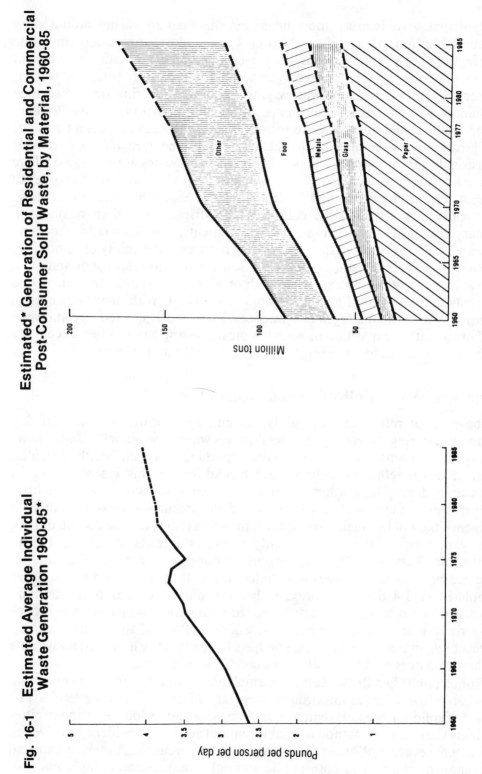

Fig. 16-1   Estimated Average Individual Waste Generation 1960-85*

Estimated* Generation of Residential and Commercial Post-Consumer Solid Waste, by Material, 1960-85

*Projections assume no major new federal policies to reduce waste generation.
Source: Analysis by Franklin Associates, Ltd. for U.S. Environmental Protection Agency, Office of Solid Waste.

Municipal waste is much more heterogeneous than are wastes produced by agriculture, mining, or specific industries. Paper and paper products constitute the single largest portion of household rejects, but an examination of a typical garbage container would also reveal glass, metal, and plastic containers; rubber, leather, and cloth items; food wastes; grass clippings, tree trimmings, discarded appliances, and numerous other items. Although proportionately smaller than the agricultural and mining waste sectors, municipal wastes represent perhaps our greatest waste management challenge (with the possible exception of industrial hazardous wastes). This is because urban wastes are generated where people live and must be quickly removed and properly disposed of in order to prevent serious environmental health problems. Since the late 19th century, Americans have regarded the collection and disposal of urban wastes as a primary responsibility of municipal governments. Unfortunately, the ever-growing volume of such wastes is beginning to surpass the ability of some cities to cope with the problem, while at the same time more stringent state and federal requirements for sounder methods of waste management have increased the costs of disposal and have presented city officials with new challenges to improve their waste management practices. Many a beleaguered city manager, confronted with the question of what his most pressing environmental concern might be, would probably reply, "Where to put all that garbage!"

Municipal Waste Collection and Disposal

The piles of refuse and unsightly, unsanitary conditions which quickly accumulate during the garbage workers' strikes which occasionally plague some cities provide dramatic illustration of the importance to public health of regular, frequent urban refuse collection. Any breakdown in this essential service, particularly during the warmer months of the year, can result in odor and litter problems or in the rapid growth of fly and rat populations. To prevent such problems, the Public Health Service recommends that refuse be collected twice weekly in residential areas and daily from restaurants, hotels, and large apartments. This is particularly important during the peak of the summer fly-breeding season when eggs may hatch in less than a day and larval stages completed in 3-4 days. Historically, because the public has been far more concerned that refuse be regularly removed than with what happens to it once the garbage truck rounds the nearest corner (the "out of sight, out of mind" philosophy), municipal solid waste budgets have generally allocated about 80% of their resources to refuse collection, only 20% to disposal.

From a public health and environmental quality standpoint, proper disposal of urban refuse is just as important as regular collection. Until the 1970's this aspect of solid waste management was given scant attention, resulting in cities utilizing the cheapest method available, with little or no consideration given to the often severe pollution problems thereby created. A new ecological awareness on the part of both public and policymakers has brought many of these long-established practices into disfavor and some are now legally prohibited or are gradually being phased out. Some of the once-common municipal waste disposal methods now regarded as environmentally unacceptable include the following:

Hog Feeding

From ancient times until the 19th century, freely-roaming pigs, goats, cows, and poultry scavenged garbage from city streets; however, since they left behind their droppings while removing food wastes, it might be argued that public thoroughfares were scarcely any cleaner for their efforts. Eventually regulations prohibiting livestock within city limits were enacted, but municipal governments frequently found it expedient to sell, or even donate, food wastes to nearby farmers for use as hog fodder. This practice was most prevalent in parts of New England (at the turn of the century, 61 towns in Massachusetts disposed of at least a portion of their garbage in this manner), but was employed profitably in several Midwestern and Western cities as well.[5] As late as 1941, a survey of American cities whose populations exceeded 25,000 revealed that more than 25% of the garbage collected was used for feeding hogs.[6] The popularity of this method was diminished, however, by the recognition that garbage-fed hogs were frequently unfit for human consumption because they harbored the parasite which produces the disease trichinosis in people eating the pork. In addition, the practice often resulted in outbreaks of diseases such as hog cholera and vesicular exanthema among herds of swine fed on raw garbage. By the late 1950s the U.S. Public Health Service and some state health departments passed regulations prohibiting the feeding of uncooked garbage to hogs. Since cooking the wastes made the practice uneconomical, this method of urban refuse disposal has by now virtually disappeared.

Ironically, since the late 1980s the practice has enjoyed a minor resurgence, thanks to the desperate shortage of landfill space in some areas. In southern New Jersey about 50 farmers have been licensed to feed their hogs food wastes collected from the tourist resorts and gambling casinos of Atlantic City and Cape May. The scraps are first ground and steam-cooked, then mixed with grain before feeding to livestock. While only 10% of New Jersey's hog farmers are currently taking advantage of the free feed, the potential for expanding the practice is great and state officials are enthusiastic about the utilization of this disposal alternative. So far it appears to be a win-win situation: restaurant owners get rid of their wastes, farmers obtain free feed (and are sometimes paid to carry it away), and the state saves desperately-needed landfill space. And the pigs?—a USDA extension agent, commenting on the gourmet scraps being channeled to the hog farms, remarked that, "These hogs eat better than most of the people in Third World countries."[7]

Water Dumping

Another widely condemned and now largely abandoned practice was the dumping of municipal wastes into the nearest body of water. Until 1933 New

York City relied on ocean dumping as a primary method of garbage disposal, a practice bitterly resented by New Jersey shoreline residents whose beaches were regularly littered with Manhattan's cast-off mattresses, old shoes, banana peels and sewage sludge. In the late 1800s, Chicago dumped much of its waste into Lake Michigan about 3 miles from the mouth of the Chicago River; New Orleans utilized the Mississippi River in a similar manner. Gradual recognition that such dumping was damaging to the aquatic environment and was generating serious shoreline nuisances caused the method to fall into disfavor in most communities or led to legal prohibitions against its continuance. A court suit filed against New York by several New Jersey coastal cities in 1933 resulted in the U.S. Supreme Court's 1934 ban on municipal waste dumping at sea (certain industrial and commercial wastes were exempted from this ruling, however). By the end of the 1960s, 50 million tons of wastes annually were still being dumped into the ocean off U.S. shores, most consisting of dredging wastes from harbor-deepening activities and sewage sludge. The 1972 Marine Protection, Research, and Sanctuaries Act calls for strict limitations on the

Fig. 16-2

GROSS DISCARDS OF MSW MATERIALS, 1986

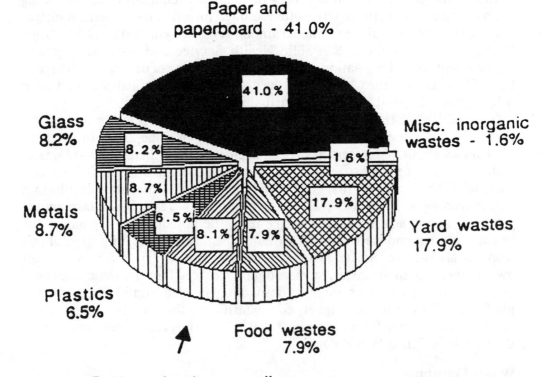

Paper and
paperboard - 41.0%

Glass
8.2%

Misc. inorganic
wastes - 1.6%

Metals
8.7%

Yard wastes
17.9%

Plastics
6.5%

Food wastes
7.9%

Rubber, leather, textiles,
wood - 8.1%

Source: U.S. Environment Protection Agency

ocean dumping of any material which will adversely affect human health or the marine environment, but a complete cessation of ocean dumping in the near future does not appear likely.

Open Dumping

By far the most common method of urban refuse disposal until quite recently, open dumping epitomizes the problems which can arise when solid wastes are mismanaged. Employed primarily because they are cheap and convenient, open dumps support large populations of rats, flies, and cockroaches which frequently invade nearby dwellings. They contaminate adjacent surface or groundwater supplies when *Leachates* (liquids resulting from the interaction of water with wastes) containing dissolved pollutants run off or seep downward through the soil from the dumpsite. If burned over to prevent litter from blowing about or to reduce the volume of wastes, open dumps can pose air quality problems. They are odorous, unsightly, and have a negative impact on property values of adjacent lands. There is a concerted effort underway today to phase out all open dumping in the U.S. The practice is already illegal in many states. Under federal regulations adopted in the late 1970s, state agencies are to identify environmentally unacceptable dumps and either to upgrade them to sanitary landfill status or to phase them out within 5 years from the date of identification.

Current Waste Disposal Alternatives

In recent decades, most municipalities seeking an economically feasible yet environmentally-acceptable alternative to open dumping have opted for sanitary landfills as their refuse disposal method of choice. A sanitary landfill differs from an open dump in that collected refuse is spread in thin layers and compacted by bulldozers. When the compacted layers are 8-10 feet deep, they are covered with about 6 inches of dirt, which is again compacted. At the end of each working day another thin layer of soil is placed over the fill to prevent litter from blowing about, to keep away insect and rodent pests, and to minimize odor problems. When the landfill has reached its ultimate capacity, a final earth cover 2 feet deep is placed over the entire area and the land can then be used for a park, golf course, or other kinds of recreational facilities.

When properly sited, well-designed, and efficiently operated, a sanitary landfill can be a perfectly adequate means of urban refuse disposal, free from offensive odors, vermin, or pollution problems. Unfortunately, however, many so-called "sanitary" landfills are not well-sited, well-planned, or well-run. In the mid-1970s it was estimated that 94% of 17,000 land disposal sites surveyed failed to meet the minimum requirements of a sanitary landfill.[8]

Landfills, of course, are not trouble-free: uneven settling of the land may occur, making it unsuitable as a site for constructing buildings after operations have ceased; anaerobic decomposition of landfilled materials may result in the accumulation of dangerous amounts of methane gas which can cause explosions

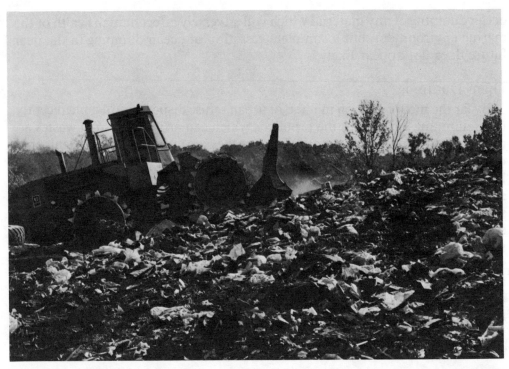

Sanitary landfill: approximately 80% of urban wastes generated in the U.S. currently are disposed of in sanitary landfills. Rapidly dwindling capacity at existing facilities and the difficulty of siting new landfills has created a national "garbage crisis", causing many cities to consider alternative disposal methods. [*Author's Photo*]

or fires if it migrates into nearby structures; perhaps the most serious environmental impact associated with landfills is their potential for polluting nearby surface streams or underlying aquifers with leachates. This problem can be minimized by careful choice of a landfill site, but is a frequently neglected consideration. Unfortunately, in too many communities wetland areas, once considered "worthless" because of the cost of developing them for residential purposes, have been utilized as cheap landfill sites. Since wetlands are extremely productive in biological terms, are important for flood control, and are usually in hydrologic contact with groundwater deposits, choice of a wetland area as a sanitary landfill site is highly inappropriate.

Today 80% of all municipal solid wastes are being buried in sanitary landfills, but the future viability of this option is very much in doubt. From an environmental perspective, landfilling is the least desirable legal method for disposing of refuse because of the threat of water contamination by migrating leachates. Increasingly stringent federal regulations mandating the use of double liners as well as leachate collection and treatment systems will ensure that future landfills will pose less of an environmental hazard, but they won't eliminate the problem entirely and compliance with such requirements will erode the cost advantage which landfills have enjoyed over other disposal alternatives until now. However, the main reason why communities coast-to-coast find themselves in a near-crisis situation, scrambling to find innovative ways of managing their ever-mounting piles of refuse, is that current landfills are near capacity, few sites for establishing new ones are available at affordable prices, and those that are frequently generate intense public opposition to siting such facilities. It is estimated that in the U.S. as a whole, existing landfill capacity is approximately 10 years; in many densely-populated urban areas it is considerably less than that: over half of all American cities expect their landfill capacity to be exhausted by 1990.[9] The immediate results of this crunch are sharply escalating tipping fees at existing facilities and intensive efforts by city and state officials to develop new, more sustainable waste management strategies for the decades ahead. Rather than focus on one "technological fix" or single disposal alternative to solve every community's problems, most waste management experts view the solution as a combination of approaches, tailored to the specific needs and realities of individual municipalities. While recognizing that there will always be a need for some amount of landfilling to accommodate specific wastes which can't be handled in any other manner, current philosophy regards landfilling as the method of last resort, to be replaced to the greatest extent possible by a mix of the following alternatives:

Waste Reduction

The best—and cheapest—way of managing wastes is not to produce them in the first place. Accordingly, policies of waste reduction are ranked #1 in every priority listing of waste management options. First raised as a possible approach for dealing with U.S. solid waste problems at a 1975 EPA-sponsored Conference on Waste Reduction, the goal of conserving materials and energy through waste prevention or by reduction of the quantity of wastes generated was given little more than lip service until recently. The present sense of urgency to relieve pressures on existing disposal facilities has prompted a more serious look at the potential for waste reduction strategies, which most advocates estimate could cut present urban waste streams by about 5%. A prime focus of such efforts would be the reduction of excess packaging (approximately 34% of household waste consists of various packaging materials and 9 cents of every dollar spent on groceries go for wrappings which end up in the wastebasket); other approaches include substituting reusable consumer items for single-use throwaway products—cloth napkins and terry towels instead of paper ones; china or plastic dishes instead of paper plates; handkerchiefs instead of Kleenex; cloth diapers in lieu of Pampers; refillable pens in place of disposable Bics. Still another approach would be to enact legislation requiring that appliances, automobiles, tires, etc., be designed for easier repair and increased durability, thereby moving away from a manufacturing policy of "planned obsolescence".

Dirty Diapers

While not commonly a topic of polite conversation, disposable diapers offer a prime target for any serious national waste reduction effort. Dwindling American landfill capacity is currently being inundated with a deluge of Pampers, Luvs, and Huggies at the rate of approximately 18 billion every year. Indeed, it is now estimated that fully 2% of the entire municipal waste stream in the U.S. consists of disposable diapers. The statistics are mind-boggling: the chubby bottoms of 80% of all American infants today are swathed in single-use diapers; one baby uses 3000 diapers in his/her first 6 months of life; the durable plastics employed to resist deterioration in the presence of uric acid and ammonia may remain intact for 5 centuries after burial in a landfill! From a sanitation perspective, the stream of dirty diapers from changing table to garbage can prompts some disquieting thoughts related to the potential presence of over 100 different intestinal pathogens. Surveys indicate that, contrary to package directions, 99% of users discard waste-laden diapers into the trash can rather than flushing fecal material down the toilet. In doing so, they are inadvertently exposing refuse collectors to possible enteric illness and, contrary to existing laws, sending raw sewage to the landfill. Improper disposal of diapers can cause other problems as well; when diaper liners are flushed down toilets (again contrary to instructions), they may clog home plumbing, necessitating a not-inexpensive house call by the Roto-Rooter man. In homes with septic tanks, toilet disposal of diapers can eventually lead to failure of the whole system.

At a time when disposable diaper manufacturers are coming out with newer, jazzier products every year (Ultra-Pampers is now trumpeting the "driest diaper ever!"), is there any hope of weaning convenience-oriented American mommies and daddies to a less wasteful, less-polluting way of attending to baby's needs? The recent renaissance of diaper services across the country offers promise of becoming the epitomy of recycling. Providing the convenience of disposables (the diaper service does all the work, collecting dirty diapers and delivering clean ones) at significantly lower cost (7-11 cents/diaper as compared with 13-31 cents for disposables), diaper services are steadily winning new converts. Promotional efforts such as the "Cotton is Better for your Baby" campaign and the growing interest in all things natural—natural childbirth, breast-feeding, natural fibers—are prompting more and more parents to consider diaper services as an environmentally and economically attractive alternative to continued use of disposables.

Such policies of waste reduction would, admittedly, entail a different national lifestyle, though not necessarily a less enjoyable one. While the concept has yet to capture the hearts and minds of most Americans and has encountered outright opposition from certain industries which would be directly affected by such policies, one particular source reduction strategy has generated a great deal of interest. *"Bottle Bills"*, laws requiring consumers to pay a refundable deposit on beer and soft drink containers, have been enacted in ten states and have been introduced in many state legislatures. In some states, non-refillable containers and flip-top openers on cans have been flatly prohibited. Bottle bills have been vigorously opposed by the bottling industry, by retail merchants' associations (many store managers don't want to be bothered with handling a flood of returnables), and by labor unions fearing job layoffs, but bottle bill proponents can point to some notable accomplishments in states where bottle bills are already in effect. Reduction in total volume of litter in such states averages 40%, while the number of beverage containers discarded along roadsides has dropped by 75-86% from pre-deposit days (although some slovenly individuals persist in tossing cans and bottles away even in bottle bill states, there is now financial motivation for others to retrieve them). Litter cleanup costs have correspondingly fallen—in Maine such expenditures were cut in half following implementation of that state's bottle bill in 1978. While nationwide Americans recycle 54% of all beverage cans, the return rate on both cans and bottles in deposit law states is 90%. (One problem looming on the horizon in this respect, however, is the growing trend among soft drink manufacturers to switch from glass bottles to less-easily recycled plastic. One study in New York showed that fully half the plastic bottles returned for deposit ultimately ended up in landfills.) Although some jobs in container manufacturing may have been lost, states which adopted bottle bills have witnessed a net employment gain as additional workers were hired to handle and transport returned containers. That the U.S. public believes the advantages of beverage container deposit legislation far outweigh any disadvantages is reflected in statistics indicating that nearly 75% of all Americans support enactment of bottle bills.

Fig. 16-3

"BOTTLE BILL" STATES	EFFECTIVE DATE
Oregon	1972
Vermont	1973
Maine	1978
Michigan	1979
Iowa	1979
Connecticut	1980
Massachusetts	1983
Delaware	1983
New York	1983
California	1987

Resource Recovery

Dramatizing Americans' wasteful habits is the fact that of the 160 million tons of municipal refuse currently generated each year, only 10% is recovered for productive use—a far lower figure than that prevailing in most other industrialized countries. Since finding a way to get rid of the remaining 90% is becoming increasingly difficult and expensive, a growing number of citizens and municipal policymakers are focusing renewed interest on programs of resource recovery—any productive use of what would otherwise be a waste material requiring disposal.

The highest rates of resource recovery witnessed in this nation occurred during World War II, when saving valuable resources to aid in the war effort was widely regarded as a patriotic duty. However, interest in resource conservation waned during the prosperous '50s and '60s and only revived with the emergence of the ecology movement and the energy "crisis" of the 1970s. At

Fig. 16-4

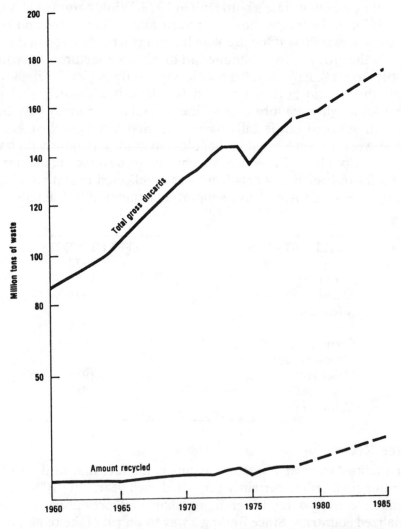

Estimated U.S. Post Consumer Solid Waste Generated and Recycled, 1960-85*

*Projections assume no major new federal policies to reduce waste generation.

Source: Analysis by Franklin Associates, Ltd. for U.S. Environmental Protection Agency, Office of Solid Waste.

that time increased emphasis on resource recovery was promoted primarily for its very real ecological benefits:

1. **resource conservation**—recycling reduces pressure on forest resources and extends the nation's supply of non-renewable mineral ores.
2. **energy conservation**—recycling consumes 50-90% less energy than manufacturing the same item from virgin materials.
3. **pollution abatement**—manufacturing products from secondary rather than virgin materials significantly reduces levels of pollutant emissions. For example, recycling scrap metal, as opposed to processing iron ore in a coke oven, reduces particulate emissions by 11 kg/metric ton and eliminates the mining wastes generated in extracting iron ore and coal. Recycling aluminum has an even greater environmental impact—both air pollution and energy use are thereby cut by 95%.

In recent years, while acknowledging the environmental advantages of recycling, advocates point to a more direct impact municipal resource recovery programs could have in their own communities: by diverting a portion of the urban waste flow, such efforts could have a significant impact on extending the lifespan of existing landfills and help to reduce the cost of waste disposal through the sale of recyclables. The USEPA advocates a nationwide goal of 25% municipal recycling by 1992; some cities are even more ambitious—Berkeley, CA, is aiming at diverting 50% of its waste stream by the early 1990s. Since the mid-1980s, hundreds of local governments and a number of states have launched resource recovery initiatives as an important element in their overall waste management strategy (such efforts are in addition to the estimated 4,000 non-governmental recycling programs, most of them staffed by dedicated volunteers, which have proliferated in towns and cities across the country). Rhode Island passed the nation's first mandatory recycling law in 1986 and has implemented an array of programs aimed at achieving a 25% solid waste recycling goal within the next 15 years. New Jersey, the state with perhaps the most urgent solid waste disposal dilemma in the nation, also has taken a leading role in implementing an ambitious statewide resource recovery effort. In 1987 New Jersey state legislators passed the Mandatory Recycling Act which requires counties to recycle 25% by weight of all municipal solid wastes, pledges that the state government will preferentially purchase recycled products, mandates composting of yard wastes, and is striving to develop new markets for secondary materials. Another state in the forefront of recycling initiatives, Oregon now requires that each city of more than 4,000 people provide curbside pickup of recyclable items at least once a month for those who wish to take advantage of the service. By mid-1988, 7 additional states had adopted mandatory recycling programs similar to those pioneered by Rhode Island, Oregon, and New Jersey. Pennsylvania, the largest and most recent state to jump on the bandwagon, will undoubtedly not be the last, as elected officials nationwide begin to recognize recycling's potential for easing their waste disposal woes. Curbside collection programs are now proliferating across the

Solid and Hazardous Wastes   471

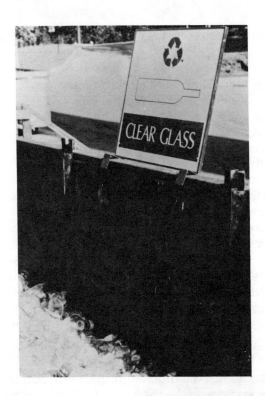

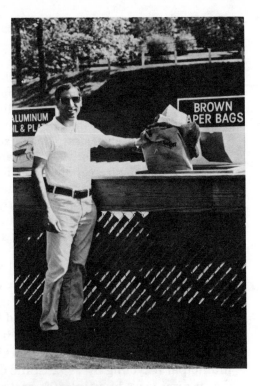

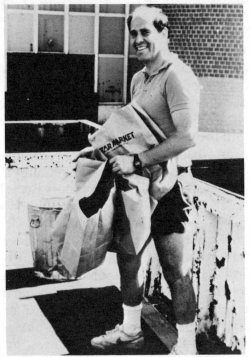

A community recycling facility in Wellesley, MA. Town residents bring paper, glass, metals, etc., to a municipal drop-off center. Many city governments are relying on increased resource recovery efforts such as this to prolong the lifespan of existing sanitary landfills. [*Author's Photo*]

country also, as governments striving to boost the percentage of materials recovered try to make household participation in recycling efforts as easy as possible.

Although public response to the concept of resource recovery has generally been enthusiastic (it's as difficult to argue against the virtues of recycling as it is to oppose motherhood or apple pie!), several obstacles have prevented Americans from realizing the full potential of "turning garbage into gold". While increasing the percentage of households actually participating in recycling programs is one challenge, an even greater one is developing strong, reliable markets for secondary materials. Unfortunately, collection is not synonymous with recycling; if the tons of paper, glass, and metal brought to a drop-off center or set out for curbside pickup have no market, or if the prevailing price for such items is less than the cost of transporting materials to the buyer, resource recovery efforts are doomed to fail. Reasons for this low market demand include:

1. virgin materials are generally cost-competitive with, or cheaper than, secondary materials and are usually perceived by manufacturers as superior in quality.
2. the composition of virgin materials is usually more homogeneous than that of secondary materials.
3. technology to utilize virgin materials is well-established, while that to process waste materials is not perfected to the same extent.
4. synthetics are often combined with natural materials, making it difficult or impossible to recycle the latter.
5. artificial economic barriers (e.g. tax depletion allowances, differential freight rates, government subsidies to producers of virgin materials) discriminate against secondary materials.

Fortunately, a growing demand for U.S. secondary materials in such countries as Mexico, South Korea, and Taiwan (scrap steel and wastepaper comprise over 40% of cargoes shipped out of the Port of New York), as well as a concerted effort on the part of many state governments to develop new markets for recycled products, offers hope that resource recovery will, in the not-too-distant future, become a way of life in the U.S. and will constitute an important element in American waste management strategies.[10]

Waste-to-Energy Incineration

Prior to passage of the 1970 Clean Air Act, burning of urban refuse at large municipal incinerators was the waste disposal method of choice in a number of communities where the high cost of land, unavailability of suitable sites, or neighborhood opposition to siting made landfilling an unfeasible option. By the 1960s, almost 300 municipal incinerators were operating in the United States. As the decade of the '70s ushered in an era of strict air quality control regulations, however, most of these incinerators closed down, unable to comply with the new emission standards. Studies indicated that in some large cities, close to 20% of all particulate pollutants were coming from municipal incinerators.[11]

Today only about 10% of U.S. urban solid waste is incinerated. However, within the past few years, as the nation's garbage woes continue to mount, interest in burning as an attractive waste disposal option has been revived by the advent of a new generation of incinerators—waste-to-energy (WTE) plants. These facilities not only burn refuse, thereby reducing its volume by 80-90%, but also capture the heat of combustion in the form of salable electricity or process steam. Hundreds of municipalities have already committed themselves to this new technology as the most feasible alternative to disappearing landfill space; it is estimated that by the mid-1990s as much as 25% of urban refuse may be incinerated and EPA officials predict the figure may reach 40% by the turn of the century (already in Europe and Japan approximately 30-40% of municipal solid wastes are burned in WTE incinerators).

Most WTE plants are "mass burn" facilities, accepting unsegregated wastes loaded onto a moving grate which feeds into the furnace; some mass burn plants combine recycling activities with incineration, separating out glass and metals prior to burning. Units come in various sizes; large facilities built on site have capacities ranging up to 3300 tons/day, while modular types can be supplied to be economically feasible for communities producing as little as 100 tons of refuse per day. Refuse-derived fuel (RDF) plants, by contrast, first remove

---

Box 16–2

Turning Garbage Into Topsoil

It may not be quite the equivalent of turning "garbage into gold", but European cities have long recognized the positive impact which composting of organic household wastes can have on reducing the amount of refuse requiring disposal. Dutch tulips and French vineyards benefit from applications of municipal compost; in Sweden 25% of all urban solid wastes are composted, and in West Germany, Belgium, Italy, and Austria large composting operations turn garbage into a valuable soil conditioner.[12] Serious consideration of composting as a viable waste management alternative in the United States, however, is a much more recent phenomenon. Even though readily decomposible food and yard wastes make up about 30% of the U.S. urban waste stream (considerably more during the warmer months of the year, less during the winter), perceived lack of demand for the finished product, plus the ease and low cost of landfilling led city officials to dismiss composting as an impractical venture. Suddenly that attitude is changing, as planners realize it makes little sense to devote valuable landfill space to grass clippings and autumn leaves. In several states (e.g. New Jersey, Minnesota, Illinois) recent legislation prohibiting the landfilling of yard wastes has given a boost to interest in municipal composting.

One form of resource recovery, composting utilizes natural biochemical decay processes to convert organic wastes into a humus-like material, suitable for use as a soil conditioner. Although its nutrient content is too low to consider it a fertilizer, compost greatly improves soil structure and porosity, aids in water infiltration and retention, increases soil aeration, and slows erosion. Co-composting of yard wastes with municipal sewage sludge (another increasingly difficult-to-dispose-of waste product), now being practiced in a number of

---

communities, enhances the nitrogen content of the finished product and makes it more valuable for agricultural uses.

Industries also are beginning to look at composting as a solution to their waste disposal problems—and as a method of avoiding escalating landfill charges. In Maine, several pilot projects have been launched to demonstrate the feasibility of composting organic industrial wastes such as papermill sludge, wood by-products, wool fibers, potato processing wastes, and the tons of fish scraps and seafood shells which constitute a significant percentage of the solid waste load along the state's mid-coast region. In North Carolina, the potential for composting sludge from a hardboard processing plant is being explored, while in the heart of the Illinois Corn Belt, experimental efforts at composting food processing wastes such as corn stalks, corncobs, silks, and shucks are underway. Even certain hazardous wastes may be feasible targets for composting. A hazardous waste remediation firm in Massachusetts has successfully demonstrated that certain petroleum-contaminated soils can be detoxified by the application of composting technologies.[13]

A variety of methods for converting wastes to compost are currently in use, ranging from the relatively simple windrow technique, where long rows of wastes are piled outdoors and mechanically turned periodically to aerate the mass, to relatively sophisticated methods, carried out inside specially-designed structures, which utilize a forced-air system for supplying oxygen to the process. Whatever the technology, the composting process consists of 4 basic steps:

1. **preparation**—incoming wastes are shredded to a relatively uniform size; in most composting operations, non-biodegradable materials such as glass, metal, plastics, tires, etc., are separated from the compostable wastes, but one process developed by a Florida-based corporation is designed to handle any municipal wastes that are not too large to pass through the hammermills. In some composting operations, sewage sludge or animal manures are added to the refuse at this point.

2. **digestion**—microbes naturally present in the waste materials or special bacterial inoculants sprayed on the refuse are utilized to break down organic waste materials. While digestion may be either aerobic or anaerobic, aerobic systems are generally preferred due to shorter time periods required and minimal odor problems. In aerobic decomposition, heat given off by microbial respiration raises the temperature in the windrows well above the 140°F necessary to kill fly eggs, weed seeds, or pathogenic organisms. In enclosed systems with forced draft aeration, digestion may be complete in as little as 2-5 days; in outdoor windrows where piles are mechanically turned, the process takes many months.

3. **curing**—after the digestion of simpler carbonaceous materials is complete, additional curing time is allowed to permit microbes to break down cellulose and lignin in the waste.

4. **finishing**—to produce an acceptable finished product, compost may be put through screens and grinders to remove non-digested materials and create a uniform appearance. Some composting facilities bag or package the finished product to facilitate marketing or distribution.

In the past, the difficulty of finding outlets for municipal compost was a major stumbling-block in convincing local officials to consider composting as a waste management strategy. In recent years, however, cities' marketing efforts and increased public awareness of compost's desirability as a soil conditioner have created sufficient demand among landscaping firms, nurseries, parks departments, and home gardeners to provide a ready outlet. This growing willingness to use compost, coupled with improvements in composting technology and a national need to curtail the flood of urban refuse destined for steadily-dwindling landfill space, suggests that municipal composting will constitute an increasingly significant waste management alternative in the years ahead.

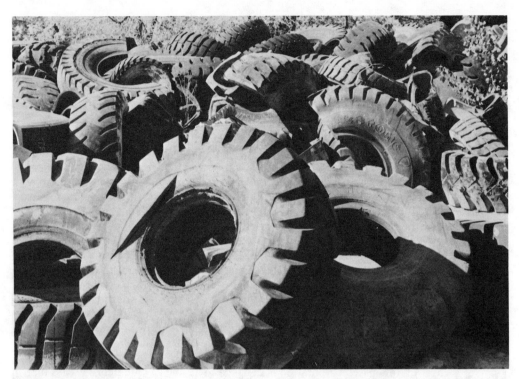

Discarded tires litter the American landscape and pose one of our more difficult solid waste disposal problems. [*Author's Photo*]

non-combustibles, then process the remaining wastes by shredding them with hammermills to produce a pelletized fuel which can be mixed with coal and burned in ordinary boilers.

The euphoria which just a few years ago welcomed WTE incinerators as the ideal solution to our disposal dilemmas is now giving way to a more cautious appraisal, as concerns are raised about possible toxic air emissions, especially dioxins and furans, and hazardous substances in incinerator ash which would require tighter regulation of ash disposal. Proponents of the technology insist such problems can be minimized through good emission control devices and proper plant operation; opponents remain wary, fearing that cities jumping on the WTE bandwagon are going to find they've simply traded one set of environmental problems for another. Perhaps the major question mark regarding the future of WTE incineration, however, is financing their construction and operation. Costs have been much greater than many cities expected and anticipated revenues from energy sales may be less than projected if electricity prices decline. Adapting European incinerator technology to accommodate the somewhat different U.S. household waste stream has been tricky and expensive. Perhaps most worrisome to local officials is the possibility that due to heavy metal residues, incinerator ash will be defined as hazardous waste, requiring disposal at specially-engineered facilities, and thus greatly increasing operating costs.

The Tire Dilemma

The blaze that ignited on Halloween night, 1983, in Winchester, VA, was no bonfire for toasting marshmallows; the unintended fuel was a stockpile of 7 million tires which continued to burn and spew noxious pollutants over the surrounding area until the following June. This incident provided dramatic evidence of the problems posed by one of modern society's most difficult waste disposal challenges—what to do with the more than 240 million car and truck tires which are discarded every year? When landfilled, tires inevitably work their way up through the soil and pop out at the surface; when piled in waste tire dumps they constitute a fire hazard and mosquito breeding habitat; thoughtlessly scattered about the countryside on rural back roads or along streambanks they constitute a visual blight.

In former years when tires were made almost entirely of natural rubber, worn out tires were generally reprocessed and used to make new tires. However, with the advent of synthetic rubber and steelbelted radial tires, reprocessing declined and stockpiles of old tires increased dramatically in volume. It is estimated that the U.S. is currently littered with more than 2 billion old tires, but relief may be on the horizon with the development of several innovative new approaches to tire recycling.

Energy recovery is the focus of a $41 million whole-tire incinerator near Modesto, CA, about 80 miles east of San Francisco. Built by Oxford Energy in partnership with General Electric, the plant is located adjacent to the world's largest tire pile—an incredible mass estimated at 42 million, with 20,000 more arriving daily. Commencing operations in the spring of 1988, the Modesto facility incinerates tires at the rate of 700 per hour, generating 13 megawatts of electricity for Pacific Gas & Electric. Plans for other waste tire-to-energy plants in Connecticut and New York are being considered, and if citizens' objections to potential air quality problems can be resolved, such facilities could help ease tire disposal problems in the Northeast as well.

Tire-derived fuel—processed, wire-free tire chips which can be used in solid fuel industrial boilers—offers another possibility for converting waste tires into useful energy. Tire shredding plants in Portland, OR, and Houston, TX, process several million tires annually, producing rubber chips to be used as fuels. A proposed facility in Camden, NJ, designed to handle 10 million tires per year, would, if built, be the largest tire processing plant in the U.S.

Incineration is not the only resource recovery method for used tires. Interest has been expressed in using recycled rubber for road surfaces and bridge decking. The U.S. Dept. of Energy is funding a study of the feasibility of using scrap rubber as a substitute for virgin polymers. Perhaps most exciting to environmentalists concerned about the air quality impact of burning tires for energy recovery is a product called "Tirecycle", developed by a Minnesota-based firm. Capable of processing 3 million tires a year, the Tirecycle system grinds the used rubber into small particles which are then coated with a proprietary polymer which enables the particles to bond together as effectively as virgin rubber. The Tirecycle product is half as expensive as virgin rubber, cheaper than plastic, and can be readily combined with both. Because the process uses no water and consumes only electrical energy, the plant in Babbitt, MN, generates no pollutant air emissions or contaminated effluent. The Tirecycle system appeared sufficiently promising to attract financing from the State of Minnesota for construction of the Babbitt facility and its record of operation since opening in 1987 has prompted state officials in Michigan and Massachusetts to opt for the process in their states as well.[14]

Hazardous Wastes

Late in the summer of 1978 the name of a small residential subdivision in the city of Niagara Falls, NY, entered the American vocabulary and became a household word almost overnight, symbolizing the dangers of our chemical age. The tragic sequence of events which unfolded at *Love Canal* epitomizes the dangers facing millions of citizens in thousands of communities across the nation as a result of our indiscriminate use and careless disposal of hazardous chemicals.

The Love Canal Story

The origin of the chemical dumpsite which became the focus of worldwide attention in the late 1970s can be traced to the mid-1890s when William T. Love began construction of a canal intended to serve as a navigable power channel, connecting the Upper Niagara to the Niagara Escarpment about 7 miles downstream, thereby bypassing the Falls. At the point where Mr. Love's canal was intended to re-enter the river, the intention was to construct a model industrial city which would be provided with cheap, abundant hydroelectric power. Unfortunately for Mr. Love, his development company went bankrupt shortly after construction of the canal had begun; the project was abandoned, leaving a waterway approximately 3000 feet long, 10 feet deep, and 60 feet wide. For many years, residents of this area on the outskirts of town used the canal for recreational fishing and swimming; in 1927 the land was annexed by the city. In 1942 Hooker Chemical Company (now a subsidiary of Occidental Petroleum), one of several major chemical industries located in Niagara Falls, received permission to dump chemical wastes into the canal, which it proceeded to do from that time until 1952 (in 1947 Hooker purchased the canal, along with two 70-feet-wide strips of land adjacent to the canal on each side). During this time more than 21,000 tons of chemical wastes—acids, alkalis, solvents, chlorinated hydrocarbons, etc.—were disposed of at this site. Only a few homes were present in the area at that time, but old-time residents recall the offensive odors, noxious vapors, and frequent fires which accompanied the dumping. By 1953 the canal was full and so was topped with soil and eventually acquired a covering of grass and weeds. Hooker then offered to sell the land to the Niagara Falls School Board for the token fee of $1. At the same time company officials pointedly advised school and city administrators that although the site was suitable for a school, parking lot, or playground, any construction activities involving excavation of the area should be avoided to prevent rupturing the dumpsite's clay lining, thereby allowing escape of the impounded chemicals. In 1955 an elementary school and playground were constructed on the site; in 1957 the city began laying storm sewers, roads, and utility lines through the area, disregarding the warnings received a few years earlier. In the years that followed, several hundred modest homes were built in the neighborhood parallel to the banks of the now-invisible canal. Most of the newer residents had no knowledge of the site's past history and, in spite of occasional chemical odors (not considered unusual in a city where chemical manufacturing was a leading industry), few outward signs of trouble were apparent. Unusually heavy precipitation in the mid-1970s, however, was accompanied by some alarming phenomena. Strange-looking, viscous chemicals began oozing through basement walls, floors, and sump holes. Vegetation in yards withered and appeared scorched. Large puddles became permanent backyard features. Holes began to open up in the field which had once been a dumpsite and the tops of corroded 55-gallon drums leaking chemicals could be seen in places protruding from the soil surface. Complaints and fears expressed by citizens were generally downplayed by local authorities who assured them there was nothing about which to be concerned.

By early 1978 pressure from a local Congressman and regular critical coverage of events in the *Niagara Gazette* prompted the U.S. Environmental Protection Agency to undertake a program of air sampling in the basements of Love Canal homes. New York State authorities also began conducting soil analyses and taking samples of residues in sump pumps and storm sewers. The results of these studies indicated that the area was extremely contaminated with more than 200 different chemicals, including 12 known or suspected carcinogens.

Box 16–4

Beyond Love Canal

While Love Canal has dominated media reports focusing on hazardous waste problems, a large and still growing number of other horror stories highlight the diversity of chemical waste situations facing communities throughout the country. A sampling of the more notorious of such incidents must include:

The Valley of the Drums

In the spring of 1978 a 7-acre rural site about 25 miles south of Louisville, Kentucky, was discovered to have been used as a dumpsite for approximately 17,000 drums, 6000 of which were full of toxic chemicals, corroding through the metal and oozing onto the ground and into the soil. Soil and water analyses revealed the presence of about 200 different organic chemicals and 30 metals. It was subsequently learned that the owner of the land, by that time deceased, had been paid by industrial firms in the Louisville area to haul their wastes to an approved disposal site; instead he pocketed the money and dumped the drums on his own land, frequently emptying the contents on the ground in order to reuse the containers.

Woburn, Massachusetts

Between 1968 and 1979, twelve children in this Boston suburb of 36,000 people were diagnosed as suffering from leukemia; from 1979-1985, 26 more cases were diagnosed and of these, 15 had died by the summer of 1985. Although a certain number of leukemia cases can be expected in any population, the incidence in Woburn was unusually high and the fact that most of the victims lived in East Woburn, many within walking distance of one another, seemed more than coincidental. In 1979 a reporter for the Woburn Daily Times revealed the startling news that 300 acres of toxic chemical wastes had been discovered buried near the site of an industrial complex in Woburn; subsequent revelations of high

---

levels of chromium, arsenic, and lead contaminating soils and groundwater there caused the site to be named one of the ten most dangerous waste dumps in the nation. In the meantime, city wells serving the East Woburn area where most of the leukemia cases had occurred were found to be polluted with high concentrations of cancer-causing industrial chemicals such as trichloroethylene (TCE), perchloroethylene (PCE), and chloroform. The wells were quickly shut down, but suspicion grew that the toxic waste dumping, drinking water contamination, and childhood leukemia deaths were somehow interrelated. Groundwater studies undertaken by state environmental agencies eventually identified the source of wellwater contamination as property owned by the W.R. Grace Company, where test wells revealed the presence of TCE and other contaminants. In 1986 the company agreed to an $8 million out-of-court settlement with eight Woburn families who had sued W.R. Grace, alleging that industrial solvents from its Cryovac Division plant in Woburn had contaminated wells and caused their children's leukemia deaths.

Stringfellow Quarry, California

Excavated in steplike fashion up the sides of Pyrite Canyon near Riverside, CA, a series of shallow pits served as the repository for a witches' brew of hazardous effluents from southern California industries from 1956-1972. About 34 million gallons of sulfuric, nitric, and hydrochloric acid wastes, as well as organic solvents, heavy metals, and pesticides were dumped into the Stringfellow pits before public pressures resulted in closure of the site. Complaints of choking odors and accidental spills were commonplace during the years the pits were receiving wastes. Since 1972, the Stringfellow Quarry has continued to generate controversy regarding future use of the pits and the fate of chemicals already buried there. By the mid-1980s it had become apparent that a toxic plume of contaminants had leaked from the pits and was slowly moving in the direction of the aquifer which serves as a drinking water source for half a million people in Los Angeles and Riverside Counties. Now a federal Superfund site, the Stringfield Quarry is so contaminated that regulatory officials estimate that cleanup efforts will go on for decades.

Rocky Mountain Arsenal, Colorado

For over 40 years this U.S. Army facility northeast of Denver has been the site of multiple incidents of hazardous waste mismanagement which have severely polluted area groundwater, surface streams, and air. Among the contaminants deposited on arsenal grounds are chemical warfare agents, nerve gas wastes, pesticides, toxic metal sludges from rockets, and incendiary bomb wastes. Migration of carelessly dumped or accidentally spilled pollutants beyond arsenal boundaries were reported as early as 1951 when local farmers complained of damage to crops grown near the base. Over the next 25 years, citizens' complaints blaming arsenal operations for pollution of private wells were brushed off by Army officials who assured nearby residents there was no cause for worry. During the 1960s, public anxieties were rekindled by a series of earthquakes caused by the Army's injection of hazardous liquids into deepwells on arsenal land, as well as by an explosion at a nerve gas plant in 1968. These incidents contributed to a decision to remove or detoxify the chemical warfare agents at the arsenal, but no thought was given at the time to cleaning up existing pollution problems. Not until the mid-1970s did mounting evidence of chemical contamination of water supplies beyond arsenal boundaries combine with growing environmental awareness nationwide to prompt Army officials to consider cleanup efforts onsite. A hopeful public looking for a "quick fix" of problems at Rocky Mt. Arsenal is likely to be disappointed, however. The site was among the first to be nominated for National Priority List status, qualifying it for inclusion in the federal Superfund program, but the complexity and cost of the project ensure that progress will be slow. Estimates for cleanup range from $360 million to $2.5 billion and completion of this massive effort is not anticipated before the year 2000.[15]

Benzene, known to be a potent human cancer-causing agent, was readily detected in the air inside many of the houses sampled. Dioxin was subsequently found in high concentrations in some of the soil samples analyzed. State officials in New York estimate that as many as 10% of the chemicals buried at Love Canal may be mutagens, teratogens, or carcinogens. On August 2, 1978, the Health Commissioner of New York publicly proclaimed "the existence of a great and imminent peril to the health of the general public" at Love Canal and advised all pregnant women and families with children under the age of 2 to leave the area if they could do so. Five days later, President Carter officially declared Love Canal a national emergency. The months that followed witnessed mass relocation at public expense of residents living closest to the dumpsite, as well as openly expressed fears by those left behind on adjacent streets that their health was similarly endangered. A number of health studies whose methodology and conclusions remain highly controversial, suggest that Love Canal residents have experienced statistically significant elevated rates of miscarriage, birth defects, and chromosomal abnormalities. Ultimately 1,004 families were evacuated from Love Canal, their homes purchased by the state. Over 300 of the residences closest to the canal were demolished and the area covered with a protective layer of clay and a synthetic liner to exclude rainwater. Most of the remaining homes were boarded up, awaiting a pending EPA assessment of whether they could ever again be inhabited. Trenches have been dug around the old canal site to capture contaminated groundwater which is then pumped to a treatment center for detoxification. Nearby creeks where high levels of dioxin seepage were detected have been fenced off to protect children and animals. Combined federal and state expenditures for relocating residents, investigating environmental damage, and halting chemical seepage from the site total $150 million, and an additional $32 million is being spent to clean up contaminated creeks and sewers and to determine the future habitability of the neighborhood (the Congressional Office of Technology Assessment estimates that if Hooker had employed current disposal standards and practices, its wastes could have been safely managed for about $2 million in 1979 dollars). Hooker, now renamed Occidental Chemical, has paid $20 million in out-of-court settlements to affected residents and is appealing a 1988 court ruling holding it liable for the cost of previous, ongoing, and future cleanup of the Love Canal site—a figure which could eventually total several hundred million dollars. Finally, in the fall of 1988, after reviewing a 5-year habitability study of the affected area, New York State Health Commissioner David Axelrod declared that most of the Love Canal neighborhood can be safely resettled by former residents. A local taskforce is now in the process of developing plans to aid in the resettlement effort and to assist with the renovation of homes that suffered deterioration during the 10-year evacuation period.[16]

The events which transpired at Love Canal cannot be shrugged off as a unique tragedy which unfortunately victimized a few thousand people in western New York State but left the rest of the nation unscathed. Health authorities and environmental agency officials regard Love Canal as but the "tip of the iceberg" in alerting society to the widespread nature of the hazardous waste problem. EPA is currently aware of more than 16,000 hazardous waste dumps scattered across the U.S. and fear that many of these may be exposing citizens to dangers as serious as those which surfaced at Love Canal. Little wonder that public opinion polls show citizens ranking hazardous waste management issues among their top environmental quality concerns.

What Is "Hazardous" Waste?

In the 1976 Resource Conservation and Recovery Act (RCRA), Congress legally defined hazardous waste as "any discarded material that may pose a substantial threat or potential danger to human health or the environment when improperly handled". The EPA has established a 2-tier system for determining whether a specific waste is subject to regulation under current hazardous waste management laws:

1) If the substance in question is among the approximately 400 wastes or waste streams itemized in Parts 261.31-33 of the Code of Federal Regulations, it will automatically be subject to regulation as a hazardous waste. Wastes may be placed on the list because of their ability to induce cancer, mutations, or birth defects, because of their toxicity to plants, or because even low doses are fatal to humans. However, the Administrator of USEPA can exercise a wide measure of discretion in deciding whether or not to list a particular waste, so a number of potential carcinogens, mutagens, and teratogens are not yet listed as officially "hazardous".

2) In addition to the wastes listed in the federal Code, any waste which exhibits one or more of the following characteristics is defined as hazardous and subject to regulation:

Toxic—wastes such as arsenic, heavy metals, or certain synthetic pesticides are capable of causing either acute or chronic health problems.

Ignitable—organic solvents, oils, plasticizers, and paint wastes are examples of wastes which are hazardous because they have a flashpoint less than 60°C (140°F) or because they tend to undergo spontaneous combustion. The resultant fires are dangerous not only because of heat and smoke, but also because they can disseminate toxic particles over a wide area.

Corrosive—substances with a pH of 2 or less or 12.5 and above can eat away at standard container materials or living tissues through chemical action and are termed corrosive. Such wastes, which include acids, alkaline cleaning agents, and battery manufacturing residues, present a special threat to waste haulers who come into bodily contact with leaking containers.

Reactive—obsolete munitions, wastes from the manufacturing of dynamite or firecrackers, and certain chemical wastes such as picric acid are hazardous because of their tendency to react vigorously with air or water or to explode and generate toxic fumes.

Two other categories of wastes which might logically be considered hazardous—radioactive wastes, and infectious wastes from hospitals and clinics—are not presently regulated under the same laws as the groups listed above. Radioactive wastes are managed according to regulations adopted by the Nuclear Regulatory Commission under the Atomic Energy Act, while biomedical waste disposal laws vary from state to state. Flagrant incidents of illegal ocean dumping of such wastes during the summer of 1988 attracted widespread media attention, as beaches from Cape Cod to the Carolinas were littered with such unsavory debris as used syringes and blood vials, some of which tested positive for AIDS virus antibodies and hepatitis B antigens. Public outrage generated by this situation resulted in passage of the 1988 Medical Waste Tracking Act, which sets up a 2-year pilot project to attempt regulation of biomedical wastes through a system similar in nature to the manifest system currently required for off-site shipments of hazardous wastes.

Generation of Hazardous Wastes

USEPA estimates that the U.S. currently generates approximately 275 million metric tons of industrial hazardous wastes annually, a figure which does not take into account those wastes which are managed illegally. (Note: statistics on annual hazardous waste generation vary somewhat, depending on how estimates are made. Figures from the Congressional Budget Office, based on employment data, at 266 million metric tons are slightly lower than EPA estimates, but are not significantly different).[17] Production of these wastes is not evenly distributed among industries, however. Over 85% of all hazardous wastes are produced by just 3 major categories of generators (see following figure). Geographic location of these industries, as well as population density, are major determinants of which states are the leading hazardous waste generators.

Fig. 16-5 Distribution of Industrial Hazardous Waste Generation, by Major Industrial Group, 1983

(thousand metric tons)

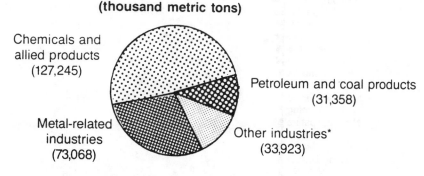

Chemicals and allied products (127,245)

Petroleum and coal products (31,358)

Metal-related industries (73,068)

Other industries* (33,923)

* Includes rubber and plastic products, miscellaneous manufacturing, motor freight transportation, wood preserving, drum reconditioning industries, nonelectrical machinery, transportation equipment, and electric and electronic machinery.

Source: Congressional Budget Office.

Fig. 16-6

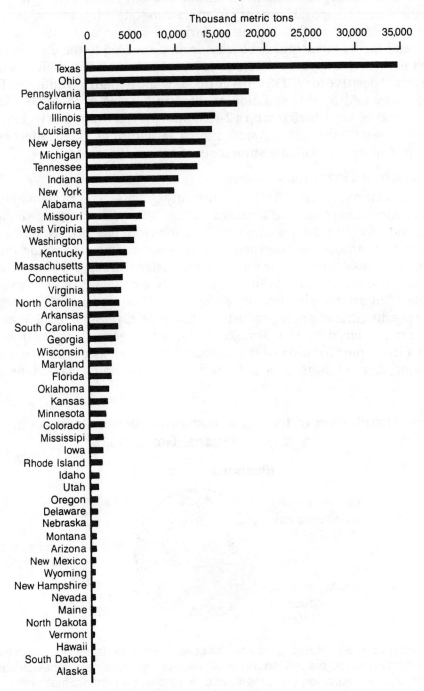

Estimated Generation of Hazardous Waste
in the United States, by State, 1983

Source: Congressional Budget Office.

Fig. 16-7 Estimated Generation of Hazardous Waste per Capita in the United States, by State, 1983

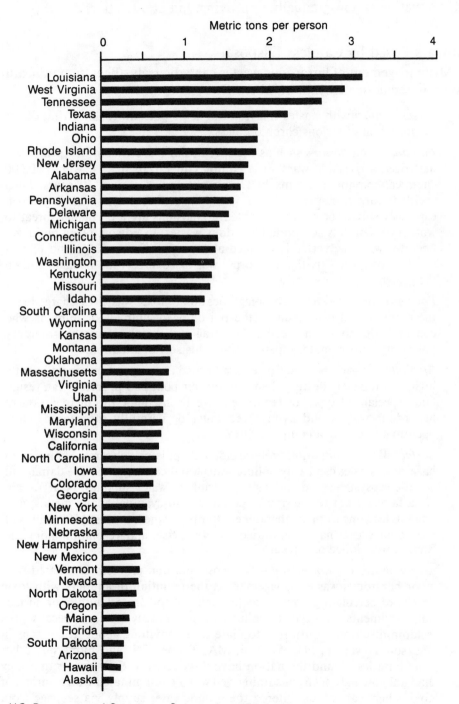

Source: U.S. Department of Commerce; Congressional Budget Office.

At the time when new federal waste management regulations went into effect in November, 1980, EPA estimated that fully 90% of all hazardous wastes were being disposed of by methods which would not meet government standards. That situation is now gradually improving, but at a relatively slow pace.

Threats Posed by Careless Disposal

Mismanagement of hazardous wastes can adversely affect human health and environmental quality in a number of ways:

Direct Contact with wastes can result in acute poisoning, skin irritation, or the initiation of serious chronic illness.

Fire and/or Explosions such as the spectacular blaze which, in April, 1980, destroyed a riverside warehouse complex in Elizabeth, NJ, where 50,000 chemical-containing drums had been sitting for almost 10 years. Such accidents are a constant threat when hazardous wastes are in transit, carelessly stored, or roughly handled. Explosions are a particular threat to workers at landfills accepting hazardous wastes. In Edison, NJ, a bulldozer operator who inadvertently crushed a container of flammable phosphorus was burned so quickly that his corpse was discovered with his hand still on the gearshift.

Poison via the Foodchain—biomagnification of toxic wastes discharged into the environment can result in the poisoning of animals or humans who consume the toxin indirectly. The tragic outbreak of methyl mercury poisoning at Minamata, Japan, typifies this sort of situation.

Air Pollution—when toxic wastes are burned at temperatures insufficiently high to completely destroy them, serious air pollution problems can result. Only specialized types of equipment are licensed for the incineration of hazardous wastes and even these must be carefully monitored while operating to ensure a complete burn.

Surface Water Contamination—accidental spills or deliberate dumping of hazardous wastes can easily pollute waterways, causing extensive damage to aquatic ecosystems and endangering drinking water supplies. Near Byron, IL, a farm stream was seriously polluted with cyanide, heavy metals, and phenols leaching from an abandoned dumpsite where at least 1500 drums of hazardous wastes had been buried. Wildlife, fish, and vegetation along the stream were killed as a result.

Groundwater Contamination—the most common problem associated with poor hazardous waste management is the pollution of aquifers with toxic leachates percolating downward through the soil from landfills or surface impoundments. This type of pollution is particularly insidious because it is seldom discovered until it is too late to do anything about it. Citizens in Jackson Township, NJ, Woburn, MA, Toone, TN, and numerous other communities around the nation have discovered to their horror that they had unknowingly been consuming well water contaminated with a variety of toxic chemicals which entered the groundwater supply via seepage from disposal sites.

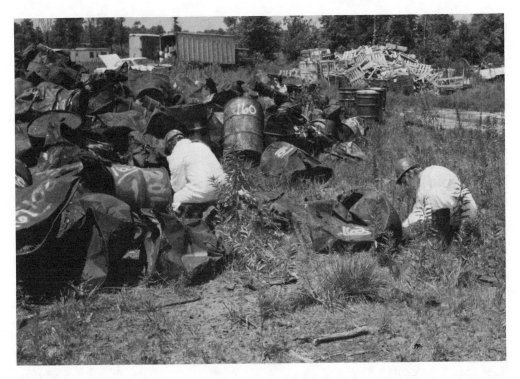

Abandoned hazardous waste dump site where hundreds of corroding drums leak their toxic contents onto the ground, endangering drinking water aquifer below the surface. [*Illinois Environmental Protection Agency*]

Methods of Hazardous Waste Disposal

Historically, the largest percentage of hazardous wastes have been disposed of on land, primarily because land disposal, particularly prior to government regulation of hazardous waste management, was by far the cheapest disposal option. During the mid-1970s, for example, almost half of all hazardous wastes, the majority of which were in the form of liquids or sludges, were simply dumped into unlined surface impoundments, technically referred to as "pits, ponds, or lagoons", located on the generators' property (even today, approximately 96% of all hazardous wastes generated in this country is treated or disposed of at the site where it is generated; only 4% of all hazardous wastes are sent off-site for management). These wastes eventually evaporated or percolated into the soil, often resulting in groundwater contamination. Other wastes, about 30% of the total, were buried in sanitary landfills, easily subject to leaching, and another 10% were burned in an uncontrolled manner. None of these methods would be in compliance with current regulations.

Although many citizens are convinced that no methods exist for the safe disposal of hazardous wastes, a number of new technologies have been developed which avoid most of the shortcomings inherent in past hazardous waste management practices. All such methods, not surprisingly, are consid-

Fig. 16-8 Hazardous Waste Management Methods, United States, 1983

Management Method	Share of Total Waste Managed
	(percent)
Land disposal[1]	67
Discharge to sewers, rivers, streams	22
Distillation for recovery of solvents	4
Burning in industrial boilers	4
Chemical treatment by oxidation	1
Land treatment of biodegradable waste	1
Incineration	1
Recovery of metals through ion exchange	—[2]
Total	100

[1]Includes injection wells (25 percent of total), surface impoundments (19 percent), hazardous waste landfills (13 percent), and sanitary landfills (10 percent).
[2]Less than 1 percent.

Source: U.S. Congressional Budget Office, *Hazardous Waste Management: Recent Changes and Policy Alternatives* (Washington, D.C.: U.S. Government Printing Office, 1985).

erably more expensive than simply dumping wastes in a pit or a municipal landfill, and thus were not widely utilized until strict regulatory action was taken by Congress. A listing of legal hazardous waste disposal options would include:

Secure Chemical Landfill—generally the cheapest method of hazardous waste disposal is the so-called "secure" chemical landfill, a specially-designed earthen excavation constructed in such a way as to contain dangerous chemicals and to prevent them from escaping into the environment through leaching or vaporization. In the past, secure landfills frequently differed from sanitary landfills only in that they were topped with a layer of clay to keep water out of the trenches in which chemical drums had been placed. This of course did not prevent chemical seepage from contaminating water supplies. Under current RCRA standards, a secure chemical landfill must be located above the 100-year floodplain and away from fault zones; it must contain double liners of clay or synthetic materials to keep leaching to a minimum; a network of pipes must be laid to collect and control polluted rainwater and leachate accumulating in the landfill; and monitoring wells must be installed to check the quality of any groundwater deposits in the area (surface water supplies must also be monitored by the landfill operator). In spite of these precautions, most experts agree that there is no way to guarantee that sometime in the future contaminants will not migrate from the landfill site. Liners eventually crack, soil can shift or settle. Since many chemical wastes remain hazardous more or less indefinitely, serious pollution problems can occur many years after a secure chemical landfill has been closed and forgotten. Many authorities feel that although chemical landfills are legal, they are the least acceptable method of managing hazardous wastes.

Since 1984 when more stringent requirements for groundwater monitoring, minimum technology standards, and financial guarantees for post-closure activities took effect, the number of operating facilities dropped substantially. Today there are approximately 100 hazardous waste landfills in the U.S., one-third of which are commercial facilities. Within the past few years, the list of wastes for which disposal in landfills is prohibited has been steadily growing; federal legislation enacted in 1984 calls for a ban on the landfilling of virtually all hazardous wastes by May 8, 1990, unless such materials undergo prior treatment to minimize their toxicity and ability to migrate. The explicit intent of such legislation is to reduce reliance on land disposal and to encourage the use of alternative technologies to the greatest extent possible.

Fig. 16-9

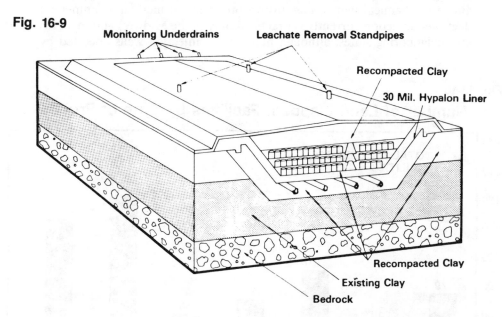

A SECURE LANDFILL

Various Chemical, Physical, or Biological Processes which reduce the volume or change the nature of the waste have been used successfully by a number of industries.

Physical methods include evaporation to concentrate corrosive brines, sedimentation to separate solids from liquid wastes, and carbon adsorption to remove certain soluble organic wastes.

Chemical techniques involve processes such as neutralization to render wastes harmless, sulfide precipitation to extract certain toxic metals, oxidation-reduction processes to convert some metals from a hazardous to a non-hazardous state, and solidification, in which the waste material is combined with a cement-like material, encapsulated in plastic, blended with organic polymers, or combined with silica to form a solid, inert substance which can be disposed of safely in a landfill.

Biological treatment, based on the ability of microbes to decompose toxic organic compounds, focuses on the use of activated sludge for soluble organic wastes and a process called "land spreading", in which nonchlorinated organic wastes such as oil residues and oil-based solvents are mechanically mixed into the upper layers of soil (generally on industry-owned land, removed from any drinking water source) where they are quickly broken down by ordinary soil bacteria, generally within one season.

Deep Well Injection—the use of deep wells for waste disposal dates back to the late 19th century when the petroleum industry employed this method to get rid of salt brine, but its use for liquid hazardous waste disposal began only during the 1940s. A number of industries, most notably petroleum refineries and petrochemical plants, now utilize this disposal method. Commercial deep well injection currently is practiced only in the Midwest and in Texas and neighboring states, although many other injection wells operated by

Fig. 16-10

Number of Land Disposal Facilities by Type of Process

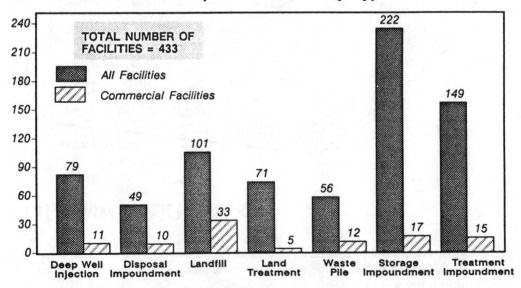

Note: Some facilities have more than one process.
Source: National Screening Survey, U.S. EPA, Office of Solid Waste (1986).

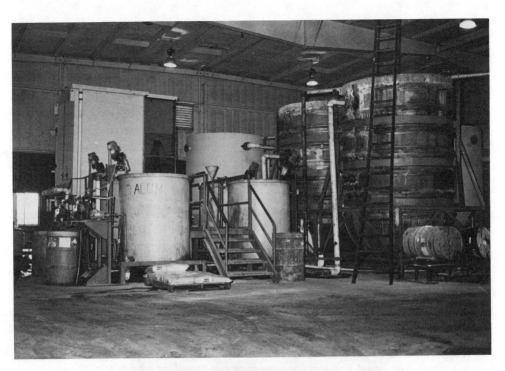

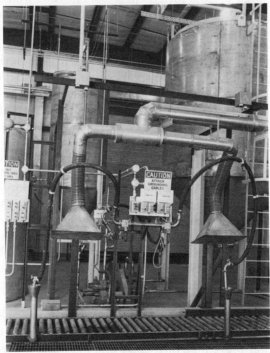

Hazardous waste treatment processes can render wastes innocuous; the increasing number of legal restrictions against land disposal of hazardous wastes is causing many waste generators today to look with favor on the various methods of waste treatment. [*Illinois Environmental Protection Agency*]

private firms solely for the disposal of their own wastes are widely scattered across the U.S. Of the total amount of hazardous waste managed each year, the largest portion—about 25% of all such wastes—is disposed of by deepwell injection. The process involves pumping liquid wastes through lined wells into porous rock formations deep underground, well below any drinking water aquifers. Some critics point out that cracks in the well casing or undetected faults in the earth which intersect the disposal zone could result in outward migration of wastes. EPA contends that deep wells are safe, provided that they are constructed, operated and maintained in accordance with Agency regulations.

Controlled Incineration—because burning at very high temperatures actually destroys hazardous wastes (as opposed to storing them out of sight underground as is essentially the case with various land disposal methods), most hazardous waste management experts regard controlled incinceration as the best and, in some cases, the only environmentally acceptable means of disposal. However, due to its relatively high cost compared to other waste management options, incineration until recently accounted for only 1% of all hazardous wastes managed. It is expected that this situation will change dramatically in the years ahead, as land disposal laws become increasingly restrictive and as generators, fearful of legal liability if their wastes migrate from a land disposal site, opt for a management method which ensures waste destruction. A controlled incinerator burns at temperatures ranging from 750-3000°F, with wastes, air, and fuel being thoroughly mixed to ensure complete combustion. Afterburners which are part of the incineration system destroy any gaseous hydrocarbons which may have survived the initial incineration process, while scrubbers and electrostatic precipitators remove pollutant emissions from the stack gases. Capable of handling solid, liquid, and gaseous wastes, incineration has several distinct advantages over other disposal methods: a) it can convert toxic compounds to harmless ones; b) it greatly reduces waste volume; c) by destroying wastes rather than isolating them, it eliminates future problems; and d) it offers the potential of energy recovery during combustion of wastes. Several different types of incinerators are currently being used, each having its own advantages and disadvantages for combustion of specific waste categories. One of the more interesting of these is the incinerator ship, which burns toxic wastes at sea, thereby having minimal environmental impact—and avoiding public protests. The incinerator ship Vulcanus was commissioned by the U.S. Air Force in 1977 to destroy large quantities of the dioxin-tainted herbicide Agent Orange and in 1981 successfully burned large U.S. stockpiles of PCBs and other toxic chemicals in the Gulf of Mexico.

Waste Exchanges—the ideal way to manage hazardous materials would be to recycle them, thus preventing their entry into the waste stream and eliminating the disposal problem. This is the idea which prompted the establishment of waste exchanges which act as helpful third parties in establishing contact between waste generators and potential waste users. For example, a paint manufacturer, faced with the problem of how to dispose of hazardous sludges from a mixing operation, contacts a waste exchange and is referred to another company which willingly purchases the sludge to use as a filler coat on cement

Fig. 16-11

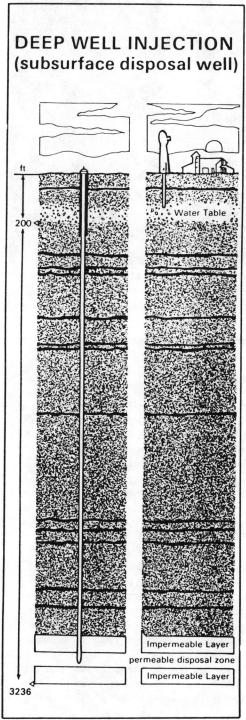

DEEP WELL INJECTION
(subsurface disposal well)

ft

200◄

Water Table

Impermeable Layer

permeable disposal zone

Impermeable Layer

3236

blocks. Not only does the paint manufacturer thereby avoid the high cost of disposal in a secure chemical landfill or controlled incinerator—he also makes a modest profit on the sale of his waste. The buyer, too, is pleased with the arrangement because he has been able to obtain a needed raw material for a lower price than unused filler would have cost; and society is well served because a potentially hazardous substance has been prevented from entering the environment. The waste exchange concept originated in Europe where the first such program began in the Netherlands in 1972. The Midwest Industrial Waste Exchange, started in 1975 in St. Louis, was the first U.S. program, with more than 40 waste exchanges being established in this country since that time. The most common type of waste exchange is basically an information clearinghouse which publishes monthly, bimonthly, or quarterly coded listings of waste items available or desired. Interested parties then contact the clearinghouse and negotiations between potential buyers and sellers are initiated. A smaller proportion of waste exchanges act as a direct brokerage service, sometimes actively seeking a buyer or seller for a particular waste material. As hazardous waste disposal costs continue to rise and as industries become more familiar with the opportunities for waste recycling, utilization of the services provided by waste exchanges is expected to increase significantly.[18]

Solid and Hazardous Wastes   493

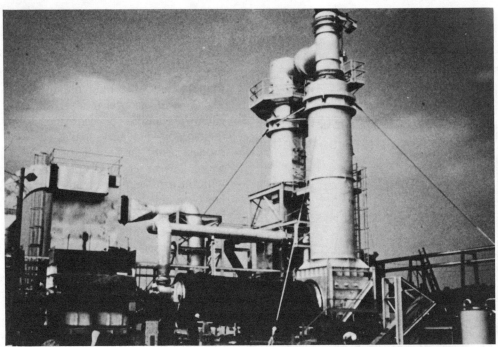

A "mobile" incinerator for destroying hazardous wastes. This equipment can be disassembled and moved from site to site on flatbed trucks. Use of such incinerators is becoming more common as a result of SARA requirements to minimize off-site transport of hazardous wastes from Superfund cleanup projects.[*Author's Photo*]

Box 16–5

Hazardous Waste Reduction

Just as municipal waste management strategies emphasize the value of waste prevention as opposed to cleanup, so does national policy for hazardous waste management stress the importance of reducing amounts of waste generated as quickly as possible. In its 1984 Hazardous and Solid Waste Amendments to RCRA, Congress decreed that "the generation of hazardous waste is to be reduced or eliminated as expeditiously as possible". EPA was told to issue waste minimization regulations designed to increase awareness among industrial managers of waste reduction possibilities and to encourage voluntary initiatives aimed at lowering the amounts of waste generated.

To date, creative efforts at waste minimization have proven that opportunities for significantly reducing the waste stream are numerous. Methods used include such practices as:

1. **changing manufacturing processes**—by switching from an acid spray to a mechanical scrubber using pumice and rotating brushes to clean copper sheeting at its electronics plant in Columbia, MO, the 3M Corporation reduced its generation of liquid hazardous wastes by 40,000 lbs. annually.
2. **reformulating the product**—in a plastics factory in New Jersey, Monsanto changed the formula for an industrial adhesive it was producing; in doing so, it eliminated the need for filtering the product and thus no longer had any hazardous filtrate or filters requiring disposal.
3. **substituting a non-hazardous chemical for a hazardous one in the manufacturing process**—in Memphis, TN, Cleo Wrap, the world's largest producer of holiday gift-wrapping paper, switched from using solvent-based printing inks to

water-based materials. In so doing, the company virtually eliminated its generation of hazardous wastes.

4. **changing equipment**—simply by adding a condenser to an existing piece of equipment, a USS Chemicals plant in Ohio was able to capture escaping emissions of cumene, returning them to the phenol process unit. By so doing, the company solved an air quality problem and recaptured a major raw material.

5. **altering the way hazardous wastes are handled in-plant**—basically housekeeping changes, efforts at minimizing spills and using chemicals more conservatively can make a considerable difference in the amount of hazardous wastes generated. Segregating wastes to reduce contamination can also have a major impact. In Fremont, CA, the Borden Chemical Company has reduced the phenol content of its wastewater by 93% simply by separately collecting and reusing rinsewaters used to clean resin-contaminated filters. Formerly the company had allowed this rinsewater to flow into floor drains where it contaminated all the wastewater which flowed from the factory to a sewage treatment plant.

Not only do the approaches described above reduce the amounts of hazardous waste requiring disposal—they also save the companies which utilize them a great deal of money. The catch-phrase "Pollution Prevention Pays", coined by the 3M Corporation, rings true in case after case. In one year after changing its process for cleaning copper sheeting, 3M saved $15,000 in raw materials and in waste disposal and labor costs; by switching to water-based inks, Cleo Wrap recouped $35,000 annually in waste disposal costs; by recovering 400,000 pounds of cumene after installation of a $5000 condenser, USS Chemicals saved $100,000 in raw materials.

In spite of these encouraging success stories, however, there is as yet no solid evidence of widespread, comprehensive hazardous waste reduction efforts in the U.S. Even at the government level, waste minimization gets more verbal support than funding. While federal, state, and local governments spend about $16 billion each year to clean up pollution, only about $4 million is directed toward efforts at reducing those solid, liquid, and gaseous wastes which are causing environmental degradation. Until both government and industry can break loose from the traditional approach of dealing with wastes after they have been generated, the potential offered by waste reduction strategies will remain largely untapped.[19]

Siting Problems: the "NIMBY" syndrome

Everyone wants hazardous wastes to be managed in ways which present the least possible threat to health or the environment, but no one wants to live near the site chosen for such storage, treatment, or disposal. Get rid of such wastes in the next county, a neighboring state, out in the desert, anyplace else—but "Not in my back yard!" (referred to as the *"NIMBY"* problem in agency jargon). This, in essence, is the siting dilemma which represents one of the most difficult obstacles faced by those trying to deal with hazardous waste management in a safe and responsible manner. Certainly waste disposal horror stories from Love Canal, Jackson Township, the Valley of the Drums, and countless other places across the nation have made citizens understandably nervous at the prospect of seeing hazardous waste management facilities locate in their communities. Nevertheless, if society desires to continue using products whose manufacture entails the production of hazardous wastes, improved waste

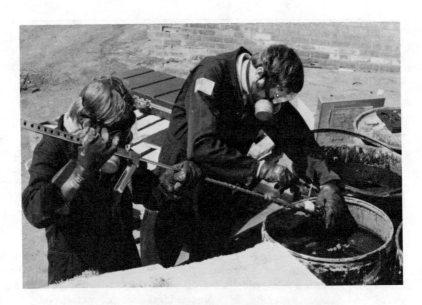

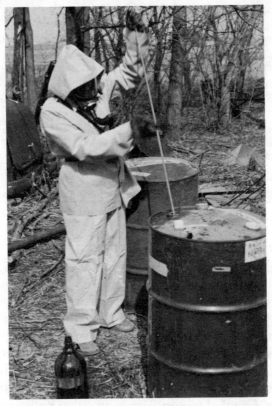

Cleanup of hazardous waste dump sites begins with careful sampling and identification of the abandoned material so that an appropriate disposal method can be chosen. Personnel carrying out the investigation wear protective "moon suits" and respirators to guard against personal injury. [*Illinois Environmental Protection Agency*]

handling facilities are urgently needed. Inevitably, the best location for some of those facilities will be in someone's "back yard". Responsible decision-making demands that citizens carefully evaluate the pros and cons of a site under consideration before automatically rejecting it. Laws governing the siting of hazardous waste facilities provide for public information and public participation programs during the siting process, though the scope for public input into the decision-making process varies widely from state to state. Before opposing or supporting a proposed facility, citizens should gather information on the following points:

characteristics of the wastes involved

nature of the proposed waste management process

the design and manner of operation of the proposed facility

the topographical, hydrogeological, and climatic characteristics of the site

transportation routes to the site

safeguards to be employed at the facility

potential for human or ecological exposure to hazardous chemicals released into the air, water, or soil

location of the site in reference to population centers, farmland, or valuable natural areas (e.g. wetlands, endangered species' habitat, etc.)

possible uses of site after closure

Public opposition has brought acquisition of new hazardous waste management sites to a virtual standstill in recent years. Even such new technologies as at-sea incineration (originally envisioned as a way to avoid the NIMBY problem, since sharks and porpoises can't voice protests) meet with opposition. Residents along the Gulf and Atlantic coasts, fearful of the effects of possible spills or airborne contamination on marine life, have stymied efforts by Waste Management, Inc., to obtain an EPA permit for the incinerator ship Vulcanus. In our ever-shrinking world, not even the oceans are regarded as sufficiently remote to escape the not-in-my-back-yard response. With waste volumes continuing to increase, protection of public health requires a new willingness on the part of citizens to sanction the siting of new facilities when a thorough review of site and operational considerations indicate that such facilities will not present serious environmental health problems.

Hazardous Waste Management Legislation: RCRA

An evaluation of the types of hazardous waste incidents which have occurred indicate that we are basically dealing with two different categories of hazardous waste problems: how to manage the new volumes of chemical wastes being generated daily by American industry and what to do about wastes improperly disposed of years ago which are only now beginning to make their presence known.

"Chemical Wastes?—Not in My Back Yard!"

The extent to which public passions and community resistance can be aroused when a hazardous waste facility moves into the vicinity was nowhere more obvious than in the small town of Wilsonville, Illinois, 30 miles northeast of St. Louis. Here on 130 acres overlying an abandoned underground coal mine a private firm was issued a state permit to develop a facility for the recovery, treatment, storage, and containment of hazardous wastes. About 70% of the area to be used for a chemical landfill was located within the village boundaries, adjacent to a residential area and just 4 blocks from the center of town. Initially the townspeople welcomed the development, having been told that the materials to be buried were "industrial residues" and receiving promises of the creation of numerous jobs in this economically depressed community. All went smoothly for the first four months of operations until the townspeople learned that the industrial wastes being landfilled included PCB-contaminated soil from Missouri. An immediate uproar ensued, with some residents bringing out weapons and threatening to blockade the landfill or to blow it up with dynamite. Some residents admitted they would launch an armed rebellion if necessary to halt operations. A local priest managed to avert violence by persuading a retired judge to serve as a special attorney for the town, and an injunction was obtained to bar further disposal of PCBs at the site. The State Attorney General, noted for pressing cases against polluters, became involved on the side of the town and filed suit to close the site completely. During the many months of litigation which ensued, evidence was presented showing extremely poor operating procedures at the site, with hazardous materials being transported directly through the village (often falling off trucks en route) and chemicals in leaking drums being carelessly handled. The disposal company could scarcely have been more inept at public relations; in the early days of the controversy the site manager was quoted by the local newspaper as saying he couldn't understand all the fuss about PCBs, because worse things than that were buried there! The company then invoked legal rights to confidentiality to prevent citizens from learning what those "worse things" might be.

Throughout the proceedings the Illinois Environmental Protection Agency, the Illinois Geological Survey, and the USEPA continued to insist that from a geological perspective, the Wilsonville site was one of the best places in the country for a chemical landfill. However, some months after the trial ended, it was found that contaminants had migrated farther off-site in 60 months than they had been expected to move in 500 years.

Ultimately the court ruled that the landfill be closed permanently and ordered that all materials buried there must be dug up and taken elsewhere—the first time a legal waste facility has ever been subject to such an action.

The people of Wilsonville, victorious in their efforts to banish a perceived threat to their town, were largely responsible for the 1981 passage of a state law granting local governments virtual veto power over the siting of waste disposal facilities within their jurisdictions. Nevertheless, while citizen involvement in environmental decision-making is both desirable and commendable, the disquieting implication of this situation is that wherever there is a proposal to establish a hazardous waste facility, emotionalism will hold sway and the local response, as in Wilsonville, will be *Not in My Back Yard!"*

In order to tackle the first of these issues, the problem of newly-created wastes, Congress in 1976 enacted the ***Resource Conservation and Recovery Act*** (RCRA—pronounced "rickra" in bureaucratese) which mandates that EPA:

define which wastes are hazardous

institute a "manifest system" to track the movement of hazardous wastes from the place they were generated to any off-site storage, treatment, or disposal facility.

set performance standards to be met by owners and operators of hazardous waste facilities

issue permits for operation of such facilities only after technical standards have been met (operating licenses specify which types of wastes may be managed at that facility; thus most hazardous waste disposal sites are authorized to accept only certain classes of wastes)

help states to develop hazardous waste management programs of their own which may be more stringent than the federal program, but which cannot be less so

RCRA took effect in 1980 when EPA finally issued its generator and transporter regulations (i.e. manifest requirements) and marked an important step forward in responsible hazardous waste management. However, it soon became apparent that the 1976 law featured some glaring loopholes which needed to be plugged. There was also mounting sentiment in Congress and elsewhere that land disposal of hazardous wastes is the least desirable method of managing these substances and that legislation should encourage reliance on alternatives. Accordingly, when RCRA came before Congress for reauthorization in 1984, the original legislation was substantially strengthened with the enactment of the **Hazardous and Solid Waste Amendments (HSWA)**. Among the key provisions of this law are mandates which 1) significantly reduce the types of hazardous wastes which can be buried in landfills; 2) strengthen requirements for landfill design and operation; 3) bring into the regulatory framework hundreds of thousands of previously-exempt "small quantity generators"—those who produce 100 kg (220 lbs.) per month or more of hazardous wastes (under the original law, only those generators producing 1000 kg or more per month were subject to regulation); and 4) create a whole new program for detecting and controlling leakage of hazardous liquids (mainly petroleum products) from underground storage tanks. Implementation of these new requirements, while making hazardous waste management considerably more expensive than it has been in the past, should give new impetus to safer, more environmentally responsible waste management strategies.

While confronting the issue of newly-generated wastes with an array of regulatory approaches, RCRA does nothing to deal with the serious problem posed by leaking abandoned dumpsites. Even in the relatively few cases where the owner can be found, he usually lacks the financial resources to clean up the site, making litigation a futile exercise. Since the EPA estimates there may be anywhere between 30,000-50,000 abandoned hazardous waste dumps in the U.S. over 2000 of which are thought to present public health risks, the potential for future problems is obviously very great.

Fig. 16-12 Who is responsible for hazardous wastes?

At the national level there are a variety of agencies responsible for the control of hazardous wastes. Which agency is responsible and under what legislation is dependent upon whether the wastes are being transported, stored, disposed of, the type of wastes, and where they were found in the ecosystem.

The following is a brief summary of federal waste responsibilities:

FEDERAL HAZARDOUS WASTES REGULATION

AREA	AGENCY	LEGISLATION	PROVISIONS
TRANSPORTATION	Department of Transportation	Hazardous Materials Transportation Act P.L. 93-633	Regulates interstate commerce of hazardous materials
	U.S. Environmental Protection Agency	Resource Conservation and Recovery Act of 1976 P.L. 94-580	Sets standards for manifests (shipping tickets and transporters)
	U.S. Coast Guard	Ports and Waterways Safety Act of 1972	The question of bulk shipment of oil and other hazardous materials on the lakes
WASTE DISPOSAL	U.S. Environmental Protection Agency	Resource Conservation and Recovery Act of 1976 P.L. 94-580	Sets standards and issues, permits for producers, transporters, and disposal sites
AIR QUALITY	U.S. Environmental Protection Agency	Clean Air Act of 1970 P.L. 91-604 Amended 95-95	Sets emission standards for 5 hazardous air pollutants
WATER QUALITY	U.S. Environmental Protection Agency	Clean Water Act of 1977 P.L. 95-217	Sets standards for toxic discharges through NPDES permits to achieve fishable and swimmable water
SPILLS	U.S. Environmental Protection Agency	Clean Water Act of 1977 P.L. 95-217	Prepares national contingency plan for spills, coordinates spill response, levies penalties and recovers costs

Category	Agency	Act / Law	Description
NUCLEAR WASTES	Nuclear Regulatory Agency	Atomic Energy Act P.L. 83-703	Sets standards and licenses nuclear waste disposal sites
DRINKING WATER	U.S. Environmental Protection Agency	Safe Drinking Act of 1974 P.L. 93-523	Sets national standards for safe drinking water Regulates the underground injection of wastes which could contaminate drinking water
FOOD	Food and Drug Administration	Food, Drug, and Cosmetic Act P.L. 75-717	Sets, enforces tolerances for contaminants in food for interstate commerce, bans unsafe foods
OTHER CONSUMER PRODUCTS	Consumer Product Safety Commission	P.L. 92-573 Consumer Product Safety Act Hazardous Substances Act	Sets and enforces tolerances for household products, requires labelling, bans unsafe products
FISH AND WILDLIFE	Department of the Interior Fish and Wildlife Service	Fish and Wildlife Coordination Act of 1965	Research, technical assistance spill response, monitoring for contaminants and effects on fish and wildlife
OCCUPATIONAL SAFETY	Occupational Safety and Health Administration	Occupational and Safety Health Act P.L. 91-596	Sets and enforces standards for worker exposure
CHEMICALS	U.S. Environmental Protection Agency	Toxic Substances Control Act P.L. 94-469	Obtains industry data on product use and health effects of chemicals Regulation of manufacturer, use, distribution, and disposal of chemical substances
PESTICIDES	U.S. Environmental Protection Agency	Federal Insecticide, Fungicide and Rodenticide Act as amended in 1975 P.L. 94-140	Registration and classification of all pesticides

Midnight Dumping

In August of 1978, residents along 210 miles of rural highways in North Carolina discovered an unwelcome gift—31,000 gallons of waste oil containing high levels of PCBs had been deliberately discharged by a tank truck whose driver had simply opened its back spigot while driving along country roads. The pervasive odor caused nausea and headaches among nearby residents and killed vegetation along the roadside. Farmers were advised not to eat or sell vegetables or beef grown within 100 yards of contaminated areas and the Governor offered a $2500 reward for information leading to the arrest of the "midnight dumpers." Within a few weeks three Pennsylvania men, a father and two sons, were arrested and confessed to having accepted $75,000 from a transformer company in Raleigh, the state capital, to haul away the PCB-laden wastes. Since the nearest PCB disposal site happened to be in Alabama, the men decided to maximize their profits by illegally draining the waste along the road where they hoped it wouldn't be noticed.[20]

Although this case was unusual in the volume of waste discarded—and in the fact that the perpetrators were apprehended—midnight dumping (illegal, clandestine disposal of wastes in gullies, fields, streams, abandoned buildings, etc.) has become a common phenomenon. Many midnight dumpers are involved with organized crime networks; few are arrested, and those who are seldom receive punishment which comes close to matching the public expense of repairing the damage they have caused.

Midnight dumping flourishes because of the scarcity of approved disposal sites, the high cost of legal disposal, and because, until recently, generators of wastes were not required to document the final disposition of their waste materials (for example, at a time when Illinois had 22 licensed disposal sites, 2 million tons of chemical wastes were legally disposed of annually, but 12 million additional tons could not be accounted for). The manifest system required by RCRA is designed primarily to amend this situation. Under manifest requirements, off-site shipments of wastes are tracked from "cradle to grave." The waste generator is required to complete an official form describing the amount and composition of the waste material, where it originated, where it is to be taken, and the transportation route to be followed. He must package the material in approved containers with proper labelling and hire a registered hauling company to transport the waste. The vehicle carrying the wastes must be properly placarded and a description of the wastes provided to the transporter. After the waste material reaches the intended waste facility, the completed manifest is returned to the waste generator and must be kept on file for 3 years. If for any reason the manifest is not returned by the waste management facility, the generator is required to notify state environmental authorities who then launch an investigation into the matter. If the experience of states like California, which has had its own mandatory record-keeping program for a number of years, is any example, institution of national manifest regulations may cramp the style of those who unscrupulously endanger public health and safety through illicit dumping.

"Superfund"

Spurred by public demands that something be done to alleviate problems caused by old, leaking dumpsites, Congress in December of 1980 enacted the **Comprehensive Environmental Response, Compensation, and Liability Act (CERCLA**, dubbed the **"Superfund"**), authorizing the expenditure of $1.6 billion over the next 5 years for emergency cleanup activities and for the more long-term containment of hazardous waste dump sites (the legislation, however did *not* include funds to compensate victims for health damage incurred by exposure to such sites—an issue which was the focus of considerable debate). The EPA, in cooperation with the states, was charged with compiling a **National Priority List (NPL)** of sites considered to be sufficiently threatening to public health or environmental quality to make them eligible for Superfund cleanup dollars. These funds can be used either to remove hazardous substances from the site (a process which may also include temporary relocation of people in the area and provision of alternative water supplies) or for remedial measures such as storage and confinement of wastes, incineration, dredging, or permanent relocation of residents (such as occurred at Times Beach, MO).

The original Superfund bill expired in September, 1985, and in spite of public demands for speedy reauthorization so that cleanup work could proceed without interruption, the law was not renewed until late the following year. Extreme Congressional dissatisfaction with the excruciatingly slow rate of progress during Superfund's first 5 years led to several significant changes in the **1986 Superfund Amendments and Reauthorization Act (SARA).** Realizing that 1980 funding levels were inadequate, Congress in 1986 increased Superfund allocations to $9 billion to be spent over the next 5 years. EPA was given mandatory deadlines for initiating site-specific cleanup plans and remediation activities. Concerned that previous cleanup actions represented little more than moving contaminated wastes from one site to another site, which would itself then become eligible for Superfund status (a modern version of the old "shell

Fig. 16-13　　　　National Distribution of Superfund Sites, June 1986

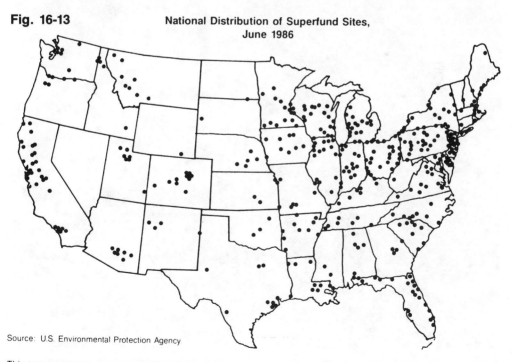

Source: U.S. Environmental Protection Agency

This map represents an approximation of the number and location of sites on the National Priority List.

Solid and Hazardous Wastes　　**503**

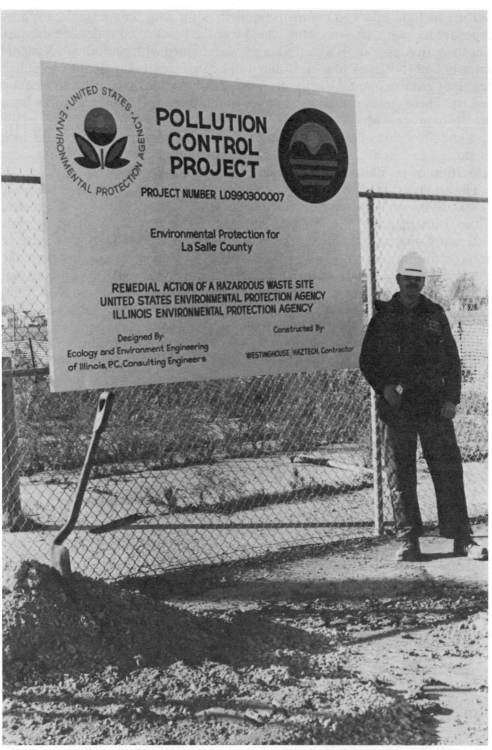

Superfund cleanup activities are currently underway at hundreds of abandoned hazardous waste sites across the country. [*Author's Photo*]

game"!), Congress specified a preference for cleanup actions which "permanently and significantly" reduce the volume, toxicity, or mobility of hazardous substances. This mandate has given a major impetus to development of treatment or disposal technologies (e.g. mobile incinerators which can be moved from one Superfund site to another) which permit hazardous wastes to be destroyed or detoxified on site, thereby avoiding the risks of transporting such wastes to another facility where they might cause future problems.

While the American public has indicated its strong support for the concept of cleaning up its hazardous waste mistakes of the past, it is obvious that the cost of such efforts will be considerable. There are currently about 1200 sites on the NPL, and the Congressional Office of Technology Assessment (OTA) estimates that number will eventually reach 10,000. Depending on how thorough a cleanup is carried out ("How clean is clean enough?" is a question currently bedeviling policymakers), remediation costs at each site are likely to average tens of millions of dollars. Although Superfund legislation mandates that 10% of site cleanup costs be paid by the state in which the site is located and requires that an attempt be made to locate the owner of the abandoned site and to recover removal or remedial costs through litigation if at all possible, the federal government will continue to bear the major financial burden for cleanup efforts. OTA estimates that the ultimate cost of Superfund cleanup may well reach $100 billion; the success of this undertaking obviously will depend on taxpayers' continued willingness to support the detoxification of America's hazardous waste dumpsites.

Household Hazardous Wastes

Comforting references to "Home Sweet Home" and the assertion that "A Man's Home is his Castle" are slightly less reassuring today than in years past. The invisible hazards posed by radon and other indoor air pollutants make us wonder if we'd be safer inhaling deeply at a busy intersection than in our panelled family room. More recently, our righteous indignation directed at corporate polluters who disregard public well-being by careless disposal of their toxic by-products is being tempered somewhat by the realization that all of us—whatever our occupations—contribute to the nation's hazardous waste woes through our use, misuse, and thoughtless disposal of hundreds of potentially dangerous household chemicals.

It is estimated that the average American generates about 160 pounds of household hazardous waste each year. Typical examples of such discarded materials include pesticides, paints and varnishes, brush cleaners, ammonia, toilet bowl cleaners, bleaches and disinfectants, oven cleaners, furniture polish, swimming pool chemicals, batteries, motor oil, outdated medicines, and many others. Although these substances may be every bit as toxic, corrosive, flammable, or explosive as the industrial wastes regulated under RCRA, federal and state hazardous waste laws do not apply to the comparatively minor household sources. Nevertheless, the cumulative environmental impact of even small amounts of these materials being carelessly discarded by millions of individuals can be significant.

Household hazardous waste disposal practices present a variety of concerns:

1) Stored inside the home, hazardous chemicals pose poisoning risks, particularly for children; some, such as paints and solvents, pose problems of indoor air pollution; others, ammonia and chlorine bleach, for example, can result in highly toxic emissions when inadvertently mixed; still others pose serious fire hazards.

2) The welfare of public employees can be threatened by hazardous household products. Home fires involving hazardous chemicals can result in explosions or the generation of toxic fumes which can kill or seriously injure firefighters. Refuse collectors frequently suffer injury when they throw garbage bags into compactor trucks, unaware that they contain corrosive or flammable materials.

3) The environment itself can be seriously degraded when householders pour hazardous liquids into drains and flush them down toilets or into septic systems. People who pour waste motor oil into storm sewers or dump paint cans in the woods can cause long-lasting damage to ground and surface water supplies. Throwing such materials in the trash may ultimately result in the threat of contaminated incinerator ash and air pollution or in the formation of toxic leachates at municipal landfills.

In an effort to raise public awareness about these problems and to provide concerned citizens with a safe and responsible way of getting rid of hazardous household wastes, an increasing number of communities and public interest groups have been sponsoring household hazardous waste collection programs in recent years. Since 1981, over 650 such events have been held in 40 different states.[21] These events have attracted large numbers of householders who are happy to take advantage of the opportunity to clean out the basement or garage and safely get rid of those old bottles of pesticides, paints, even ammunition (!) that may have been sitting on a shelf gathering dust for 20 years or more. Once wastes are brought to a collection center, they must be separated by type, packaged and manifested as RCRA hazardous wastes by trained personnel (usually licensed hazardous waste transporters), and taken to a licensed facility for treatment, disposal, or recycling. The cost of such programs, as well as concerns about legal liability, have limited their more widespread adoption. Nevertheless, these widely-publicized efforts have had an impact far beyond the city limits of their sponsoring communities, enhancing public awareness of the fact that each one of us is a part of America's solid waste problem and pointing the way toward safer, more responsible ways of managing the hazardous by-products of our national lifestyle.

REFERENCES

[1]Melosi, Martin V., *Garbage in the Cities: Refuse, Reform, and the Environment, 1880-1980,* Texas A&M University Press, 1981.

[2]Mantell, C.L., *Solid Wastes: Origin, Collection, Processing, and Disposal,* John Wiley & Sons, 1975.

[3]"Solid Waste—It Won't Go Away", *Current Focus,* League of Women Voters Education Fund, Pub. No. 675, April 1971.

[4]Lehman, John P., *Growth Potential in the Hazardous Waste Management Service Industry,* U.S. Environmental Protection Agency, 1976.

[5]Melosi, op. cit.

[6]Stolting, W.H., *Food Waste Material, A Survey of Urban Garbage Production, Collection, and Utilization,* U.S. Department of Agriculture, 1941.

[7]"Impact of Hogs on an Ecological Crisis", *Biocycle,* vol. 29, no. 5, May/June 1988.

[8]Melosi, op. cit.

[9]*The Solid Waste Dilemma: An Agenda for Action,* Office of Solid Waste, USEPA, September 1988; Morris, David, and Neil Seldman, "New Ways to Keep a Lid on America's Garbage Problem", *Wall Street Journal,* April 15, 1986.

[10]Pollock, Cynthia, "Mining Urban Wastes: the Potential for Recycling", *Worldwatch Paper 76,* Worldwatch Institute, April 1987.

[11]Melosi, op. cit.

[12]Pollock, op. cit.

[13]Logsdon, Gene, "Composting Industrial Wastes Solves Disposal Problems", *Biocycle,* vol. 29, no. 5, May/June 1988.

[14]Powell, Jerry, "Tire recycling bounces along", *Resource Recycling,* July 1988; Tonge, Peter, "Old tires bounce back as new rubber products", *The Christian Science Monitor,* August 9, 1988; Poole, Claire, "Burn This", *Forbes,* April 25, 1988.

[15]Brown, Michael, *Laying Waste: the Poisoning of America by Toxic Chemicals,* Pantheon Books, 1980; Di Perna, Paula, *Cluster Mystery: Epidemic and the Children of Woburn, Mass.,* The C.V. Mosby Company, 1985; Wiley, Karen, and Steven L. Rhodes, "Decontaminating Federal Facilities: the Case of Rocky Mountain Arsenal", *Environment,* vol. 29, no. 3, April 1987.

[16]Levine, Adeline G., *Love Canal: Science, Politics, and People,* Lexington Books, D.C. Heath & Company, 1982; Brown, Michael, "Love Canal Revisited", *Amicus Journal,* vol. 10, no. 3, Summer 1988.

[17]"*The Hazardous Waste System*", USEPA, Office of Solid Waste and Emergency Response, 1987.

[18]Hertzberg, Richard, and Delyn Kies, "A Primer on Waste Exchanges", *Resource Recycling,* vol. 1, no. 6, January/February 1983.

[19]"*State of the Environment: A View toward the Nineties*", Conservation Foundation, 1987.

[20]Brown, op. cit.

[21]Duxbury, Dana, "Home is Where the Hazards Are", *RE : SOURCES,* Environmental Task Force, vol. 7, no. 2.

Appendix A

Federal Environmental Laws

During recent years increasing public concern about environmental degradation and toxic pollutants has led to the enactment by the U.S. Congress of a number of key environmental laws which have played a very significant role in the national effort to clean up America's air, water, and land resources. It is the author's conviction that a general understanding of the legislation which underlies the national effort to improve health and environmental quality is a necessary first step for citizens determined to see that the goals of such laws are achieved. Passage of a law does not, of course, result in immediate improvement of the situation with which that law was meant to deal. Regulations and standards must be proposed and approved—a process which not uncommonly takes several years; interim deadline dates must be established and achieved; monitoring of progress toward defined goals must be carried out to ensure compliance; and funding for the staff and equipment essential to carrying out regulatory programs must be provided. Thus progress toward a cleaner, healthier American environment has not been as rapid as most of us would have desired, but gradual, steady improvement is being made nevertheless.

Although a few pieces of environmental health legislation, such as the 1938 Food, Drug, and Cosmetic Act, have been on the books for many years, most current laws are of much more recent origin, spawned as an outgrowth of the environmental activism of the late 1960s and 1970s. While several of the major anti-pollution laws are discussed in some detail within the chapters pertaining to specific environmental issues, a brief description of a number of recent laws involving environmental health or general ecological issues is given below.

1969—National Environmental Policy Act (NEPA)

This law for the first time established that protection and restoration of the environment is a national policy and directed all agencies of the federal government to interpret and administer their programs in accordance with these goals. NEPA's mandate that all federal agencies file an environmental impact statement (EIS) prior to initiating any action which might significantly affect the environment meant that thenceforth public officials had to consider and publicly discuss the ecological consequences of proposed projects. NEPA has thus had a very significant impact on a wide variety of programs as diverse as highway construction, housing development, dam-building, and oil drilling.

1970—Clean Air Act Amendments

The first comprehensive national program for attacking air pollution, the Clean Air Act Amendments of 1970 established uniform national ambient air quality standards; set auto emission standards and performance standards for new or modified stationary sources; required state implementation plans (SIPs) to ensure compliance with standards; and set deadline dates and penalties for non-compliance. Further amendments to the Clean Air Act in 1977 provided for the prevention of significant air quality deterioration in areas cleaner than required by federal standards and established methods (e.g. "offset policy") for improving air quality in nonattainment areas.

1972—Federal Water Pollution Control Act (FWPCA)

Subsequently renamed the "Clean Water Act", this landmark water quality law rejected the use of waterways as convenient dumping places for industrial and municipal wastes. The Clean Water Act called for restoration and maintenance of the integrity of America's streams, lakes, and rivers—goals to be achieved largely through uniform, enforceable regulation of discharges. The law is complex and comprehensive, dealing not only with effluents from industry and sewage treatment plants, but also with those nonpoint sources (primarily runoff from farmlands, urban streets, construction sites, etc.) which contribute about half of all water pollutants. Amendments to the Act in 1977 included an increased emphasis on the control of toxic pollutants, a postponement of deadline dates for industrial and municipal compliance with federal regulations, and the introduction of incentives for adoption of innovative ways of treating sewage.

1972—Marine Protection, Research, and Sanctuaries Act

More commonly referred to as the "Ocean Dumping Act", this law regulates the dumping of dredging wastes, industrial chemicals, and sewage sludge into the ocean environment.

1972—Noise Control Act

Under this legislation, EPA is authorized to set maximum allowable noise levels for construction and transportation equipment (except aircraft) and for all engines, motors, and electrical equipment manufactured after 1972. It also permits the Agency to require manufacturers to label their products by the amount of noise they generate (something which has not been done to any large extent) and authorizes EPA to conduct noise control research.

1972—Environmental Pesticide Control Act

Basically a revision of the 1947 Federal Insecticide, Fungicide, and Rodenticide Act (FIFRA) which provided for registration of pesticides marketed in interstate commerce, the 1972 law extended federal registration and regulation to cover all pesticides, including those used and distributed within a single state. The law also transferred regulatory authority over pesticides from the Department of Agriculture to the Environmental Protection Agency.

1973—Endangered Species Act

One of the most stringent—and controversial—federal environmental laws, this bill prohibits the killing, collecting, wounding, hunting, harming, shooting, or pursuing of any animal (including eggs or dead body parts) officially listed as "endangered". Equally significant is the requirement that no federal agency may act in such a way as to destroy or modify the critical habitat of any listed species, including endangered plants as well as animals.

1974—Safe Drinking Water Act (SDWA)

Since implementation of SDWA, all public water supply systems—including municipal systems, motels, restaurants, factories, campgrounds, etc.—must comply with EPA primary regulations regarding maximum contaminant levels for impurities in drinking water. The Safe Drinking Water Act also provides for EPA regulation of deep well injection of liquids which potentially could contaminate drinking water aquifers. Included in SDWA are provisions for the technical training of water treatment plant operators and requirements for studies on ways to deal with potential public health hazards and rural drinking water needs and problems.

1976—Toxic Substances Control Act (TSCA)

An effort to achieve more comprehensive control over toxic chemicals, TSCA requires that the manufacturer of a new chemical bear the costs of testing and the "burden of proof" regarding safety. It also requires manufacturers to give EPA 90 days notice of intent and background information before beginning production of any new chemical and gives EPA authority to collect information on new and existing chemicals and to establish an information system for both the public and the Agency to use.

1976—Resource Conservation and Recovery Act (RCRA)

A law which replaced the Solid Waste Disposal Act of 1965 and the Resource Recovery Act of 1970, RCRA greatly expanded the federal role in solid waste management by providing for joint federal/state regulation of hazardous wastes, the phaseout of open dumping, more technical assistance to states and regions for solid waste management, and new methods for enhancing resource conservation and recovery efforts.

1977—Surface Mining Control and Reclamation Act

An attempt to ameliorate the severe land degradation problems which accompany the strip mining of coal, this Act requires that before mine operators are issued a mining permit they must prove they can restore the land in such a manner that it can be used for the same purposes it served before it was mined. After operations are complete, the mine operator must restore the contour of the land, removing all wastes, replacing topsoil, and replanting with grass and trees. Miners must utilize the best available technology to minimize the impact of the mining operation on local water quality.

1980—Comprehensive Environmental Response, Compensation, and Liability Act (CERCLA)

Congressional response to toxic waste disposal problems such as those at Love Canal resulted in the enactment of so-called "Superfund" legislation. This bill created a $1.6 billion fund, financed largely by taxes on chemical feedstocks and crude oil, to be used for emergency cleanup of abandoned hazardous waste dumps.

1980—Low-Level Radioactive Waste Policy Act

Responding to complaints by South Carolina, Nevada, and Washington (sites of the nation's only LLW disposal facilities) that they were becoming the "nuclear dumping grounds" for the whole country, Congress passed this legislation assigning states the responsibility for safe management of low-level radioactive wastes generated within their jurisdictions. Realizing that a LLW facility in each of the 50 states was neither feasible nor necessary, the Act provides for the formation of regional compacts among consenting states. While the original legislation mandated Jan. 1, 1986, as the date by which regional facilities were to be ready to receive low-level radioactive wastes for disposal, a subsequent amendment to the Act extended the deadline to Jan. 1, 1993.

1982—Nuclear Waste Policy Act

Addressing the issue of what should be done with ever-increasing amounts of commercially-generated high-level nuclear wastes, Congress mandated that the federal government, with DOE acting as lead agency, select a site and establish a permanent repository for these intensely radioactive by-products of nuclear power production.

1984—Hazardous and Solid Waste Amendments (HSWA)

Intended to plug loopholes in the 1976 RCRA legislation, HSWA provisions are aimed at encouraging alternatives to land disposal of wastes by imposing stringent standards for design and operation of new landfills and by flatly prohibiting the land disposal of certain listed wastes. HSWA brought hundreds of thousands of "small quantity generators" into the RCRA regulatory framework and created an entirely new program to deal with problems of leaking underground storage tanks.

1985—Food Security Act

The farm bill enacted in 1985 brought concerns about environmental quality and resource preservation into the mainstream of U.S. agricultural policy by linking USDA program benefits to farmers with broad conservation goals. One of the most important provisions in this bill was the Conservation Reserve Program, which pays farmers to take highly erodable lands out of production. The Act also contains two provisions—the Sodbuster Policy and the Swampbuster Policy—intended to discourage cultivation of certain fragile or environmentally important lands not yet in crop production by denying farm program benefits to those who convert such lands to agricultural use.

1986—Superfund Amendments and Reauthorization Act (SARA)

Reflecting Congressional dissatisfaction with the pace of Superfund cleanup, SARA substantially increased funding for the CERCLA program but also imposed binding schedules for USEPA initiation of cleanup planning and remedial action. It also specified cleanup standards, giving priority to remediation methods which reduce the toxicity, volume, and mobility of wastes, and strongly discourages off-site transport of untreated wastes. In addition, SARA incorporates the Emergency Planning & Community Right-to-Know Act, a provision aimed at helping communities meet their responsibilities regarding potential chemical emergencies and giving the public access to information on the presence of hazardous chemicals in their communities.

1986—Asbestos Hazard Emergency Response Act (AHERA)

Enacted as Title II under TSCA, this law requires that school districts inspect their facilities for the presence of asbestos and that they file and carry out a hazard abatement plan if asbestos is found.

Appendix B

Environmental Agencies of the Federal Government

National policy-making regarding environment health issues has been delegated among several different federal agencies and cabinet-level departments. Among the more important groups dealing with issues discussed in this book are:

United States Environmental Protection Agency (USEPA)
401 M Street, N.W., Washington, D.C. 20460

Created by President Nixon in December, 1970, the USEPA is an independent agency formed to coordinate the administration of a wide range of environmental programs which, prior to that time, had been scattered among a number of governmental agencies and departments, several of which frequently worked at cross-purposes. USEPA has been charged with setting and enforcing standards pertaining to air and water pollution, solid and hazardous waste management, noise, public water supplies, pesticides, and radiation (excluding that associated with nuclear power plants). The Agency also administers the municipal sewage treatment plant construction grant program authorized by Congress in the 1972 Clean Water Act. All USEPA actions are published in the *Federal Register* as "proposed regulations", with time being allowed for public comment prior to their adoption as legally enforceable "final regulations".

The Administrator of the USEPA is appointed by the President of the U.S., as are 5 assistant administrators who head the 5 major divisions within the Agency: the Office of Planning and Management, the Office of Enforcement, the Office of Air and Waste Management, the Office of Water and Hazardous Substances, and the Office of Research and Development. All six Presidential appointments must be confirmed by the U.S. Senate. Although USEPA headquarters are in the nation's capital, the Agency has 10 regional offices, each with its own regional administrator, responsible for the states within its region.

The Council on Environmental Quality (CEQ)
722 Jackson Place, Washington, D.C. 20006

Established by the National Environmental Policy Act signed by President Nixon on Jan. 1, 1970, the CEQ operates within the Executive Office of the President. Consisting of 3 members appointed by the President, one of whom functions as chairman, the CEQ employs a professional staff of scientists and attorneys. Prior to the Reagan Administration, this professional staff consisted of about 30 people; all were dismissed by Reagan (the first time any staff member had been discharged by an incoming administration) and replaced by approximately 6 new staff people. The CEQ coordinates the environmental impact statements required by the National Environmental Policy Act and assists the President in preparing environmental legislation. It also had conducted extensive studies on the environmental effects of governmental policies and is charged with preparing annual reports for the President on the current state of the nation's environmental quality. Unfortunately, the drastic budget cuts imposed on the CEQ and the dismissal of all experienced staff members under the Reagan Administration seriously limited the Council's previously valuable activities.

Nuclear Regulatory Commission (NRC)
1717 H Street, N.W., Washington, D.C. 20555

A 5-member civilian board, created in 1974 by the National Energy Reorganization Act which broke up the old Atomic Energy Commission (AEC) into the research-oriented Energy Research and Development Administration (ERDA—subsequently absorbed by the Department of Energy) and the NRC. The Nuclear Regulatory Commission has jurisdiction over the licensing and regulation of nuclear reactors and also over the processing, transportation, and security of nuclear materials.

Office of Science and Technology Policy
Executive Office Building, Washington, D.C. 20500

Established within the Executive Office of the President, this agency advises the President on scientific and technological considerations involved in a wide range of national concerns, including health and the environment.

Office of Technology Assessment (OTA)
600 Pennsylvania Ave., S.E., Washington, D.C. 20510

An agency within the legislative branch of the government, OTA provides independent, objective information on the impacts of technological applications and identifies policy alternatives for technology–related issues. The main function of the OTA is to provide Congressional committees with studies which define a broad range of both social and physical consequences of various policy choices affecting the uses of technologies.

Consumer Product Safety Commission
1111 Eighteenth Street, N.W., Washington, D.C. 20207

This independent regulatory agency seeks to reduce unreasonable risks of injury associated with consumer products by encouraging the development of voluntary standards related to consumer product safety, requiring the reporting of hazardous consumer products and, if justified, recall for corrective action of hazardous products already on the market. The Commission conducts research on consumer product hazards, can establish mandatory standards, and, if necessary, has the authority to ban hazardous consumer products.

Public Health Service
200 Independence Ave., S.W., Washington, D.C. 20201

An office within the Department of Health and Human Services, the U.S. Public Health Service assists states and communities in developing local health resources, conducts and supports medical research, and overseas other public health functions. Among the various subdivisions within the Public Health Service which are of particular environmental health interest are

Centers for Disease Control (CDC)
1600 Clifton Road, N.E., Atlanta, GA 30333

This agency is charged with protecting public health by providing leadership and direction in the prevention and control of disease. It administers programs related to communicable and vectorborne diseases, urban rat control, control of childhood lead-based paint poisoning, and a range of other environmental health problems. CDC also participates in a national program of research, information, and education regarding smoking and health. The 9 major offices of the CDC are those dealing with epidemiology, international health, laboratory improvement, prevention services, environmental health, occupational safety and health, health promotion and education, professional development and training, and infectious diseases.

Food and Drug Administration (FDA)
5600 Fishers Lane, Rockville, MD 20857

The FDA's activities are aimed at protecting public health against impure and unsafe foods, drugs, cosmetics, and other possible hazards such as radiation. In carrying out its responsibilities, the FDA conducts research and develops standards for food, drugs, medical devices, veterinary medicines, and biologic products. Through its National Center for Toxicological Research, the FDA studies the biologic effects of potentially toxic chemicals in the environment.

Occupational Safety and Health Administration (OSHA)

Operating within the Department of Labor, OSHA develops and promulgates safety and health standards and regulations for the American workforce. It conducts investigations and inspections of workplaces to ensure compliance with those regulations and can issue citations and propose penalties for employers who violate such standards.

Fish and Wildlife Service

A bureau within the Department of the Interior, the Fish and Wildlife Service has jurisdiction over matters regarding endangered species, certain marine mammals, wild birds, inland sports fisheries, and wildlife research. The bureau carries out biological monitoring for effects of pesticides, heavy metals, and thermal pollution; it maintains wildlife refuges, enforces game laws, and carries out programs to control livestock predators and pest species. The bureau maintains a number of fish hatcheries, conducts environmental education and public information programs, and provides both national and international leadership regarding endangered fish and wildlife species.

Office of Surface Mining Reclamation and Enforcement

Another agency within the Interior Department, this office is charged with assisting states in developing a nationwide program to protect society and the environment from the harmful effects of coal mining, while simultaneously ensuring an adequate coal supply to meet the nation's energy needs.

Bureau of Land Management (BLM)

The BLM is responsible for managing the nation's 341 million acres of public lands, most of which are located in the Far West. In doing so, the Bureau manages the timber, minerals, rangeland vegetation, wild and scenic rivers, wilderness areas, endangered species, and energy resources of these lands. BLM also is involved in watershed protection, development of recreational opportunities, and programs to protect and manage wild horses and burros. The Bureau provides for the protection, orderly development, and use of public lands and resources under principles of multiple use and sustained yield. Criticism in recent years has focused on the Bureau's over-emphasis on permitting exploitation of public resources for private gain and insufficient protection and conservation of these resources.

Soil Conservation Service (SCS)

An agency of the Department of Agriculture, the SCS develops and carries out soil and water conservation programs in cooperation with landowners and operators, land developers, and community planning agencies. SCS also is active in programs aimed at controlling agricultural pollution and in effecting environmental improvement.

Appendix C

Environmental Organizations

Individuals wishing to influence environmental policy have been greatly helped by public participation provisions in almost all recent federal and state environmental legislation. Prior to adoption of proposed regulations, advertised public hearings offer an opportunity for ordinary citizens to make their views known. However, although a dedicated and informed person can have a surprising amount of influence, one's personal impact can be significantly enhanced by joining forces with one of many environmental organizations operating at the local, state, or national level to inform their members on environmental issues and, in the case of many such groups, to lobby their elected representatives to support the causes they espouse. Quite commonly the national organizations publish informative newsletters, bulletins, or magazines to keep their membership up-to-date on current environmental issues and many people affiliate with such groups simply to receive their attractive and interesting publications. The following list includes the names and addresses of many of the most prominent national environmental organizations which the interested student may wish to contact for further information on membership or publications:

American Lung Association
1740 Broadway, New York, NY 10019
(212) 315-8720

The Acid Rain Foundation, Inc.
1630 Blackhawk Hills Road, St. Paul, MN 55122
(612) 454-2621 or (617) 455-7719

Acid Rain Information Clearinghouse
33 South Washington Street, Rochester, NY 14608
(716) 546-3796

Citizens for a Better Environment
59 East VanBuren St., Suite 1600, Chicago, IL 60605
(312) 939-1530

Citizens' Clearinghouse for Hazardous Wastes
P.O. Box 926, Arlington, VA 22216
(703) 276-7070

The Conservation Foundation
1250 24th St., NW, Washington, DC 20037
(202) 293-4800
Publication: *Conservation Foundation Letter*

Environmental Action, Inc.
1525 New Hampshire Ave., NW, Washington, DC 20036
(202) 745-4870
Publication: *Environmental Action*

Environmental Defense Fund, Inc.
257 Park Ave. South, New York, NY 10010
(212) 505-2100

Environmental Policy Institute
218 D St., SE, Washington, DC 20003
(202) 544-2600

Freshwater Foundation
2500 Shadywood Road, P.O. Box 90, Navarre, MN
(612) 471-8407

Friends of the Earth
530 7th St., SE, Washington, DC, 20003
(202) 543-4312

Greenpeace
1432 U St., NW, Washington, DC 20009
(202) 462-1177

League of Conservation Voters
320 Fourth St., NE, Washington, DC 20002
(202) 547-7200

League of Women Voters of the United States
1730 M St., NW, Suite 1000, Washington, DC 20036
(202) 429-1965

National Audubon Society
950 Third Ave., New York, NY 10022
(212) 832-3200
Publications: *Audubon, American Birds, Audubon Activist*

National Coalition Against the Misuse of Pesticides
530 7th St., SE, Washington, DC 20003
(202) 543-5450

National Council on Radiation Protection and Measurements
7910 Woodmont Ave., Suite 1016, Bethesda, MD 20814
(301) 657-2652

National Environmental Health Association
720 S. Colorado Blvd., Suite 970 South Tower
Denver, CO 80222
(303) 756-9090
Publication: *Journal of Environmental Health*

National Wildlife Federation
1412 16th St., NW, Washington, DC 20036
(202) 797-6800
Publications: *National Wildlife, International Wildlife, Ranger Rick*

Natural Resources Defense Council
40 West 20th St., New York, NY 10011
(212) 727-2700
Publications: *Amicus Journal* and *NRDC Newsline*

Population Reference Bureau, Inc.
777 14th St., NW, Suite 800, Washington, DC 20005
(202) 639-8040
Publications: *Population Bulletin, Population Today*

Resource Recovery Institute
2045 N. 15th St., Suite 310, Arlington, VA 22201
(703) 528-5756
Publication: *Resource Recovery Magazine*

Sierra Club
730 Polk St., San Francisco, CA 94109
(415) 776-2211
Publication: *Sierra Club Bulletin*

The Skin Cancer Foundation
245 Fifth Ave., Suite 2402, New York, NY 10016
(212) 725-5176

The Wilderness Society
1400 I St., NW, Washington, DC 20005
(202) 842-3400

Worldwatch Institute
1776 Massachusetts Ave., NW, Washington, DC 20036
(202) 452-1999
Publications: *Worldwatch Papers, World Watch Magazine, State of the World* (annual report published by W.W. Norton Co., New York

Zero Population Growth, Inc.
1400 Sixteenth St., NW, Suite 320, Washington, DC 20077
(202) 332-2200

INDEX